AF616715

PROGRESS IN CLINICAL AND BIOLOGICAL RESEARCH

RECENT TITLES

Vol 311: **Molecular and Cytogenetic Studies of Non-Disjunction,** Terry J. Hassold, Charles J. Epstein, *Editors*

Vol 312: **The Ocular Effects of Prostaglandins and Other Eicosanoids,** Laszlo Z. Bito, Johan Stjernschantz, *Editors*

Vol 313: **Malaria and the Red Cell: 2,** John W. Eaton, Steven R. Meshnick, George J. Brewer, *Editors*

Vol 314: **Inherited and Environmentally Induced Retinal Degenerations,** Matthew M. LaVail, Robert E. Anderson, Joe G. Hollyfield, *Editors*

Vol 315: **Muscle Energetics,** Richard J. Paul, Gijs Elzinga, Kazuhiro Yamada, *Editors*

Vol 316: **Hemoglobin Switching,** George Stamatoyannopoulos, Arthur W. Nienhuis, *Editors*. Published in two volumes: Part A: *Transcriptional Regulation*. Part B: *Cellular and Molecular Mechanisms*.

Vol 317: **Alzheimer's Disease and Related Disorders,** Khalid Iqbal, Henryk M. Wisniewski, Bengt Winblad, *Editors*

Vol 318: **Mechanisms of Chromosome Distribution and Aneuploidy,** Michael A. Resnick, Baldev K. Vig, *Editors*

Vol 319: **The Red Cell: Seventh Ann Arbor Conference,** George J. Brewer, *Editor*

Vol 320: **Menopause: Evaluation, Treatment, and Health Concerns,** Charles B. Hammond, Florence P. Haseltine, Isaac Schiff, *Editors*

Vol 321: **Fatty Acid Oxidation: Clinical, Biochemical, and Molecular Aspects,** Kay Tanaka, Paul M. Coates, *Editors*

Vol 322: **Molecular Endocrinology and Steroid Hormone Action,** Gordon H. Sato, James L. Stevens, *Editors*

Vol 323: **Current Concepts in Endometriosis,** Dev R. Chadha, Veasy C. Buttram, Jr., *Editors*

Vol 324: **Recent Advances in Hemophilia Care,** Carol K. Kasper, *Editor*

Vol 325: **Alcohol, Immunomodulation, and AIDS,** Daniela Seminara, Ronald Ross Watson, Albert Pawlowski, *Editors*

Vol 326: **Nutrition and Aging,** Derek M. Prinsley, Harold H. Sandstead, *Editors*

Vol 327: **Frontiers in Smooth Muscle Research,** Nicholas Sperelakis, Jackie D. Wood, *Editors*

Vol 328: **The International Narcotics Research Conference (INRC) '89,** Rémi Quirion, Khem Jhamandas, Christina Gianoulakis, *Editors*

Vol 329: **Multipoint Mapping and Linkage Based Upon Affected Pedigree Members: Genetic Analysis Workshop 6,** Robert C. Elston, M. Anne Spence, Susan E. Hodge, Jean W. MacCluer, *Editors*

Vol 330: **Verocytotoxin-Producing *Escherichia coli* Infections,** Martin Petric, Charles R. Smith, Clifford A. Lingwood, James L. Brunton, Mohamed A. Karmali, *Editors*

Vol 331: **Mouse Liver Carcinogenesis: Mechanisms and Species Comparisons,** Donald E. Stevenson, R. Michael McClain, James A. Popp, Thomas J. Slaga, Jerrold M. Ward, Henry C. Pitot, *Editors*

Vol 332: **Molecular and Cellular Regulation of Calcium and Phosphate Metabolism,** Meinrad Peterlik, Felix Bronner, *Editors*

Vol 333: **Bone Marrow Purging and Processing,** Samuel Gross, Adrian P. Gee, Diana A. Worthington-White, *Editors*

Vol 334: **Potassium Channels: Basic Function and Therapeutic Aspects,** Thomas J. Colatsky, *Editor*

Vol 335: **Evolution of Subterranean Mammals at the Organismal and Molecular Levels,** Eviatar Nevo, Osvaldo A. Reig, *Editors*

Vol 336: **Dynamic Interactions of Myelin Proteins,** George A. Hashim, Mario Moscarello, *Editors*

Vol 337: **Apheresis,** Gail Rock, *Editor*

Vol 338: **Hematopoietic Growth Factors in Transfusion Medicine,** Jerry Spivak, William Drohan, Douglas Dooley, *Editors*

Vol 339: **Advances in Cancer Control: Screening and Prevention Research,** Paul F. Engstrom, Barbara Rimer, Lee E. Mortenson, *Editors*

Vol 340: **Mutation and the Environment,** Mortimer L. Mendelsohn, Richard J. Albertini, *Editors*. Published in five volumes: Part A: *Basic Mechanisms*. Part B: *Metabolism, Testing Methods, and Chromosomes*. Part C: *Somatic and Heritable Mutation, Adduction, and Epidemiology*. Part D: *Carcinogenesis*. Part E: *Environmental Genotoxicity, Risk, and Modulation*.

Vol 341: **Chronobiology: Its Role in Clinical Medicine, General Biology, and Agriculture,** Dora K. Hayes, John E. Pauly, Russel J. Reiter, *Editors*. Published in two volumes.

Vol 342: **Progress in Comparative Endocrinology,** August Epple, Colin G. Scanes, Milton H. Stetson, *Editors*

Vol 343: **Horizons in Membrane Biotechnology,** Claude Nicolau, Dennis Chapman, *Editors*

Vol 344: **Isozymes: Structure, Function, and Use in Biology and Medicine,** Zen-Iichi Ogita, Clement L. Markert, *Editors*

Vol 345: **Sleep and Respiration,** Faiq G. Issa, Paul M. Suratt, John E. Remmers, *Editors*

Vol 346: **Recent Progress in Research on Nutrition and Cancer,** Curtis J. Mettlin, Kunio Aoki, *Editors*

Vol 347: **Mutagens and Carcinogens in the Diet,** Michael W. Pariza, Hans-Ulrich Aeschbacher, James S. Felton, Shigeaki Sato, *Editors*

Vol 348: **EORTC Genitourinary Group Monograph 9: Basic Research and Treatment of Renal Cell Carcinoma Metastasis,** C.G. Bollack, D. Jacqmin, *Editors*

Vol 349: **Cytokines and Lipocortins in Inflammation and Differentiation,** Marialuisa Melli, Luca Parente, *Editors*

Vol 350: **Uro-Oncology: Current Status and Future Trends,** H.G.W. Frohmüller, Manfred Wirth, *Editors*

Vol 351: **Taurine: Functional Neurochemistry, Physiology, and Cardiology,** Herminia Pasantes-Morales, David L. Martin, William Shain, Rafael Martìn del Rio, *Editors*

Vol 352: **The Biology of Hematopoiesis,** Nicholas Dainiak, Eugene P. Cronkite, Ronald McCaffrey, Richard K. Shadduck, *Editors*

Vol 353: **Neoadjuvant Chemotherapy in Invasive Bladder Cancer,** Ted A.W. Splinter, Howard I. Scher, *Editors*

Vol 354: **Effects of Therapy on Biology and Kinetics of the Residual Tumor,** Joseph Ragaz, Linda Simpson-Herren, Marc Lippman, Bernard Fisher, *Editors*. Published in two volumes: Part A: *Pre-Clinical Aspects*. Part B: *Clinical Aspects*.

Vol 355: **Radiolabelled Cellular Blood Elements,** Helmut Sinzinger, Mathew L. Thakur, *Editors*

Vol 356: **Molecular Biology and Differentiation of Megakaryocytes,** Janine Breton-Gorius, Jack Levin, Alan T. Nurden, Neil Williams, *Editors*

Vol 357: **EORTC Genitourinary Group Monograph 7: Prostate Cancer and Testicular Cancer,** W.G. Jones, Donald W.W. Newling, *Editors*

Vol 358: **Treatment of Post Surgical Adhesions,** Gere S. diZerega, L. Russell Malinak, Michael P. Diamond, Cary B. Linsky, *Editors*

Vol 359: **EORTC Genitourinary Group Monograph 8: Treatment of Prostatic Cancer—Facts and Controversies,** Fritz H. Schröder, *Editor*

Please contact publisher for information about previous titles in this series.

THE BIOLOGY OF HEMATOPOIESIS

THE BIOLOGY OF HEMATOPOIESIS

Proceedings of the 15th Annual Frederick Stohlman, Jr., M.D., Memorial Symposium: An International Symposium on the Biology of Hematopoiesis, Held in Cambridge, Massachussetts, October 15–20, 1989

Editors

Nicholas Dainiak
Departments of Medicine and Lab Medicine
University of Connecticut Health Center
Farmington, Connecticut

Eugene P. Cronkite
Medical Department
Brookhaven National Laboratory
Upton, New York

Ronald McCaffrey
Department of Medical Oncology
Boston University Medical Center
Boston, Massachusetts

Richard K. Shadduck
Department of Medicine
Hematology/Oncology Unit
Montefiore Hospital
Pittsburgh, Pennsylvania

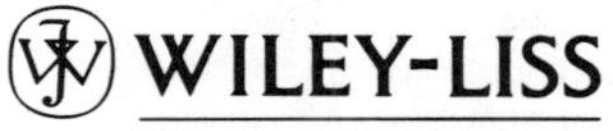

A JOHN WILEY & SONS, INC., PUBLICATION
NEW YORK • CHICHESTER • BRISBANE • TORONTO • SINGAPORE

Address all Inquiries to the Publisher
Wiley-Liss, Inc., 41 East 11th Street, New York, NY 10003

Printed in United States of America

The publication of this volume was facilitated by the authors and editors who submitted the text in a form suitable for direct reproduction without subsequent editing or proofreading by the publisher.

Library of Congress Cataloging-in-Publication Data

International Symposium on the Biology of Hematopoiesis (1989 : Cambridge, Mass.)
The biology of hematopoiesis : proceedings of the 15th Annual Frederick Stohlman, Jr., M.D., Memorial Symposium : an International Symposium on the Biology of Hematopoiesis, held in Cambridge, Massachusetts, October 15-20, 1989 / editors, Nicholas Dainiak ... [et al.].
p. cm. -- (Progress in clinical and biological research ; v. 352)
Includes bibliographical references.
ISBN 0-471-56820-1
1. Hematopoiesis--Congresses. I. Dainiak, Nicholas. II. Title. III. Series.
[DNLM: 1. Hematopoiesis--congresses. 2. Hematopoietic Stem Cells--congresses. W1 PR668E v. 352 / WH 140 I614b]
QP92.I58 1989
612.4'1--dc20
DNLM/DLC
for Library of Congress 90-12242
CIP

Contents

Contributors .... **xiii**

Preface
Nicholas Dainiak, Eugene P. Cronkite, Ronald McCaffrey, and Richard K. Shadduck .... **xxi**

Acknowledgments .... **xxiii**

Dedication
Richard K. Shadduck .... **xxv**

DEFINED TISSUE CULTURE SYSTEMS AND PURIFIED STEM CELLS

Culture of Purified Pluripotent Haemopoietic Stem Cells
J.W.M. Visser, M.G.C. Hogeweg-Platenburg, P. de Vries, J. Bayer, and R.E. Ploemacher **1**

Growth of Highly Purified Human CFU-E in Serum-Free Medium
Sanford B. Krantz and Ken-Ichi Sawada **9**

The Regulation of Hematopoiesis in the Human Fetal Liver
Stephen G. Emerson **21**

Characterization of Human Hematopoietic Stem Cells
J.E. Brandt, E.F. Srour, K. van Besien, and R. Hoffman **29**

Some Observations on the Growth Requirements of Multipotent Stem Cells Under Defined Culture Conditions
Francis C. Monette and George Sigounas **37**

SURFACE MOLECULES AND CELLULAR DIFFERENTIATION

Cell Membrane Family of Growth Regulatory Factors
Nicholas Dainiak **49**

Membrane Bound Forms of Human Macrophage Colony Stimulating Factor (M-CSF, CSF-1)
Douglas P. Cerretti, Janis Wignall, Dirk Anderson, Robert J. Tushinski, Byron Gallis, and David Cosman **63**

Cell-Surface Heparan-Sulfate Proteoglycan Regulates the Expression of a Membrane-Associated Neuronal Mitogen
N. Ratner . . . 71

A Protein (NRP) That Negatively Regulates Erythroid Stem Cell Proliferation: Antagonism to IL-3 Stimulation
Arthur A. Axelrad, Mona M. Shreeve, Denise Eskinazi, and Fred G. Pluthero . . . 79

MATRIX COMPONENTS AND STROMAL REGULATION OF HEMATOPOIESIS

Molecular Mechanism of Hematopoietic Stem Cell Binding to the Supportive Stroma
Mehdi Tavassoli, Cheryl L. Hardy, Shin Aizawa, Takashi Matsuoka, and Jose Minguell . . . 87

Hemonectin: A Novel Hematopoietic Adhesion Molecule
Alan Campbell, Brent Sullenberger, Wadie Bahou, David Ginsberg, Michael Long, and Max Wicha . . . 97

Stromal Regulation of Hemopoiesis
Peter J. Quesenberry, Kotteazeth Srikumar, Daniel S. Temeles, Helen E. McGrath, and Rowena Crittenden . . . 107

Role of Stromal Cell Factors (Restrictins) in Microorganization of Hemopoietic Tissues
Dov Zipori . . . 115

MEGAKARYOCYTOPOIESIS

***In Vitro* Regulation of Human Megakaryocyte Maturation**
Alan M. Gewirtz . . . 123

Megakaryocyte Size and Ploidy in Thrombocytopenic or Megakaryocytopenic Mice
Shirley Ebbe . . . 133

HEMATOPOIETIC GROWTH FACTOR RECEPTORS

Biology and Biochemistry of the Erythropoietin Receptor
Stephen T. Sawyer . . . 145

Structure of the Erythropoietin Receptor in Stable Fibroblast Transfectants
Alan D. D'Andrea, Gerald D. Fasman, Leonard I. Zon, Jing-Po Li, and Harvey F. Lodish . . . 153

Dimethyl Sulfoxide Amplification of the Erythropoietin Response: Clues to the Signal Transduction Pathway
Yijuang E. Chern, Shuji Yonekura, and Arthur J. Sytkowski . . . 161

The Mechanism of Action of Murine Interleukin-3: Current Status
Alice L-F Mui, Sudish C. Murthy, Poul H.B. Sorensen, and Gerald Krystal . . . 169

Structure and Function of Interleukin-2 Receptors
Warren J. Leonard, Michael Sharon, and James R. Gnarra **179**

Characterization of Hematopoietic Growth Factors Receptors
Linda S. Park and Steven Gillis **189**

SECOND MESSENGER SIGNALING SYSTEMS

Control of Lymphokine Production by Protein Kinase C
Julianne J. Sando, E. Chris Homan, and David E. Jensen **197**

Phorbol Esters, Lipopolysaccharides and Colony Stimulating Factor Production
Dov H. Pluznik and Matthias Bickel **205**

Synergistic Interactions Between Two Signal Transduction Pathways During Megakaryocyte Proliferation
Michael W. Long **215**

TRANSCRIPTIONAL AND TRANSLATIONAL CONTROL OF HEMATOPOIESIS

Regulation of Erythropoietin Gene Expression
Eugene Goldwasser and Nega Beru **225**

Erythropoietin Structure-Function Relationships
Jean-Paul Boissel and H. Franklin Bunn **227**

Interleukin-1 Stimulation Stabilizes GM-CSF mRNA in Human Vascular Endothelial Cells: Preliminary Studies on the Role of the 3′ AU Rich Motif
G.C. Bagby, G. Shaw, M.C. Heinrich, S. Hefeneider, M.A. Brown, T.G. DeLoughery, G.M. Segal, and L. Band **233**

Activator Proteins Which Regulate Immunoglobulin Heavy Chain Gene Transcription in B Lymphocytes
Christopher Roman, Karen Riggs, Kevin Merrell, and Kathryn Calame **241**

Topoisomerase Inhibitors Suppress Release of Globin Sequences Into Small Soluble DNA in Erythroblasts
Phyllis R. Strauss **249**

Control of Hematopoietic Growth Factors
Makoto Akashi, H. Phillip Koeffler **257**

Lymphohematopoietic Factors and Biological Control Mechanisms
William L. Farrar and Diana Linnekin **269**

Cytogenetic and Molecular Analysis of the Deletions of Chromosome 5 in Myeloid Disorders
Michelle M. Le Beau **277**

GENE TRANSFER AND EXPRESSION IN HEMATOPOIETIC CELLS

The Combination of IL-3 and IL-6 Enhances Retrovirus Mediated Gene Transfer Into Hematopoietic Stem Cells
David M. Bodine, Nancy Seidel, Stefan Karlsson, and Arthur W. Nienhuis **287**

Retroviral Gene Transfer: Applications to Human Therapy
Eli Gilboa **301**

Developmental Control of Human Globin Gene Expression
Bernard G. Forget **313**

Globin Gene Switching: Insights From Studies in Somatic Heterospecific Hybrids and in Transgenic Mice
Thalia Papayannopoulou, Martha Brice, Tariq Enver, and George Stamatoyannopoulos **323**

Insertional Mutagenesis and Transformation of Hematopoietic Stem Cells
James N. Ihle, Kazuhiro Morishita, Takayas Matsugi, and Christopher Bartholomew **329**

ETHICAL CONSIDERATIONS REGARDING POTENTIALS OF HUMAN GENE THERAPY

Human Gene Therapy—Playing God?
Frank D. Seydel **339**

An Ethical Analysis of Gene Therapy as Molecular Surgery
Matthew J. Temple **347**

Ethical Considerations Regarding Potentials of Human Gene Therapy: Ethical Dilemmas in Serendipity
Terry R. Bard **355**

BIOLOGY OF HEMATOPOIESIS AND IMPLICATIONS FOR THERAPY

Biological Effects of Recombinant Human GM-CSF
Richard K. Shadduck, Sandra S. Kaplan, Theresa L. Whiteside, and Edward J. Wing **365**

The Biology of Human Granulocyte-Macrophage Colony-Stimulating Factor (GM-CSF)
Judith C. Gasson, Gayle C. Baldwin, Kathleen M. Sakamoto, and John F. DiPersio **375**

Growth Factors Controlling the Development of Hemopoietic Cells
Frank Lee **385**

Kinetic Response of Haemopoietic Cell Lineages to Growth Factors *In Vivo*: Their Relationship to the Microarchitecture of the Tissue and Its Microenvironment
Brian I. Lord **391**

Terminal Transferase as a Therapeutic Target in Leukemia Cells
Ronald McCaffrey, Robert Duff, Kyran Bulger, Zachary Spigelman, Karl Flora, Raymond Schinazi, and C.K. Chu **409**

Developmental Regulation of Normal and Leukemic Human B Cell Precursors
Tucker W. LeBien **417**

Surviving Hematological Malignancies: Stress Responses and Predicting Psychological Adjustment
Lynna M. Lesko ... **423**

RADIATION INJURY AND BONE MARROW FUNCTION

Is Natural Background or Radiation From Nuclear Power Plants Leukemogenic?
Eugene P. Cronkite ... **439**

Bone Marrow Proliferation After Passage Through an Irradiated Host
G. Brecher, S. Neben, and M. Yee ... **449**

Prediction of Clinical Outcome of Radiation Accident Victims
T.M. Fliedner, M. Maiwald, W. Weinsheimer, and T. Szepesi ... **459**

Radioprotection and Therapy of Radiation Injury With Cytokines
Ruth Neta ... **471**

Factors Influencing Reconstitution by Bone Marrow Transplantation
D.W. van Bekkum, J.J. Wielenga, F. van Gils, and G. Wagemaker ... **479**

CLINICAL TRIALS OF HEMATOPOIETIC GROWTH FACTORS

Serum Immunoreactive Erythropoietin in Patients With End Stage Renal Disease
L.F. Gimenez, A.J. Watson, and J.L. Spivak ... **493**

The Use of Recombinant Human Erythropoietin (rHuEpo) in Man
J.W. Adamson and J.W. Eschbach ... **505**

Target Cells for GM-CSF and Kinetics of Response
M. Aglietta, F. Bussolino, W. Piacibello, F. Aprá, F. Sanavio, A. Stacchini, C. Monzeglio, F. Carnino, A.C. Stern, and F. Gavosto ... **519**

Hematopoietic Growth Factors in Bone Marrow Transplantation for Hematologic Malignancies
Hillard M. Lazarus ... **531**

Index ... **539**

Contributors

J.W. Adamson, New York Blood Center, New York, NY 10021 **[505]**

M. Aglietta, Clinica Medica A, Dipartimento di Scienze Biomediche ed Oncologia Umana, Universitá di Torino, Torino, Italy 10126 **[519]**

Shin Aizawa, Department of Veterans Affairs, University of Mississippi School of Medicine, Jackson, MS 39216 **[87]**

Makoto Akashi, Division of Hematology/Oncology, UCLA School of Medicine, Los Angeles, CA 90024 **[257]**

Dirk Anderson, Department of Molecular Biology, Immunex Corporation, Seattle, WA 98101 **[63]**

F. Aprá, Dipartimento di Scienze Biomediche ed Oncologia Umana, Clinica Medica A, Universitá di Torino, Torino, Italy 10126 **[519]**

Arthur A. Axelrad, Department of Anatomy, University of Toronto, Toronto, Canada, M5S 1A8 **[79]**

G.C. Bagby, Division of Hematology and Medical Oncology, Oregon Health Sciences University, Portland, OR 97201 **[233]**

Wadie Bahou, Department of Internal Medicine, University of Michigan Medical Center, Ann Arbor, MI 48109 **[97]**

Gayle C. Baldwin, Department of Medicine, UCLA School of Medicine, Center for the Health Sciences, Los Angeles, CA 90024 **[375]**

Louise Band, Molecular Hematology Laboratory, Portland Veterans Administration Medical Center, Portland, OR 97201 **[233]**

Terry R. Bard, Department of Pastoral Services, Beth Israel Hospital, and Department of Psychiatry, Harvard Medical School, Boston, MA 02215 **[355]**

Christopher Bartholomew, Department of Biochemistry, St. Jude Children's Research Hospital, Memphis, TN 38105 **[329]**

J. Bayer, Radiobiological Institute TNO, Rijswijk 2288 G, The Netherlands **[1]**

Nega Beru, Department of Medicine, Section of Hematology/Oncology, University of Chicago, Chicago, IL 60637 **[225]**

The numbers in brackets are the opening page numbers of the contributors' articles.

Matthias Bickel, Division of Cytokine Biology, Center for Biologics, Evaluation and Research, Food and Drug Administration, Bethesda, MD 20892 **[205]**

David M. Bodine, Clinical Hematology Branch, NHLBI, National Institutes of Health, Bethesda, MD 20892 **[287]**

Jean-Paul Boissel, Department of Medicine, Division of Hematology, Brigham and Women's Hospital, Harvard Medical School, Boston, MA 02115 **[227]**

J.E. Brandt, Department of Medicine, Indiana University School of Medicine, Indianapolis, IN 46202 **[29]**

G. Brecher, Cell and Molecular Biology Division, University of California, Lawrence Berkeley Laboratory, Berkeley, CA 94720 **[449]**

Martha Brice, Department of Medical Genetics, University of Washington, Seattle, WA 98195 **[323]**

Melissa A. Brown, Division of Hematology and Medical Oncology, Oregon Health Sciences University, Portland, OR 97201 **[233]**

Kyran Bulger, Department of Medical Oncology, Boston University Medical Center, Boston, MA 02118 **[409]**

H. Franklin Bunn, Department of Medicine, Division of Hematology, Brigham and Women's Hospital, Harvard Medical School, Boston, MA 02115 **[227]**

F. Bussolino, Dipartimento di Genetica, Biologia e Chimica Medica, Universitá di Torino, Torino, Italy 10126 **[519]**

Kathryn Calame, Department of Microbiology, Columbia University College of Physicians and Surgeons, New York, NY 10032 **[241]**

Alan Campbell, Department of Internal Medicine, Ann Arbor VA Medical Center, Ann Arbor, MI 48109 **[97]**

O. Carm, Department of Biology, Nazareth College of Rochester, Rochester, NY 14610 **[347]**

F. Carnino, Divisione di Ginecologia C, Ospedale S. Anna di Torino, Torino, Italy 10126 **[519]**

Douglas P. Cerretti, Department of Molecular Biology, Immunex Corporation, Seattle, WA 98101 **[63]**

Yijuang E. Chern, Laboratory for Cell and Molecular Biology, New England Deaconess Hospital, Boston, MA 02215 **[161]**

C.K. Chu, University of Georgia, Athens, GA 30602 **[409]**

David Cosman, Department of Molecular Biology, Immunex Corporation, Seattle, WA 98101 **[63]**

Rowena Crittenden, Department of Internal Medicine, University of Virginia Health Sciences Center, Charlottesville, VA 22908 **[107]**

Eugene P. Cronkite, Medical Department, Brookhaven National Laboratory, Upton, NY 11973 **[xxi, 439]**

Nicholas Dainiak, Departments of Medicine and Lab Medicine, University of Connecticut Health Center, Farmington, CT 06032 **[xxi, 49]**

Alan D. D'Andrea, Department of Biology, Whitehead Institute for Biomedical Research, Massachusetts Institute of Technology, Cambridge, MA 02142 **[153]**

Thomas G. DeLoughery, Division of Hematology and Medical Oncology, Oregon Health Sciences University, Portland, OR 97201 **[233]**

P. de Vries, Radiobiological Institute TNO, Rijswijk 2288 G, The Netherlands **[1]**

John F. DiPersio, Department of Medicine, UCLA School of Medicine, Center for Health Sciences, Los Angeles, CA 90024 **[375]**

Robert Duff, Department of Medical Oncology, Boston University Medical Center, Boston, MA 02118 **[409]**

Shirley Ebbe, Lawrence Berkeley Laboratory, University of California, Berkeley, Berkeley, CA 94720, and Department of Laboratory Medicine, University of California, San Francisco, San Francisco, CA 94143 **[133]**

Stephen G. Emerson, Departments of Internal Medicine and Pediatrics, and Program in Cell and Molecular Biology, University of Michigan, Ann Arbor, MI 48109 **[21]**

Tariq Enver, Department of Medical Genetics, University of Washington, Seattle, WA 98195 **[323]**

J.W. Eschbach, University of Washington, Seattle, WA 98195 **[505]**

Denise Eskinazi, Department of Anatomy, University of Toronto, Toronto, Canada M5S 1A8 **[79]**

William L. Farrar, Laboratory of Molecular Immunoregulation, National Cancer Institute, Frederick Cancer Research Facility, Frederick, MD 21701-1013 **[269]**

Gerald D. Fasman, Department of Biology, Whitehead Institute for Biomedical Research, Massachusetts Institute of Technology, Cambridge, MA 02142 **[153]**

T.M. Fliedner, Institute of Occupational and Social Medicine, University of Ulm, D-7900 Ulm, Federal Republic of Germany **[459]**

Karl Flora, National Cancer Institute, Bethesda, MD 20892 **[409]**

Bernard G. Forget, Department of Internal Medicine, Yale University School of Medicine, New Haven, CT 06510 **[313]**

Byron Gallis, Department of Biochemistry, Immunex Corporation, Seattle, WA 98101 **[63]**

Judith C. Gasson, Department of Medicine and Biological Chemistry, UCLA School of Medicine, Center for Health Sciences, Los Angeles, CA 90024 **[375]**

F. Gavosto, Dipartimento di Scienze Biomediche ed Oncologia Umana, Clinica Medica A, Universitá di Torino, Torino, Italy 10126 **[519]**

Alan M. Gewirtz, Departments of Medicine, Pathology, and Thrombosis Research, and the Fels Cancer Research Institute, Temple University School of Medicine, Philadelphia, PA 19140 **[123]**

Eli Gilboa, Program in Molecular Biology, Memorial Sloan-Kettering Cancer Center, New York, NY 10021 **[301]**

Steven Gillis, Department of Science Administration, Immunex Corporation, Seattle, WA 98101 **[189]**

L.F. Gimenez, Divisions of Nephrology and Hematology, The Johns Hopkins University School of Medicine, Baltimore, MD 21205 **[493]**

David Ginsberg, Department of Internal Medicine, University of Michigan Medical Center, Ann Arbor, MI 48109 **[97]**

James R. Gnarra, Cell Biology and Metabolism Branch, National Institute of Child Health and Human Development, National Institutes of Health, Bethesda, MD 20892 **[179]**

Eugene Goldwasser, Department of Biochemistry and Molecular Biology, University of Chicago, Chicago, IL 60637 [**225**]

Cheryl L. Hardy, Department of Veterans Affairs, University of Mississippi School of Medicine, Jackson, MS 39216 [**87**]

Steven Hefeneider, Department of Immunology Research, Portland V.A. Medical Center, Portland, OR 97201 [**233**]

Michael C. Heinrich, Division of Hematology and Medical Oncology, Oregon Health Sciences University, Portland, OR 97201 [**233**]

R. Hoffman, Department of Medicine, Indiana University School of Medicine, Indianapolis, IN 46202 [**29**]

M.G.C. Hogeweg-Platenburg, Radiobiological Institute TNO, Rijswijk 2288 G, The Netherlands [**1**]

E. Chris Homan, Department of Pharmacology and Cancer Center, University of Virginia, Charlottesville, VA 22908 [**197**]

James N. Ihle, Department of Biochemistry, St. Jude Children's Research Hospital, Memphis, TN 38105 [**329**]

David E. Jensen, Department of Pharmacology and Cancer Center, University of Virginia, Charlottesville, VA 22908 [**197**]

Sandra S. Kaplan, Department of Pathology, Children's Hospital, Pittsburgh, PA 15213 [**365**]

Stefan Karlsson, Developmental and Metabolic Neurology Branch, NINDS, National Institutes of Health, Bethesda, MD 20892 [**287**]

H. Phillip Koeffler, Division of Hematology/Oncology, UCLA School of Medicine, Los Angeles, CA 90024 [**257**]

Sanford B. Krantz, Department of Medicine, Division of Hematology, Veterans Administration Medical Center and Vanderbilt University School of Medicine, Nashville, TN 37232 [**9**]

Gerald Krystal, Department of Pathology, University of British Columbia, and the Terry Fox Laboratory, Vancouver, British Columbia, Canada V5Z 1L3 [**169**]

Hillard M. Lazarus, Department of Medicine, Ireland Cancer Center, University Hospitals of Cleveland, Case Western Reserve University, Cleveland, OH 44106 [**531**]

Michelle M. Le Beau, Department of Medicine, Section of Hematology/Oncology, University of Chicago, Chicago, IL 60637 [**277**]

Tucker W. LeBien, Department of Laboratory Medicine and Pathology, University of Minnesota Medical School, Minneapolis, MN 55455 [**417**]

Frank Lee, Department of Molecular Biology, DNAX Research Institute of Molecular and Cellular Biology, Palo Alto, CA 94304-1104 [**385**]

Warren J. Leonard, Cell Biology and Metabolism Branch, National Institute of Child Health and Human Development, National Institutes of Health, Bethesda, MD 20892 [**179**]

Lynna M. Lesko, Department of Neurology, Psychiatry Service, Memorial Sloan-Kettering Cancer Center, New York, NY 10021 [**423**]

Jing-Po Li, Department of Biology, Whitehead Institute for Biomedical Research, Massachusetts Institute of Technology, Cambridge, MA 02142 [**153**]

Diana Linnekin, Laboratory of Molecular Immunoregulation, National Cancer Institute, Frederick Cancer Research Facility, Frederick, MD 21701-1013 **[269]**

Harvey F. Lodish, Department of Biology, Whitehead Institute for Biomedical Research, Massachusetts Institute of Technology, Cambridge, MA 02142 **[153]**

Michael W. Long, Department of Pediatrics, Division of Hematology/ Oncology, University of Michigan, Ann Arbor, MI 48109 **[97, 215]**

Brian I. Lord, Department of Experimental Hematology, Paterson Institute for Cancer Research, Christie Hospital and Holt Radium Institute, Manchester M20 9BX, United Kingdom **[391]**

M. Maiwald, Institute of Occupational and Social Medicine, University of Ulm, D-7900 Ulm, Federal Republic of Germany; present address: Staatliches Medizinal-, Lebensmittel- und Veterinäruntersuchungsamt Südhessen, Abt. I: Allgemeine Seuchen- und Umwelthygiene, D-6100 Darmstadt, Federal Republic of Germany **[459]**

Takayas Matsugi, Department of Biochemistry, St. Jude Children's Research Hospital, Memphis, TN 38105 **[329]**

Takashi Matsuoka, Department of Veterans Affairs, University of Mississippi School of Medicine, Jackson, MS 39216 **[87]**

Ronald McCaffrey, Department of Medical Oncology, Boston University Medical Center, Boston, MA 02118 **[xxi, 409]**

Helen E. McGrath, Department of Internal Medicine, University of Virginia Health Sciences Center, Charlottesville, VA 22908 **[107]**

Kevin Merrell, Department of Microbiology, Columbia University College of Physicians and Surgeons, New York, NY 10032 **[241]**

Jose Minguell, Department of Veterans Affairs, University of Mississippi School of Medicine, Jackson, MS 39216 **[87]**

Francis C. Monette, Department of Biology, Boston University, Boston, MA 02215 **[37]**

C. Monzeglio, Divisione di Ginecologia, Ospedale S. Anna di Torino, Torino, Italy 10126 **[519]**

Kazuhiro Morishita, Department of Biochemistry, St. Jude Children's Research Hospital, Memphis, TN 38105 **[329]**

Alice L-F Mui, Department of Pathology, University of British Columbia, and the Terry Fox Laboratory, Cancer Control Agency of British Columbia, Vancouver, British Columbia, Canada V5Z 1L3 **[169]**

Sudish C. Murthy, Department of Pathology, University of British Columbia, and the Terry Fox Laboratory, Cancer Control Agency of British Columbia, Vancouver, British Columbia, Canada V5Z 1L3 **[169]**

S. Neben, Cell and Molecular Biology Division, University of California, Lawrence Berkeley Laboratory, Berkeley, CA 94720; present address: Joint Center for Radiation Therapy, Harvard Medical School, Boston, MA 02115 **[449]**

Ruth Neta, Department of Experimental Hematology, Armed Forces Radiobiology Research Institute, Bethesda, MD 20814 **[471]**

Arthur W. Nienhuis, Clinical Hematology Branch, NHLBI, National Institutes of Health, Bethesda, MD 20892 **[287]**

Thalia Papayannopoulou, Department of Hematology, University of Washington, Seattle, WA 98195 **[323]**

Linda S. Park, Department of Biochemistry, Immunex Corporation, Seattle, WA 98101 **[189]**

W. Piacibello, Dipartimento di Scienze Biomediche ed Oncologia Umana, Clinica Medica A, Universitá di Torino, Torino, Italy 10126 **[519]**

R.E. Ploemacher, Department of Cell Biology, Erasmus University, Rotterdam 3000 DR, The Netherlands **[1]**

Fred G. Pluthero, Department of Anatomy, University of Toronto, Toronto, Canada M5S 1A8 **[79]**

Dov H. Pluznick, Division of Cytokine Biology, Center for Biologics, Evaluation and Research, Food and Drug Administration, Bethesda, MD 20892 **[205]**

Peter J. Quesenberry, Department of Internal Medicine, University of Virginia Health Sciences Center, Charlottesville, VA 22908 **[107]**

N. Ratner, Department of Anatomy and Cell Biology, University of Cincinnati Medical School, Cincinnati, OH 45267 **[71]**

Karen Riggs, Department of Microbiology, Columbia University College of Physicians and Surgeons, New York, NY 10032 **[241]**

Christopher Roman, Department of Microbiology, Columbia University College of Physicians and Surgeons, New York, NY 10032 **[241]**

Kathleen M. Sakamoto, Department of Pediatrics, Children's Hospital of Los Angeles, Los Angeles, CA 90027 **[375]**

F. Sanavio, Dipartimento di Scienze Biomediche ed Oncologia Umana, Clinica Medica A, Universitá di Torino, Torino, Italy 10126 **[519]**

Julianne J. Sando, Department of Pharmacology and Cancer Center, University of Virginia, Charlottesville, VA 22908 **[197]**

Ken-Ichi Sawada, The Second Department of Internal Medicine, Hokkaido University School of Medicine, Sapporo 060, Japan **[9]**

Stephen T. Sawyer, Division of Hematology, Vanderbilt University School of Medicine, Nashville, TN 37232 **[145]**

Raymond Schinazi, Emory University, Atlanta, GA 30033 **[409]**

Gerald M. Segal, Division of Hematology and Medical Oncology, Oregon Health Sciences University, Portland, OR 97201 **[233]**

Nancy Seidel, Clinical Hematology Branch, NHLBI, National Institutes of Health, Bethesda, MD 20892 **[287]**

Frank D. Seydel, Department of Obstetrics and Gynecology, Georgetown University School of Medicine, Washington, DC 20007 **[339]**

Richard K. Shadduck, Department of Medicine, Hematology/Oncology Unit, Montefiore Hospital, Pittsburgh, PA 15213 **[xxi, xxv, 365]**

Michael Sharon, Cell Biology and Metabolism Branch, National Institute of Child Health and Human Development, National Institutes of Health, Bethesda, MD 20892 **[179]**

Gray Shaw, Genetics Institute, Cambridge, MA 02140 **[233]**

Mona M. Shreeve, Department of Anatomy, University of Toronto, Toronto, Canada M5S 1A8 **[79]**

George Sigounas, Department of Biology, Boston University, Boston, MA 02215; present address: Experimental Hematology Unit, Armed Forces Radiobiology Research Unit, Bethesda, MD 20814 **[37]**

Poul H.B. Sorensen, Department of Pathology, University of British Columbia, and the Terry Fox Laboratory, Vancouver, British Columbia, Canada V5Z 1L3 **[169]**

Zachary Spigelman, Department of Medical Oncology, Boston University Medical Center, Boston, MA 02118 **[409]**

J.L. Spivak, Divisions of Nephrology and Hematology, The Johns Hopkins University School of Medicine, Baltimore, MD 21205 **[493]**

Kotteazeth Srikumar, Department of Internal Medicine, University of Virginia Health Sciences Center, Charlottesville, VA 22908 **[107]**

E.F. Srour, Department of Medicine, Indiana University School of Medicine, Indianapolis, IN 46202 **[29]**

A. Stacchini, Dipartimento di Scienze Biomediche ed Oncologia, Clinica Medica A, Universitá di Torino, Torino, Italy 10126 **[519]**

George Stamatoyannopoulos, Department of Medical Genetics, University of Washington, Seattle, WA 98195 **[323]**

A.C. Stern, Clinical Research Department Sandoz, Ospedale S. Anna di Torino, Basel, Switzerland 4002 **[519]**

Phyllis R. Strauss, Department of Biology, Northeastern University, Boston, MA 02115 **[249]**

Brent Sullenberger, Department of Internal Medicine, Ann Arbor VA Medical Center, Ann Arbor, MI 48109 **[97]**

Arthur J. Sytkowski, Laboratory for Cell and Molecular Biology, New England Deaconess Hospital, Boston, MA 02215 **[161]**

T. Szepesi, Institute of Occupational and Social Medicine, University of Ulm, D-7900 Ulm, Federal Republic of Germany; present address: Allgemeines Krankenhaus der Stadt Wien, Abt. für Strahlentherapie und Strahlenbiologie, A-1090 Wien, Austria **[459]**

Mehdi Tavassoli, Department of Veterans Affairs, University of Mississippi School of Medicine, Jackson, MS 39216 **[87]**

Daniel Temeles, Department of Internal Medicine, University of Virginia Health Sciences Center, Charlottesville, VA 22908 **[107]**

Matthew J. Temple, Department of Biology, Nazareth College of Rochester, Rochester, NY 14610 **[347]**

Robert J. Tushinski, Department of Experimental Hematology, Immunex Corporation, Seattle, WA 98101 **[63]**

D.W. van Bekkum, Radiobiological Institute, 2280 HV Rijswijk, The Netherlands, and Department of Radiobiology, Erasmus University, Rotterdam, The Netherlands **[479]**

K. van Besien, Department of Medicine, Indiana University School of Medicine, Indianapolis, IN 46202 **[29]**

F. van Gils, Department of Radiobiology, Erasmus University, Rotterdam, The Netherlands **[479]**

J.W.M. Visser, Radiobiological Institute TNO, Rijswijk 2288 G, The Netherlands **[1]**

G. Wagemaker, Department of Radiobiology, Erasmus University, Rotterdam, The Netherlands **[479]**

A.J. Watson, Divisions of Nephrology and Hematology, The Johns Hopkins University School of Medicine, Baltimore, MD 21205 **[493]**

W. Weinsheimer, Institute of Occupational and Social Medicine, University of Ulm, D-7900 Ulm, Federal Republic of Germany **[459]**

Theresa L. Whiteside, Department of Pathology and Clinical Immunopathology, Pittsburgh Cancer Institute, Pittsburgh, PA 15213 **[365]**

Max Wicha, Department of Internal Medicine, University of Michigan Medical Center, Ann Arbor, MI 48109 **[97]**

J.J. Wielenga, Radiobiological Institute, 2280 HV Rijswijk, The Netherlands **[479]**

Janis Wignall, Department of Molecular Biology, Immunex Corporation, Seattle, WA 98101 **[63]**

Edward J. Wing, Department of Infectious Disease, Montefiore Hospital, Pittsburgh, PA 15213 **[365]**

M. Yee, Cell and Molecular Biology Division, University of California, Lawrence Berkeley Laboratory, Berkeley, CA 94720 **[449]**

Shuji Yonekura, Laboratory for Cell and Molecular Biology, New England Deaconess Hospital, Boston, MA 02215; present address: Department of Internal Medicine, Tokai University School of Medicine, Kanagawa 259-11, Japan **[161]**

Dov Zipori, Department of Cell Biology, Weizmann Institute of Science, Rehovot 76100, Israel **[115]**

Leonard I. Zon, The Children's Hospital, Dana-Farber Cancer Institute, Department of Pediatrics, Harvard Medical School, Boston, MA 02115 **[153]**

Preface

In October 1984, the First International Colloquium on Hematopoietic Stem Cell Physiology was held in Boston in honor of the memory of Frederick Stohlman, Jr., M.D. Since that time, the application of new cellular and molecular biology techniques has greatly expanded our knowledge of how hematopoiesis is regulated. The development of better defined tissue culture systems has permitted study of humoral and intercellular processes that govern stem cell self-renewal. They are now being used to investigate intracellular mechanisms involved in growth factor signal recognition and transduction. The ability to transfect cells with genes has been realized, giving rise to an evolving subspeciality within the field of molecular genetics. Availability of recombinant hematopoietic growth factors by the private sector has resulted in initiation of clinical phase I, II, and III trials in man. Utilization of such factors in protecting against radiation injury to the bone marrow is now being studied, an area of renewed interest inasmuch as the Chernobyl nuclear accident reinforced the conviction that we are all vulnerable in today's nuclear world.

The Fifteenth Annual Frederick Stohlman, Jr., M.D. Memorial Symposium (and the Second International Symposium) was organized to review progress made in hematopoiesis research in a complete and comprehensive fashion. The proceedings of this five-day symposium held on October 15–20, 1989 are organized in this volume according to five major themes. The first theme addresses hematopoietic tissue culture systems, including humoral and cellular requirements for stem cell differentiation and growth. Specific areas of study (represented here as the twelve section titles of this volume) include Defined Tissue Culture Systems and Purified Stem Cells (Section I), Surface Molecules and Cellular Differentiation (Section II), Matrix Components and Stromal Regulation of Hematopoiesis (Section III), and Megakaryocytopoiesis (Section IV). The second major theme addresses receptors for growth factors and signal peptides, and intracellular mechanisms that are involved in mediating growth factor effects. Specific areas covered include Hematopoietic Growth Factor Receptors (Section V), Second Messenger

Signalling Systems (Section VI), and Transcriptional and Translational Control of Hematopoiesis (Section VII). The third major area addresses the transfer and expression of mammalian genes in hematopoietic stem cells. Two specific areas are identified: Gene Transfer and Expression in Hematopoietic Cells (Section VIII) and Ethical Considerations Regarding Potentials of Human Gene Therapy (Section IX). The fourth major area addresses what is known about the biology and physiology of hematopoietic growth control and potential ways such knowledge may be used therapeutically in the treatment of leukemia and other disorders of hematopoietic cell growth: Biology of Hematopoiesis and Implications for Therapy (Section X). The final theme concerns the pathogenesis and therapy of impaired hematopoiesis that can be associated with radiation exposure or hematologic malignancies. Two specific areas are identified: Radiation Injury and Bone Marrow Function (Section XI) and Clinical Trials of Hematopoietic Growth Factors (Section XII). Included in Section XI is the 1989 Robert de Villiers Award lecture, given by Eugene P. Cronkite, M.D. This award is the highest scientific honor of the Leukemia Society of America.

The editors have assembled this volume in an effort to disseminate the great deal of information that was presented and discussed at the symposium. In addition, abstracts presented at this meeting are published in the journal *Leukemia*, Vol. 3, No. 10, October 1989. It is hoped that the information published herein, together with that available in abstract form, will serve as a catalyst to further development of the rapidly changing field of hematopoiesis.

The editors express their sincere gratitude to Dr. Alan S. Levine, Ph.D. (Chief, Blood Diseases Branch, NHLBI) and David G. Badman, Ph.D. (Hematology Program Director, NIDDK) for their advice and encouragement regarding organizational aspects of the symposium. They also express their appreciation for the outstanding organizational and secretarial assistance offered by Bernadette Stohlman-Trenholm (Stohlman Foundation), Janis Biermann (Leukemia Society of America), Donald Howard (St. Elizabeth's Hospital), and Sandra Sorba and Tracy Arnone (University of Connecticut Health Center).

Nicholas Dainiak
Eugene P. Cronkite
Ronald McCaffrey
Richard K. Shadduck

Acknowledgments

The organizers of the Fifteenth Annual Frederick Stohlman, Jr., M.D. Memorial Symposium gratefully acknowledge the following institutions, agencies, and companies for their generous support, without which this symposium would not have been possible:

Department of Energy, USA
Leukemia Society of America
National Institute of Allergy and Infectious Diseases
National Heart, Lung and Blood Institute
National Institute of Diabetes and Digestive and Kidney Diseases
St. Elizabeth's Hospital of Boston
Sandoz Pharmaceuticals and Schering-Plough
Stohlman Foundation
Tufts University School of Medicine

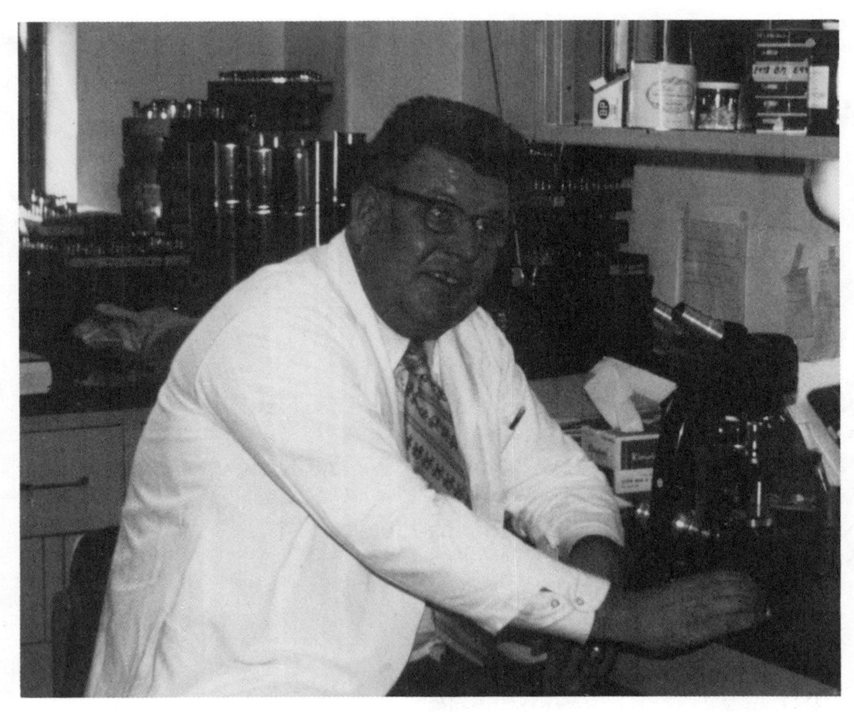

FREDERICK STOHLMAN, JR., M.D.

(1926 - 1974)

Dedication

Fred Stohlman entered the field of hematology and blood cell research in the 1950s following his graduation from Georgetown Medical School and training at the Boston City Hospital. At that point, very little was known about hematopoiesis. Several investigators had described recovery from lethal irradiation in animals by infusion of splenic or marrow homogenates. There was also reason to believe that erythropoiesis might be influenced by a circulating factor. With this information, Fred Stohlman joined Dr. George Brecher at the National Institutes of Health, where he began an illustrious career. His initial studies explored whether erythropoiesis was controlled by a circulating or humoral factor. Fred Stohlman had shown previously that a patient with a patent ductus ateriosus with reversed flow had marked erythrocytosis. The interesting finding was that of hypercellularity of the iliac crest marrow that was exposed to hypoxia. With this careful observation in one patient, he pursued studies to detect a potential humoral factor, particularly one that was released from organs or tissues located below the diaphragm. He perfected new assays for erythropoietin and, in a series of careful studies, delineated the kinetics of erythroid cell production.

During the 1950s, Fred Stohlman also followed up on observations by Osgood of in vitro cultures of hematopoietic cells. He, in fact, demonstrated that lymphocytes and not hematopoietic stem cells were responsive to mitogens in culture; this provided some of the background for our present understanding of lymphopoiesis. Fred Stohlman developed a close scientific and personal friendship with Dr. Eugene P. Cronkite, who was at the Naval Research Laboratory across the street from the NIH. During this time, Brecher, Cronkite, and Stohlman developed many of the concepts and techniques upon which further ideas and research were founded.

During the 1960s, Fred Stohlman:

1. Developed a unifying concept for microcytosis and macrocytosis
2. Described the effects of erythroid perturbation on the stem cell (CFU-S)

3. Expanded studies of granulopoiesis by early use of in vitro colony techniques
4. Helped, with Shirley Ebbe, to define the mechanism of megakaryocyte production
5. Developed the concept of committed stem cells (progenitor cells) for myeloid, erythroid, and megakaryocytic cells
6. Provided extensive descriptions of fetal hematopoiesis

During this period of explosive productivity, Fred Stohlman had a series of associates and fellows, both at the NIH and at St. Elizabeth's Hospital in Boston, where he moved in 1962. These associates and fellows listed, have gone on to distinguish themselves in academic and clinical pursuits in many corners of the globe.

Alberto Carmena	Guido Lucarelli	Keven Rickard
Claudio Carnevale	John McBride	Vittorio Rizzoli
Jeffrey Devon	Marilyn Miller	August Salvado
Shirley Ebbe	Francis Monette	Richard K. Shadduck
Luigi Ferrari	Alex Morely	Judith Sides
Sandra Gilmore	Bernard Morse	Michael Symann
Joan Goldberg	Eero Niskanen	William Tyler
Harry Jacob	Adolfo Porcellini	Julio Vimo
Bernard Kubanek	Peter Quesenberry	Sheila Weinberg
Brigid Leventhal	Nicholas Rencricca	

Each of them owes a special debt of gratitude to Frederick Stohlman, Jr., an excellent investigator, compassionate physician, skilled administrator, and ultimate scholar.

In the 1970s Frederick Stohlman was clearly in an exponential growth phase of his career. He was at the leading edge of defining physiologic and pharmacologic effects of the hematopoietic growth factors. He was appointed editor of the journal *Blood* in 1970 and in many respects was recognized as the leading figure in hematology at that time. Clearly, Frederick Stohlman exerted a major influence in the field of hematopoiesis.

Since the untimely death of Fred and his wife Bernadette at the hands of terrorists, we have witnessed dramatic changes in our field. We have seen the development of cloned growth factors. Erythropoietin, granulocyte-macrophage colony-stimulating factor, granulocyte colony-stimulating factor, macrophage colony-stimulating factor, and interleukin-3 or multi-colony-stimulating factor are all active in clinical trials. The field of bone marrow transplantation is expanding dramatically. We see further understanding of the cellular and humoral mechanisms that regulate hematopoiesis. We gather here at the Fifteenth Annual Frederick Stohlman, Jr. Memorial Symposium to honor the man and to hear further about the exciting developments that will lead us into new understandings of hematopoietic control mechanisms.

I want to acknowledge the continuing strong support of the Stohlman Foundation and particularly the Stohlman children and the Leukemia Society of America for sponsoring this important and timely conference.

Richard K. Shadduck

The Biology of Hematopoiesis, pages 1–8

CULTURE OF PURIFIED PLURIPOTENT HAEMOPOIETIC STEM CELLS

J.W.M. Visser, M.G.C. Hogeweg-Platenburg, P. de Vries, J. Bayer and R.E. Ploemacher,

Radiobiological Institute TNO,Rijswijk,and Erasmus University,Rotterdam,(R.E.P.),The Netherlands.

INTRODUCTION

The regulation of the proliferation and differentiation of the pluripotent haemopoietic stem cells (PHSC) has been the subject of intensive studies aimed at the improvement of bone marrow transplantation and at the treatment of immunological and haematological diseases. A variety of cell culture systems has been developed in order to enumerate the PHSC, to detect steps in their differentiation, and to support their proliferation without differentiation increasing the number of the crucial long term repopulating cells in bone marrow grafts. More recently, *in vitro* proliferation of PHSC has become of practical importance also for gene therapy protocols which employ the haemopoietic system. Retroviral vectors are inserted efficiently only in DNA synthesizing cells. However, up to now, induction of proliferation of PHSC *in vitro* also induced differentiation, so that the reconstitution of recipients of manipulated stem cells was only temporary. On the other hand, since the PHSC are co-cultured during transfection, and, since the culture of PHSC on stromal cell layers as yet seems to be the only method to make them self renew *in vitro*, the development of a successful co-culture combination can be envisaged. Therefore, the interactions between the PHSC and specific stromal cells, adherence molecules, growth factors and inhibitors have to be known in more detail. Purification of PHSC seems to be of use for such studies, however, culture of purified stem cells on stromal layers has not been successful in the past (Spooncer et al., 1985).

The availability of purified and recombinant growth factors has facilitated the culture of haemopoietic progenitor cells in recent years. In addition, well defined, serum-free culture media could be developed for those cells. The only regulatory components in these cultures which are not defined and controled, are the co-cultured more mature bone marrow cells, many of which are capable of producing growth factors and inhibitors. Therefore, we study the regulation of the growth of the PHSC *in vitro* using isolated stem cells (Visser et al., 1984; Migliaccio and Visser, 1986; Miggliaccio et al., 1988; Hagenaars et al., 1989). The purification of the PHSC from mouse bone marrow revealed that the stem cell compartment is heterogeneous. The cells which repopulate the thymus and the marrow and which provide radioprotection, could be separated from the majority of the spleen colony forming cells (Bertoncello et al., 1985; Mulder et al., 1985; Mulder and Visser, 1987; Ploemacher et al., 1989). Therefore, the spleen colony (CFU-S) assay can not be regarded any more as a reliable method for the enumeration of pluripotent stem cells. The investigations with murine PHSC now need new assays to quantitate the pluripotent cells, and to distinguish them from the committed ones. One new assay makes use of long-term bone marrow culture techniques, which have been shown to allow the proliferation and probably self-renewal of PHSC (Toksoz et al., 1980). We have therefore reinvestigated the growth of different subpopulations of purified stem cells on stromal cultures. A subpopulation of PHSC could be isolated which gave rise to long-term chimaerism after transplantation into lethally irradiated recipients and also to efficient and long-term cobblestone area formation in stromal layers.

RESULTS

Purification of stem cells using wheat germ agglutinin, monoclonal antibody 15-1.1 and the dye rhodamine 123.

Mouse (male B/CBA, 7 weeks old) bone marrow cells were separated using equilibrium density centrifugation and light-activated cell sorting for wheat germ agglutinin (WGA) positive cells with medium forward and low perpendicular light scatter intensities as described previously (Visser and Bol, 1981; Visser et al., 1984). After removal of the WGA using N-acetyl-D-glucosamine, the sorted cells were incubated with the monoclonal antibody 15-1.1, which labels mature and immature myeloid cells, and which does not bind to PHSC (Vries et al., 1988). The 15-1.1 negative cells were incubated with the mitochondria-specific dye rhodamine 123 (Rh123), and sorted again as described previously (Visser and de Vries, 1988). Two subpopulations of stem cells could be separated with this dye: Rh123-bright ones, which gave spleen colonies both at 8 and 12 days after transplantation (200-fold enriched for CFU-S, Table 1) and Rh123-dull ones, which gave only late appearing spleen colonies (Table 1) and which are known to have marrow and thymus repopulating ability. They may be regarded as pre-CFU-S (Bertoncello et al., 1985; Mulder and Visser, 1987; Ploemacher and Brons, 1989). Fig. 1 shows that the marrow repopulating cell (MRA, determined as described by Bertoncello et al., 1985) is 200-fold enriched in the Rh123-dull fraction, and virtually absent in the bright cells.

Sorted cells were also transplanted into female recipients and chimaerism was analysed using fluorescent in situ hybridisation with a murine Y-chromosome specific probe (kindly provided by Dr. L.Singh,

Singh et al., 1987) as described by Pinkel et al. (1986, see also Van Dekken and Bauman, 1988). In mice which received Rh123-dull sorted cells, male cells could be observed in the peripheral blood at eleven weeks after transplantation (Table 2), transplanted Rh123-bright cells gave no long-term reconstitution.

These results indicate that CFU-S, even day-12 ones, do not represent long-term repopulating PHSC, and they confirm that the spleen colony forming cells can be separated from the PHSC using rhodamine 123. Enrichments of 200-fold can be obtained, both for CFU-S and for MRA cells. However, now that we do not have a clonal assay, the absolute purity of the sorted suspensions is unknown (Visser and de Vries, 1988).

TABLE 1. Spleen colony formation by sorted stem cells.

Cell type	# CFU-S per 10^5 transplanted cells	
	day 8	day 12
unfractionated bone marrow	38±4	42±4
$WGA^+/15\text{-}1.1^-/Rh123^-$	160±40	5600±800
$WGA^+/15\text{-}1.1^-/Rh123^+$	7200±900	9100±900

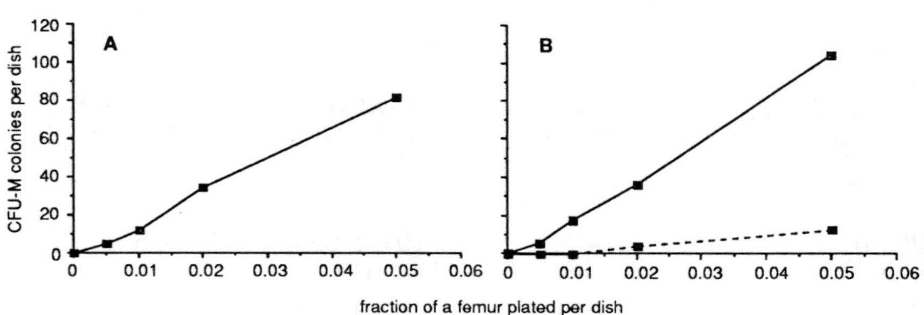

Fig. 1. Marrow repopulating ability (MRA) of (A) unfractionated control, and of sorted Rh123-dull (B, solid line) and -bright (B, dashed line) bone marrow cells. Recipient mice were given 2 x 10^5 unfractionated bone marrow cells, 10^3 purified Rh123-dull or 10^3 sorted Rh123-bright cells. Their femoral bone marrow was plated at day 14.

TABLE 2. Long term (11 weeks) chimaerism after transplantation of purified stem cells as revealed by Y-chromosome in situ hybridisation of peripheral blood cell nuclei.

Cell type	Number of cells transplanted	% male cells
unfractionated bone marrow	5 x 10^4	61± 9
WGA$^+$/15-1.1$^-$/Rh123$^-$	500	92±10
WGA$^+$/15-1.1$^-$/Rh123$^+$	725	2± 1

98 % of controle male blood cells were positive, whereas 0 out of 100 female blood cells hybridised with the probe.

In vitro colony formation by purified stem cells.

The sorted fractions were plated in semisolid agar containing 20 % serum with colony stimulating factors added as described before (Visser et al., 1984). Table 3 indicates that colony formation by the Rh123-dull cells is poor, except when combinations of growth factors are present. Rh123-bright cells responded to both IL-3 and PMUE (pregnant mouse uterus extract, which contains M-CSF) without an enhancement by IL-1, whereas

TABLE 3. *In vitro* colony formation by sorted stem cells in agar.

	Colonies per 10^5 cells		
Growth factor added	unfractionated marrow	WGA$^+$/15-1.1$^-$ Rh123-dull	WGA$^+$/15-1.1$^-$ Rh123-bright
PMUE	140±13	1010± 630	3350±1810
IL-1	2± 1	0	0
IL-3	107±12	1100± 630	11950±2620
IL-1+IL-3	121±12	2470± 920	15670±3160
IL-1+PMUE	160±14	1990± 880	4890±1480
IL-3+PMUE	174±15	7100±1840	20330±3010
IL-1+IL-3+PMUE	183±13	14170±2790	21410±5130

PMUE, pregnant mouse uterus extract; IL, interleukin.

the latter cytokine contributed significantly to the growth of the Rh123-dull cells. The sorted suspensions were devoid of monocytes and lymphocytes (due to the use of 15-1.1 and WGA), and the addition of such cells to the stem cell cultures did not affect the results, indicating that the enhancement of colony formation by IL-1 is due to a direct effect on the PHSC.

Similar studies with fractions of purified stem cells were performed using serum-free methylcellulose cultures (Merchav and Wagemaker, 1986) and new combinations of growth factors. Under those conditions no enhancement by IL-1 was observed, and the highest colony numbers from Rh123-dull cells were obtained with IL-3 *plus* CSF-1, added together, giving 14±2 colonies per 100 cells plated. Rh123-bright sorted cells could be cultured serum-free with a plating efficiency of up to 50 % with a combination of IL-1 *plus* IL-3 *plus* CSF-1.

In another series of experiments, sorted stem cells were first cultured serum-free in suspension in the presence of added growth factors, and next plated with other growth factors. IL-1 was found to enhance the formation of CFU-GM, CFU-M, and BFU-E in cultures of sorted Rh123-dull cells, but not in cultures of bright ones. Enhancement by IL-1 of the growth of Rh123-dull cells which had been sorted and deposited at one per well in serum-free liquid culture, has been described earlier (Hagenaars et al.,1989). Whereas the Rh123-dull fraction contained 6 CFU-M per 1,000 cells at the onset of the suspension culture, the tube contained 1,280 of those progenitors at day 4 in the presence of IL-1 *plus* IL-3 *plus* CSF-1. For the Rh123-bright fraction these figures were 84 CFU-M at the onset, and 6440 at day 4 of culture.

All results regarding the culture of the purified stem cells indicate that the Rh123-dull cells need combinations of factors for colony formation, and still then, that they respond poorly to the known growth factors, whereas the Rh123-bright ones form colonies efficiently even with single growth factors. It could be that the Rh123-dull cells are in a special quiescent state, not using mitochondria, with condensed chromatin, and that therefore they are hard to culture. Ikebuchi et al. (1987) have shown that the induction of quiescent PHSC to a responsive state requires IL-6. We did not observe enhancement by that cytokine. However, this may be due to a difference in preparation or concentration. In our experiments IL-1 and CSF-1 both seemed to be activating the PHSC, without inducing colony formation by themself.

Growth of purified stem cells on stromal layers.

A new limiting dilution assay for long-term repopulating haemopoietic stem cells using stroma-dependent bone marrow cultures in microtiter wells (Ploemacher et al., 1989), was employed to further characterize the sorted stem cell fractions. Fig. 2 shows the time course of the appearance and disappearance of cobblestone areas of unfractionated bone marrow cells and of the two fractions of sorted stem cells. At the onset of the culture the Rh123-dull cells could be observed to home in the

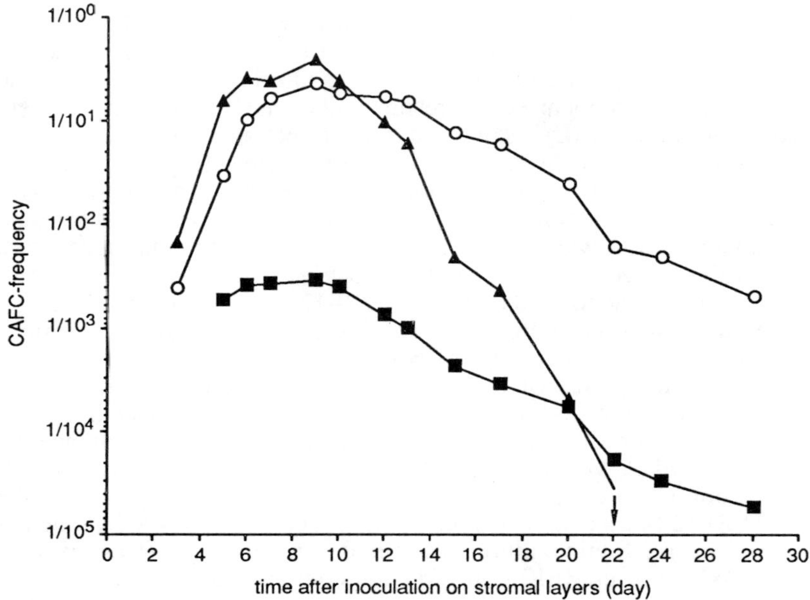

Fig. 2. Cobblestone area formation by purified hematopoietic stem cells. Squares, unfractionated bone marrow cells; circles, purified Rh123-dull stem cells; and, triangles, Rh123-bright sorted stem cells, containing 48, 7500, and 9250 day-12 CFU-S per 10^5 cells, respectively.

stromal layer, and to produce daughter cells which migrated to other sites in the layer, whereas the Rh123-bright cells also homed within the layer, but started to make a cobblestone area without further migration. In agreement with earlier observations (Ploemacher et al., 1989), the Rh123-bright cells gave rise to cobblestone areas which disappeared before day 21 of culture, whereas the Rh123-dull cells formed cobblestone areas which persisted longer. A 100- to 200-fold enrichment for cobblestone area forming cells (CAFC) was obtained by the sorting procedure (Fig. 2). By daily examination of the wells, the total clonogenicity of the sorted cells in the stromal layers was found to be 27 % for the Rh123-dull fraction, and 52 % for the Rh123-bright cells.

DISCUSSION

The purification of PHSC from mouse bone marrow yields several subpopulations which differ by their response to growth factors *in vitro*.

Rh123-dull cells have a poor response, whereas they are the ones that provide long-term haemopoietic reconstitution *in vivo*, and in stromal layers *in vitro*. The Rh123-bright cells can give many colonies with the known cytokines, but they do not give long-term reconstitution. In view of this it seems justified to state that the Rh123-bright cells are no PHSC, in spite of their efficient formation of spleen colonies and cobblestone areas.

In many respects the Rh123-dull sorted stem cells resemble PHSC of 5-FU treated mice. In an elegant experiment using ^{89}Sr-treated animals Van Zant (1984) showed that these PHSC home in the bone marrow to produce daughter cells which may give spleen colonies. Therefore, adherence to specific sites seems to be the key event in the regulation of early stem cell proliferation, and it may be speculated that the low plating efficiency of the sorted Rh123-dull cells is due to the absence of adherence sites in the culture. Indeed, improved growth of purified stem cells was obtained in stromal layers. As was shown earlier by Ploemacher et al. (1989) Rh123-dull cells give rise to long-living cobblestone areas in Dexter cultures, whereas Rh123-bright cells give cobblestones for only a short period of time. This indicates that cobblestone formation by itself is not a measure of PHSC, rather the ongoing formation of cobblestone areas is a sign of PHSC. Direct examination of the purified Rh123-dull stem cells in the stromal cultures showed that they divide and then separate several times before they produce cobblestone areas.

In view of these results it can be speculated that quiescent PHSC are dependent on specific sites or niches to remain pluripotent. Perhaps a differentiation inhibiting factor is present at those sites in high amounts. Activation and proliferation of PHSC would have to be possible at those sites, and it seems that erythropoietin (Miggliaccio et al., 1988), M-CSF (Table 3) and IL-6 (Ikebuchi et al., 1987) are capable of inducing that. Upon division normally one of the two daughter cells would need to leave the site and migrate elsewhere. This occurs rather at random, so that stochastic differentiation can be explained by stochastic migration.

REFERENCES

Bertoncello I, Hodgson GS, Bradley TR (1985). Multiparameter analysis of transplantable hemopoietic stem cells.I.The separation and enrichment of stem cells homing to marrow and spleen on the basis of rhodamine-123 fluorescence.Exp Hematol 13:999-1006.

Hagenaars CE, Kraan AAM van der, Kawilarang-de Haas EWM, Visser JWM, Nijweide PJ (1989). Osteoclast formation from cloned pluripotent hemopoietic stem cells. Bone and Mineral 6:179-189.

Ikebuchi K, Wong GG, Clark SC, Ihle JN, Hirai Y, Ogawa M (1987). Interleukin 6 enhancement of interleukin 3-dependent proliferation of multipotential hemopoietic progenitors. Proc Natl Acad Sci USA 84:9035-9039.

Merchav S, Wagemaker G (1984). Detection of murine bone marrow granulocyte/ macrophage progenitor cells (GM-CFU) in serum-free cultures stimulated with purified M-CSF or GM-CSF. Int J Cell Cloning 2:356-367.

Migliaccio AR, Visser JWM (1986). Proliferation of purified murine hemopoietic stem cells in serum-free cultures stimulated with purified stem-cell-activating factor. Exp Hematol 14:1043-1048.

Migliaccio G, Migliaccio AR, Visser JWM (1988). Synergism between erythropoietin and interleukin-3 in the induction of hematopoietic stem cell proliferation and erythroid burst colony formation. Blood 72:944-951.

Mulder AH, Visser JWM (1987). Separation and functional analysis of bone marrow cells separated by rhodamine-123 fluorescence. Exp Hematol 15:99-104.

Mulder AH, Visser JWM, Engh GJ van den (1985). Thymus regeneration by bone marrow cell suspensions differing in the potential to form early and late spleen colonies. Exp Hematol 13:768-775.

Pinkel D, Straume T, Gray JW (1986). Cytogenetic analysis using quantitative, high-sensitivity, fluorescence hybridization. Proc Natl Acad Sci USA 83:2934-2938.

Ploemacher RE, Brons NHC (1989). Separation of CFU-S from primitive cells responsible for reconstitution of the bone marrow hemopoietic stem cell compartment following irradiation: evidence for a pre-CFU-S cell. Exp Hematol 17:263-266.

Ploemacher RE, Sluijs JP van der, Voerman JSA, Brons NHC (1989). An in vitro limiting dilution assay of long-term repopulating hemopoietic stem cells in the mouse. Blood (in press).

Singh L, Matsukuma S, Jones KW (1987). The use of Y-chromosome-specific repeated DNA sequences in the analysis of testis development in an XX/XY mouse. Development 101:143-149.

Spooncer E, Lord BI, Dexter TM (1985) Defective ability to self-renew in vitro of highly purified primitive haematopoietic stem cells. Nature 316:62-64.

Toksoz D, Dexter TM, Lord BI, Wright EG, Lajtha LG (1980). The regulation of hemopoiesis in long-term bone marrow cultures.II.Stimulation and inhibition of stem cell proliferation. Blood 55:931-939.

Van Dekken H, Bauman JGJ (1988). A new application of fluorescent in situ hybridization: detection of numerical and structural chromosome aberrations with the combination of a centromeric and a telomeric DNA probe. Cytogen Cell Genet 48:188-189.

Van Zant G (1984) Studies of hematopoietic stem cells spared by 5-fluorouracil. J Exp Med 159:679-690.

Visser JWM, Bauman JGJ, Mulder AH, Eliason JF, Leeuw AM de (1984). Isolation of murine pluripotent hemopoietic stem cells. J Exp Med 59:1576-1590.

Visser JWM, Bol SJL (1981). A two-step procedure for obtaining 80-fold enriched suspensions of murine pluripotent hemopoietic stem cells. Stem Cells 1: 240-249.

Visser JWM, Vries P de (1988). Isolation of spleen-colony forming cells (CFU-s) using wheat germ agglutinin and rhodamine 123 labeling. Blood Cells 14: 369-384.

Vries P de, Pronk GJ, Visser JWM (1988). A multiple staining procedure for the flow cytometric screening of monoclonal antibodies directed against murine pluripotent stem cells (CFU-S). Blood Cells 14:561.

The Biology of Hematopoiesis, pages 9–20

GROWTH OF HIGHLY PURIFIED HUMAN CFU-E IN SERUM-FREE MEDIUM

Sanford B. Krantz and Ken-Ichi Sawada

Division of Hematology and Department of Medicine, Veterans Administration Medical Center and Vanderbilt University School of Medicine, Nashville, Tennessee

INTRODUCTION

Study of the growth requirements of normal human colony-forming units-erythroid (CFU-E) has been hampered by a lack of highly purified CFU-E and a lack of serum-free medium that would allow growth of purified CFU-E. While human marrow CFU-E have been grown in a modified Iscove's serum-free medium (Iscove et al., 1980; Casadevall et al., 1982; Akahane et al., 1987) large numbers of contaminant accessory cells may have provided necessary growth factors. In addition, the presence of burst-forming units-erythroid (BFU-E) at different levels of maturation may have contributed to the erythroid colonies that were produced. We have developed a method for harvesting highly purified CFU-E that are grown in vitro from human blood BFU-E (Sawada et al., 1987). These CFU-E have been obtained with a sufficient yield to define the necessary requirements for their growth and to demonstrate direct interaction of the cells with recombinant human erythropoietin (rEp), insulin-like growth factor (IGF)-I, and insulin.

MATERIALS AND METHODS

Purification of Human CFU-E

Approximately 400 ml of normal peripheral blood was collected in preservative-free sodium heparin, 20 U/ml final concentration, after obtaining informed consent. The blood was layered on Ficoll-Hypaque (FH;1.077 g/ml) and centrifuged at 400 g for 25 min at 24°C as previously described (Sawada et al., 1987). The interface mononuclear cells were collected and were depleted of T lymphocytes by sheep erythrocyte rosetting and B cells by incubation, at 4°C, on plastic dishes coated with affinity-purified sheep anti-human IgG specific for the $F(ab)_2$ fragment. Monocytes were removed by adherence to polystyrene plastic at 37°C overnight and the remaining cells were incubated for 60 min, 4°C, with four monoclonal antibodies CD11b/OKM*1 (Civin and Loken, 1987; McMichael, 1987), CD2/OKT*11 (Civin and Loken, 1987; McMichael, 1987), CD45R/MY 11 (Civin and Loken, 1987; McMichael, 1987; Straus et al., 1986), and MY 23 (Civin and Loken, 1987; McMichael, 1987; Knapp, 1989) to coat granulocytes, monocytes, colony-forming units granulocyte-macrophage (CFU-GM), T and B lymphocytes and natural killer cells (Sawada et al., 1987). The former two antibodies were obtained from Ortho Diagnostic Systems Inc., Raritan, NJ and the latter two were a gift of Dr. Curt Civin. Excess antibody was then washed away and these cells were removed from the cell suspension by incubation at 4°C on plastic dishes coated with affinity-purified goat anti-murine IgG. The non-adherent cells, containing BFU-E, were washed from the plates and cultured in methylcellulose (MC) with rEp as previously described (Sawada et al., 1987; 1989). After 7 d the cells were collected and washed before removing adherent cells by a 1 h incubation at 37°C. Following a 30 min incubation of the non-adherent cells in serum-free medium to remove bound rEp, the 2 ml cell suspension was layered on 2 ml FH and centrifuged at 450 g for 15 min, 24°C, to remove dead cells and debris. The interface cells (MC FH cells) were collected and assayed for CFU-E by the plasma clot method (Tepperman et al., 1974). CFU-E were defined as cells that gave rise to single colonies of 8-49 hemoglobinized cells (Ogawa et al., 1977; Eaves and Eaves, 1984) while erythroid colony-forming cells (ECFC) were defined as cells that gave rise to single colonies of two or more hemoglobinized cells. Bone marrow cells were used after separation over FH (BM FH cells) as described above.

Media

Crystalline bovine serum albumin (BSA; nuclease and protease-free; Calbiochem-Behring Corp., La Jolla, CA), human transferrin, and lipid suspension were prepared as described by Iscove et al. (1980) with minor modifications by Sawada et al. (1989). The crystalline BSA was deionized, with resin AG 501-X8(D) (Bio-Rad Laboratories,

Richmond, CA (Tepperman et al., 1974), delipidated with Dextran T40 (Pharmacia, Uppsala, Sweden) and activated charcoal (Sigma Chemical Co., St. Louis, MO) and dialyzed (C-BSA-3D) before filter-sterilization and storage at -20°C. Human transferrin (Sigma Chemical Co.) was totally saturated with $FeCl_3$ before filter-sterilization and storage at -70°C. Oleic acid, 28 mg, L-α-phosphatidylcholine, 40 mg, and cholesterol (Sigma Chemical Co.) 39 mg, were first dissolved in 0.5 ml chloroform, which was then evaporated. 50 ml of PBS, pH 7.4, with 1% C-BSA-3D, was added and the beaker was sonicated for 30 min. The contents were sterile-filtered and stored at 4°C. Human fibrinogen (grade L, coagulability 90% of total protein, KabiVitrum, Stockholm, Sweden), 100 mg protein, was dissolved in 5 ml of water and dialyzed with one liter of PBS, pH 7.4, for 1 h and with 1 liter of α-minimum essential medium (Sigma Chemical Co.) for another 2 h before filter sterilization (Sawada et al., 1989). The fibrinogen solution was stored at 24°C and used within 48 h.

Culture of CFU-E in Serum-free Medium

Purified CFU-E were plated in a 0.5 ml mixture of C-BSA-3D (10 mg/ml), transferrin (300 µg/ml), lipid suspension (oleic acid, 5.6 µg/ml; L-α phosphatidylcholine, 8.0 µg/ml; cholesterol, 7.8 µg/ml), porcine insulin (26.3 USP U/mg; Calbiochem-Behring Corp., 10 µg/ml), or recombinant human insulin (26 U/mg; Eli Lilly & Co., Indianapolis, IN; 10 µg/ml), rEp 10,000 U/mg, AMGen Biologicals, Thousand Oaks, CA; 1 U/ml), fibrinogen (2 mg/ml), thrombin (0.2U/-ml), aminocaproic acid (Elkins-Sinn, Inc., Cherry Hill, NJ; 1.5 mM), and 50% Iscove's modified Dulbecco's medium/50% F-12[Ham] (Sigma Chemical Co.). The cells were cultured for 7 d at 500 cells/ml in 24-well flat-bottomed tissue culture plates (Linbro, Flow Laboratories, Inc., McLean, VA), at 37°C in a high humidity 5% CO_2-95% air incubator and were fixed and stained with benzidine as previously described (Tepperman et al., 1974). BM FH cells were cultured in the same medium at 5 x 10^4 cells/ml.

RESULTS

Using density gradient sedimentation, sheep erythrocyte rosetting, adherence to plastic and negative panning with monoclonal antibodies, human blood BFU-E were purified

22-fold to 0.4% with a 43% yield (Sawada et al., 1987). After 7-9 d of culture in methylcellulose large erythroid bursts were evident. These cells were collected and further purified using adherence and density sedimentation, which yielded 10^7 mononuclear cells with a purity of 70 ± 18% ECFC. The relation between the number of erythroid colonies and the number of these cells plated in plasma clots was a straight line through the origin (Fig. 1A). The cells were sensitive to as little as 10 mU/ml of rEp and a plateau occurred at 1 U/ml (Fig. 1B) which is similar to the response of human marrow CFU-E (Tepperman et al., 1974)

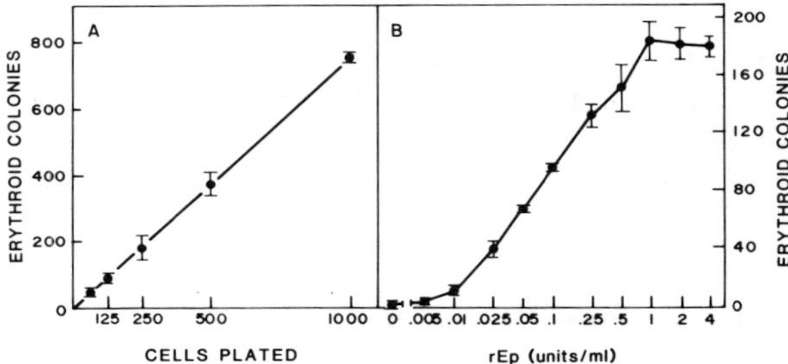

Fig. 1 Relation between the number of erythroid colonies and the number of MC FH cells plated (A), and the concentration of rEP (B). The cells were plated in 0.5 ml plasma clots at 62-1,000 cells/well with 1 U/ml of rEp (A) or 250 cells/well with increasing concentrations of rEp (B) and were incubated at 37°C for 6 d. Each value is the mean of three replicates ± SD. (Reproduced from the J Clin Invest (1987) 80:357-366 by copyright permission of the American Society for Clinical Investigation.)

The necessity for each ingredient of the serum-free medium and the optimum concentrations are shown in Figure 2. Deletion of any of these ingredients greatly reduced the number of erythroid colonies, but with the optimum combination of each the number of erythroid colonies was equivalent to the number in serum-medium.

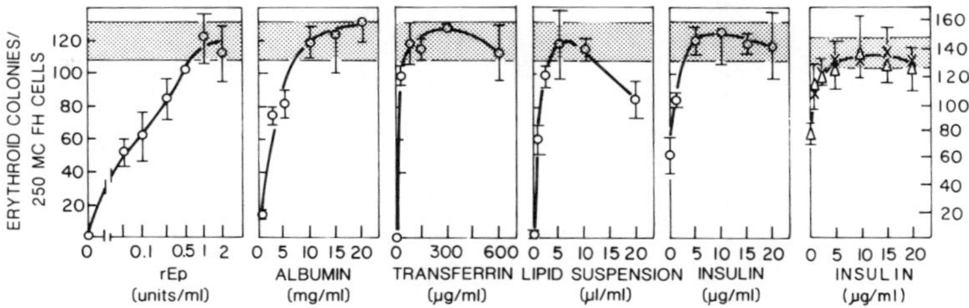

Fig. 2 Effect of increasing concentrations of individual components of serum-free medium on CFU-E growth. The complete serum-free medium consisted of 50% IMDM/50% F-12[HAM] supplemented with delipidated crystalline BSA (10 mg/ml), iron-saturated transferrin (300 μg/ml), lipid suspension (oleic acid, 5.6 μg/ml; L-α-phosphatidylcholine, 8.0 μg/ml; cholesterol, 7.8 μg/ml), insulin (10 μg/ml), rEP(1 U/ml), fibrinogen (2 mg/ml), and thrombin (0.2 U/ml). MC FH cells were plated in 0.5-ml clots at a concentration of 500 cells/ml. Each point (O) represents the mean ± SD of triplicates. Shaded areas shown the mean ± SD of triplicates observed in serum medium. In a separate experiment recombinant human insulin (X) was compared to porcine insulin (/\) under the same conditions (Reproduced from the J Clin Invest (1989) 83:1701-1709 by copyright permission of the American Society for Clinical Investigation.)

Table 1 shows the size of the erythroid colonies after 7 d of culture in serum-free medium. While both media supported the same number of erythroid colonies, the number of CFU-E colonies (8-49 cells) was 82% in serum-free medium as compared to 64% in serum-medium ($p<0.001$). This increase may be evident because of a better nutrient combination or the removal of a serum inhibitor. No BFU-E were present (data not shown) and only 1 colony of 50 or more cells was seen. BM FH cells grown in serum-free medium had only 61% of the colonies seen in serum-medium and had 22% colonies of 50 or more cells in serum-medium which did not appear in serum-free medium (Table 1). Thus BM FH cells have more immature progenitor cells (late BFU-E) and the serum-free medium constructed for CFU-E does not support these earlier cells.

Table 1. Proliferative Capacity of Erythroid Colony Forming Cells in Serum-Free Medium

Cells	Serum	Number of cells in erythroid colonies					Erythroid Colonies
		2-4	5-7	8-16	17-49	>50	
		%	%	%	%	%	Percentage of control
MC FH	(+)	26±5	13±4	53±10	11±10	1±3	100
	(-)	9±2	8±1	49±5	33±3	1±1	103±5
BM FH	(+)	31±8	9±3	24±5	19±6	22±6	100
	(-)	23±4	7±4	53±6	16±5	0.4±0.5	61±12

MC FH cells and BM FH cells were cultured in serum- and serum-free 0.5-ml clots at 500 cells/ml and 1 X 10^5 cells/ml, respectively. After 7 d of culture, clots were fixed and stained, and the number of hemoglobin-containing cells per colony was counted. Mean values±SD for three experiments are shown. The number of erythroid colonies observed in serum-free medium was compared with the number in serum-medium, and the data expressed at % (±SD) of the latter. The absolute number of erythroid colony-forming cells observed in serum-medium in these three experiments was 137±35 per 250 MC FH cells and 522±212 per 5 X 10^4 BM FH cells. (Reproduced from the J Clin Invest (1989) 83:1701-1709 by copyright permission of the American Society for Clinical Investigation.)

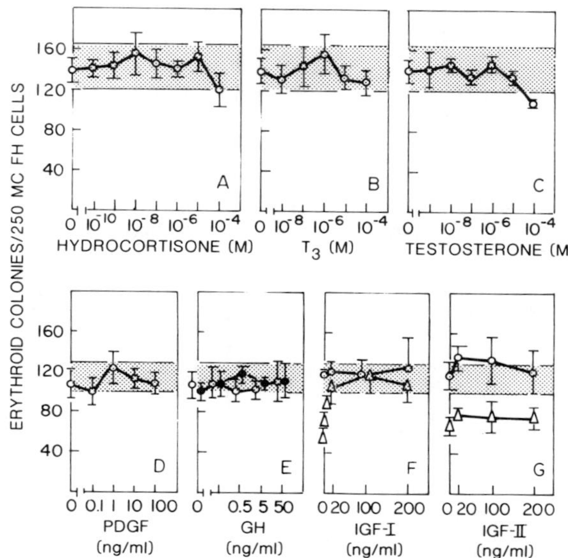

Fig. 3 Effect of a variety of hormones and growth factors on erythroid colony-forming cell growth in standard serum-free medium which contained insulin (10 μg/ml). MC FH cells were plated in triplicate and each value represents the mean ± SD (O). In some experiments, 10 ng/ml IGF-I was added (O) (E), whereas in others insulin was omitted from the culture medium (/\) F,G). Shaded areas show the mean ± SD of triplicates observed in serum-containing cultures. This figure is a composite of two individual experiments (A-C and D-G). (Reproduced from the J Clin Invest (1989) 83:1701-1709 by copyright permission of the American Society for Clinical Investigation.)

Figure 3 shows that the addition of a wide variety of other hormones to the highly purified CFU-E in this serum-free medium had no further effect on erythroid colony growth. Interleukin-3 (IL-3) and granulocyte-macrophage colony-stimulating factor (GM-CSF) also had no effect on these cells while markedly enhancing BFU-E growth (data not shown). When insulin was omitted from the same serum-free medium physiologic concentrations of IGF-I were necessary to restore normal erythroid colony growth (Fig. 3). Because the effect of IGF-I was only seen in the absence of insulin, the experiments of Figure 3 were repeated without insulin, but none of the above hormones had a stimulating effect on these CFU-E (Sawada et al., 1989). Dose-response curves with insulin or IGF-I showed increased numbers of erythroid colonies with 1 ng/ml of insulin or 1.56 ng/ml of IGF-I, which are within the physiologic range and small concentrations of each significantly enhanced the effect of small concentrations of the other. While the CFU-E reached normal growth with normal serum concentrations of IGF-I (Fig. 3), 100-fold greater concentrations of insulin, in the pharmacologic range (Fig. 2), were necessary for this effect. No colonies formed without rEp.

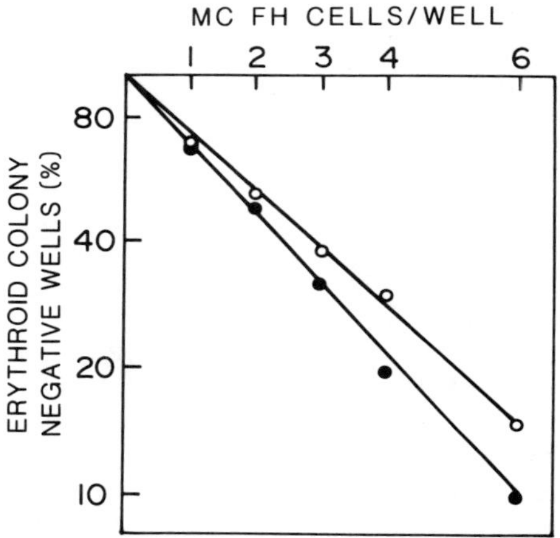

Fig. 4 Limiting dilution analysis of CFU-E growth in serum-free medium with IGF-I. MC FH cells at concentrations of 20, 40, 60, and 120 cells/ml, were suspended in serum-free medium without insulin, but with the addition of 100 ng/ml of IGF-1 (O), or in serum-medium (O). Aliquots of 50 µl were plated into 96-well tissue culture flat-bottomed plates. After 7 d of incubation, clots were fixed and stained by benzidine, and the number of clots in which erythroid colonies did not grow was counted as erythroid colony-negative wells. This was plotted against the number of MC FH cells plated into the wells. Each point represents the value obtained from 60 wells. (Reproduced from the J CLin Invest (1989) 83:1701-1709 by copyright permission of the American Society for Clinical Investigation.)

CFU-E were cultured in a limiting dilution assay in serum-free medium with IGF-I, or serum-medium, and the percentage of non-responder wells was plotted against the cell concentration (Fig. 4). Both groups demonstrated overlapping straight lines through the origin indicating that the CFU-E do not depend on accessory cells and that the effect of IGF-I is a direct effect on the CFU-E. A similar result was seen when insulin replaced IGF-I, and autoradiography confirmed specific binding of ^{125}I-insulin and ^{125}I-IGF-I to the CFU-E (Sawada et al., 1989).

DISCUSSION

This work demonstrates a capacity to produce CFU-E with a sufficient yield and degree of purity to study those factors that are necessary for the growth of these cells. Since CFU-E have had a long-standing, but arbitrary definition as cells that give rise to single colonies of 8-49 hemoglobinized cells, and since 18% of the colonies observed with this method have 2-7 cells, we have used the more general term of ECFC. However, 82% of these erythroid progenitors are classical CFU-E. The high purity of these cells markedly reduces the effects of non-erythroid cells and the serum-free medium avoids the effects of a wide variety of chemicals and hormones that are present in serum. Moreover, the lack of BFU-E avoids misinterpretation of the effects of added agents which might alter the growth of BFU-E, but not CFU-E. This is shown in the experiments of Table I where the BM FH cells produced many more erythroid colonies of greater than 50 cells, which unlike the CFU-E, did not grow in the restricted serum-free medium. Without highly purified CFU-E, it is possible to misinterpret the effect of added agents as a direct effect on CFU-E when it might be an indirect effect on the non-erythroid accessory cells or an effect on mature BFU-E which shifts these cells into the CFU-E population.

With these highly purified CFU-E we have been able to define those nutrients that are absolutely necessary for their growth and maturation: BSA, lipids, human transferrin, rEp and either insulin or IGF-I. Despite the addition of the latter, no erythroid colonies were seen without rEp. This is unlike the studies of Kurtz et al. (1982; 1983) who found that murine marrow and fetal liver CFU-E responded to IGF-I, or insulin, in a serum-free medium without Ep. The reason for this difference is not known, but murine CFU-E may have different requirements, or the adjacent murine accessory cells may have been stimulated to produce other factors that enhanced the development of erythroid colonies.

In our system, we found little effect of hydrocortisone, testosterone, thyroid or growth hormones, platelet-derived growth factor, IGF II, IL-3 or GM-CSF on erythroid colony growth . The concentrations of the first four in the serum-free medium were measured by radioimmunoassays and were less than 1% of the concentrations in normal sera (data not shown) so a high baseline concentration cannot account for this lack of effect. It is possible that the effect of these hormones on erythroid growth in vitro that have previously been reported may have occurred through an effect on accessory cells or more immature erythroid progenitor cells. The effect of thyroid hormone on human BFU-E growth has indeed been shown to occur through an effect on accessory cells (Dainiak et al., 1986) and the effect of growth hormone on human BFU-E and CFU-E growth has been shown to occur through the stimulation of monocytes to produce IGF-I (Merchav et al., 1988).

It has previously been shown that human CFU-E have Ep receptors which specifically bind rEp and that these are not present on a wide variety of other cells (Sawada et al., 1988). However, whether IGF-I and insulin act directly on the CFU-E was not clear because some contaminant cells that produce a wide variety of growth factors have always been present. For this reason we used limiting dilution analysis to determine that the system was measuring a direct effect on the CFU-E. With this analysis a straight-line through the origin represents a single hit curve which is an indication of a single limiting cell type for colony formation (Lefkovits & Waldman, 1984). Deviation from a straight line would suggest a complex interaction involving more than one cell or a deficient medium. This analysis, which clearly shows a single hit curve, indicates that IGF-I and insulin act directly on the CFU-E and that the CFU-E do not require accessory cells. However, CFU-E do require rEp, IGF-I and/or insulin for erythroid development, and some factors, previously thought to enhance CFU-E growth in vitro, have little effect on these cells.

ACKNOWLEDGEMENTS

The studies reported here were supported by VA Medical Research Funds, plus grants DK 15555, 2 T32 DK 07186, and RR-95 from the National Institutes of Health.

REFERENCES

Akahane K, Arinobu T, Urabe A, Takaku F (1987). Pure erythropoietic colony and burst formations in serum-free culture and their enhancement by insulin-like growth factor I. Exp Hematol 15:797-802.

Casadevall N, Vainchenker W, Lacombe C, Vinci G, Chapman J, Breton-Gorius J, Varet B (1982). Erythroid progenitors in polycythemia vera: demonstration of their hypersensitivity to erythropoietin using serum free cultures. Blood 59:447-451.

Civin CI and Loken MR (1987). Cell surface antigens on human marrow cells: Dissection of hematopoietic development using monoclonal antibodies and multiparameter flow cytometry. Int J Cell Cloning 5:267-288.

Dainiak N, Sutter D, Krezco S (1986). L-triiodothyronine augments erythropoietic growth factor release from peripheral blood and bone marrow leukocytes. Blood 68:1289-1297.

Eaves AC, Eaves CJ (1984). Erythropoiesis in culture. Clinics Haematol 13:371-391.

Iscove NN, Guilbert LJ, Weyman C (1980). Complete replacement of serum in primary cultures of erythropoietin-dependent red cell precursors (CFU-E) by albumin, transferrin, iron, unsaturated fatty acid, lecithin and cholesterol. Exp Cell Res 126:121-126.

Knapp W (Ed.) (1989). "Leukocyte Typing IV: White Cell Differentiation Antigens". Oxford/New York/Tokyo: Oxford University Press.

Kurtz A, Jelkmann W, Bauer C (1982). A new candidate for the regulation of erythropoiesis. Insulin-like growth factor I. FEBS (Fed Eur Biochem Soc) Lett 149:105-108.

Kurtz A, Jelkmann W, Bauer C (1983). Insulin stimulates erythroid colony-formation independently of erythropoietin. Br J Haematol 53:311-316.

Lefkovits I, Waldman H (1984). Limiting dilution analysis of the cells of immune system. I. The clonal basis of the immune response. Immunol Today 5:265-268.

McMichael AJ (Ed.) (1987). "Leukocyte Typing III: White

Cell Differentiation Antigens". Oxford/New York/Tokyo: Oxford University Press.

Merchav S, Tatarsky I, Hochberg Z (1988). Enhancement of erythropoiesis in vitro by human growth hormone is mediated by insulin-like growth factor I. Br J Haematol 70:267-271.

Ogawa M, MacEachern MD, Avila L (1977). Human marrow erythropoiesis in culture: II. Heterogeneity in the morphology, time course of colony formation, and sedimentation velocities of the colony-forming cells. Am J Hematol 3:29-36.

Sawada K, Krantz SB, Kans JS, Dessypris EN, Sawyer S, Glick AD, Civin CI (1987). Purification of human erythroid colony-forming units and demonstration of specific binding of erythropoietin. J Clin Invest 80:357-366.

Sawada K, Krantz SB, Sawyer ST, Civin CI (1988). Quantitation of specific binding of erythropoietin to human erythroid colony-forming cells. J Cell Physiol 137:337-345.

Sawada K, Krantz SB, Dessypris EN, Koury ST, Sawyer ST (1989). Human colony-forming units-erythroid do not require accessory cells but do require direct interaction with insulin-like growth factor I and/or insulin for erythroid development. J Clin Invest 83:1701-1709.

Strauss LC, Brovall C, Fackler MJ, Schwartz JF, Shaper JH, Loken MR, Civin CI (1986). Antigenic Analysis of hematopoiesis. IV. The My-11 hematopoietic cell surface antigen is expressed by myelomonocytic and lymphoid, but not erythroid, progenitor cells. Exp Hematol 14:935-945.

Tepperman AD, Curtis JE, McCulloch EA (1974). Erythropoietic colonies in cultures of human marrow. Blood 44:659-669.

The Biology of Hematopoiesis, pages 21–28

THE REGULATION OF HEMATOPOIESIS IN THE HUMAN FETAL LIVER

Stephen G. Emerson, M.D., Ph.D.

Departments of Internal Medicine and Pediatrics, and Program in Cell and Molecular Biology, University of Michigan, Ann Arbor, MI 48109

The precise and accurate delineation of the cellular and molecular regulation of hematopoiesis was for many years hindered by the extreme rarity of the critical regulatory target cells, the hematopoietic progenitor cells, in the bone marrow and blood. While many groups therefore sought methods to purify and enrich progenitor cells from these tissues, fetal liver appeared to be an equally attractive, if not superior tissue for study due to the large number of progenitor cells present (Rowley et al., 1978). Beginning with studies in the laboratory of Dr. David G. Nathan at the Dana-Farber Cancer Institute, Boston, MA. and continuing in our laboratory at Ann Arbor, we have therefore analyzed in detail the hematopoietic physiology of progenitor cells isolated from human fetal liver. These studies will be now summarized, including: the purification of fetal progenitor cells, their use as accessory cell-free target cells to analyze the activities of hematopoietic growth factors, the generation of monoclonal antibodies detecting erythropoietin responsive progenitor cells, and the possible role of immature autoimmune regulation in permitting the expansion of the hematopoietic mass in fetal life.

A. THE PURIFICATION OF FETAL HEPATIC PROGENITOR CELLS

Prior to the initiation of these studies, several approaches had been pursued to purify progenitor cells, including differential centrifugation, fluorescence activated cell sorting, immune rosetting, and combinations of these immunologic and physical techniques. However, when examined in detail, each of these techniques proved to be either too cumbersome, inefficient or both. We therefore turned to negative immunoselection by panning. In this approach, adherence depleted mononuclear cells were incubated with a panel of murine monoclonal antibodies (anti-CD2, CD5, CD10, CD11b, CD20, HLA-DQ, & glycophorin A) detecting maturing myeloid, erythroid and lymphoid cells but not progenitor cells, and then antibody-labelled cells were removed by adherence to plastic dishes coated with secondary antibody. This rapid, economical approach resulted in a thousand-fold progenitor cell purification with final cloning efficiency of 22-75%, with over 95% progenitor yield.

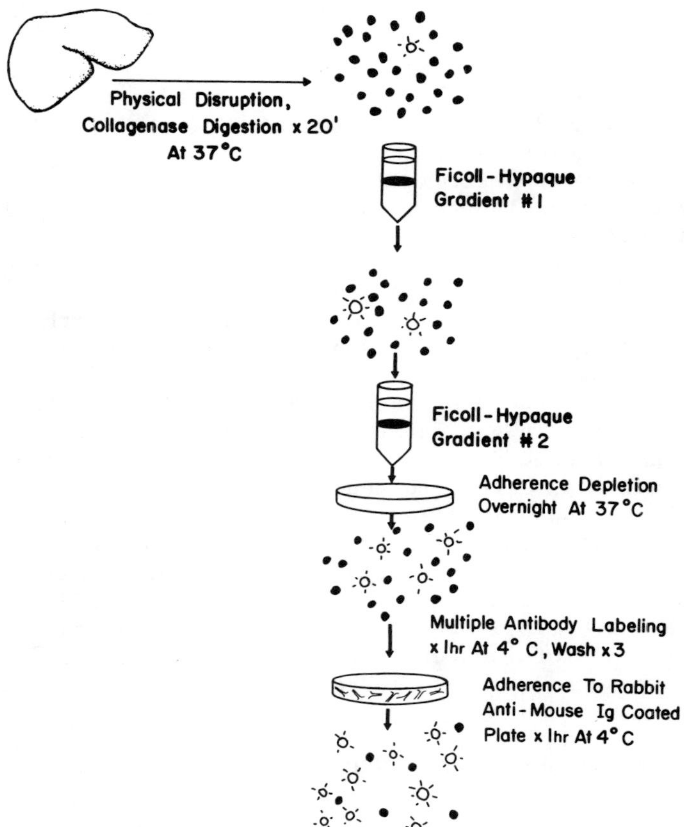

Figure 1. Purification protocol for hematopoietic progenitors from human fetal liver. (-ọ́- = progenitors, ● = others)

This high degree of purity allowed these cells to be used as target cells for the functional characterization of hematopoietic growth factors. For example, if erythropoitin is witheld from fetal progenitors for 72 hours in methylcellulose cultures, no erythroid or myeloid colonies will develop over the next two weeks despite the readdition of Epo or any source of hematopoietic growth factor (HGF). However, if graded doses, over the range of 0.1-20 ng/ml, of either GM-CSF or IL-3 are added at the outset of the culture, erythroid, myeloid and multilineage colonies are observed. (data for erythroid bursts is shown in Fig.2, below)

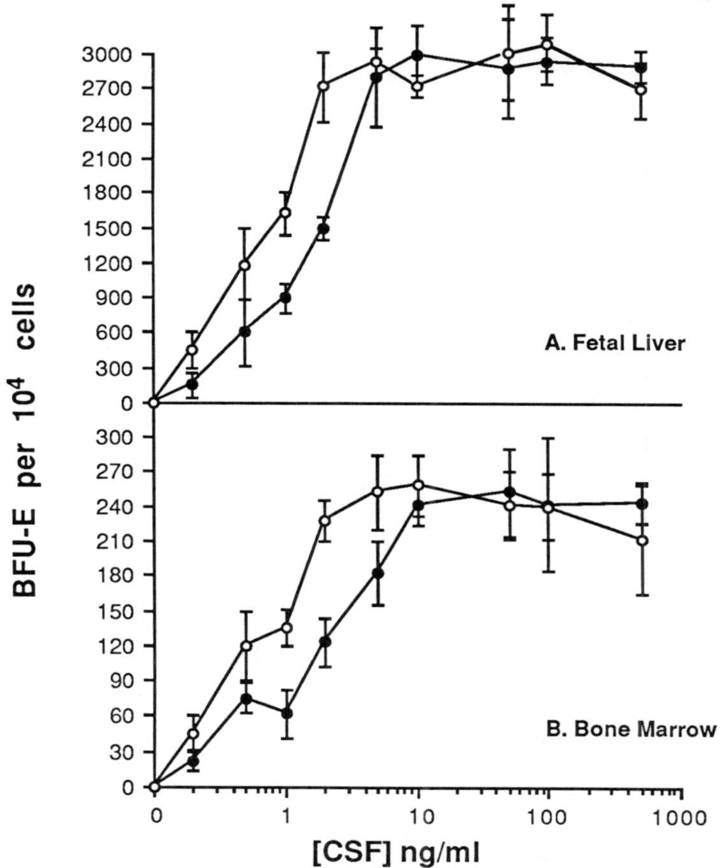

Figure 2. The response of enriched fetal hepatic versus adult marrow BFU-E to GM-CSF & IL-3 (o-o, IL-3;●-●, GM-CSF). Reprinted from Emerson et al., 1989a, courtesy of the journal BLOOD and Grune and Stratton publishers.

On the other hand, if Epo is included in fetal cultures from the outset, erythroid colonies develop whether or not GM-CSF or IL-3 is included. This is in sharp contrast to the behavior of adult bone marrow or blood BFU-E, which are highly dependent on additional so called "burst promoting activities" supplied by e.g. IL-3 or GM-CSF (Emerson et al., 1985, 1988, 1989a). This contrast suggested that Epo might function as a BPA for fetal, but not adult BFU-E. To test this hypothesis, isolated fetal or adult marrow progenitors were incubated in suspension cultures in the presence of Epo

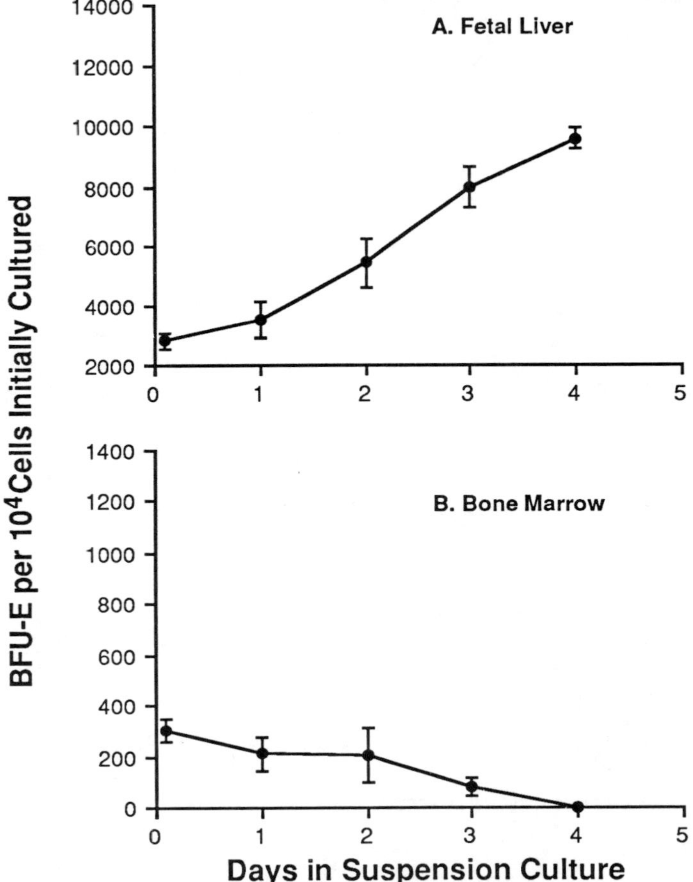

Figure 3. Burst promoting activity of Epo on fetal BFU-E. Fetal or adult progenitors were cultured in Epo for up to 4 days, and then cultured in methylcellulose for 14 days, at which time erythroid bursts were enumerated.

for up to 4 days, and then the suspended cells were plated in methylcellulose. In this assay, Epo clearly stimulated the division of fetal BFU-E, increasing the apparent cloning efficiency of the initially cultured preparation 4-500%. On the other hand, Epo had no such BFU-E proliferative effect on adult marrow BFU-E (Fig. 3, and Emerson et al., 1989a). These data indicated that fetal progenitor cells are unusually sensitive to Epo, responding to its stimulation by both division and differentiation. Under the influence of Epo, then, the fetal BFU-E mass would indeed be expected to increase in size, whereas in the adult it would remain a constant size over time.

B. GENERATION OF MONOCLONAL ANTIBODIES DETECTING EPO RESPONSIVE PROGENITOR CELLS

We then asked whether the enriched fetal progenitor preparations could be used to generate murine anti-human monoclonal antibodies specific for progenitor cells. Despite the relatively large number of progenitors that could be isolated from an individual preparation, cell numbers were insufficient to utilize normal immunization protocols. Therefore, we utilized subcapsular intrasplenic injection for the primary immunizations with 10^7 enriched fetal progenitor cells. In collaboration with Drs. James Ferrara and Julia Greenstein, we thereby repetitively immunized a balb/c mouse, harvested the splenocytes, and fused the cells with a nonsecreting NS-1 myeloma cell line. To screen the fusion, we identified wells whose supernatants detected, by complement fixation, ^{51}Cr-labelled enriched fetal progenitor cells but failed to detect similarly prepared JY lymphoblastoid cells. This selected for non-MHC antibodies, and resulted in some 35 distinct hybridoma antibodies.

To focus on progenitor-specific antibodies, we looked for antibodies that detected the smallest percentage of normal bone marrow cells. Using this approach, we identified one particulary interesting antibody, which we termed Ep 3. This IgM antibody identified 2-7% of bone marrow cells, as determined by immunofluorescence and complement fixation. When Ep 3 depleted cells were cultured in methylcellulose, a fascinating pattern emerged. First, all fetal BFU-E were

$Ep\ 3^+$. Second, a variable number of adult marrow BFU-E were $Ep\ 3^+$, varying from 20-75%. Finally, circulating BFU-E were invariably $Ep\ 3^-$. This pattern recalled the interesting earlier observations of Dr. Colin Sieff (Sieff et al., 1986) who had found that bone marrow BFU-E could functionally be divided into 2 populations: 1)those (immature) BFU-E that were BPA-dependent, and Epo-unresponsive; and 2) those (mature, CFU-E-like) BFU-E that were BPA-independent, and Epo-responsive.

We therefore repeated the GM-CSF deprival and Epo delay experiments of Sieff et al. on $Ep\ 3^+$ and on $Ep\ 3^-$ fractions of bone marrow BFU-E, and indeed found that the Ep 3 antibody labelled only Epo-responsive, BPA-independent BFU-E. We went further then, extending these experiments to the analysis of CFU-E as detected by classical day 7 plasma clot assays. As might have been predicted, all (Epo-responsive/dependent) CFU-E were $Ep\ 3^+$. Finally, treatment of circulating BFU-E with either GM-CSF or IL-3 in liquid culture converted these BFU-E from $Ep\ 3^-$ to $Ep\ 3^+$. Thus Ep 3, within the erythroid lineage, detected all Epo-responsive BFU-E. Of note, while a tail vein heteroserum from the immunized mice inhibited erythropoiesis in methylcellulose cultures, none of the monoclonal antibodies isolated had any inhibitory or stimulatory effect whatever.

C. AUTOIMMUNE REGULATION OF CYCLING PROGENITOR CELLS IN BONE MARROW AND FETAL LIVER

One of the mysteries of hematopoiesis is why cycling progenitors are $HLA\text{-}DR^+$, not to mention DR^+/DQ^-. The existence of patients with apparently DR-specific, lineage-restricted hematopoietic suppression syndromes has lead to the speculation that such cases are abnormal expansions of normal hematoregulatory cells. We therefore wondered whether the purified fetal progenitor cells could act as a stimulator of autoreactive, autosupressive T lymphocytes _in vitro_.

In collaboration with Dr. Joseph Antin, we irradiated enriched progenitor cells from both fetal liver and adult bone marrow, and then incubated them for 2-12 days with autologous T cells, either isolated from fetal spleen or from adult peripheral blood. We then measured T cell proliferation by 16 hour ^{3}H-TdR pulses. These experiments yielded two sets of surprising results. First, isolated bone marrow CD 34^+ cells stimulated the strong proliferation of a subset of autologous T cells, which could be expanded by repetitive stimulation. This proliferative response, which we termed the "autologous proliferative T cell response (APLR)" was dependent on progenitor cell DR and LFA-3 antigens, and on T cell CD2 antigens. Moreover, once expanded, the responsive T cells, when incubated with autologous progenitor cells supressed hematopoiesis. This was in sharp contrast to unstimulated or PHA stimulated T cells, which of course stimulated hematopoiesis (Fig. 4 and Emerson and Antin, 1989.)

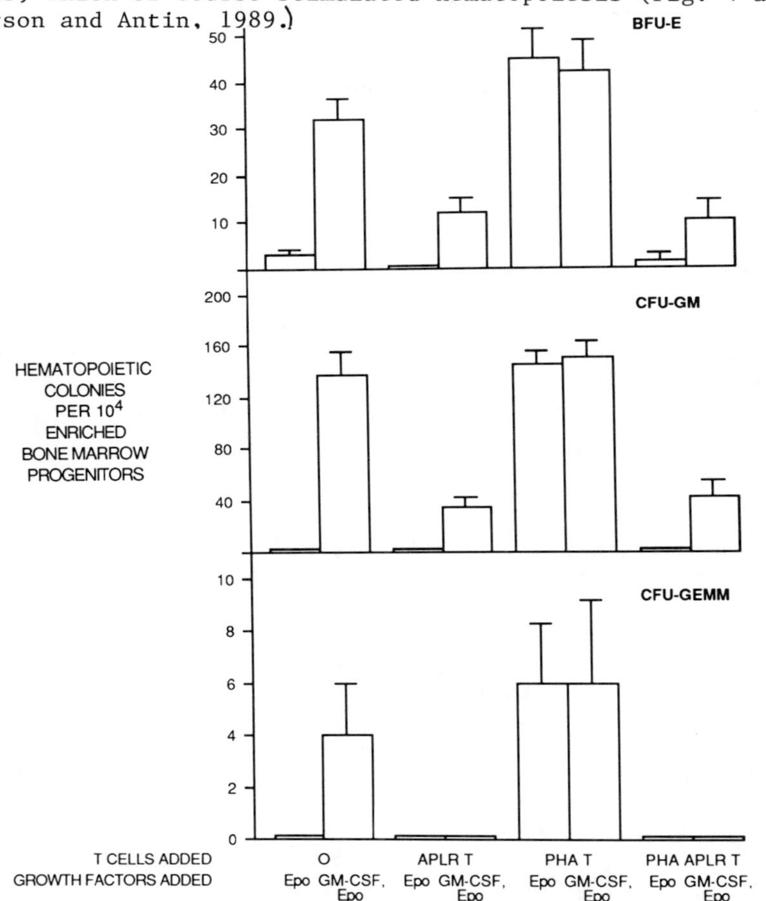

Figure 4. Suppression of autologous hematopoiesis by APLR activated T cells. Multiply APLR-activated, PHA stimulated, or PHA stimulated APLR-activated T cells were incubated with methylcellulose cultures (courtesy of Williams & Wilkins,Inc.)

The second, contrasting result was that fetal hepatic progenitors failed to stimulate an APLR. This defect seemed to be largely traceable to the apparent refractoriness of the fetal splenic T cells:

TABLE 1. Fetal Progenitors do not Stimulate a Fetal APLR

Stimulator	Responder	Mean S.I.
Adult BM Progen.	Adult T Cells	4.5*
Fetal Liver Progen.	Fetal Splenic T Cells	0.9
Fetal Liver Progen.	Adult Allogeneic Ts	10.0
Adult BM Progen.	Fetal Splenic T Cells	2.5

*Stimulation Index = ^{3}H-TdR incorporation of APLR T cells÷ ^{3}H-TdR incorporation of resting T cells.

These data suggest that a second, Epo-independent mechanism which may lead to clonal expansion in fetal life is may be the lack of adult homeostate regulatory T cell circuits, which normally serve to prevent the overgrowth of any particular hematopoietic clone.

In summary, these studies have demonstrate the utility of purified progenitor cells for elucidating the roles of HGFs and T cells in fetal and adult hematopoieisis, and have generated new antibody reagents that further assist in dissecting the physiology of hematopoiesis.

REFERENCES

Emerson SG, Sieff CA, Wang EA, et al. (1985). Purification of fetal hematopoietic progenitors and demonstration of multipotential CSA. J Clin Invest 76:1286-1290.

Emerson SG, Yang YC, Clark SC, Long MW (1988). Human IL-3 and GM-CSF have overlapping but distinct hematopoietic activities. J Clin Invest 82:1282-1287.

Emerson SG, Thomas S, Ferrara JL, Greenstein JL (1989). Developmental regulation of erythropoiesis. Blood 74:49-55.

Emerson SG, Antin JH (1989). Bone marrow progenitors induce a regulatory APLR. J Immunol 142:766-772.

Rowley PT, Ohlsson-Wilhelm BM, Farly BA (1978). Erythroid colony formation from human fetal liver. Proc Acad Nat Sci USA 75:984-988.

Sieff CA, Emerson SG, Mufson A, et al. (1986). Dependence of highly enriched bone marrow progenitors on HGFs and their response to recombinant Epo. J Clin Invest 77:74-81.

The Biology of Hematopoiesis, pages 29–36

CHARACTERIZATION OF HUMAN HEMATOPOIETIC STEM CELLS

JE Brandt, EF Srour, K van Besien and R Hoffman
Department of Medicine, Indiana University School of Medicine, Indianapolis, Indiana 46202

INTRODUCTION

Human bone marrow is composed of heterogenous populations of hematopoietic precursor and progenitor cells which are ultimately responsible for the production of the formed elements of the blood. These cell populations arise from a more primitive population of pluripotential hematopoietic stem cells which have been detected *in vivo* in the mouse by their ability to regenerate the hematopoietic and lymphoid systems of lethally irradiated recipients.[1] These cells are able to maintain a continual supply of stem cells, a process referred to as self-renewal, and also to undergo definitive lineage restricted differentiation.[1] The process of differentiation is associated with a progressive decrease in self-renewal capacity. In the 1960's, an *in vivo* spleen colony forming unit assay (CFU-S) was developed to quantitate the frequency of hematopoietic stem cells.[1] Both Visser et al and Spangrude et al have successfully used either lectin agglutination or monoclonal antibody labelling in conjunction with fluorescence activated cell sorting to purify murine hematopoietic stem cells.[2,3] The *in vivo* CFU-S assay was utilized by these investigators to test the biological behaviour of these purified cell populations. It has been estimated that these primitive murine hematopoietic stem cells represent only about 0.05% of all murine bone marrow cells.[3]

Pitfalls in Present Methodologies of Isolating Human Hematopoietic Stem Cells

A major obstacle in isolating a human equivalent of the murine CFU-S has been the lack of an available suitable human *in vivo* assay system for this purpose. Recently, several laboratories have cloned from human marrow, in an *in vitro* semisolid assay system, hematopoietic colonies which are composed of blasts and are capable of self-renewal and differentiation into multiple hematopoietic lineages.[4-6] The cells that give rise to such colonies have been termed the colony forming unit-blast or CFU-Bl. Although a great deal has been learned about the cytokine regulation of the CFU-Bl system, further analysis has proven difficult.[4-7] The CFU-Bl assay relies on subjective identification of late starting colonies and replating studies are necessary to test for the self-renewal capacity of hematopoietic stem cells. As performed in our laboratory, this assay requires 35-40 days to complete and is far too tedious to be utilized for routine purposes.[6]

An additonal methodological pitfall has been the absence of probes that are unique to the human pluripotent hematopoietic stem cell. Spangrude et al used monoclonal antibodies to the Thy-1 locus and the stem cell antigen-1 to purify the murine CFU-S.[3] Civin et al. have developed monoclonal antibodies to the human CD34 antigen.[8] This antigen appears to be present on the overwhelming majority of human hematopoietic progenitor cells and is likely expressed by human hematopoietic stem cells.[9] Additional specific probes useful for identification of the human equivalent of the mouse CFU-S are not available to date.

A growing number of cytokines that affect hematopoietic cell differentiation have been purified to homogeneity and cloned using recombinant DNA technology.[10,11] Definition of the individual cytokines or combinations of such cytokines that might permit *in vitro* proliferation of human hematopoietic stem cells has not been achieved to date. Establishment of optimal cytokine requirements for human hematopoietic stem cells is a critical component for the construction of an *in vitro* assay for this cell population.

The Blast Cell Colony System

Our laboratory has employed density centrifugation, counterflow centrifugal elutriation and monoclonal antibody staining followed by fluorescence activated cell sorting to characterize the CFU-Bl.[6] We have shown that the CFU-Bl expresses the CD34 antigen but does not express detectable amounts of the major histocompatibility class II antigen (HLA-DR).[6] The lack of expression of HLA-DR was confirmed using antibody-mediated complement-dependent cytotoxicity.[6] We next performed a series of experiments in which we attempted to determine the relationship between the CFU-Bl and the cells which are capable of initiating long term hematopoiesis _in vitro_.[6] For this purpose we utilized a modification of Dexter's method for sustaining long term hematopoiesis _in vitro_ where an increase in progenitor and precursor cell number is dependent upon close physical proximity to a preestablished stromal cell layer.[12] We have shown that $CD34^+DR^-$ cells but not $CD34^+DR^+$ are capable of initiating long term hematopoiesis for 50 days when seeded upon such irradiated stromal cell layer. By day 50, cultures initiated with $CD34^+DR^-$ cells contained 4x more assayable progenitor cells than $CD34^+DR^+$ cultures. These findings are in agreement with studies by Moore et al and Keating et al who used continuous marrow cultures to show that human bone marrow cells necessary for generation of long-term cultures were HLA-DR negative.[13,14] Such data suggest that the cells responsible for blast cell colony formation are identical to or closely related to the cell populations responsible for long term hematopoiesis _in vitro_. Andrews et al have previously demonstrated that the CD33 antigen is expressed by various classes of hematopoietic progenitor cells but not by cells responsible for long term hematopoiesis. We have shown that virtually none of the $CD34^+DR^-$ cells express the CD33 antigen (Figure 1), and that $CD34^+DR^-CD33^-$ cells are capable of both blast cell colony formation and initiating long term hematopoiesis _in vitro_.

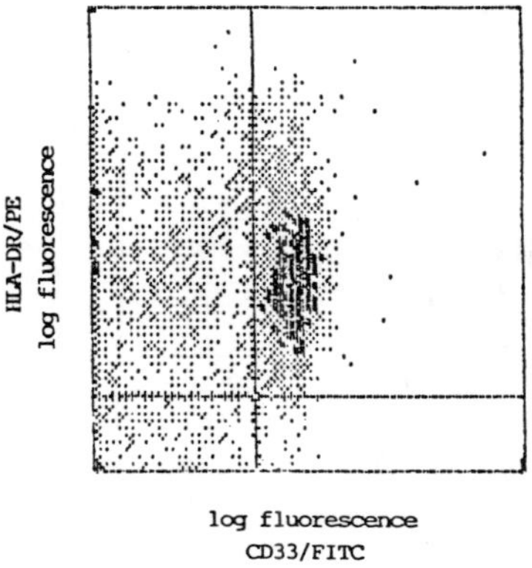

Figure 1.

Figure 1.
Dual parameter histogram representing the distribution of HLA-DR and CD33 antigens in CD34-positive bone marrow cells. Human low density mononuclear cells were obtained by density centrifugation over Ficoll-hypaque. Progenitor cells were highly enriched by counterflow centrifugal elutriation as previously described.[6] The cells were next stained using monoclonal antibodies to CD34, HLA-DR, and CD33 either directly or via second-step antibodies conjugated to either Texas red, phycoerythrin, or FITC respectively. Controls consisted of isotype matched incidental mouse antibodies and second step reagents. Stained cells were gated on positivity for TR-CD34. Positive fluorescence was defined as including those cell populations exhibiting fluorescence intensity above 99% of control cells. $CD34^{+}DR^{-}$ $CD33^{+}$ cells (lower right-hand quadrant) were present in very small numbers. The overwhelming majority of the $CD34^{+}DR^{-}$ cells did not express CD33 (lower left-hand quadrant). Analysis and sorting was performed on a Coulter Epics 753 dual laser flow cytometer.

The Suspension Culture System for Long Term Hematopoiesis.

The Dexter culture system is dependent on the establishment of an adherent cell layer which is then recharged with cell populations containing primitive hematopoietic cells. The adherent cell layer provides multiple functions in order for hematopoiesis to be sustained. Cytokines and matrix proteins are likely produced by such an adherent cell layer and important cellular interactions between accessory cells and hematopoietic cells are continuously occurring. The adherent layer based system is however inherently complex and this complexity hinders identification of cytokines that might be important for the long term maintenance of hematopoiesis.

With the hope of further identifying the cytokines which are important in sustaining long term hematopoiesis, we developed a suspension culture system for hematopoietic stem cells. Populations of marrow cells obtained after monoclonal antibody staining and fluorescence activated cell sorting were cultured in this suspension system in the absence of a pre-established stromal cell layer. Different cytokines singularly or in combination were then added every 48 hours for the duration of the culture. Weekly, the cultures were demidepopulated and cells enumerated, morphologically evaluated, and their ability to form progenitor cell derived colonies in semisolid media determined. The frequency of the various marrow cell fractions examined in this fashion are shown in Table 1. CD15 is a marker expressed by myeloid cells which was utilized with the hope of eliminating contaminating myeloid progenitor cells.[16] CD71 was used to identify cells expressing the transferrin receptor.[16] Since primitive hematopoietic stem cells are thought to be extremely quiescent, and CD71 is expressed primarily on proliferating cells, we hypothesized that they would express little if any CD71.

Frequency of Various Cell Fraction in Normal Human Bone Marrow

Cell Fraction	% of Nucleated Bone Marrow
Low density bone marrow	30
Marrow elutriated at 12-14 ml/min	3
$CD34^+$	0.2
$CD34^+DR^-$	0.07
$CD34^+DR^-CD33^-$	0.07
$CD34^+DR^-CD15^-$	0.06
$CD34^+DR^-CD71^-$	0.06

Both $CD34^+DR^-CD15^-$ and $CD34^+DR^-CD71^-$ cells represent, on average, only 0.06% of nucleated marrow cells. In the absence of added cytokine(s) these bone marrow subsets fail to expand their cell numbers. The repeated addition of interleukin-1 did not prolong effective hematopoiesis while the addition of interleukin-6 or GM-CSF alone prolonged the period during which progenitor cells were assayable to only three weeks. Hematopoietic progenitor cells were assayed from suspension cultures containing IL-3 for 4 weeks. By contrast, combinations of IL-1 and IL-3 and IL-6 and IL-3 contained assayable progenitor cells for 8 weeks. The IL-6 and IL-3 combination appeared to be the most effective for this purpose. These cultures were initiated with 5×10^3 $CD34^+DR^-CD15^-$ cells and by week seven contained 1.2×10^6 hematopoietic cells. The initial cellular innoculum contained 555 CFU-GM while by week 6 1,080 CFU-GM were assayed. Unlike long term marrow cultures utilizing preestablished stromal cell layers which are declining systems, the present system is an expanding one, indicating the tremendous proliferative potential not only of the starting cell population but also of the IL-3 and IL-6 cytokine combination. It is intriguing that Leary et al. have also reported IL-6 to be a cofactor with IL-3 in promoting the formation of blast cell colonies.[7] A confluent adherent cell layer was never established during the life of the suspension cultures after their initiation with the sorted cell populations. The ability to sustain long term hematopoiesis without such an adherent cell layer but following repeated recharging with cytokines suggests that marrow stroma is a rich source of cytokines that are important for human stem cell self renewal and differention. The observation that the suspension culture system is an expanding one indicates that stroma may also provide down regulators of hematopoietic cellular proliferation.

Summary

These data clearly indicate that suitable systems are presently available to isolate the human hematopoietic stem cell. The CFU-Bl and cells responsible for initiating long term hematopoiesis in vitro are likely identical since they share the same phenotype, $CD34^{+}DR^{-}CD33^{-}CD15^{-}C71^{-}$. The suspension culture system as indicated above has several advantages over an adherent cell based long term marrow culture system. Use of this suspension culture system with 48 hourly feeding with recombinant cytokines will facilitate definition of the cytokine requirements for the human CFU-S.

References

1. Till JE, McCulloch EA. A direct measurment of the radiation sensitivity of normal mouse bone marrow cells. Radiat Res 14:231, 1961.

2. Visser JWM, Bauman JGJ, Mulder AH, Eliason JF, deLeeuw AW. Isolation of murine pluripotent hematopoietic stem cells. J Exp Med 59: 1576, 1984.

3. Spangrude GT, Heimfeld S, Weissman LL. Purification and characterization of mouse hematopoietic stem cells. Science 211:58, 1988.

4. Rowley SD, Sharkis SJ, Hattenburg C, Sensenbrenner L. Culture of human bone marrow blast progenitor cells with an extensive proliferative capacity. Blood 69: 804, 1981.

5. Leary AG, Ogawa M. Blast cell colony assay from umbilical cord blood and adult bone marrow progenitors. Blood 69:953, 1987.

6. Brandt J, Baird N, Lu L, Srour E, Hoffman R. Characterization of a human hematopoietic progenitor cell capable of forming blast cell containing colonies in vitro. J Clin Invest 82: 1017, 1988.

7. Leary AG, Ikebuchi K, Hirai K, Wong GG, Yang YC, Clark SC, Ogawa M. Synergism between interleukin-6 and interleukin-3 in supporting proliferation of human hematopoietic stem cells. Comparison with interleukin-1 alpha. Blood 71: 1759, 1988.

8. Civin CI, Strauss LC, Brovall C, Fackler MJ, Schwartz JF, Shaper JH. Antigenic analysis of hematopoiesis III, A hematopoietic progenitor cell surface antigen defined by a monoclonal antibody KG-1a cells. J Immunol. 133:151, 1984.

9. Lu L, Walker D, Broxmeyer HE, Hoffman R, Hu W, Walker E. Characterization of adult human hematopoietic progenitors highly enriched by two color sorting with My10 and major histocompatibility class II monoclonal antibodies. J Immuno 139: 1323, 1987.

10. Sieff CA. Hematopoietic growth factors. J Clin Invest 79: 1549, 1987.

11. Clark SC, Kamen R. The human hematopoietic colony-stimulating factors. Science 236: 1229, 1987.

12. Dexter TM, Allen TD, Lajtha LG. Conditions controlling the proliferation of hematopoietic stem cell in vitro. J. Cell Physiol. 91: 335, 1977.

13. Moore MAS, Broxmeyer HE, Sheridan PA, Sheridan PA, Myers PA, Jacobsen A, Winchester RJ. Continuous human bone marrow culture. Ia antigen characterization of probable pluripotential stem cells. Blood 55: 682, 1980.

14. Keating AJ, Powell J, Takashashi M, SInger JW. The generation of human long term marrow cells from marrow depleted of Ia (HLA-DR) positive cells. Blood 64: 1159, 1989.

15. Andrews RG, Takahashi M, Segal GM, Powell JS, Bernstein ID, Singer JW. The L4F3 antigen is expressed by unipotent and multipotent colony-forming cells but not by their precursors. Blood 68: 1030, 1986.

16. Knapp W, Dorken B, Rieber P, Schmidt RE, Steen H, von dem Borne AEG Kr. CD antigens. 1989. Blood 74: 1448.

The Biology of Hematopoiesis, pages 37–48

SOME OBSERVATIONS ON THE GROWTH REQUIREMENTS OF MULTI-POTENT STEM CELLS UNDER DEFINED CULTURE CONDITIONS

Francis C. Monette and George Sigounas

Boston University, Department of Biology, Boston, Mass 02215

INTRODUCTION

It has been well over three decades since Eagle (1955) first identified some of the essential nutrients for mammalian cell culture. Although the growth-promoting properties of serum are well known (see reviews by Barnes and Sato (1980) and Dainiak (1985), it represents a very complex mixture of proteins and other factors which, until recently, have been difficult to define and/or purify to homogeneity. The recent availability of recombinant growth factors and hormones, however, has allowed an ernest attempt to better define the conditions under which mammalian cells are grown. One of the first reports of the complete replacement of serum in hematopoietic cell cultures was that of Iscove et al. (1980) who reported growing murine erythroid colony-forming units (CFU-e) with the addition of bovine serum albumin (BSA), iron-saturated transferrin, and a mixture of purified lipids to serum-depleted marrow cultures. Since then, a number of reports have appeared (Table 1) describing variously defined culture systems for hematopoietic cell progenitors. It will be the purpose of this report to review some of the major remaining obstacles to the complete definition of hematopoietic cell culture systems and to assess the growth requirements of multipotent stem cells under serum-free growth conditions.

Protein Additives

Typically, as has been the case for mammalian culture in general, two large molecular weight proteins are consistently added to serum-deprived cultures. Albumin, often as a crude preparation, is associated with fatty acids of undefined nature. In addition to serving as a carrier for essential fatty acids and some trace minerals, albumin may also have secondary functions such as transporting hormones and growth factors, act as a detoxifying agent for H_2O_2, as well as protecting cells against mechanical shear damage (Iscove and Melchers, 1978; Kan and Yamane,

TABLE 1. Summary of Reports on HSC Culture Without Exogenous Serum*

Reference	Cell	Matrix	Albumin	TF	Lipid	Other
Aye et al (1979)	BFU-E CFU-GM	MC	+	+	+	
Iscove et al (1980)	CFU-e	MC	+	+	+	
Golde et al (1980)	CFU-e BFU-E	MC	+	+		
Darfler et al (1980)	T-Lymphoma	Susp.	Casein	+	+	
Casadevall et al (1980)	CFU-e BFU-E	MC	+	+	+	
Stewart et al (1982)	CFU-e BFU-E	MC	+	+	+	
Dainiak et al (1984)	CFU-e BFU-E CFU-GM	FC	+	+		
Eliason & Odartchenko (1985)	BFU-E CFU-Mix	MC	+	+	+	Hemin
Suda et al (1986)	CFU-GEMM	MC	+	+	+	
Monette & Sigounas (1988)	CFU-GEMM	MC	+			Hemin

*Adapted from Dainiak (1985). MC, methylcellulose; Susp., suspension culture; FC, fibrin clot culture; HSC, hematopoietic stem cell.

1982; Darfler and Insel, 1983; Lambert and Birch, 1985; Glassy et al. 1988). Attempts to purify albumin to homogeneity have largely been unsuccessful although the protein can be delipitated to some extent by passing it over dextran-coated activated charcoal (Iscove et al. 1980). Recently, however, the complete amino acid sequences for human, bovine, and rat serum albumins have been determined and the three-dimensional structure of human serum albumin has been detailed (Carter et al. 1989).

In an attempt to circumvent albumin's drawbacks, there have been several reports of hematopoietic cell culture either in the absence of albumin (Sinclair et al., 1988; Patel et al., 1989) or with the supplementation of other purified proteins (e.g., casein, Darfler et al., 1980). Nevertheless, the presence of up to 2% exogenous protein in cultures otherwise deprived of other proteins is a potentially serious drawback when one is striving to totally define a culture system. The spectrum of potential interactions between exogenous protein and other culture components is extensive and has been detailed elsewhere (Dainiak, 1985).

A second major protein additive to serum-deprived cultures is transferrin, an iron-binding glycoprotein which has a principal role in facilitating the transport of iron across the plasma membrane (Trowbridge and Omary, 1981). Other sources of protein include hormones and growth factors which, if not pure, can prove misleading in an otherwise "defined" culture system. Clearly, as long as partially-purified serum proteins are added to such cultures they can not truly be defined as "serum-free."

Lipids

Bovine serum albumin contains both high and low affinity binding sites for fatty acids (Jonas, 1976) and thus is an efficient source of lipids which are required for the proliferation and differentiation of mammalian cells in culture (Chen and Kandutsch, 1981). This has caused some investigators to suggest that the main role of BSA in cell culture might be as a supplier of lipids or lipid precursors. The earlier work of Iscove (Guilbert and Iscove, 1976; Iscove et al., 1980) and Aye et al. (1979) suggested that lipoproteins were essential for hematopoietic colony growth in culture. Lipids are presumably essential for the biogenesis of cell membranes. One early study (Aye et al., 1979) identified a low density lipoprotein (LDL) fraction as the most potent stimulator of both erythroid and granulocytic colony growth in culture. Recently, Konwalinka et al. (1988) have systematically assessed the effects of highly purified fractions of all the major human lipoproteins on early (BFU-E) and late (CFU-e) erythroid progenitors. Their results suggest that although all lipid fractions stimulated erythropoiesis, LDL fractions were most effective and very-LDL were the least effective. Since the ability of lipoproteins to stimulate cell growth was correlated with the amount of cholesterol in the lipoprotein, Konwalinka et al. (1988) have suggested that lipoproteins exert their stimulatory effect by providing cells with cholesterol. In contrast, the work of Dainiak's group (Armstrong et al., 1989) suggests that although purified phospholipids support colony formation under serum-free conditions, lipoproteins negatively regulate the release of growth factors from accessory cells in culture and may thereby prove inhibitory to hematopoietic cell growth overall. Inhibition by LDL of cell function has been noted in other systems as well (Waddell et al., 1976; Curtiss et al., 1980). The reason for the discrepancy between these two laboratories is not clear but it should be noted that not all reagents utilized in these studies were homogeneous and thus some of these findings may be open to further interpretation.

Water Quality

One culture component often taken for granted is the quality of water for suspension. The method of preparation of pure water is important since different types of water purification systems as well as storage methods can fail to remove classes of contaminants or can actually increase the contaminants in the water (Mather et al., 1986). For example, stills do not remove volatile organics and liquid droplets can be carried over to the condensate along with the original water contaminants. On the other hand, ion exchange resins can add particulates and/or bacteria to water which is also true of activated carbon. Long-term storage also results in the degradation of water quality (Gabler et al., 1983). In a comprehensive analysis of the effects of trace organic and inorganic contaminants in tissue culture water on the growth of a variety of rodent cell lines in serum-free culture, Mather et al. (1986) found that the organic (humic acid, phenol, chloroform, phthalate ester) rather than the inorganic contaminants were more deleterious to cell growth. Small amounts (<10 ppb) of cadmium had the most marked effect on cell growth while the other inorganics tested (magnesium, copper, and lead) exibited variable effects. The need to utilize fresh, high purity water, free of both organic and inorganic compounds in serum-free cultures which are devoid of proteins which might otherwise reduce the toxicity of these compounds therefore seems highly advisable.

Oxygen Tension

Although most culture systems involve exposing cells to ambient oxygen tension (~19–20%), the oxygen levels in normal human tissues is more in the range of 2 to 5% (15–40 mmHg) (Cater and Silver, 1960). Therefore, the use of an ambient oxygen atmosphere for cell culture may result in oxygen toxicity and low cell plating efficiencies. This has been shown to be true for established rodent and human cell lines (Richter et al., 1972; Balin et al., 1982). Table 2 summarizes some of the published reports on the enhancement in hematopoietic colony growth secondary to reduced oxygen tension (to 5 or 10%). Consistent enhancement in colony plating efficiency has been noted by a number of laboratories from a low of 35–50% to a greater than two-fold enhancement. Not only is an enhancement of growth observed for most

TABLE 2. Hematopoietic Colony Growth Under Reduced Oxygen Tension

Colony Type	Species	Colony Enhancement§ 10% Oxygen	Colony Enhancement§ 5% Oxygen	Reference
CFU-GM	human		+	1, 4, 5, 7
	mouse		+	1
CFU-F (endosteal)	mouse	+	+	6
BFU-E	mouse		+	2
	human		+	3, 5, 7
		+		4
CFU-e	mouse		+	2
		+		4
CFU-Meg	human		+	7
CFU-Mix (CFU-GEMM)	human	+		4
			+	5, 7

References: 1, Bradley et al., 1978; 2, Rich & Kubanek, 1982; 3, Lu & Broxmeyer, 1985; 4, Maeda et al., 1986; 5, Smith & Broxmeyer, 1986; 6, Gupta et al., 1987;7, Katahira & Mizoguchi, 1987.
§, Relative to growth under ambient oxygen (19%). '+' indicates an observed significant enhancement in colony numbers.

of the cell types studied but stimulated growth is observed over a wide spectrum of growth factor/hormone concentrations (Rich and Kubanek, 1982; Maeda et al., 1986). This has led to the speculation that reduced oxygen enhances the sensitivity of cells to mitogens (Maeda et al.) whereas others have emphasized the reduced formation of free oxygen radicals (Rich and Kubanek, 1982; Smith and Broxmeyer, 1985). In contrast, the work by Allalunis-Turner et al. (1987), who compared the growth of murine CFU-GM under ambient and reduced oxygen tension (0.2 to 18%) suggests that other factors (such as pH), in addition to reduced oxygen, influence clonogenicity. Since it is well known that oxygen radicals are formed intracellularly in proportion to oxygen concentration (Freeman et al., 1982) and that in turn, these oxygen metabolites promote lipid peroxidation that potentially disturbs membrane functions (Fridovich, 1975), the oxygen radical hypothesis must be taken very seriously. Although serum-supplemented culture systems may indirectly (or directly) reduce the effective levels of oxygen-induced toxic molecules, cells grown in serum-free culture systems may be highly vulnerable to such toxicity.

Observations on the Behavior of Multipotent Stem Cells (CFU-GEMM) in Serum-Deprived Cultures

We have observed that murine bone marrow-derived CFU-GEMM exhibit a substantially reduced requirement for exogenous serum when grown in the presence of optimal levels of the lymphokine interleukin-3, the hormone erythropoietin, and iron protoporphyrin IX (hemin) (Monette and Sigounas, 1988). Although these cultures contained 1% BSA, they were not supplemented with exogenous lipid or transferrin. Optimum colony growth was observed at 5% serum, however a substantial level of colony formation occurred without serum (Fig. 1). This observation raised the possibility that an essentially simple "serum-deprived" semi-solid culture system could be established for the growth of murine hematopoietic stem cells. In order to optimize the growth

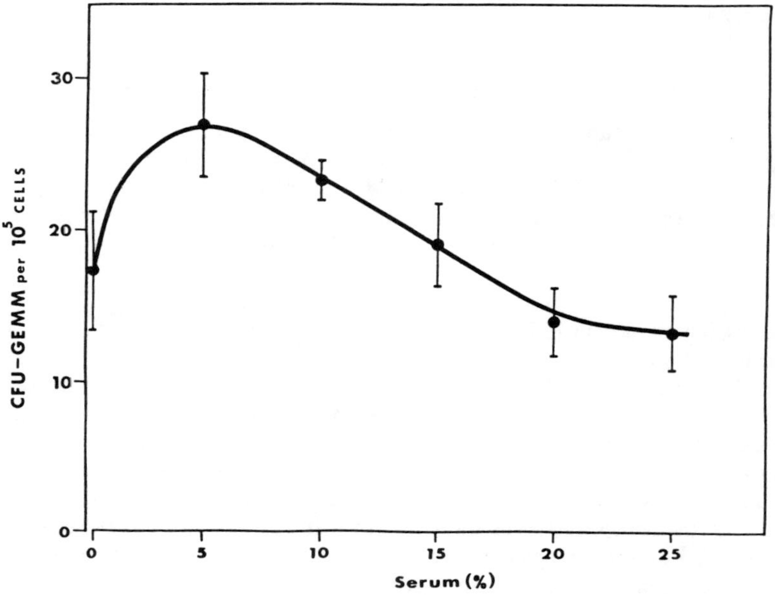

Figure 1. Fetal Bovine serum titration of murine marrow CFU-GEMM. Results were averaged from 4 separate studies employing two different serum lots. Cultures contained 30 μ/ml Il-3, 2 μ/ml r-EPO, 200 μM hemin, and 1% BSA. Reproduced with permission from Monette & Sigounas,1988.

factor requirements for this system, titrations of interleukin-3 (Il-3), erythropoietin (EPO), and hemin were performed. Figure 2 shows that in contrast to the high Il-3 requirement observed in serum-containing cultures, optimal CFU-GEMM growth was observed at an Il-3 concentration of ~5 units per ml. This represents a >four-fold reduction in the optimal Il-3 concentration. Likewise, the EPO requirement was

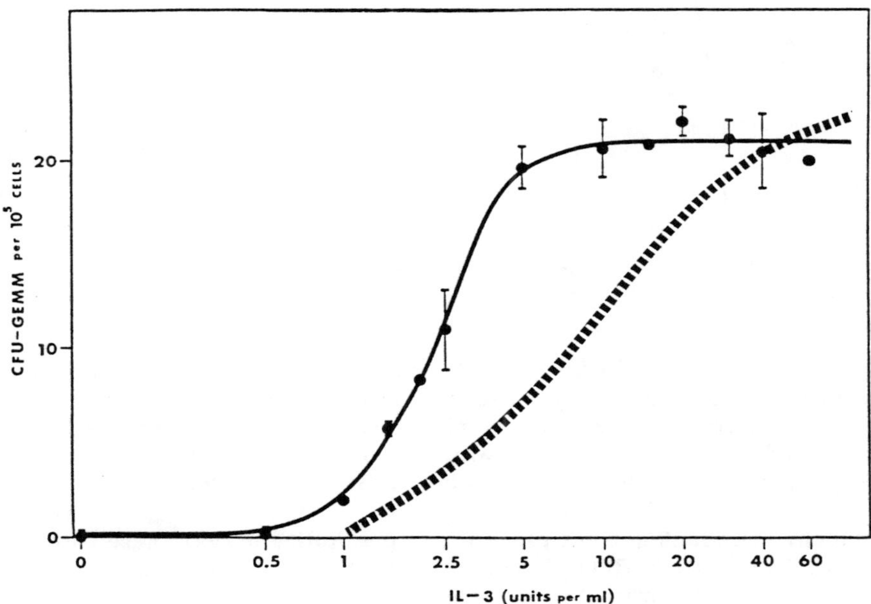

Figure 2. Growth of CFU-GEMM in "serum-free" methylcellulose cultures titered against murine interleukin-3 and expressed as $\pm$ 1 standard deviation. Results are from two (no error bars) to eight separate studies. Cultures contained 2.0 µ/ml r-EPO and 200 µM hemin. Dashed line = serum-containing culture.

reduced by a factor of 3 or more when serum-containing cultures were compared to serum-deprived cultures (Fig. 3). A slight reduction in the optimal hemin requirement was also observed in serum-depleted marrow cultures (Monette and Sigounas, 1988). The simplest interpretation for these "shifts-to-the-left" in the titration curves when cells are grown without exogenous serum is the reduction in non-specific adsorption of growth factors with the elimination of exogenous protein. In other words, there appears to be an increase in the cell sensitivity to growth factors when the overall protein load is

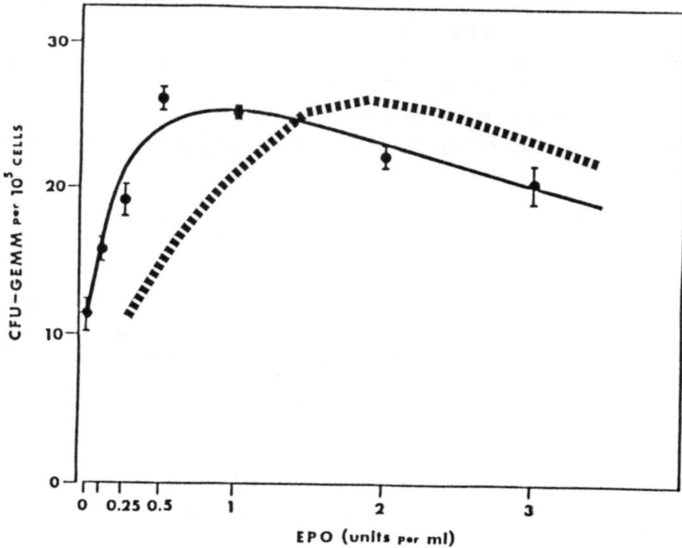

Figure 3. Growth of CFU-GEMM in "serum-free" methylcellulose cultures titered against human recombinant EPO (r-EPO). Results are from three separate studies and are expressed as the mean $\pm$ 1 standard deviation. Cultures contained 20 to 30 units/ml Il-3 and 200 μM hemin. Dashed line = serum-containing culture.

reduced. Although not yet proven, one possibility is that these three growth factors (Il-3, EPO, & hemin) do not require exogenous protein carriers for their optimal effectiveness.

The Role of Serum Albumin

As discussed above, albumin may serve as a carrier for a number of factors required for cell growth in vitro, one obvious candidate being phospholipids. Since the above studies utilized a standard, partially purified preparation of bovine serum albumin (BSA, Cohn fraction V) the effectiveness of crystalline and delipidated preparations was examined (Fig. 4). The results of six studies suggest that both purified (crystalline) and delipidated serum albumin are capable of supporting colony formation in serum-deprived marrow cultures to a level ranging from 36 to 58%, respectively, of the fraction V control. One possible suggestion is that the phospholipid transport role of exogenous serum albumin in serum-deprived cultures is minimal at best. Other roles for albumin will therefore need to be examined. For example, albumin is known to bind the metabolized protoporphyrins hemin and hematin (Adams and Berman, 1980). The

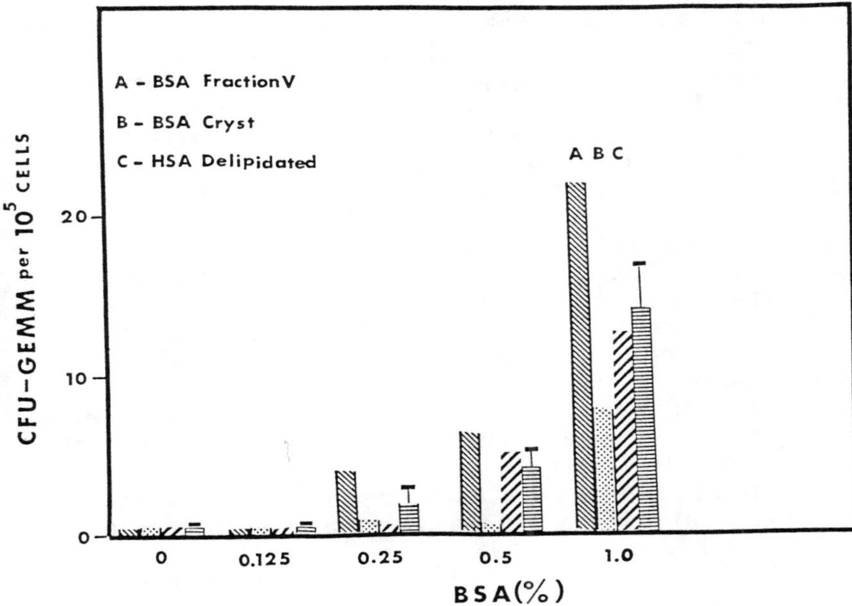

Figure 4. Titration of three preparations of serum albumin in serum-depleted marrow cultures. A, partially purified deionized BSA, Cohn fraction V. B, crystalline BSA obtained from commercial sources, lyophillized and deionized. C, highly purified human serum albumin. Purified from whole human plasma by affinity chromatography and delipidated and determined to be essentially pure by one-dimensional electrophoresis and virtually free of cholesterol (this preparation was kindly supplied by N. Dainiak. See Dainiak et al., 1985 for methods).

role of albumin in the efficacy of hemin and other stimulators of colony growth in serum-deprived cultures remain to be determined.

REFERENCES

Adams PA, Berman MC (1980). Kinetics and mechansim of the interaction between human serum albumin and monomeric haemin. Biochem J 191: 95-102.

Allalunis-Turner MJ, Koch CJ, Chapman JP (1987). Growth of murine bone marrow under various oxygen conditions in media buffered with HEPES. Internat J Cell Clon 5: 315-321.

Armstrong MJ, Warren HB, Davies PF, Dainiak N (1989). Nutrition requirements for mammalian cells and hematopoietic growth factor production. Annals N Y Acad Sci 554: 66-74.

Aye MT, Seguin JA, McBurney JP (1979). Erythroid and granulocytic colony growth in cultures supplemented with human serum lipoproteins. J Cell Physiol 99: 233-238.

Balin AK, Goodman DPB, Rasmussen H, Caristofalo VJ (1976). The effect of oxygen tension on the growth and metabolism of WI-38 cells. J Cell Physiol 89: 235-250.

Barnes D, Sato G (1980). Serum-free cell culture: a unifying approach. Cell 22: 649-655.

Bradley TR, Hodgson GS, Rosendaal M (1978). The effects of oxygen tension on hematopoietic and fibroblast proliferation in vitro. J Cell Physiol 97: 517-522.

Carter DC, He X-M, Munson SH, Twigg PD, Gernert KM, Broom MB, Miller TY (1989). Three-dimensional structure of human serum albumin. Science 244: 1195-1198.

Cater DB, Silver IA (1960). Quantitative measurements of oxygen tension in normal tissues and in the tumors of patients after radiotherapy. Acta Radiol 53: 233-256.

Chen HW, Kandutsch AA (1981). Cholesterol requirements for cell growth: endogenous synthesis versus exogenous sources. In Weymouth C, Ham RG, Chapple PJ (eds): "The Growth Requirements of Vertebrate Cells In Vitro," New York: Cambridge University Press, pp 327-342.

Curtiss LK, Deheer DH, Edington TS (1980). Influence of the immunoregulatory serum lipoprotein LDL-In on the in vivo proliferation and differentiation of antigen-binding and antibody-secreting lymphocytes during a primary immune response. Cell Immunol 49: 1-11.

Dainiak N (1985). Role of defined and undefined serum additives to hematopoietic stem cell culture. In Cronkite EP, Dainiak N, McCaffrey RP, Palek J, Quesenberry PJ (eds): "Hematopoietic Stem Cell Physiology," New York: Alan R. Liss, pp 59-76.

Darfler FJ, Insel PA (1983). Clonal growth of lymphoid cells in serum-free media requires elimination of H_2O_2 toxicity. J Cell Physiol 115: 31-36.

Darfler FJ, Murakami H, Insel PA (1980). Growth of T-lymphoma cells in serum-free medium: lack of involvement of the cyclic AMP pathway in long-term cultures. Proc Natl Acad Sci USA 77: 5993-5997.

Eagle H (1955). Nutritioin needs of mammalian cells in tissue culture. Science 122: 501-504.

Freeman BA, Topolosky MK, Crapo JD (1982). Hyperoxia increases oxygen radical production in rat lung homogenates. Arch Biochem Biophys 216: 477-484.

Fridovich I (1975). Superoxide dismutases. Ann Rev Biochem 44: 147-159.

Gabler R, Hegde R, Hughes D (1983). Degradation of high purity water on storage. J Liquid Chromatog 6: 2565-2570.

Glassy MC, Tharakan JP, Chau PC (1988). Serum-free media in hybridoma culture and monoclonal antibody production. Biotechnol Bioengineering 32: 1015-1028.

Guilbert LJ, Iscove NN (1976). Partial replacement of serum by selenite, transferrin, albumin, and lecithin in haemopoietic cell cultures. Nature 263: 594-595.

Gupta U, Rajaraman S, Costanzi JJ (1987). Effect of oxygen on the clonal growth of adherent cells (CFU-F) from different compartments of mouse bone marrow. Exptl Hematol 15: 1153-1157.

Iscove NN, Melchers F (1978). Complete replacement of serum by albumin, transferrin, and soybean lipid in cultures of lipopolysaccharide-reactive B lymphocytes. J Exptl Med 147: 923-933.

Iscove NN, Guilbert LJ, Weyman C (1980). Complete replacement of serum in primary cultures of erythropoietin-dependent red cell precursors (CFU-E) by albumin, transferrin, iron, unsaturated fatty acid, lecithin and cholesterol. Exptl Cell Res 126: 121-126.

Jonas A (1976). Interaction of phosphatidylcholine with bovine serum albumin. Biochim Biophys Acta 427: 325-336.

Kan M, Yamane I (1982). In vitro proliferation and lifespan of human diploid fibroblasts in serum-free BSA-containing medium. J Cell Physiol 111: 155-162.

Katahira J, Mizoguchi H (1987). Improvement of culture conditions for human megakaryocytic and pluripotent progenitor cells by low oxygen tension. Internat J Cell Clon 5: 412-420.

Konwalinka G, Breier C, Geissler D, Peschel C, Wiedermann CJ, Patsch J, Braunsteiner H (1988). Proliferation and differentiation of human erythropoiesis in vitro: effect of different human lipoprotein species. Exptl Hematol 16: 125-130.

Lambert KJ, Birch JR (1985). In "Animal Cell Biotechnology," Spier RE, Griffiths JB (eds), Vol. 1, New York: Academic Press, pp 85-122.

Lu L, Broxmeyer HE (1985). Comparative influences of phytohemagglutinin-stimulated leukocyte conditioned medium, hemin, prostaglandin E, and low oxygen tension on colony formation by erythroid progenitor cells in normal human bone marrow. Exptl Hematol 13: 989-993.

Maeda H, Tomomitus H, Yamada H (1986). Enhanced colony formation of human hemopoietic stem cells in reduced oxygen tension. Exptl Hematol 14: 930-934.

Mather J, Kaczarowski F, Gabler R, Wilkins F (1986). Effects of water purity and addition of common water contaminants on the growth of cells in serum-free medium. Biotechnol 4: 56-63.

Monette FC, Sigounas G (1988). Growth of murine multipotent stem cells in a simple "serum-free" culture system: role of interleukin-3, erythropoietin, and hemin. Exptl Hematol 16: 250-255.

Patel JM, Keene PAC, Ross FP, Loubser MD, Mendelow BV (1989). Selective culture of primate marrow-derived macrophages in medium devoid of protein additives. Exptl Hematol 17: 96-101.

Rich IV, Kubanek B (1982). The effect of reducecd oxygen tension on colony formation of erythropoietic cells in vitro. Brit J Haematol 52: 579-588.

Richter A, Sanford KK, Evans VS (1972). Influence of oxygen and culture media on plating efficiency of some mammalian tissue cells. J Nat Ca Inst 49: 1705-1712.

Sinclair J, McClain D, Taetle R (1988). Effects of insulin and insulin-like growth factor I on growth of human leukemia cells in serum-free and protein-free medium. Blood 72: 66-72.

Smith S, Broxmeyer HE (1986). The influence of oxygen tension on the long term growth in vitro of haematopoietic progenitor cells from human cord blood. Brit J Haematol 63: 29-34.

Trowbridge IS, Omary MB (1981). Human cell surface glycoprotein related to cell proliferation is the receptor for transferrin. Proc Natl Acad Sci USA 78: 3039-3043.

Waddell CC, Taunton OD, Twomey JJ (1976). Inhibition of lymphoproliferation by hyperlipoproteinemic plasma. J Clin Invest 58: 950-954.

Acknowledgments

The work described herein was supported by PHS grants DK 35325 and DK 37366 from the N.I.H.

The Biology of Hematopoiesis, pages 49–61

CELL MEMBRANE FAMILY OF GROWTH REGULATORY FACTORS

Nicholas Dainiak

Departments of Medicine and Lab Medicine
University of Connecticut Health Center
Farmington, CT 06032

INTRODUCTION

Plasma membrane proteins can be associated with the lipid bilayer in a number of ways. Transmembrane proteins pass as a single alpha helix or as multiple helices across the bilayer (see Figure 1). They are amphipathic, having hydrophobic regions that interact with the hydrophobic tails of lipid molecules within the bilayer, as well as hydrophilic regions that are exposed to water at either surface of the membrane. Other integral membrane proteins may be anchored to the bilayer via covalently attached lipids. Sometimes this linkage occurs via phosphotidylinositol groups to which may be attached carbohydrate units. In contrast to these proteins which are deeply imbedded in the bilayer, peripheral membrane proteins are bound by non-covalent (hydrogen bond or electrostatic) interactions with other membrane components (Alberts et al, 1989). All membrane proteins bind assymetrically to the lipid bilayer, a characteristic that is essential to the function of biological membranes.

Membrane proteins may be partially or selectively solubilized by a number of methods. Integral membrane proteins are released by disrupting the bilayer with organic solvents or detergents. In contrast, peripheral membrane proteins are released by relatively gentle extraction procedures, including manipulation of ionic strength and pH. Many membrane proteins have been identified and purified using these methods in an effort to understand membrane processes. Some of these proteins remain biologically active in detergent solution, such as rhodopsin and calsequestrin (Stryer, 1988). Others require reconstitution in a membrane to express function.

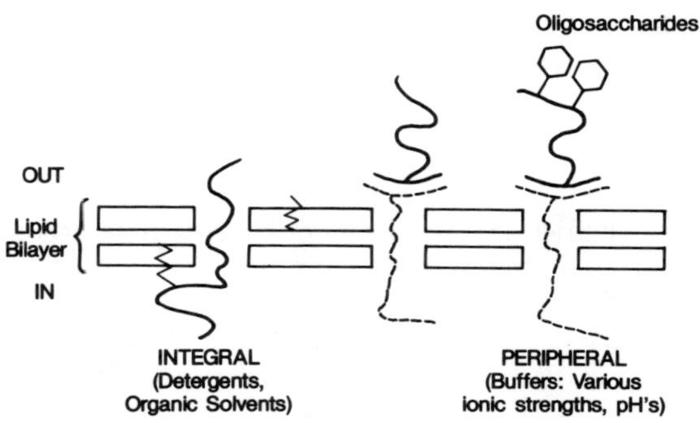

Figure 1: Membrane-associated proteins. Tightly bound integral membrane proteins may extend across the lipid bilayer (transmembrane) and may have covalently attached fatty acyl chains inserted into the monolayer. They are extracted with detergents or organic solvents. Other proteins do not extend into the hydrophobic interior of the lipid bilayer, but rather attach via noncovalent interactions with other membrane proteins. These peripheral membrane proteins are removed from the membrane by gentle extraction procedures.

Over the past five years, several growth regulators have been identified in association with the plasma membrane. These factors include membrane-associated erythroid burst-promoting activity (mBPA), an integral membrane component purified in my laboratory; a neurite mitogen for Schwann cells and possibly erythroid progenitor cells that is a peripheral membrane protein (Ratner et al, 1987); a negative regulator of DNA synthesis in erythroid BFU-Es that may be loosely associated with the cell surface (Del Rizzo et al, 1988); and multiple forms of membrane M-CSF, several of which appear to be transmembrane proteins that may be proteolyzed at the cell surface (Rettenmier et al, 1987; Cerretti et al, 1988). The location of these factors relative to the lipid bilayer is presented schematically in Figure 2.

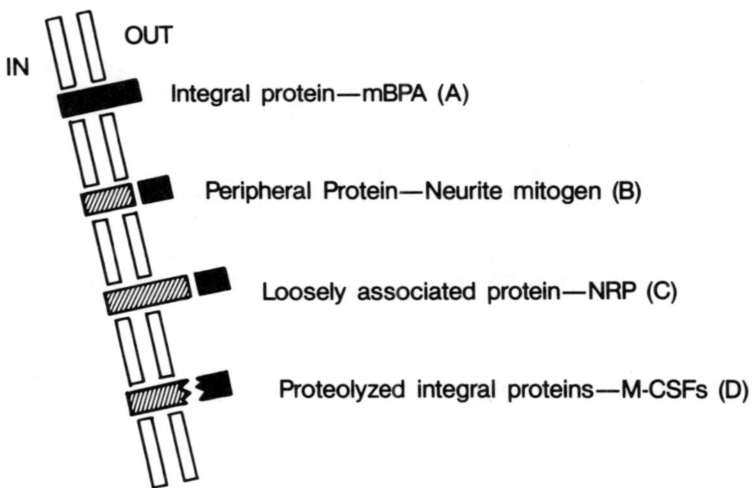

Figure 2: Surface molecules and cellular differentiation. Positive and negative regulators of cell proliferation have been identified in association with the plasma membrane. These include an integral lymphocyte membrane protein which is extracted with non-ionic detergents (A); a peripheral neurite membrane protein which is removed by extraction with salt and/or EGTA in the absence (and to a greater degree in the presence) of OG (B); a washable a protein that negatively regulates DNA synthesis in early erythroid progenitors which may be loosely attached to the cell surface (C), and a series of transmembrane proteins expressing M-CSF which may function at the membrane or may be proteolytically cleaved from the surface (D).

EXTRACTION AND PURIFICATION OF mBPA

When a partially purified preparation of lymphocyte plasma membranes is added to serum-free human marrow culture, a dose-related increase in erythroid burst formation is observed (Dainiak et al, 1982). Stimulatory activity is expressed not only by vesicles of the intact plasma membranes, but also by extracellular vesicles which are shed into serum-free liquid culture medium. In both cases a saturable dose-response curve is evident. The source of this activity (termed mBPA) appears to be the B-lymphocyte (Dainiak et al, 1987). Whereas mBPA remains associated with the pelletable fraction of membrane vesicles following incubation with potassium chloride, EDTA, sodium hydroxide, HEPES and PBS, it is solubilized when membrane vesicles are incubated with the non-ionic detergent ocytl-beta-D-glucopyranoside (OG). This behavior provides strong evidence that mBPA is an integral membrane component (Helenius and Simons, 1975).

Membranes that were isolated from light-density peripheral mononuclear cells were sequentially extracted with sodium hydroxide (as a negative selection step) and OG (as a positive step), and subjected to gel filtration chromatography on Sephacryl S300. mBPA eluted in fractions containing proteins with an Mr approximate 28,000 daltons. When the active fractions were pooled and applied to a DE-52 column, activity eluted as a sharp peak with either 20 mM phosphate or 0.2 M sodium chloride. mBPA-containing fractions from the latter eluant were applied to a TSK-240 HPLC column, and activity eluted as a single sharp peak (Feldman et al, 1987).

INTERACTION OF mBPA WITHIN THE LIPID BILAYER

To examine how deeply mBPA is associated with the lipid bilayer, intact plasma membrane and shed extra-cellular vesicles were incubated with Triton X-114. This nonionic detergent was selected since it is homogeneous at 0-4° C but partitions into aqueous and detergent phases at temperatures greater than 20° C. Therefore, it was possible to separate membrane hydrophilic and amphiphilic proteins of the membrane. Figure 3 outlines the protocol followed wherein intact membranes or shed vesicles were separated into detergent phase molecules containing amphiphilic proteins and aqueous phase molecules containing hydrophilic proteins.

PHASE SEPARATION OF MEMBRANE PROTEINS WITH TRITON X-114

1. Principle: Non-ionic detergent existing as single phase at 0-4°C, two phases at >20°C.

   Detergent phase amphiphilic proteins
   Aqueous phase hydrophilic proteins

2. Experiment;

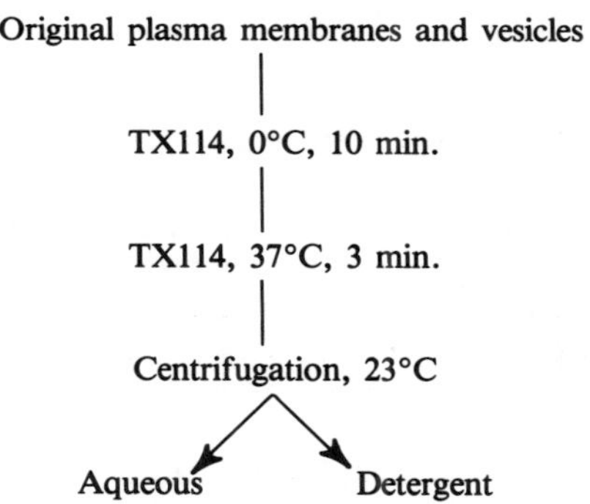

Figure 3: Partially purified plasma membranes and shed extracellular vesicles were solubilized in Triton-X114. During solubilization, nonionic detergents replace most lipids in contact with the hydrophobic domain of integral membrane proteins. Heating of TX-114 solubilized proteins to 37° C partitions the proteins into an aqueous phase (consisting of a large, clear, upper layer with approximately 20% of plasma membrane protein and 40% of shed vesicle protein), and a detergent phase (containing a small, turbid, lower layer with the remainder of extracted protein).

mBPA was localized by immunoreactivity with IgG purified from a monospecific rabbit antimembrane anti-serum which was found to adsorb the factor from solution (Dainiak et al, 1985a). Compared to the original preparation of shed vesicles and membranes, the detergent-soluble proteins contained significantly more cross-reactive material than did the aqueous proteins. Furthermore, bioactivity assessed in serum-free marrow cultures was present in preparations of the unextracted plasma membranes and detergent-soluble proteins to which synthetic phospholipids were added and the detergent removed in order to return the membrane proteins to the bilayer. In contrast, aqueous phase fractions similarly treated expressed no activity (see Table 1). These data suggest that mBPA is deeply imbedded in the lipid bilayer, and they raise the possibility that extensive interactions occur between the factor and lipid molecules within the bilayer.

RELATIONSHIP OF mBPA AND A NEURITE MEMBRANE-DERIVED MITOGEN

Recently, it has been reported by Ratner et al (1988) that a neurite plasma membrane mitogen which stimulates the proliferation of Schwann cells also binds to heparin. Since a number of hematopoietic growth factors are heparin-binding glycoproteins (Roberts et al, 1988), we explored the possibility that this mitogen may be related to mBPA. When added to serum-free human marrow culture, a crude extract of bovine Schwann cell mitogen stimulated BFU-E proliferation in a fashion analogous to lymphocyte plasma membranes. Furthermore, the activity was immunoprecipitated from solution with a monoclonal antibody which we previously prepared against mBPA (Dainiak et al, 1988), and which reacted with the surface membrane of B-lymphocytes (see Figure 4).

TABLE 1: EXPRESSION of mBPA by TX-114 SOLUBLE MEMBRANE PROTEINS

Membrane Preparations	Protein Concentration (μg/ml)	*No. Bursts/6 x 10^4 cells (Mean ± SD)
Plasma Membranes:		
Original Preparation	10,25	+15 ± 2, +20 ± 3
Detergent Phase	10,25	+18 ± 2, +19 ± 2
Aqueous phase	10,25	8 ± 4, 9 ± 1
Shed Extracellular Vesicles:		
Original Preparation	10,25	+17 ± 3, +21 ± 2
Detergent Phase	10,25	+28 ± 2, +35 ± 2
Aqueous Phase	10,25	9 ± 1, 10 ± 3

*No. of BFU-E derived colonies in 125 μl serum-free fibrin clots (Dainiak et al, 1985b). Control cultures without added membrane preparations contained 8 ± 2 bursts/125 μl.
+Relative to control, $p < 0.05$ or less.

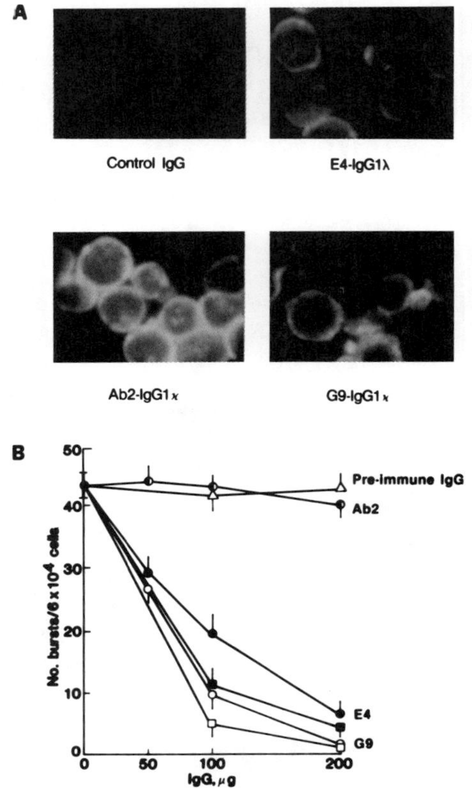

Figure 4: Fluoresent antibody staining of mBPA protein present on the lymphocyte surface. A: In contrast to control IgG, 3 monoclonal antibodies (E4, G9 and Ab2) react with surface components of B-cells. B: Two of the monoclones (E4 and G9) impair BFU-E proliferation in a dose-dependent fashion. The latter monoclones react similarly whether prepared from monoclonal supernatants (circles) or ascites fluid (squares). Additional testing by immunoabsorption revealed that E4 recognizes mBPA (Dainiak et al, 1988).

In addition, medium containing extracellular lymphocyte-derived vesicles stimulated Schwann cell proliferation as well (see Ratner in this volume). Accordingly, although the cell

TABLE 2: COMPARISON OF CELL SURFACE GROWTH FACTORS

Cell Source	B-Lymphocyte	Neurite
Bioactivity	Erythroid Progenitors Schwann Cells (?)	Schwann Cells Erythroid Progenitors (?)
Induction	Spontaneous	Spontaneous
Biochemical properties:		
extraction	OG	NaCl, EGTA, OG
glycoprotein	YES	?
Mrapp	28Kd	30Kd (60Kd)
Temp. stability:		
-70° C	YES	YES
56° C, 10 min	YES	NO
Stability to:		
DDT	YES	?
Neuraminidase	NO	YES
Castanospermine	?	NO
Heparin binding	?	YES
Immunologic behavior	Reacts with and adsorbed by anti (lymph)-membrane IgG	Reacts with and adsorbed by anti (lymph)-membrane IgG (?)

sources of these membrane bound growth factors are distinct, bioactivity may be shared. A comparison of the similarities and dissimilarities of biochemical properties and immunologic behavior of these two factors is provided in Table 2. It is possible that while distinct, these factors are conserved as growth factors for neuronal cells as well as hematopoietic cells. Additional studies with purified materials will be required to investigate the possibility that these factors are part of a family of membrane-associated growth factors.

SUMMARY

Both negative and positive regulators of cell growth and differentiation have been found in association with the surface of a variety of cell types, including fibroblasts, lymphocytes, undifferentiated components of the slug, neuronal cells, monocytes and mesenchymal cells (see Table 3). These molecules have been implicated in mediating contact inhibition, suppression of lymphopoiesis, inhibition of DNA synthesis in erythroid progenitors, induction of differentiation in Dictyostellium, stimulation of Schwann cell proliferation, and stimulation of the proliferation of a variety of hematopoietic cells, including myeloid (Price et al, 1975), erythroid and macrophage progenitor cells. In some cases, families of membrane bound growth factors have been described or are currently being appreciated. The importance of cell surface-associated regulators in mediating close cell-cell interactions in vitro and in vivo as well is under active investigation.

TABLE 3: Cell Surface-Associated Growth Regulators

Function	Cell Type	References
Negative Growth Regulators	Fibroblasts	Todaro et al, J Cell Comp Physiol 66:325, 1965 Abercrombie, Nature 281:259, 1979 Vale et al, J Cell Biol 98:1129, 1984 Whittenberger & Glaser, PNAS 74:2251, 1987
	Lymphocytes	Stallcup et al, J Cell Biol 99:1227, 1984 Del Rizzo et al, PNAS 85:4320, 1988
Positive Growth Regulators and Cell Differentiation Inducers	Dictyostelliium	Chung et al, Cell 24:785, 1981
	Neurites	Salzer et al, J Cell Biol 84:767, 1980 Ratner et al, PNAS 85:6992, 1988
	Lymphocytes, Monocytes Mesenchyme	Price et al, Exp Hematol 3:227, 1975 Dainiak et al, Blood 60:583, 1982 Feldman et al, PNAS 84:6775, 1987 Kurt-Jones et al, PNAS 82:1204, 1985 Nara & McCulloch, J Exp Med 162:1435, 1985 Kawasaki et al, Science 230:291, 1985 Rettenmier et al, Mol Cell Biol 7:2378, 1987 Cerretti et al, Mol Immunol 25:761, 1988

REFERENCES

1. Alberts B, Bray D, Lewis J, Raff M, Roberts K, Watson JD (1989). "Molecular Biology of the Cell". New York: Garland Publishing, pp 275-340.

2. Cerretti DP, Wignall J, Anderson D, Tushinski RJ, Gallis BM, Stya M, Gillis S, Urdal DL, Cosman D (1988). Human macrophage-colony stimulating factor: alternative RNA and protein processing from a single gene. Molecular Immunology 25:761-770.

3. Dainiak N, Cohen CM (1982). Surface membrane vesicles from mononuclear cells stimulate erythroid stem cells to proliferate in culture. Blood 60:583-594.

4. Dainiak N, Feldman L, Cohen CM (1985a). Neutralization of erythroid burst-promoting activity in vitro with antimembrane antibodies. Blood 65:877-885.

5. Dainiak N, Kreczko S, Cohen A, Pannell R, Lawler J (1985b). Primary human marrow cultures for erythroid bursts in a serum-substituted system. Exp Hematol 13:1073-1079.

6. Dainiak N, Najman A, Kreczko S, Baillou C, Mier J, Feldman L, Gorin NC, Duhamel G (1987). B-lymphocytes as a source of cell surface growth-promoting factors for hematopoietic progenitors. Exp. Hematol 15: 1086-1096.

7. Dainiak N, Warren G, Sutter D, Kreczko S, Howard D (1988). A monoclonal antibody to exfoliated surface vesicles that recognizes a membrane-associated erythroid burst-promoting activity. Blood 72:989-994.

8. Del Rizzo DF, Eskinazi D, Axelrad AA (1988). Negative regulation of DNA synthesis in early erythropoietic progenitor cells (BFU-E) by a protein purified from the medium of C57BL/6 mouse marrow cells. Proc Natl Acad Sci USA 85:4320-4324.

9. Feldman L, Cohen CM, Riordan MA, Dainiak N, (1987). Purification of a membrane-derived human erythroid growth factor. Proc Natl Acad Sci USA 84:6775-6779.

10. Helenius A, Simons K (1975). Solubilization of membranes by detergents. Biochim Biophys Acta 415:29-79.

11. Price GB, McCulloch EA, Till JE (1975). Cell membranes as sources of granulocyte colony stimulating activities. Exp Hematol 3:227-233.

12. Ratner N, Wood PW, Bunge RP, Glaser L (1987). In Althaus HH, Seifert W, eds: "Glial Neuronal Communication in Development and Regeneration". New York: Springer-Verlag.

13. Ratner N, Hong D, Lieberman MA, Bunge RP, Glaser L (1988). The renewal cell-surface molecule mitogenic for Schwann cells is a heparin-binding protein. Proc Natl Acad Sci USA 85:6992-6996.

14. Rettenmier CW, Roussel MF, Ashmuu RA, Ralph P Price K, Sherr CJ (1987). Synthesis of membrane-bound colony-stimulating factor 1 (CSF-1) and downmodulation of CSF-1 receptors in NIH 3T3 cells transformed by cotransfection of the human CSF-1 and c-fms (CSF-1 receptor) genes. Mol Cell Biol 7:2378-2387.

15. Roberts R, Gallagher J, Spooncer E, Allen TD, Bloomfield F, Dexter TM (1988). Heparin sulfate bound growth factors: a mechanism for stromal cell mediated haemopoiesis. Nature 332:376-378.

The Biology of Hematopoiesis, pages 63–70

MEMBRANE BOUND FORMS OF HUMAN MACROPHAGE COLONY STIMULATING FACTOR (M-CSF, CSF-1)

Douglas P. Cerretti, Janis Wignall, Dirk Anderson, Robert J. Tushinski, Byron Gallis, and David Cosman

Departments of Molecular Biology, Biochemistry and Experimental Hematology, Immunex Corporation, 51 University St., Seattle, Washington 98101

INTRODUCTION

Macrophage colony stimulating factor (M-CSF, CSF-1) is a subclass of colony stimulating factors that is thought to be required for the proliferation and differentiation of macrophages from immature hematopoietic progenitor cells(Clark and Kamen, 1987). In addition M-CSF can also induce effector functions of the mature cells such as increased secretion of cytokines and superoxide (Warren and Ralph, 1986; Wing *et al.*, 1985). Unlike the other colony stimulating factors, which are small monomeric glycoproteins, M-CSF is a more complex protein. Natural M-CSF is a glycosylated, disulfide-linked homodimer with molecular weights reported from 45-90 kDa. Dimerization is required for biological activity (Das and Stanley, 1982). Recently, three different but related M-CSF cDNA clones have been isolated that encode proteins of 256 (Kawasaki *et al.*, 1985), 554 (Wong *et al.*, 1987), and 438 (Cerretti *et al.*, 1988) amino acids, which we have termed M-CSFα M-CSFβ, and M-CSFγ, respectively. In this report, we show that all three cDNAs secrete proteins which are biologically active and that these proteins are processed from membrane bound precursors.

RESULTS AND DISCUSSION

The sequence of the cDNAs , as illustrated in Fig. 1, reveal that the proteins encoded by these clones share a common amino-terminus of 149 amino acids, including a 32 amino acid signal sequence and a common 75 amino acid carboxyl-terminus including a membrane spanning region. The additional amino acids encoded in M-CSFβ and M-CSFγ lie in between these regions of identity and are encoded by alternatively spliced mRNA species (Cerretti *et al.*, 1988). The coding regions for M-CSFα, M-CSFβ and M-CSFγ were inserted into the mammalian expression vector, pDC201 (Cerretti *et al.*, 1988) and the resulting plasmids were transfected into COS-7 monkey kidney cells. After 72 hr, the cultures were labeled for 24 hr with ^{35}S-Met and ^{35}S-Cys and M-CSF specific proteins were immunoprecipitated from the supernatents with a rabbit anti-M-CSF polyclonal antiserum. This antiserum was made against the amino-terminal 149 amino acids of M-CSFα. Immunoprecipitates were subjected to SDS-PAGE under reducing conditions and protein bands visualized by autoradiography.

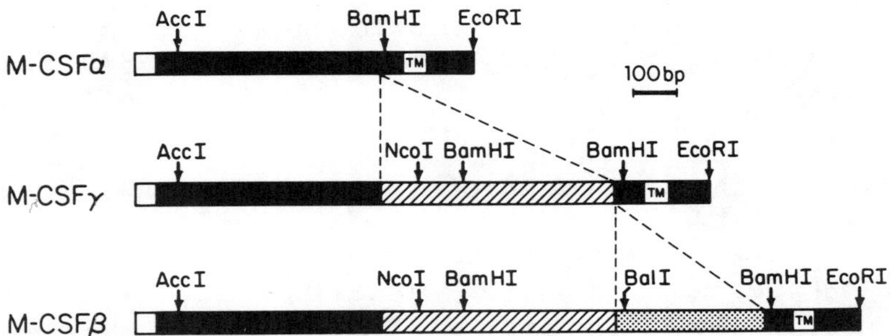

Figure 1. Schematic representation of the coding regions of human M-CSF cDNAs, M-CSFα, M-CSFβ and M-CSFγ. Open boxes and TM represent the signal sequence and transmembrane region.

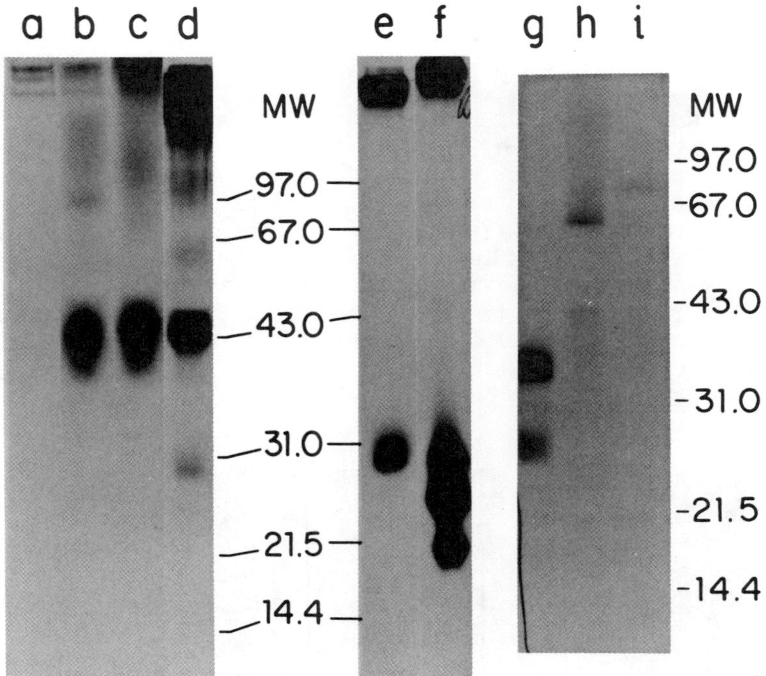

Figure 2. Autoradiogram of SDS-PAGE of M-CSF specific proteins synthesised by COS-7 cells transfected with pDC201 (lane a) M-CSFγ (lane b and h), M-CSFβ (lane c and i), genomic M-CSF (lane d), M-CSFα (lane e and g) and [s]M-CSFα (lane f). Proteins were immunoprecipitated from culture supernatents (lanes a-f) or from membranes (lanes g-i) with rabbit anti-M-CSF antiserum.

As can be seen from Fig. 2, proteins synthesized and secreted by M-CSFβ and M-CSFγ have a molecular size of 44 kDa (lanes b and c) while M-CSFα synthesized a protein of molecular size 28 kDa (lane e). Thus, even though the M-CSFβ precursor is 116 amino acids larger than that of M-CSFγ, proteins of similar size are secreted. As a comparison, COS-7 cells, transfected with a genomic clone of M-CSF, synthesized proteins of 44 and 28 kDa (lane d) indicating that these proteins are the predominant extracellular forms of M-CSF.

The cell surface localization of M-CSF proteins were analyzed by staining transfected COS-7 cell with the rabbit anti-M-CSF antiserum followed by treatment with goat anti-rabbit antiserum conjugated with fluorescein isothiocyanate. Fig. 3 shows that COS-7 cells, transfected with each the three M-CSF cDNAs, have a uniform cell surface staining indicating the

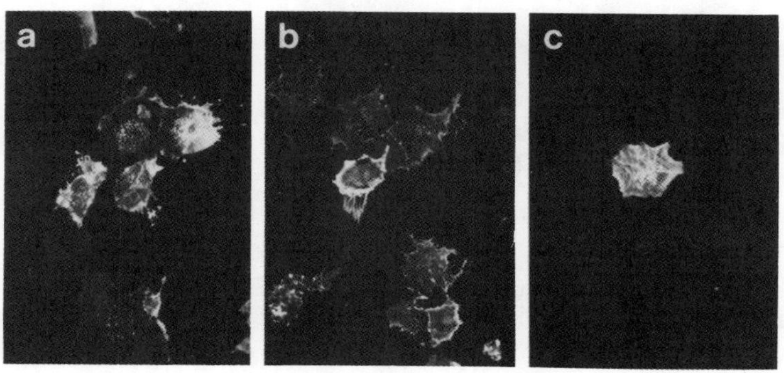

Figure 3. Fluorescent antibody staining of M-CSF protein expressed on the cell surface of COS-7 cells transfected with M-CSFα (panel a), M-CSFγ (panel b) and M-CSFβ (panel c).

membrane localization of the M-CSF protein. Analysis of these membrane proteins on SDS-PAGE after radiolabeling and immunoprecipitation demonstrates that M-CSFα, M-CSFβ and M-CSFγ synthesize proteins with molecular sizes of 33, 70, and 60 kDa (Fig. 2, lanes g, h, and i). These bands probably represent full length translation products including contributions from N-linked glycosylation.

The precursor nature of the membrane bound protein was tested by construction of a truncated form of M-CSFα, [s]M-CSFα, that lacks the carboxyl-terminal 66 amino acids of M-CSFα including the transmembrane region. COS-7 cells, transfected with this cDNA, were analysed as above. SDS-PAGE (Fig. 2, lane f) of secreted M-CSF reactive proteins, shows that a protein is synthesized (28 kDa) similar in size to that secreted by cells transfected with full length M-CSFα . In addition, no cell surface staining with anti-M-CSF antiserum was seen. This indicates that the membrane bound proteins are precursors to the secreted forms of M-CSF. The smaller molecular size bands in Fig. 2, lane f represent heterogenous glycosylation.

Supernatants from the M-CSF cDNA transfections were tested for M-CSF activity in

TABLE 1. BONE MARROW ASSAYS OF RECOMBINANT M-CSF EXPRESSED IN COS-7 CELLS

	Proliferation Units/ml		Monocytic Colony Formation Units/ml	
Plasmid	Murine	Human	Murine	Human
pDC201	0	0	0	0
M-CSFα	3,177	0	19,140	238
M-CSFβ	5,375	0	35,863	280
M-CSFγ	3,991	0	16,240	392
[s]M-CSFα	16,443	0	114,260	1,092
genomic M-CSF	63	0	1815	120
GM-CSF (human)	0	130,876	0	111,531

murine and human bone marrow proliferation and colony formation assays.As can be seen from Table 1, the three M-CSF cDNAs as well as genomic M-CSF and [s]M-CSFα clones produce proteins that were active on murine bone marrow cells in proliferation and monocytic colony assays. This indicates that the transmembrane region, absent in [s]M-CSFα, is not required for biological activity. In human bone marrow, however, none of the M-CSF clones were active in the proliferation assay and only weakly active in the colony assay. The colonies that were formed are fewer in number and much less dense (<100 cells) when compared to the colonys formed in the murine assay. This dichotomy of activity, greater activity in murine bone marrow than in human bone marrow, is not seen in other human CSFs such as GM-CSF, G-CSF and IL-3 and raises the question of the role of M-CSF in human hematopoiesis. In murine hematopoiesis it is clear that M-CSF is a potent colony stimulating factor required for growth, survival and differentiation of the mononuclear macrophage lineage (Tushinski *et al.*, 1982). It is possible that in humans, M-CSF has lost many of these functions and its main role is as an effector of mature macrophages. Alternatively, perhaps its main role is not that of a soluble cytokine but that of a cell membrane family of molecules, the expression of which may direct cell to cell interactions important to the regulation of hematopoiesis.

CONCLUSIONS

1. The gene for human M-CSF transcribes at least three mRNA species. These multiple mRNAs are probably a result of alternative RNA splicing.

2. The three M-CSF cDNAs, which we have termed M-CSFα, M-CSFβ and M-CSFγ encode primary translation products of 256, 554 and 438 amino acids respectively. The proteins share a common

N-terminus of 149 amino acids and a common C-terminus of 75 amino acids including a transmembrane region. They differ only by the length of an internal amino acids sequence.

3. When expressed in mammalian cells, M-CSF cDNAs produce multiple M-CSF proteins. The two largest clones M-CSFβ and M-CSFγ secrete a 44 kDa protein while M-CSFα secretes a 28 kDa protein. All three clones produce a membrane bound form of M-CSF.

4. All M-CSF clones, including a version lacking the transmembrane region, cause proliferation and differentiation of murine bone marrow but only differentiation of human bone marrow. The differentiation effect on human bone marrow is not very strong when compared to the differentiation effect on murine bone marrow. These results also indicate that the transmembrane region, present in all three cDNAs is not required for biological activity.

5. Since M-CSF exists as a membrane bound molecule, it may function in the context of cell-cell interactions.

ACKNOWLEDGEMENTS

We thank Iris Bachmann for preparation of the manuscript, Steve Gimpel, Eric Spoor, Jana Jackson and Vickie Craig for excellent technical assistance. This work was made possible by an ongoing collaboration between Immunex Corporation and Behringwerke A.G.

REFERENCES

Cerretti DP, Wignall J, Anderson D, Tushinski RJ, Gallis BM, Stya M, Gillis S, Urdal DL, Cosman D (1988). Human macrophage-colony stimulating factor: alternative RNA and protein processing from a single gene. Molecular Immunology

25:761-770.

Clark SC and Kamen R (1987). The human hematopoietic colony-stimulating factors. Science 236:1229-1237.

Das SK and Stanley ER (1982) Structure-function studies of a colony stimulating factor (CSF-1). J Biol Chem 257:13679-13684.

Kawasaki EE, Ladner MB, Wang AM, Van Arsdell J, Warren MK, Coyne MY, Schweichart VL, Lee MT, Wilson KJ, Boosman A, Stanley ER, Ralph P, Mark DF (1985). Molecular cloning of a complementary DNA encoding human macrophage-specific colony stimulating factor (CSF-1). Science 230:291-296.

Rettenmier CW, Roussel MF, Ashmun RA, Ralph P, Price K, Sherr CJ (1987). Synthesis of membrane-bound colony-stimulating factor 1 (CSF-1) and downmodulation of CSF-1 receptors in NIH 3T3 cells transformed by cotransfection of the human CSF-1 and c-fms (CSF-1 receptor) genes. Mol Cell Biol 7:2378-2387.

Tushinski RJ, Oliver IT, Guilbert LJ, Tynan PW, Warner JR, Stanley ER (1982). Survival of mononuclear phagocytes depends on a lineage-specific growth factor that the differentiated cells selectively destroy. Cell 28:71-81.

Warren MK, Ralph P (1986). Macrophage growth factor CSF-1 stimulates human monocyte production of interferon, tumor necrosis factor and colony stimulating activity. J Immunol 137:2281-2285.

Wing EJ, Ampel NM, Waheed A, Shadduck RK (1985). Macrophage colony-stimulating factor (M-CSF) enhances the capacity of murine macrophages to secrete oxygen reduction products. J Immunol 135:2052-2056.

Wong GG, Temple PA, Leary AC, Witek-Giannoti JS, Yang YC, Ciarletta AB, Chung M, Murtha P, Kriz R, Kaufman RJ, Ferenze CR, Sibley BS, Turner KJ, Hewick RM, Clark SC, Yanai N, Yokota H, Yamada M, Saito M, Motoyoshi K, Takaku F (1987). Human CSF-1: molecular cloning and expression of a 4 kb cDNA encoding the human urinary protein. Science 235:1504-1508.

The Biology of Hematopoiesis, pages 71–78

CELL-SURFACE HEPARAN-SULFATE PROTEOGLYCAN REGULATES THE EXPRESSION OF A MEMBRANE-ASSOCIATED NEURONAL MITOGEN

N. Ratner

Dept of Anatomy and Cell Biology, Univ of

Cincinnati Medical School, Cincinnati, OH

INTRODUCTION

A number of lines of evidence strongly suggest that a membrane-associated mitogen plays a physiologically important role in the stimulation by neurons of proliferation of their sheath cells, Schwann cells. A tissue culture system has been developed in which neurons and Schwann cells can be purified, separated and recombined (Wood, 1976) for analysis of cell-cell interactions; this culture system has been used to characterize the neuronal cell surface molecule mitogenic for Schwann cells (Neuron-Derived Growth Factor, NDGF).

In contrast, although a number of mitogens, including colony-stimulating factor-1, interleukin-1α, transforming growth factor-α, epidermal growth factor, and vaccinia virus growth factor, are synthesized in both soluble and membrane-associated forms (Cerretti *et al*. 1988, and references therein) the function of the membrane-associated form is not understood; it has been suggested that membrane-associated CSF-1 could direct cell-cell interactions which regulate hematopoeisis.

PRELIMINARY CHARACTERIZATION OF NDGF

Schwann cell proliferation is tightly regulated *in vivo* and *in vitro*. A burst of Schwann cell division occurs during early postnatal life in rodents, and Schwann cells exhibit very low basal proliferation thereafter (Asbury, 1967). However, Schwann cells can be stimulated to re-enter the cell cycle in the adult in reaction to injury and during peripheral nerve regeneration. In tissue culture, Schwann cells also divide at a very low level, even in the presence of serum (<1% of cultured Schwann cells incorporate S-phase markers in 24h), unless provided with specific mitogenic stimuli (Wood & Bunge, 1976; Raff et al., 1978).

Both *in vivo* and *in vitro* evidence suggest that the neuron itself provides the mitogenic stimulus for Schwann cells. *In vivo*, Schwann cell numbers expand as neuronal outgrowth occurs and experimental manipulations leading to reduced numbers of axons lead to decreases in Schwann cell number, implying that the size of the Schwann cell population is proportional to axonal number (Aguayo *et al.*, 1976). Neuronal stimulation of Schwann cell proliferation has been shown directly in tissue culture (Figure 1), where Schwann cells proliferate only when in contact with neurons, and not in the presence of neuronal conditioned medium or when separated from neurons by a membrane permeable to molecules of up to at least 100,000 daltons (Wood and Bunge, 1975; Salzer *et al.*, 1980a).

Interactions of Neurons and Schwann Cells *In Vitro*

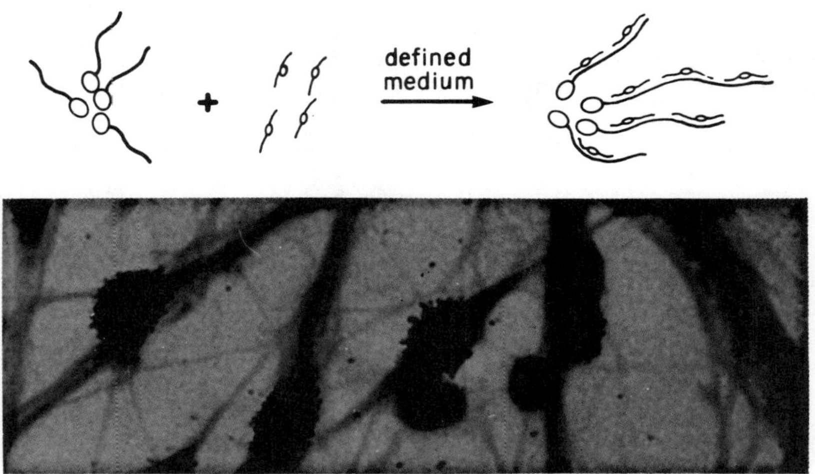

Figure 1: Dorsal root ganglion neurons from embryonic day 15 rat embryos are dissociated enzymatically and plated onto collagen-coated substrata. In the presence of antimitotic agents these cells survive and grow neurites free of non-neuronal cells. Embryonic or neonatal Schwann cells are

purified separately and added to these networks. In serum-free medium Schwann cells adhere to neurites and proliferate; within a few weeks Schwann cells fill the cultures. The lower panel shows autoradiograph of such a culture showing ^{3}H-thymidine labelled (proliferating) Schwann cells associated with neuronal processes.

Similarly, neuronal membranes stimulate Schwann cell proliferation *in vitro* while cytosolic fractions from neurons do not (Ratner *et al.*, 1987). Schwann cells are refractory to a number of other mitogens including serum proteins, membranes from a variety of tissues, and a large number of soluble growth factors, reflecting the fact that Schwann cells proliferate only when associated with neurons in the developing nerve (Salzer *et al.*, 1980b; Raff *et al.*, 1978).

Partial biochemical characterization of the neuronal mitogen has been carried out. The activity is trypsin-sensitive, sensitive to heat treatment (56°C x 10 minutes), and to glutaraldehyde fixation, suggesting that it is a protein (Salzer *et al.*, 1980). Solubilization of the mitogen from the cell surface can be accomplished under conditions consistent with the idea that the mitogen is peripherally associated with the neuronal membrane (0.5M NaCl + 2mM EGTA) (Ratner *et al.*, 1988). Although the mitogen may be a glycoprotein, specific N-linked sugars are not essential for its activity; inhibitors of N-linked sugar processing (swainsonine, castanospermine) added to neuron-Schwann cell cultures do not inhibit Schwann cell proliferation, even after 2 weeks under conditions that remove >80% of mature N-linked sugars from the cell surface. (Ratner *et al.*, 1986).

Several lines of evidence suggest that the neuronal mitogen is associated in the neuronal membrane with a heparan sulfate proteoglycan (HSPG). 1) Competitive inhibitors of proteoglycan biosynthesis added to neurons *in vitro* render the neurons non-mitogenic for Schwann cells; mitogenic activity is decreased 80-90% in the presence of 1mM 4-methyl umbelliferyl-β-D-xyloside, but not by inactive xylosides such as α-xylosides or 4-methyl umbelliferyl-β-D-arabinoside. 2) Digestion of the neuronal cell surface with heparitinase, which degrades glycosaminoglycans of the heparan-sulfate class, but not with chondroitinase or heparinase prior to isolation of neuronal membranes causes a large decrease in the ability of purified membranes to stimulate Schwann cell proliferation (Ratner *et al.*, 1987). 3) Heparin-Sepharose chromatography can be used to enrich mitogenic activity from membrane extracts (Ratner *et al.*, 1988). These data have led us to propose that a neuronal heparan sulfate proteoglycan is required for transport of the mitogen to the neuronal surface and/or for proper presentation of the mitogen to Schwann cells.

HEPARIN-LIKE MOLECULES AS REGULATORS OF THE MITOGENIC RESPONSE

Unresolved questions concern the mechanisms by which membrane-associated neuronal mitogen (and other membrane-associated mitogens) stimulate cell proliferation: does mitogen dissociate from the membrane before binding to target cells? Is mitogenic activity regulated and if so, how? The recognition that NDGF is complexed to a HSPG in the neuronal membrane has led us to consider the possibility that HSPGs regulate the mitogenic signal. One area of intensive investigation is the regulation of soluble growth factors (and other bioactive molecules) by heparin and heparin-like molecules. One or more of these mechanisms may regulate the activity of the membrane-associated neuronal mitogen, and possibly other membrane-associated growth factors.

For example, basic fibroblast growth factor (bFGF) is stored in the extracellular matrix (ECM) and active bFGF can be released from the ECM by addition of heparin (Flaumenhaft et al., 1989); bFGF is mitogenic for endothelial cells and smooth muscle cells and is thought to play an important role in neovascularization and wound repair. Association with HSPG protects extracellular bFGF from degradation (Saksela *et al.*, 1988), and may restrict this potent mitogen to specific sites from which it is released when needed by displacement from the matrix by a heparin-like molecule for which it has higher affinity. Thrombospondin, an autocrine growth factor for smooth muscle cells, binds to a cell surface receptor (syndecan) which is a proteoglycan, from which it can be released by heparin; only cell-associated thrombospondin enhances cell growth (Sun *et al.*, 1989 and references therein). It has been suggested that internalization of thrombospondin, together with the HSPG receptor, might provide a signal for cell proliferation in this system. Proliferation of stem cells in the bone marrow stimulated by granulocyte-macrophage colony-stimulating factor may be activated by binding to a HSPG, since treatment with heparitinase results in loss of stem cell proliferation *in vitro* (Gordon *et al.*, 1987; Roberts *et al.*, 1988). These are examples in which heparin or heparin-like molecules protect, activate, and localize soluble mitogens. Heparin also releases a number of heparin-binding coagulation factors and lipolytic enzymes into the circulation (where they carry out their physiological functions) from cell-surface proteoglycan binding sites (Bengtsson-Olivecrona *et al.*, 1986).

Can heparin or HSPG regulate the function of membrane-associated growth factors? We have shown that a HSPG is required for expression of NDGF in the neuronal membrane. In addition, heparin (but not chondroitin sulfate) inactivates partially purified NDGF in a dose-dependent fashion (1/2 maximal inhibition at ~1 μg/ml) (Ratner *et al.*, 1988), suggesting that heparin-like molecules can modulate the ability of NDGF to stimulate Schwann cell division.

It is possible that altered interaction of NDGF with a HSPG in the adult inactivates NDGF, explaining the very low Schwann cell division in adult nerves. NDGF-like activity can be extracted from adult axonal membranes by heparin (DeCoster *et al.*, 1989), suggesting that the mitogen is bound to a HSPG from which it can be displaced by heparin. The identification of specific HSPGs from fetal and adult neuronal membranes and the characterizations of the interactions of these proteoglycans with NDGF will define the regulatory properties of HSPG in this system.

PURIFICATION OF NDGF FROM CNS TISSUE

We have recently purified NDGF from fetal cow brain membranes, after showing that a variety of rat CNS neurons, including retinal and spinal cord neurons are mitogenic for Schwann cells *in vitro*. (Ratner *et al.*, 1987). The ability of central nervous system membranes to stimulate peripheral glial cells suggests that a normal target of the mitogen is present in the central nervous system. The myelin-forming cells of the CNS, oligodendrocytes, can be stimulated to proliferate by contact with neurons, suggesting that these cells may be one target of the neuronal mitogen (Wood and Williams, 1984). NDGF migrates at 50,000 daltons in non-reducing Laemmli gels; a minor active component is also observed at 30,000 daltons. Purification results from a combination of extraction of membranes using high salt, heparin-affinity chromatography, ion exchange, and elution from non-reducing gels. Active protein eluted from gel slices is applied to reverse-phase columns, and resulting activity is apparently homogeneous (Ratner *et al.*, in preparation).

An obstacle to the characterization of several membrane-associated growth factors has been the purification of these molecules in sufficient quantities to enable sequence analysis for comparison of the membrane-bound factors and for detailed studies of their interaction with the cell membrane and with target cells. An advantage of the neuronal mitogen, as purified from fetal brain, is that sufficient mitogen can be purified from this source to obtain sequence information and begin to address these issues.

POSSIBLE SIMILARITY OF NDGF TO HEMATPOIETIC MITOGENS

Interestingly, it has been reported that activated lymphocytes secrete mitogen for Schwann cells (Lisak *et al.*, 1985); we have shown that lymphocyte conditioned medium containing membrane-associated erythroid-burst promoting activity (BPA) is also mitogenic for Schwann cells *in vitro*. T-cell factors also stimulate the proliferation of central nervous system glial cells *in vitro* (Beneviste *et al.*, 1985,1988; Fontana *et al.*, 1981). Lymphocytes might directly influence the development of glial cells, or specific lymphokines could be expressed in the nervous system. In pathological conditions lymphoctyes do invade the nervous system, and it has been shown that T-cell derived B-cell growth factor (BCGF) is mitogenic for brain astoglial cells, which react to injury by proliferating (Beneviste *et al.*, 1988). Since under normal conditions blood cells are kept out of the nervous system, it is possible that the stimulatory effects of lymphocyte factors on developing glial cells reflects conservation of mitogens on both hematopoetic and neuronal cells which have different targets in the different tissues; studies of the interaction of NDGF with HSPG may lend insight into the mechanism of control of hematopoeitic cell growth.

ACKNOWLEDGEMENTS

The contributions of Drs. Richard Bunge, Luis Glaser, Patrick Wood, Betty Fei, Dingming Hong and of Mr. Michael Nordlund to this work are gratefully acknowledged. This work was supported by a Harry Weaver Junior Faculty Award from the Multiple Sclerosis Society, and grants from the National Neurofibromatosis Foundation.

REFERENCES

Aguayo AJ, Peyronnard JM, Terry LC, Romine JS, Bray GM (1976). Neonatal neuronal loss of rat superior cervical ganglia: Retrograde effects on developing preganglionic axons and Schwann cells. J Neurocytol 5:137-155.

Asbury AK (1967). Schwann proliferation in developing mouse sciatic nerve. A radioautographic study. J Cell Biol 34:735-743.

Bengtsson-Olivecrona G, Olivecrona T, Jörnvall H (1986). Lipoprotein lipases from cow, guinea-pig and man. Structural characterization and identification of protease-sensitive internal regions. Eur J Biochem 161:281-288.

Benveniste EN, Buter JL, Gibbs DA, Chen A, Whitaker JN (1988). Rat astrocyte proliferation by human B-cell growth factors. Ann NY Acad Sci 540:392-395.

Benveniste EN, Merrill JE, Kaufman SE, Golde DW, Gasson JC (1985). Purification and characterization of a human T-lymphocyte-derived glial growth-promoting factor. Proc Natl Acad Sci USA 82:3930-3934.

Cerretti DP, Wignal J, Anderson D, Tushinski RJ, Gallis BM, Stya M, Gillis S, Urdal DL, Cosman D (1988) Human macrophage-colony stimulating factor: Alternative RNA and protein processing from a single gene. Mol Immunol 25:761-770.

DeCoster MA, DeVries GH (1989). Evidence that the axolemmal mitogen for cultured Schwann cells is a positively charged, heparan sulfate proteoglycan bound, heparin-displaceable molecule. J Neurosci Res 22:283-288.

Flaumenhaft R, Moscatelli D, Saksela O, Rifkin DB (1989). Role of extracellular matrix in the action of basic fibroblast growth factor: Matrix as a source of growth factor for long-term stimulaton of plasminogen activator production and DNA synthesis. J Cell Physiol 140:75-81.

Fontana A, Otz U, DeWeck AL, Grob PJ (1981). Glia cell stimulating factor (GSF): A new lymphokine. J Neuroimmunol 2:73-81.

Gordon MY, Riley GP, Watt SM, Greaves MF (1987). Compartmentalization of a haematopoietic growth factor (GM-CSF) by glycosaminoglycans in the bone marrow microenvironment. Nature 326:403-405.

Lisak RP, Gobue G, Kuchmy D, Burns JB, Pleasure DE (1985). Products of activated lymphocytes stimulate Schwann cell mitosis *in vitro*. Neurosci Let 57:105-111.

Raff MC, Abney E, Brockes JP, Hornby-Smith A (1978). Schwann cell growth factors. Cell 15:813-822.

Ratner N, Elbein A, Porter S, Bunge MB, Bunge RP, Glaser L (1986). Specific asparagine-linked oligosaccharides are not required for certain neuron-neuron and neuron-Schwann cell interactions. J Cell Biol 103:159-170.

Ratner N, Glaser L, Bunge RP (1984). A neuronal cell surface heparan sulfate proteoglycan is required for dorsal root ganglion neuron stimulation of Schwann cell proliferation. J Cell Biol 98:1150-1155.

Ratner N, Hong D, Lieberman MA, Bunge RP, Glaser L (1988). The neuronal cell-surface molecule mitogenic for Schwann cells is a heparin-binding protein. Proc Natl Acad Sci USA 85:6992-6996.

Ratner N, Wood PW, Bunge RP, Glaser L (1987). In Althaus HH, Seifert W. eds: "Glial Neuronal Communication in Development and Regeneration" Springer-Verlag, NY.

Roberts R, Gallagher J, Spooncer E, Allen TD, Bloomfield F, Dexter TM (1988). Heparan sulphate bound growth factors: a mechanism for stromal cell mediated haemopoiesis. Nature 332:376-378.

Saksela O, Moscatelli D, Sommer A, Rifkin DB (1988). Endothelial cell-derived heparan sulfate binds basic fibroblast growth factor and protects it from proteolytic degradation. J Cell Biol 107:743-751.

Salzer JL, Bunge RP, Glaser L (1980a). Studies of Schwann cell proliferation. III. Evidence for the surface localization of the neurite mitogen. J Cell Biol 84:767-778.

Salzer JL, Williams AK, Glaser L, Bunge RP (1980b). Studies of Schwann cell proliferation. II. Characterization of the stimulation and specificity of the response to a neurite membrane fraction. J Cell Biol 84:753-766.

Sun X, Mosher DF, Rapraeger A (1989). Heparan sulfate-mediated binding of epithelial cell surface proteoglycan to thrombospondin. J Biol Chem 264:2885-2889.

Wood P (1976). Separation of functional Schwann cells and neurons from peripheral nerve tissue. Brain Res 115:361-375.

Wood PM, Bunge RP (1975). Evidence that sensory axons are mitogenic for Schwann cells. Nature 256:662-664.

Wood PM, Williams AK (1984). Oligodendrocyte proliferation and CNS myelination in cultures containing dissociated embryonic neuroglia and dorsal root ganglia neurons. Dev Brain Research 314:225-241.

The Biology of Hematopoiesis, pages 79–86

A PROTEIN (NRP) THAT NEGATIVELY REGULATES ERYTHROID STEM CELL PROLIFERATION: ANTAGONISM TO IL-3 STIMULATION

Arthur A. Axelrad, Mona M. Shreeve, Denise Eskinazi and Fred G. Pluthero
Department of Anatomy, University of Toronto
Toronto, Canada, M5S 1A8

INTRODUCTION

We have reported that DNA synthesis of the erythroid stem cell BFU-E can be controlled by an inhibitory growth factor which we have named Negative Regulatory Protein or NRP (Axelrad et al., 1981; Del Rizzo et al., 1988). NRP was obtained from supernatant of fresh marrow cells from C57BL/6 ($\underline{Fv\text{-}2}^{rr}$) mice, or from conditioned medium of a C57BL/6 mouse bone marrow-derived cell line called Pan B6. We were able to show that the inhibition of DNA synthesis by NRP took place within minutes, was reversible when NRP was washed away, appeared to be specific to the BFU-E as its target cell, and was opposed by the stimulatory action of Interleukin-3 (IL-3)(Axelrad et al., 1987; Del Rizzo et al., 1989).

Because of the low frequency of BFU-E in the hemopoietic tissues (∿1/3000 cells in mouse marrow), the proportion of BFU-E that were engaged in DNA synthesis under various conditions could not be determined directly. It had to be done with the help of the cell suicide technique, in which the proportion of BFU-E killed by exposure to an S-phase-specific cytotoxic agent, ^{3}H-thymidine or hydroxyurea, was used as a measure of the proportion of BFU-E that were synthesizing DNA. In order to investigate the molecular mechanism of negative regulation by NRP, it would be useful to have a more direct measure of cell proliferation.

Branch, Turc and Guilbert (1987) have claimed that the

cell line DA-1, which is critically dependent for its growth on IL-3, represents a transformed (immortalized) BFU-E. The cells of this line proliferate in suspension in liquid culture and their growth can be monitored by serial cell counts or tritiated thymidine incorporation. Since NRP and IL-3 were known from our earlier work to be antagonistic to one another with respect to DNA synthesis of the BFU-E, we wondered whether NRP would inhibit the growth of DA-1 cells.

MATERIALS AND METHODS

The term NRP is used here for convenience to signify any preparation known to have negative regulatory activity as judged by BFU-E suicide assay. The DA-1 cell line, kindly provided by Dr. L. Guilbert, University of Alberta, Edmonton, was maintained in Iscove's Modified Dulbecco's Medium (IMDM) with 20% WEHI-3 conditioned medium and 10% fetal calf serum (FCS, Bocknek Labs, Inc., Toronto) at 37oC in a humidified atmosphere with 5% CO_2 in air. For experiments, the cells were washed twice and resuspended in IMDM plus 5% FCS together with purified murine IL-3 (a gift of J.N. Ihle, Frederick Cancer Research Facility or purchased from ICN), and with or without NRP at 1×10^5 cells/0.5 ml medium in 24-well plates (Nunc) or at 2×10^4 cells/0.1 ml medium in 96-well plates (Micro Test II, Falcon). Dosages of IL-3 are given in units quoted from the source. Cell counts were made in the presence of 0.1% trypan blue.

RESULTS

When NRP alone was given to cultures of DA-1 cells, no growth was detected. This however was also true of DA-1 cells that were deprived of IL-3 without being exposed to NRP. Since IL-3 was evidently essential for the survival and proliferation of DA-1 cells, we tested the effect of NRP in the presence of IL-3. The results (Fig. 1) show that NRP inhibited the growth of DA-1 cells. The inhibitory effect of NRP given at the initiation of culture took 24 to 48 hours to become manifest.

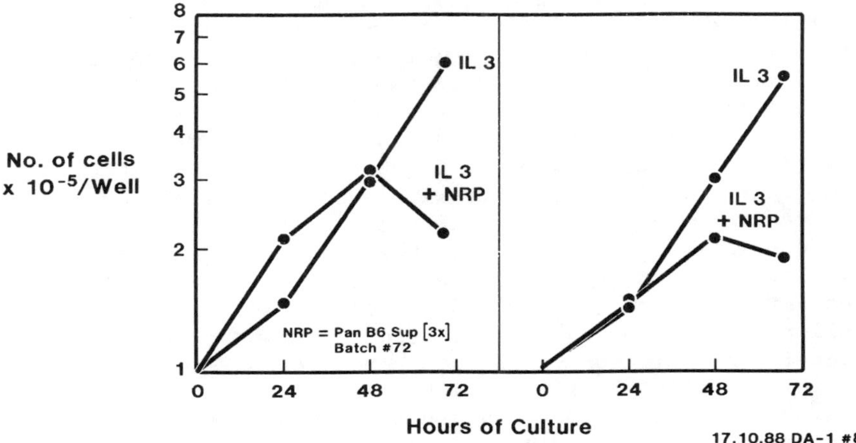

Figure 1. Results of two experiments are shown. Control: DA-1 cells exposed to IL-3 (1 U/ml) given as a single dose at time zero. Experimental: the same cells exposed to IL-3 plus Pan B6 cell supernatant concentrated 3-fold (NRP [3x]) over that at which it was harvested from culture.

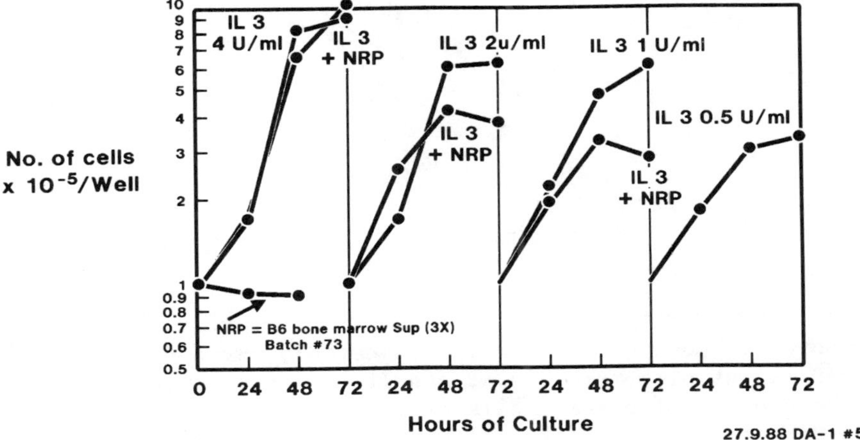

Figure 2. Control: DA-1 cells exposed to IL-3 at various concentrations (0.5 to 4.0 U/ml). Experimental: The same cells exposed to IL-3 plus B6 bone marrow supernatant concentrated 3-fold (NRP [3x]), or the same cells exposed to NRP [3x] alone.

Theoretically this effect could have been entirely due to toxicity of NRP. To investigate this possibility, we tested the reversibility of the effect of NRP on proliferation of DA-1 cells in two ways. First, DA-1 cells were grown in the presence of IL-3 at various concentrations administered as a single dose at the initiation of culture, or in the presence of IL-3 at the same concentrations together with a fixed dose of NRP (concentrated 3-fold). The results (Fig. 2) show that as the concentration of IL-3 was increased, the rate of proliferation of DA-1 cells increased. While at low concentrations of IL-3 (1 and 2 U/ml) inhibition of DA-1 cell proliferation by NRP was readily demonstrated, at the higher concentration of IL-3 (4 U/ml) the NRP-induced inhibition of DA-1 cell proliferation was entirely overcome. It was also found in these experiments that the proportion of trypan-blue stained (non-viable) cells was not increased by exposure to NRP at concentrations that effectively inhibited growth (data not shown).

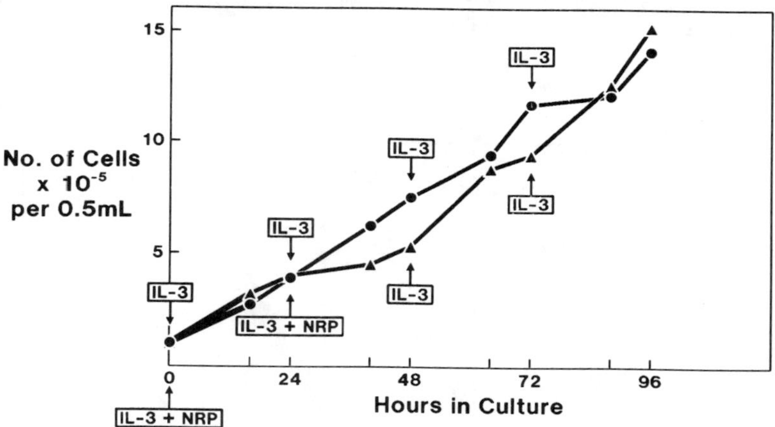

Figure 3. Control: DA-1 cells repeatedly exposed to IL-3 (5 U/ml) at time zero, 24,48 and 72 hrs in culture. Experimental: The same cells exposed to IL-3 (5 U/ml) plus B6 Pan cell supernatant concentrated 3-fold (NRP [3x]) at time zero and at 24 hrs, followed by IL-3 (5 U/ml) alone at 48 and 72 hrs in culture.

Next we tested the effect of delayed administration of IL-3 alone to DA-1 cells that had been exposed to NRP in the presence of IL-3. As seen in Fig. 3 with IL-3 alone given repeatedly as control, the cells showed the expected growth, and with IL-3 and NRP they showed growth inhibition. At 48 hrs, when the growth inhibited cells were given IL-3 alone, the cells began to grow again and grew at about the same rate as controls. Thus the effect of NRP could be completely reversed by the delayed addition of IL-3 to cells that were already on the plateau of the growth curve as a result of the action of NRP.

These results show by direct assay that NRP inhibits cell proliferation, and does so in a reversible manner.

As a basis for the assay of DA-1 cell growth inhibitory activity we have used the percentage reduction in DA-1 cell number per well after 3 days of growth in the presence of NRP plus IL-3 as compared to the cell number in control cultures given IL-3 alone. We have also determined the proportion of dead cells as judged by trypan blue staining. Fractions were considered to have NRP activity if they showed significant inhibition of cell proliferation together with insignificant toxicity. This may underestimate the level of NRP activity if the antagonistic effect of NRP on the action of IL-3 is sufficient to effectively deprive the DA-1 cells of the IL-3 activity necessary for survival.

The assay method is being used to localize DA-1 cell growth-inhibitory activity in Mono Q anion exchange fractions of Pan B6 conditioned medium and of B6 marrow supernatants that are known to contain NRP, as previously determined by BFU-E suicide assay (Pluthero et al., Submitted).

Relation between IL-3 dependence and response to growth inhibition by NRP.

To investigate the specificity of the growth-inhibitory effect, we exposed the cells of 7 different cell lines to Pan B6 supernatant known to contain NRP, and measured the growth of these cells. As shown in Table 1, three of the cell lines, DA-1, B6.SUt and FDC-P1, were IL-3 dependent and the growth of all three was inhibited by NRP. The cells of WEHI-3, an autocrine, IL-3-producing cell line, were also growth inhibited. But NRP had no effect on the growth of three cell lines, V2, JG6 and Pan B6; the cells of all three are IL-3 independent, and one of them, Pan B6, is a producer of NRP. Thus NRP appears to inhibit specifically that cell growth which is dependent on IL-3.

TABLE 1. Relation between IL-3 dependence and response to growth inhibition by NRP.

Cell line	Note or reference	Characteristic	Growth inhibition by NRP (%)
DA-1	a	IL-3 dependent	29.3 ± 9.3 (M±S.D.)
B6.S UtA	b	IL-3 dependent	50; 42.2
FDC-P1	c	IL-3 dependent	77; 100
WEHI-3	d	Autocrine, IL-3 producing	20.5; 19.5
V2	e	IL-3 independent	0
JG6	f	IL-3 independent	0
Pan B6	g	IL-3 independent, NRP producing	0

Cells of each line were washed twice and incubated in IMDM with 2 or 5% FCS ± IL-3 and ± NRP at 2×10^4 cells/0.1 ml medium and counted at 48 hrs.

[a] Branch et al., 1987.
[b] Greenberger et al., 1983.
[c] Dexter et al., 1980.
[d] Dexter et al., 1980.
[e] V2 is a REDS cell line, selected by passage of C57BL/6 non-adherent bone marrow cells in pokeweed mitogen-stimulated spleen cell conditioned medium (Wendling et al., 1985) (on which it was totally dependent) and infected with MPLV (Wendling et al., 1989), which rendered it factor independent and able to produce erythropoietin-independent erythroid colonies and bursts.
[f] JG6 is an FV-P-transformed Friend erythroleukemia cell line originally isolated by Dr. J. Gusella from subclones of line 745 established by Dr. C. Friend and obtained through the courtesy of Dr. A. Bernstein, Mount Sinai Research Institute, Toronto, Canada.
[g] Pan B6 or Pan cell is a cell line that was developed by D.S. Vaithilingam (Thesis, University of Toronto, 1983) by panning of normal C57BL/6 mouse marrow cells.

DISCUSSION

The present work shows that preparations containing NRP (which inhibit DNA synthesis of BFU-E, as shown indirectly by protection against ^{3}H-thymidine or hydroxyurea suicide) are capable of giving true, reversible inhibition of hemopoietic cell proliferation, as determined directly by cell counting. If it can be shown unequivocally that the two methods measure exactly the same inhibitory molecules, the present work would offer the basis of an assay method for NRP that is objective, simple, rapid and free of animal-generated variability. It would permit many more samples to be assayed per unit time and thus facilitate further purification.

These experiments also show that IL-3 and NRP are antagonistic to one another in their actions on the growth of DA-1 cells, just as they were on the DNA synthesis of BFU-E in marrow cell cultures (Axelrad et al., 1987; Del Rizzo et al., 1989). The antagonistic effect of IL-3 and NRP on cell growth seen in the present experiments re-emphasizes the dual control of hemopoietic cell proliferation (Axelrad, in press). An arrangement of positive and negative regulators in equilibrium would, under normal steady state conditions, permit cells to remain in a non-proliferative state, and yet respond rapidly with DNA synthesis and proliferation on increased hemopoietic demand. This could result from either an increase in positive regulation or a decrease in negative regulation, or a combination of both. It would also permit a rapid return to the steady state once the increased demand was satisfied. The level at which these opposing controls operate and their molecular mechanisms will be interesting problems for the future.

ACKNOWLEDGMENTS

This work was supported by a grant of the National Cancer Institute of Canada.

REFERENCES

Axelrad AA, Croizat H, Eskinazi, D (1981). A washable macromolecule from Fv-2[rr] marrow negatively regulates DNA synthesis in erythropoietic progenitor cells BFU-E. Cell 26: 233-244.

Axelrad AA, Croizat H, Del Rizzo D, Eskinazi D, Pezzutti G, Stewart S, Van der Gaag H (1987). Properties of a protein NRP that negatively regulates DNA synthesis of the early erythropoietic progenitor cells BFU-E. In Najman A, Guigon M et al., (eds): "The Inhibitors of Hematopoiesis," Paris: John Libby Eurotext, Colloque INSERM 162: 79-92.

Axelrad AA Some hemopoietic negative regulators. Exp Hemat. In press.

Branch D, Turc JM, Guilbert L (1987). Identification of an erythropoietin-sensitive cell line. Blood 69: 1782-1785

Del Rizzo DF, Eskinazi D, Axelrad AA (1988). Negative regulation of DNA synthesis in early erythropoietic progenitor cells (BFU-E) by a protein purified from the medium of C57BL/6 mouse marrow cells. Proc Natl Acad Sci USA 85: 4320-4324.

Del Rizzo DF, Eskinazi D, Axelrad AA (1989). Interleukin-3 opposes the action of negative regulatory protein (NRP) and of Transforming Growth Factor-β (TGF-β) in their inhibition of DNA synthesis of the erythroid stem cell BFU-E. Exp Hemat. In press.

Dexter TM, Garland J, Scott D, Scolnick E, Metcalf, D (1980). Growth of factor-dependent hemopoietic precursor cell lines. J Exp Med 152: 1036-1047.

Greenberger JS, Eckner RJ, Sakakeeny M, Marks P, Reid D, Nabel G, Hapel A, Ihle JN, Humphries KC (1983). Interleukin 3-dependent hematopoietic progenitor cell lines. Fed Proc 42: 2762-2770.

Pluthero FG, Shreeve MM, Eskinazi D, Axelrad AA An antagonist to Interleukin-3 produced by mouse marrow cells. Submitted.

Wendling F, Shreeve M, McLeod D, Axelrad AA (1985). A self-renewing, bipotential erythroid/mast cell progenitor in continuous cultures of normal murine bone marrow. J Cell Physiol 125: 10-18.

Wendling F, Pencioletti, JF, Charon M, Tambourin, P (1989). Factor-independent erythropoietic progenitor cells in leukemia induced by the Myeloproliferative Leukemia Virus. Blood 73:1161-1167.

The Biology of Hematopoiesis, pages 87–96

MOLECULAR MECHANISM OF HEMATOPOIETIC STEM CELL BINDING TO THE SUPPORTIVE STROMA

Mehdi Tavassoli, Cheryl L. Hardy, Shin Aizawa, Takashi Matsuoka, Jose Minguell

Department of Veterans Affairs and University of Mississippi School of Medicine, Jackson, Mississippi 39216

During marrow transplantation, progenitor cells are introduced intravenously in anticipation of their selective recognition and "homing" to hemopoietic tissues. For the past two decades, evidence has emerged that the molecular basis of this recognition involves an interaction between a membrane lectin and appropriate configuration of certain carbohydrate groups of membrane glycoconjugates, leading to recognition and selective binding of circulating stem cells to marrow stroma.

Synthetic Neoglycoprotein Probes

To systematically investigate this area, we synthesized a group of probes by covalently linking various biologically active monosaccharides in pyranose form to bovine serum albumin (BSA). This generates large molecules, not diffusible into the cell, but capable of being labeled with ^{125}I. There are other theoretical considerations in their synthesis that have been described elsewhere in detail (Kataoka and Tavassoli, 1984). The probes can then compete with naturally-occurring glycoconjugates in their interactions with membrane lectins. This competition prevents lectin-glycoconjugate interactions and the biological consequences that may arise from them. Another essential characteristic of these probes is their lack of toxicity (Aizawa and Tavassoli, 1987a). Not only are they harmless to animals when injected intravenously, but they also lack toxicity in cell culture systems and, in particular, they lack inhibitory and stimulatory activities in hemopoietic cell systems.

Inhibition of Homing

To investigate the molecular basis of homing of intravenously transplanted stem cells to the marrow, transplantation was done in the presence or absence of various synthetic neoglycoproteins in inhibiting concentrations. Concentrations of stem cells (CFU-S) and progenitor cells (CFU-GM) were then measured in the tibia at 2 h, and 24 h and then weekly after transplantation. It was found that among the biologically active sugars, galactose- and mannose-specific probes (galactosyl-BSA, G-BSA and mannosyl-BSA, M-BSA) inhibit homing of stem cells to the marrow. Consequently, the seeding efficiency of stem cells (defined as the concentration of stem cells in the bone marrow, 2 h and 24 h after intravenous transplantation of isologous stem cells into lethally-irradiated mice) declined. Reconstitution of hemopoiesis (defined by the cellularity of marrow and concentration of CFU-S and CFU-GM after a week) was prevented and the dose-dependent survival of animals was thus compromised. This type of observation then supported previous suggestions that homing is mediated by a lectin-carbohydrate interaction and further assigned the specificity of carbohydrate to galactosyl and mannosyl moieties. Neoglycoproteins with other specificities affected neither homing nor long term reconstitution of hemopoiesis (Aizawa and Tavassoli, 1987a,b, 1988a). Similar results were obtained in vitro as well, by reconstitution of hemopoiesis in standard long-term marrow cultures (Aizawa and Tavassoli, 1987a,b). In this system, too, M-BSA and G-BSA, but not fucosyl-BSA (F-BSA), inhibited the binding of progenitor cells to stroma.

The long-term marrow culture system was simplified by the use of cloned progenitor cells and stromal cells. The adherent stromal cell clone, D2X (Greenberger et al., 1984), was grown to near confluence. The progenitor cell FDCP-1, a bipotential clone not unlike CFU-GM, was used for binding to the stroma (Dexter et al., 1980). Binding may be quantitated by labeling the progenitor cells with ^{51}Cr and measuring the amount of radioactivity firmly bound to the dish in the presence or absence of neoglycoproteins. Here again, the system reproduced the results of previous observations with persistent consistency: Synthetic neoglycoproteins of galactosyl and mannosyl specificities, but not those of other specificities, inhibited the binding of progenitor cells to stroma (Hardy and Tavassoli, 1988).

Assignment of Lectins to Progenitor Cells

At this point, it was clear that an interaction between a membrane lectin on one side of the equation and a membrane glycoconjugate on the other side is responsible for the binding of progenitor cells to the stroma. It was not clear, however, on which side of the equation membrane lectins (herein referred to as homing receptors) are located. To study this question, selective agglutination of progenitor cells was attempted (Aizawa and Tavassoli, 1988b). The theoretical basis of this experiment exploits the presence of homing receptors which are able to cross-link the cells that possess them through the use of neoglycoproteins. Cross-linking was done in whole marrow cell suspensions, containing all types of progenitor cells. Cross-linked cells were then agglutinated by centrifugation onto a layer of BSA, providing differential concentrations of progenitor cells in the agglutinated and non-agglutinated fractions.

These experiments allowed us to assign homing receptors to the side of progenitor cells, since both CFU-S and CFU-GM could be selectively agglutinated by neoglycoproteins of galactosyl and mannosyl specificities. This conclusion was subsequently confirmed in cloned progenitor cells (B6SUT and FDCP-1) through the use of ^{125}I-labeled G-BSA and M-BSA in standard binding assays (Matsuoka et al., 1989). Membrane lectins with these specificities, but not those of other sugars, were found on the surface of these cells. In the cell line B6SUT (Greenberger et al., 1983) Scatchard analyses indicated Kd of 2.3×10^{-7} M and 1.0×10^{-7} M respectively for G-BSA and M-BSA with receptor numbers being respectively 10^6 and 3.7×10^5 per cell. Comparable data were also obtained for FDCP-1. ^{125}I-labeling and binding assays also indicated that stromal cells lack this lectin. The absence of membrane lectin on stromal cells was confirmed not only in the adherent stroma of long term marrow culture which may be heterogenous in nature, but also in cloned stromal cell line D2X.

Purification of Homing Receptors

Availability of cloned progenitor cells permitted work on purification of homing receptors. Cell membrane fraction was obtained from these cells, solubilized in Triton X-100, and the membrane proteins were then labeled with ^{125}I. An affinity column was constructed with either galactosyl or mannosyl groups covalently bound to CNBr-activated Sepharose 4B. Elution of cell membrane proteins was undertaken with buffer only until all the unbound radioactivity was eluted. Subsequent competitive elution with buffer containing either galactosyl or mannosyl sugars in correct form (but not other sugars) led to the elution of a sharp peak of radioactivity. The sharpness of this peak suggested that only a single molecular species was involved. Elution of this peak could be obtained not only with homologous sugar, but also with heterologous sugar (e.g. galactosyl-containing buffer on mannosyl column), suggesting that the glycoconjugate ligand also involved a single molecular species and contained both galactosyl and mannosyl groupings. It is the configuration of these two sugars in the molecule that is being recognized by the lectin. This information may be helpful in purifying the glycoconjugate.

The peak obtained by affinity chromatography was subjected to polyacrylamide gel electrophoresis followed by autoradiography. Under nonreducing conditions a major band with a Mr of 110,000 and two lesser bands with a Mr of 87,000 and 23,000 were seen. Only the latter two bands were seen under reducing conditions. Experiments with endoglycosidase F treatment indicated a 5% carbohydrate content. Thus, we concluded that the receptor is a glycoprotein heterodimer, disulfide-bonded, with two chains of 87 Kd and 23 Kd for a total mass of 110 Kd.

This finding is quite consistent with the wealth of recent information on membrane lectins with a biological recognition function. A major group of these lectins, known as C-lectins, are calcium - dependent in their interaction with carbohydrates (as is the hemopoietic homing receptor), are disulfide-bonded and their recognition function depends on this bonding. They are usually components of the cell membrane and are highly glycosylated (Drickamer, 1988). In these characteristics, homing receptor protein is in the mainstream of C-lectins. Similarities also exist between this homing receptor in hemopoietic progenitors and the homing receptor in lymphocytes (Butcher et al., 1979; Gallatin et al., 1983; Gallatin et al., 1986; Siegelman et al., 1989; Stoolman, 1989). Although carbohydrate specificity is somewhat different, preliminary work in our laboratory suggests that both of these lectins may belong to a single group of peptides that have evolved with the evolution of blood cells (Siegelman and Weissman, 1989).

The Role of Extracellular Matrix

The binding of homing receptors to their putative ligand is of relatively low affinity (vide supra). This low affinity binding attracted our attention to the extracellular matrix and, in particular, proteoglycans as an additional mechanism of homing (Giancotti et al., 1986; Virtanen et al., 1987; Coulombel et al., 1988; Weinstein et al., 1989). In this role proteoglycans may provide, if not high specificity (as is the case with homing receptors) at least strengthening of the bond between progenitor cells and stroma.

Proteoglycans are a group of matrix-associated molecules consisting of a core protein to which a repeating sequence of usually sulfated glycan structures is attached (Wight et al., 1986). They are synthesized by cells of hemopoietic tissues, mostly by stromal cells, and released into the extracellular space. Proteoglycans have recently received considerable attention, because emerging evidence indicates that some are involved in regulation of hemopoiesis. One line of evidence indicates that they selectively extract and bind hemopoietic growth factors (Gordon et al., 1987; Roberts et al., 1988). Other proteoglycans may be instrumental in homing of hemopoietic stem cells (Campbell et al., 1987) while yet another class may be related to the developmental regulation of erythoid cells (Patel and Lodish, 1986; Tsai et al., 1987). This latter class is preferentially membrane associated.

In the course of studying proteoglycans produced by

hemopoietic progenitors, we found that these cells synthesize a considerable amount of chondroitin sulfate (CS) that is first associated with the membrane, but subsequently is released into the extracellular space. When these progenitor cells are layered on top of stromal cells so that they bind (home) to stromal cells, their homing is associated with stabilization of membrane-associated CS. The life span of these molecules on the membrane is also prolonged (Minguell and Tavassoli, 1989). Recent work in our laboratory has indicated that membrane-associated CS can also mediate the binding of progenitor cells to stromal cells. This binding occurs via the interaction between membrane-associated CS on progenitor cells and membrane-associated fibronectin (FN) on stromal cells. This interaction subsequently stabilizes membrane-associated CS (Minguell and Tavassoli, 1989). The presence of FN on the stromal cell membrane has been well-documented (Kirby and Bentley, 1987). That membrane-associated CS may be involved in the binding of progenitor cells is derived from studies where enzymatic removal of CS abolishes the binding.

CONCLUSION

Homing is likely to be a complex phenomenon involving multiple interactions at the molecular level. Membrane-associated molecules as well as extracellular matrix may be involved. From the studies described here, we can, however, conclude that the molecule responsible for selective recognition of progenitor cells by stroma is probably homing receptor. Interaction of CS and FN is too commonplace to provide for selectivity in recognition. Nonetheless, this interaction can serve to strengthen and stabilize the binding that has occurred via homing receptors.

REFERENCES

Aizawa S, Tavassoli M (1987a). In vitro homing of hemopoietic stem cell is mediated by a recognition mechanism with galactosyl and mannosyl specificity. Proc Natl Acad Sci USA 84:4485-4489.

Aizawa S, Tavassoli M (1987b). Interaction of murine

granulocyte-macrophage progenitors and supporting stroma involves a recognition mechanism with galactosyl and mannosyl specificities. J Clin Invest 80:1698-1705.
Aizawa S, Tavassoli M (1988a). Molecular basis of the recognition of intravenously transplanted hemopoietic cells by bone marrow. Proc Natl Acad Sci USA 85:3180-3183.
Aizawa S, Tavassoli M (1988b). Detection of membrane lectins on the surface of hemopoietic progenitor cells and their changing pattern during differentiation. Exp Hematol 16:325-329.
Badley RA, Woods A, Carruthers L, Rees DA (1980). Cytoskeleton changes in fibroblast adhesion and detachment. J Cell Sci 43:379-390.
Butcher EC, Scollay RG, Weissman IL (1979). Lymphocyte adherence to high endothelial venules: characterization of a modified in vitro assay, and examination of the binding of syngeneic and allogeneic lymphocyte populations. J Immunol 123:1996-2003.
Campbell AD, Long, MW, Wicha MS (1987). Haemonectin, a bone marrow adhesion protein specific for cells of granulocytic lineage. Nature 329:744-746.
Coulombel MH, Vuillet C, Leroy C, Tchernia G (1988) Lineage- and stage-specific adhesion of human hematopoietic progenitor cells to extracellular matrices from marrow fibroblasts. Blood 71:329-334.
Dexter TM, Garland J, Scott D, Scolnick E, Metcalf D (1980). Growth of factor-dependent hemopoietic precursor cell lines. J Exp Med 152:1036-1047.
Drickamer K (1988). Two distinct classes of carbohydrate-recognition domains in animal lectins. J Biol Chem 263:9557-9560.
Gallatin WM, Weissman IL, Butcher EC (1983). A cell-surface molecule involved in organ-specific homing of lymphocytes. Nature 304:30-34.
Gallatin M, St. John TP, Siegelman M, Reichert R, Butcher EC, Weissman IL (1986). Lymphocyte homing receptors. Cell 44:673-680.
Giancotti FG, Comoglio PM, Tarone G (1986). Fibronectin-plasma interaction in the adhesion of hemopoietic cells. J Cell Biol 103:429-437.
Gordon MY, Riley GP, Watt SM, Greaves MF (1987). Compartmentalization of a haematopoietic growth factor (GM-CSF) by glycosaminoglycans in the bone marrow microenvironment. Nature 326:403-405.
Greenberger JS, Sakakeeny MA, Humphries RK, Eaves CJ,

Eckner RJ (1983). Demonstration of permanent factor-dependent multipotential (erythroid/neutrophil/basophil) hematopoietic progenitor cell lines. Proc Natl Acad Sci USA 80:2931-2935.

Greenberger JS, Sakakeeny MA, Davis LM, Maloney WC, Reid D (1984). Biologic properties of factor-independent non-adherent hematopoietic and adherent preadipocyte cell lines derived from continuous bone marrow culture. Leuk Res 8:363-375.

Hardy C, Tavassoli M (1988). A test system for analysis of hemopoietic progenitor cell homing. Exp Hematol 16:550.

Kataoka M, Tavassoli M (1984). Synthetic neoglycoproteins: a class of reagents for detection of sugar-recognizing substances. J Histochem Cytochem 32:1091-1098

Kirby SL, Bentley SA (1987). Proteoglycan synthesis in two murine bone marrow stromal cell lines. Blood 70:1777-1782.

Matsuoka T, Hardy C, Tavassoli M (1989). Characterization of membrane homing receptors in two cloned murine hemopoietic progenitor cell lines. J Clin Invest 83:904-911.

Minguell JJ, Tavassoli M (1989). Proteoglycan synthesis by hemopoietic progenitor cells. Blood 73:1821-1827.

Patel VP, Lodish HF (1986). The fibronectin receptor on mammalian erythroid precursor cell: characterization and development regulation. J Cell Biol 102:449-456.

Roberts R, Gallagher J, Spooncer E, Allen TD, Bloomfield F, Dexter TM (1988). Heparan sulfate bound growth factors: a mechanism for stromal cell mediated haemopoiesis. Nature 332:376-378.

Siegelman MH, van de Rijn M, Weissman IL (1989). Mouse lymph node homing receptor (DNA) clone encodes a glycoprotein revealing tandem interaction domains. Science 243:1165-1172.

Siegelman MH, Weissman IL (1989). Human homologue of mouse lymph node homing receptor: evolutionary conservation at tandem cell interaction domains. Proc Natl Acad Sci USA 86:5562-5566.

Stoolman LM (1989). Adhesion molecules controlling lymphocyte migration. Cell 56:907-910.

Tsai S, Patel V, Beaumont E, Lodish HF, Nathan DG, Sieff CA (1987). Differential binding of erythroid and myeloid progenitors to fibroblasts and fibronectin. Blood 69:1587-1594.

Virtanen I, Ylanne J, Vartio T (1987). Human erythro-leukemia cells adhere to fibronectin: evidence

for a Mr 190,000 - receptor protein. Blood 69:578-583.
Weinstein R, Rioidan MA, Wenc K, Kreczko S, Zhou M, Dainiak N (1989). Dual role of fibronectin in hematopoietic differentiation. Blood 73:111-116.
Wight TN, Kinella MG, Keating A, Singer JW (1986). Proteoglycans in human long-term bone marrow cultures: Biochemical and ultrastructural analyses. Blood 67:1333-1343.

The Biology of Hematopoiesis, pages 97–105

HEMONECTIN: A NOVEL HEMATOPOIETIC ADHESION MOLECULE

Alan Campbell*†, Brent Sullenberger†, Wadie Bahou*, David Ginsberg*, Michael Long‡ and Max Wicha*

Departments of Internal Medicine* and Pediatrics‡
University of Michigan Medical Center and
Ann Arbor VA Medical Center†

INTRODUCTION

The maintenance of close cell-cell contact between stromal and hematopoietic cells is critical to normal of hematopoiesis (1-4). The molecular basis underlying this adhesive interaction, however, is not well understood. A variety of potentially adhesive macromolecules have been identified within the extracellular matrix of bone marrow, including fibronectin, laminin, type 4 collagen, a variety of proteoglycans and recently N-CAM and possibly ICAM-1 (2,5,6,11,12). Of these, fibronectin mediated adhesion has emerged as an important adhesion mechanism of erythroid progenitor cells (7,8). The basis for adhesion in the myeloid lineage and its relation to adhesion at the stem cell level, however, is less clear. Disturbances in the interaction of adhesion molecules on the surface of stromal cells and/or their cognate receptors on the surface of hematopoietic cells, could have an impact on a variety of processes of normal hematopoiesis including proliferation, differentiation and release, and is therefore of great interest in the study of leukemogenesis.

IDENTIFICATION OF HEMONECTIN AS A BONE MARROW SPECIFIC ADHESION PROTEIN

We have previously shown that a complex extract of extracellular matrix components derived from bone marrow could promote growth and differentiation of hematopoietic cells in long-term marrow culture (LTMC) (9), and also appeared to promote the adhesion of marrow cells when these cultures were initiated. In order to identify specific components which might be involved in adhesion promotion, we separated bone marrow matrix components by SDS gel electrophoresis, transferred them to nitrocellulose paper and incubated these blots with radiolabelled bone marrow cells. Using this technique we were able to identify a specific 60kD protein, termed hemonectin, to which these radiolabelled bone marrow cells specifically attached (10) (Figure 1).

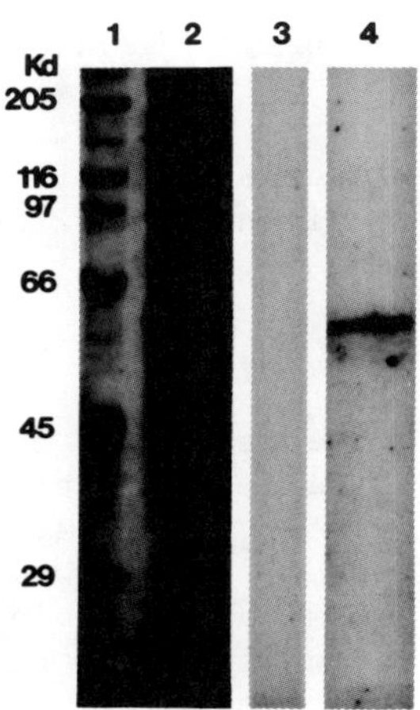

Figure 1. Cell attachment to hemonectin. High molecular weight standards (lane 1) and bone marrow ECM proteins (lane 2) were separated by 10% SDS-PAGE and visualized by silver staining. Identical gel lanes were transferred to nitrocellulose incubated with ^{51}Cr-labelled murine marrow cells, rinsed, and visualized by autoradiography (lanes 3 and 4). Cell attachment is seen only at 60kD (lane 4).

Morphological examination of the attached cells showed that the great majority of them had morphologic features of murine granulocytic cells. This 60kD protein was absent from extracellular matrix extracts derived from spleen, mammary gland and kidney by this cell attachment assay. Antihemonectin antisera was raised in a guinea pig and used to show that this 60kd band was also absent from these tissues by immunoblotting (Figure 2). Furthermore, no cross reactivity with fibronectin, laminin, type 4 collagen, vitronectin, or osteopontin was seen by immunoblotting. Immunofluorescence microscopy confirmed the presence of hemonectin in mouse bone marrow, especially along the endosteal surface of bone, and its absence in splenic tissue. The limited tissue distribution of hemonectin and its lineage specificity suggested an interesting molecular basis for the predominantly myeloid hematopoiesis of bone marrow as compared to the erythroid hematopoiesis of spleen and also suggested a mechanism by which stem cells infused during bone marrow transplantation could home preferentially to bone marrow.

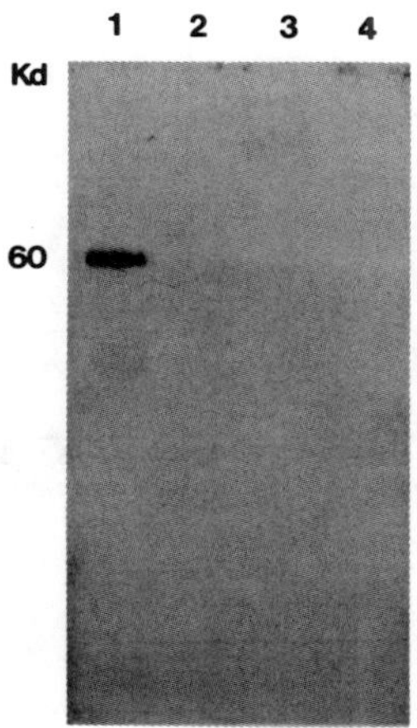

Figure 2. Tissue distribution of hemonectin. ECM was isolated (9) from bone marrow (lane 1), spleen (lane 2), mammary gland (lane 3) and kidney (lane 4) and analyzed by Western blotting for the presence of hemonectin using polyclonal anti-hemonectin antiserum. Hemonectin is detected only in bone marrow ECM (lane 1).

DEVELOPMENTALLY REGULATED BINDING OF GRANULOCYTIC CELLS TO HEMONECTIN

To further study the properties of this protein, we developed a schema for purification from homogenized rabbit bone marrow. Briefly, marrow from 6-8 week old rabbits was mechanically scraped from femurs and tibias and homogenized in a 3.4m sodium chloride buffer to precipitate ECM components. After extensive washing in the same buffer the precipitated material was then extracted with 4M guanidine and dialyzed into 6M urea. This material was then applied to a DEAE Sephacel (Pharmacia) ion exchange column which was eluted with a 0-1M sodium chloride gradient (Figure 3).Hemonectin containing fractions came off at approximately .15m sodium chloride and were then separated from lower molecular weight components by G50 Sephadex gel filtration. SDS polyacrylamide gel electrophoresis of these steps is shown in figure 4.

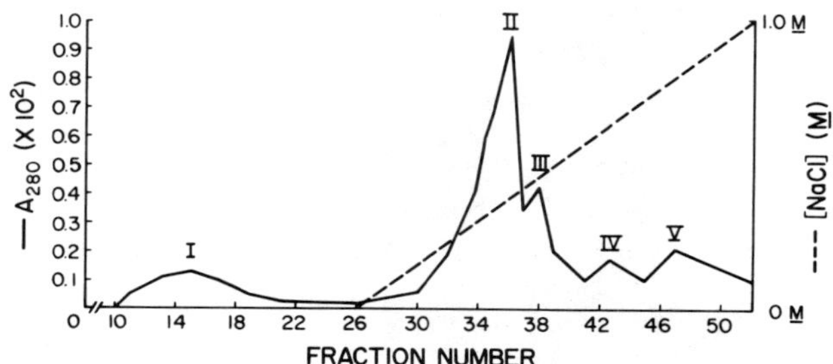

Figure 3. Anion-exchange chromatography of bone marrow ECM. Bone marrow ECM was isolated (9), dialyzed into 6M urea .05 M Na Acetate .05 M Tris pH 7.0, applied to a DEAE-Sephacel (Pharmacia) column, eluted with a linear NaCl gradient, and monitored continuously at 280 nm. Hemonectin containing fractions (Peak II) were eluted beginning at .15 M NaCl.

The final protein preparation which was judged to be 90% pure by silver stained SDS gel electrophoresis, was then tested for its ability to promote adhesion. A solution of 10ug/ml of purified hemonectin was immobilized on tissue culture plastic slides, incubated with C57/BL6 murine bone marrow cells and compared to adhesion mediated by fibronectin. Again, predominantly myeloid cells were found to attach to the hemonectin coated substrate and a greater fraction of immature granulocytic marrow cells (defined as having a central nuclear perforation less than half the diameter of the nucleus) were found attached to hemonectin as compared to fibronectin.

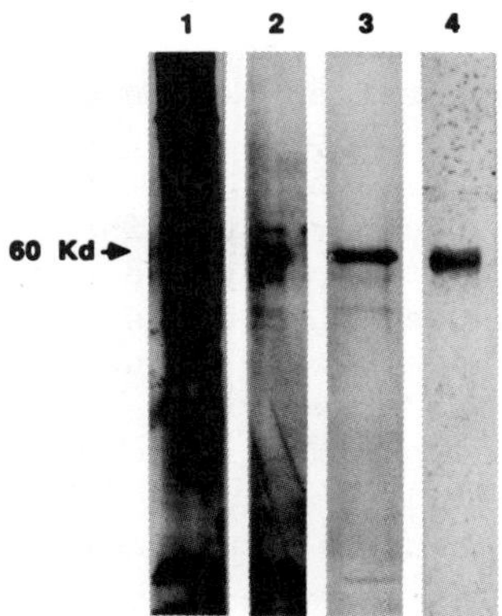

Figure 4. Gel electrophoresis of HN purification steps. SDS-PAGE was performed and visualized by silver staining (lanes 1-3) or transferred to nitrocellulose and probed with anti-hemonectin antiserum (lane 4). Lane 1, unfractionated bone marrow ECM extract; lane 2, pooled fractions from peaks II and III from DEAE Sephacel column; lane 3, pooled fractions for peaks II and III after gel filtration; lane 4, nitrocellulose replica of lane 3 stained with antihemonectin antiserum.

To develop a simple model of hemonectin mediated adhesion, we studied the ability of the granulocytic cell line HL60 to adhere to hemonectin coated substrates. In these studies, uninduced HL60 cells grown to density arrest were labelled with chromium 51 and incubated in dishes coated with 10ug/ml of purified hemonectin for 1 hour at 37 degrees in serum-free RPMI. Controls included dishes coated with 10ug/ml bovine serum albumin, and uncoated plastic dishes. Cell attachment was measured by rinsing the dishes vigorously with serum-free medium and lysing the attached cells in 2% SDS followed by quantitation of radioactivity in the lysate. Figure 5 shows the results of such an assay and demonstrate that on an average, 60% of uninduced labelled HL60 cells bind to hemoneectin coated substrates as opposed to 15% bound to uncoated plastic and less than 5% bound to BSA coated dishes.

Since cell binding to uncoated plastic was four-fold less than binding to hemonectin coated substrate, the contribution of non-specific binding to the total bound to hemonectin was not greater than 25%. This data demonstrated that hemonectin purified by the procedures described retained its adhesion promoting activity and can be used to study granulocytic cell attachment in a simple assay. To study whether HL60 binding to hemonectin is a stage specific property, we compared binding of uninduced to DMSO induced HL60 cells in this cell attachment assay. HL60 cells were induced to differentiate using 1.4% DMSO for 3 days. This figure shows data pooled from 3 different experiments each done in triplicate and shows that binding of uninduced HL60 cells is approximately 3-4 fold greater than binding of induced and differentiated HL60 cells. This data supports our earlier suggestion that binding of granulocytic cells to hemonectin is a differentiation stage dependent property and may be involved in the mechanism of release of developing bone marrow granulocytic cells from the bone marrow into the peripheral circulation.

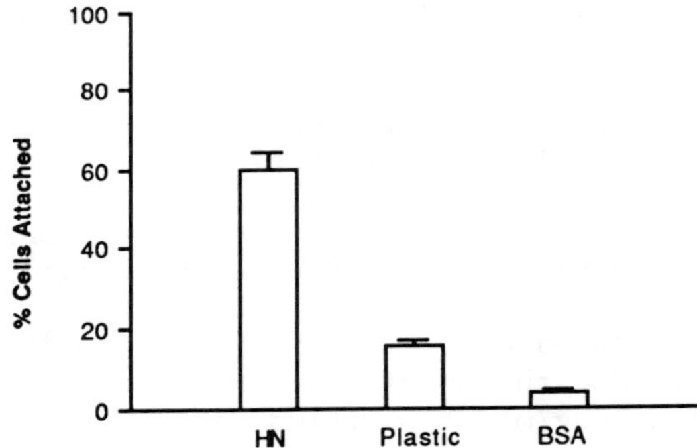

Figure 5. HL-60 cell binding to purified HN. 10ug of HN or BSA were immobilized on 35mm Petri dishes. ^{51}Cr labelled HL-60 cells were then allowed to attach in the absence of serum, non-adherent cells removed, adherent cells lysed in 2% (w/v) SDS, and cpm in the lysate determined. Values are expressed as $\frac{\text{cpm in lysate}}{\text{total cpm added}} X100$. Values are means of triplicates $\pm$ SEM.

AMINO ACID SEQUENCE DATA

We have initiated studies of the aminoacid sequence of purified hemonectin. Purified hemonectin was trypsin cleaved and the resulting tryptic peptides were separated by reverse phase HPLC and 2 short peptides were selected for sequencing by Edman degradation at the Yale School of Medicine Protein Sequencing Facility. Thusfar, a 19 residue and 13 residue peptide have been sequenced. No homology to other ECM adhesion proteins was found. The 19 residue peptide shows a 78% amino acid homology to alpha 2 HS glycoprotein (AHSG), which was described 30 years ago by Heremans and Schmid as a component of mammalian serum which is concentrated 100-fold in cortical bone. The physiologic function of this interesting protein has not been completely delineated as yet but it has been found to be chemotactic for mononuclear cells, and suggested as a mechanism for recruitment of circulating mononuclear cells to areas of bone remodelling and osteoclast formation (14). In addition, it has recently been found to have a significant sequence homology to fetuin, a plasma protein of ruminant artiodactyls which may promote cell adhesion and spreading (16). The second hemonectin peptide shows a 52% aminoacid identity with alpha 2HS glycoprotein. They can be differentiated, however, since an endothelial cell line which expresses hemonectin protein by immunoblotting does not express ASHG mRNA by Northern blotting (Dr. Wadie Bahou-personal comunication). It is interesting to speculate that HN and ASHG are members of a family of proteins involved in homing of circulating blood cells to bone and bone marrow, in a manner similar to homing of circulating lymphoid cells to different lymphoid sites mediated by the vascular addressins (15). The second hemonectin derived peptide also showed a 38% homology to N-CAM, the neural cell ahesion molecule which is involved in neuron-neuron adhesion in the nervous system and has recently been identified in bone marrow stromal cells (11). Whether this very interesting similarity will remain after further sequencing and cDNA cloning is accomplished, remains to be seen.

CONCLUSIONS

Cell-cell adhesion in bone marrow may well involve dynamic expression of a variety of adhesive glycoproteins by stromal cells, and their cognate receptors by hematopoietic cells. It is conceivable that this adhesion strategy is modulated as differentiation from stem cell to mature hematopoietic cell proceeds. Our data strongly suggests that hemonectin is an important component of this overall hematopoietic adhesion strategy.

BIBLIOGRAPHY

1. Bentley SA (1981). Close cell:cell interaction required for stem cell maintenance in continuous bone marrow culture. Exp. Hematol. 9:308-312.
2. Zuckerman KS, Wicha MS (1983). Extracellular matrix production by the adherent cells of long-term murine bone marrow cultures. Blood 61:540-547.
3. Dexter TM, Testa NG (1976) Differentiation and proliferation of hematopoietic cells in culture. Meth. Cell Biol 14:387-393.
4. Allen TD, Dexter TM (1984). The essential cells of the hematopoietic microenvironment. Exp. Hematol. 12:517-521.
5. Campbell AD, Wicha MS (1988). Extracellular matrix and the hematopoietic microenvironment. J. Lab. Clin. Med. 112:140-146.
6. Wight TN, Kinsella MG, Keating A, Suiger JW (1986). Proteoglycans in human long-term marrow cultures: biochemical and ultrastructural analyses. Blood 67:1333-1343.
7. Patel VP, Lodish MF (1984). Loss of adhesion of murine erythroleukemia cells to fibronectin during erythroid differentiation. Science 224:996-998.
8. Patel VP, Lodish MF (1986). The fibronectin receptor on mammalian erythroid cells: characterization and developmental regulation. J. Cell Biol. 102:449-456.
9. Campbell AD, Long MW, Wicha MS (1985). Extracellular matrix promotes the growth and differentiation of hematopoietic cells in long-term marrow culture. J. Clin. Invest. 75:2085-2090.
10. Campbell AD, Long MW, Wicha MS (1987). Haemonectin, a bone marrow adhesion protein specific for cells of granulocytic lineage. Nature 329:744-746.
11. Thomas PS, et. al (1988). Demonstration of neural cell adhesion molecules on stromal cells that support lymphopoiesis. Leukemia 2:171-175.
12. Makgoba MW, et al (1988) ICAM-1 a ligand for LFA-1-dependent adhesion of B, T and myeloid cells. Nature 331:86-88.
13. Schwick GH and Haupt H. Human plasma proteins of unknown function. In Putnam F (ed): "Plasma Proteins" Vol IV New York: Academic Press, 1984 pp 168-220.
14. Malone JD, and Richards M (1987). 2 HS Glycoprotein in chemotactic for mononuclear phagocytes. J. Cell. Physiol. 142:118-124.

15. Streeter PR, Berg EL, Rouse BTN, Bargatze RF, Butcher EC (1988) A tissue-specific endothelial cell molecule involved in lymphocyte homing. Nature 331:41-46.

The Biology of Hematopoiesis, pages 107–114

STROMAL REGULATION OF HEMOPOIESIS

Peter J. Quesenberry, Kotteazeth Srikumar, Daniel S. Temeles, Helen E. McGrath and Rowena Crittenden
Department of Internal Medicine, University of Virginia Health Sciences Center, Charlottesville, Virginia 22908

The introduction of the Dexter long-term murine marrow culture system has allowed for the detailed study of marrow adherent stromal elements (Dexter et al, 1977; Dexter and Lajtha, 1974; Dexter, 1979). This particular culture system is dependent upon the formation of adherent cell layers which appear to represent a model for the marrow microenvironment. Early studies with the Dexter stromal system suggested that the system was devoid of hemopoietic growth factors (Dexter, 1979; Williams et al, 1978; Dexter & Shadduck, 1980) and this was used as an argument for their lack of physiologic relevance. Subsequently Heard and colleagues (1982) and our own group investigated the capacity of Dexter stromal cells to produce hemopoietic growth factors using an agar overlay on top of stromal cells (Gualtieri et al, 1984). In this particular system target marrow cells were incorporated into agar, and media and overlaid directly upon unirradiated or irradiated Dexter stromal layers. Utilizing this type of system it became apparent that colony stimulating activities were present, and that after radiation, with removal of active hemopoiesis, multilineage colony stimulating activities were routinely observed. It appears that the difficulty in detecting colony stimulating activities in supernatants of these cultures relates in large part to the utilization and/or proteolytic degradation of the factors in the system by ongoing active hematopoiesis. Subsequent studies revealed that exposure of irradiated stromal layers to the lectin, pokeweed mitogen, resulted in high levels of colony stimulating activity induction (Alberico et al,

1987). The first of the colony stimulating factors to be defined in this conditioned media were colony stimulating factor-1 (CSF-1) by radioimmunoassay (Gualtieri et al, 1984) and GM-CSF by selective cell line stimulation and antibody blocking (Alberico et al, 1987), and later by mRNA detection (Temeles et al, 1989). GM-CSF was elevated with lectin exposure and also with lithium exposure (McGrath et al, 1987). This latter model is of particular interest since lithium is capable of stimulating virtually all hematopoietic stem cells in the Dexter culture system and provies an alternate look at hemopoietic regulation in this system (Table 1).

TABLE 1. HEMATOPOIETIC STEM/PROGENITOR CELLS INCREASED BY LITHIUM EXPOSURE IN DEXTURE CULTURES

Granulocyte-macrophage colony forming unit culture (GM-CFU-C) (Levitt & Quesenberry, 1980)

Colony forming unit spleen (CFU-S) (Levitt & Quesenberry, 1980)

Colony forming unit diffusion chamber (CFU-D) (Doukas et al, 1986)

Colony forming unit megakaryocyte (CFU-meg) (McGrath et al, 1987)

High proliferative potential colony forming cell (HPP-CFC) (Wade & Quesenberry, 1983)

Interleukin-1 was also found to be a stimulator of stromal factor production. CSF-1, while present in the system, did not appear to be elevated by these manipulations although mRNA levels were augmented with lectin exposure (Temeles et al, 1989). This would appear to be explained by the rapid binding and absorption of CSF-1 by adherent Dexter culture macrophages; thus increases in bioactivity are not seen while large increases in messenger RNA are observed. The probable explanation is that increased production of CSF-1 does occur, but that the bioactive CSF-1 molecules are rapidly bound and internalized by the large number of adherent macrophages in the system, and thus are not detected in conditioned media. Further studies utilizing Northern blot analysis for presence of various growth factor mRNAs have shown that Dexter stroma, irradiated or unirradiated, can also be induced to produce G-CSF and IL-6 mRNA by either lectin or interleukin-1. Figure 1 presents an overview of these findings. Thus, murine Dexter stroma appears to be a rich source of bioactive molecules affecting hemopoietic lineages. In addition, cell lines isolated from this stroma have been the source of other growth factors active on marrow cells. IL-7 was in fact discovered via planned studies on murine marrow stromal lines (Namen et al, 1988).

We have also investigated the nature of the cells forming these adherent layers. Our studies have shown that irradiated stromal layers which seem sufficient for reasonable short term hemopoietic marrow support consist predominantly of nonspecific esterase positive, acid phosphatase positive and alkaline phosphatase negative adherent macrophages, and another cell population which is alkaline phosphatase positive, negative for the other stains and has characteristics of a preadipocyte, ie fibroblast (Gualtieri et al, 1984; Song & Quesenberry, 1984). These two cell types appear sufficient for hemopoietic support. Utilizing an irradiated mouse explant model, stromal colony formation has also been studied. Initially it was felt that colonies of both cell types, along with single lineage colonies, were seen when murine marrow was explanted 24 hours after 1100 R in vivo whole body irradiation. These colonies would form over periods of 5-7 days. Further investigation of these phenomena, however, reveals that the colonies do not appear to have been derived from single cells but rather from large marrow aggregates which adhere and from which the colonies grow. In most cases, the aggregates either "dissolve" or release leaving a colony area (Quesenberry & Ennis, 1989). Thus it appears that these stromal colonies are not truly clonal in nature, but come from organized marrow aggregates.

We have utilized two systems to attempt to study the production of growth factors by the individual stromal components. One system involves study of an adherent marrow cell line isolated from murine Dexter culture by forced trypsin passage. This line was isolated under somewhat altered conditions in that fetal calf serum was substituted for horse serum and the temperature was raised to 37 degrees. These are conditions which begin to approach those utilized for a separate system, the Whitlock-Witte culture system (Whitlock & Witte, 1982; Whitlock et al, 1984), which supports long-term pre-B and B cell production in liquid culture. The cell line isolated by these techniques, the TC-1 cell line (Song et al, 1985), has some of the characteristics of the alkaline phosphatase preadipocyte, although it also stains variably with nospecific esterase, and thus is not identical phenotypically to the large cell characterized in explant marrow. The other cell system in which we have studied growth factor production is that described by Tushinski and colleages (Tushinski et al, 1982); explant bone marrow macrophage cultures. In this latter system, bone marrow is sequentially subcultured in the presence of CSF-1, initially discarding adherent cells and finally studying adherent cells after several subcultures. This cell population consists approximately 95% phenotypical macrophages. Studies on the TC-1 cell line have revealed that this line is capable of making GM-CSF, CSF-1, probably G-CSF and another activity which appears capable of synergizing with CSF-1 to give large macrophage colonies (Song et al, 1985; Quesenberry et al, 1987) identical in phenotype to the high proliferative potential colony forming cell described by Bradley and colleagues (Bradley et al, 1985; Bradley & Hodgson, 1979). This biologic activity has been studied extensively and appears to contain potent mitogenic activity for relatively early bone marrow stem cells. Biochemical characterization of the activity suggests that it is of relatively large molecular weight (over 120,000 dalton), a glycoprotein and quite protease resistant. A sequential biochemical separative approach, including anion exchange, Conconavalin A affinity chromatography, Sephacryl S-300 sizing chromatography and 2 FPLC steps, has still not resulted in purification of this activity. Some of the characteristics of the bioactivity studied could be that of multiple growth factors bound to a proteoglycan or other central core protein protecting them from proteolytic degradation. This suggestion is of particular interest given the demonstration that many growth factors interact synergistically to stimulate high proliferative potential colony forming cells, and in particular the fact that G-CSF, GM-CSF, CSF-1 and IL-3 coordinately interact in multiple combinations to give HPP-CFC formation (McNiece et al, 1988a; McNiece et al, 1988b). It is possible that

Stromal Growth Factor Production

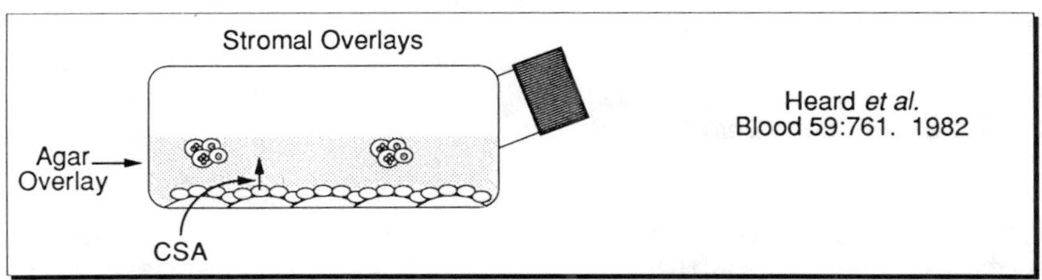

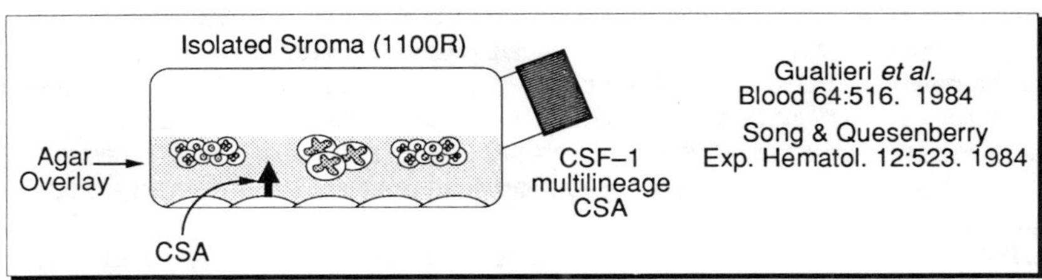

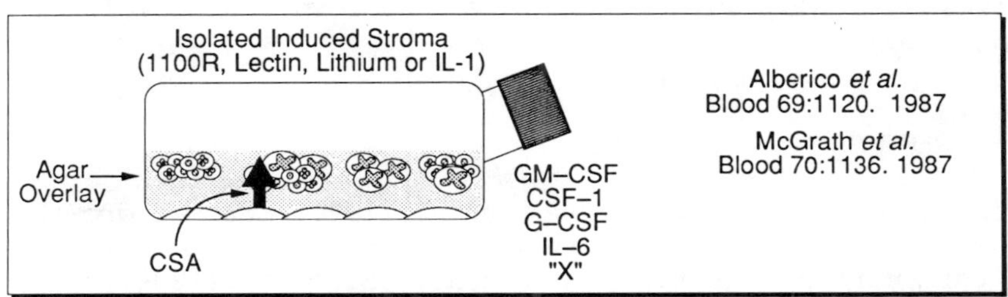

Stroma – A ***Rich*** Source of Growth Factor

Figure 1.

very low levels of multiple growth factors bound to a core protein could exert potent regulatory effects and this is presently the focus of much of the study in my laboratory.

Study of marrow macrophages has revealed that they too are potent sources of multiple growth factors. It appears that they are capable of producing CSF-1 itself (possible autocrine-type mechanism), G-CSF and IL-6 with somewhat equivocal results relating to their capacity to produce GM-CSF (Temeles et al, 1989).

Altogether these data suggest that adherent marrow stromal cells are rich sources of multiple growth factors, that probably several cells within these stromal components are capable of producing mixes of growth factors, and further, that regulation of hemopoiesis might occur via combinations of growth factors presented to target marrow cells either on cell surfaces or in the extracellular matrix. This would be consistent with data suggesting that proteoglycans may bind GM-CSF and present them to target cells (Gordon et al, 1987) and also consistent with the growing body of information on the ubiquitous synergies seen between growth factors and the fact that very low levels of some growth factors may act synergistically with other growth factors (Caracciolo et al, 1987).

REFERENCES

Alberico T, Ihle JN, Quesenberry PJ (1987) Stromal growth factor production in irradiated lectin exposed long-term murine bone marrow cultures. Blood 69:1120-1127.

Bradley TR, Hodgson GS, Bertoncello I (1985) I. Characteristics of primitive macrophage progenitor cells with high proliferative potential: relationship to cells with marrow repopulating ability in 5-fluorouracil treated mouse bone marrow. In: Experimental Hematology Today. Baum S, Ledney G, Khan A (eds), p. 285.

Bradley TR, Hodgson GS (1979) Detection of primitive macrophage progenitor cells in mouse bone marrow. Blood 54:1446-1450.

Caracciolo D, Shirsat N, Wong GG, Lange B, Clark S, Rovera G (1987) Recombinant human macrophage colony stimulating factor requires subliminal concentrations of granulocyte/macrophage (GM-CSF) for optimal stimulation of human macrophage colony formation in vitro. J Exp Med 166:1851-1860.

Dexter TM (1979) Clinical Haematology 8:453-468 (Lajtha L, ed), W.B. Saunders, Philadelphia, PA.

Dexter TM, Allen TD, Lajtha LG (1977) Conditions controlling the proliferation of haemopoietic stem cells in vitro. J Cell Physiol 91:335-344.

Dexter TM, Lajtha LG (1974) Proliferation of haemopoietic stem cells in vitro. Br J Haematol 28:525-530.

Dexter TM, Shadduck RK (1980) The regulation of hematopoiesis in long term bone marrow cultures: I. Role of L-cell CSF. J Cell Physiol 102:279-280.

Doukas M, Niskanen E, Quesenberry PJ (1986) The effect of lithium on stem cell and stromal cell proliferation in vitro. Exp Hematol 14:215-221.

Gordon MY, Riley GP, Watt SM, Geaves MF (1987) Compartmentalization of a haematopoietic growth factor by glycosaminoglycans in the bone marrow microenvironment. Nature 326:403.

Gualtieri RJ, Shadduck RK, Baker DG, Quesenberry PJ (1984) Hematopoietic regulatory factors produced in long term bone marrow cultures and the effect of in vitro irradiation. Blood 64:516-525.

Heard JM, Fichelson S, Varet B (1982) Role of colony stimulating activity in murine long term bone marrow cultures: Evidence for its production and consumption by the adherent cells. Blood 59:761-767.

Levitt L, Quesenberry PJ (1980) The effect of lithium on murine hematopoiesis in a liquid culture system. N Eng J Med 302:713-719.

McGrath HE, Liang C, Alberico T, Quesenberry PJ (1987) The effect of lithium on growth factor production in long term bone marrow cultures. Blood 70:1136-1142.

McNiece IK, Robinson BE, Quesenberry PJ (1988a) Stimulation of murine colony forming cells with high proliferative potential by the combination of GM-CSF and CSF-1. Blood 72:191-195.

McNiece IK, Stewart FM, Deacon DH, Quesenberry PJ (1988b) Synergistic interactions between hematopoietic factors as detected by in vitro murine bone marrow colony formation. Exp Hematol 16:383-388.

Namen AE, Schmierer AE, March CJ, Overell RW, Park LS, Urdal DL, Mochizuki DY (1988) B cell precursor growth-promoting activity. Purification and characterization of a growth factor active on lymphocyte precursors. J Exp Med 167:988-1002.

Quesenberry PJ, Ennis J (1989) Unpublished observations.

Quesenberry P, Song Z, McGrath HE, McNiece IK, Shadduck RK, Waheed A, Baber G, Kleeman E, Kaiser D (1987) Multilineage synergistic activity produced by a murine adherent marrow cell line. Blood 69:827-835.

Robinson BE, Quesenberry PJ (1989) Hematopoietic Growth Factors (a review) Submitted to Am J Med Sciences.

Song ZX, Quesenberry PJ (1984) Radioresistant murine marrow stromal cells: a morphologic and functional characterization. Exp Hematol 12:523-533.

Song ZX, Shadduck RK, Innes Jr DJ, Waheed A, Quesenberry PJ (1985) Hematopoietic factor production by a cell line (TC-1) derived from adherent murine marrow cells. Blood 66:273-281.

Temeles DS, McGrath HE, Bender P, Shadduck RK, Quesenberry PJ (1989) Induction of growth factor production in populations of murine stromal cells. Submitted for publication.

Tushinski RJ, Oliver LJ, Tynan PW, Warner JR, Stanley ER (1982) Survival of mononuclear phagocytes dependes upon a lineage-specific growth factor that the differentiated cells selectively destroy. Cell 28:71-81.

Wade P, Quesenberry PJ (1983) The effect of lithium chloride on high proliferative potential colony forming cells in murine Dexter cultures (abstract). J Cell Biochem Suppl 7B:30.

Whitlock CA, Witte ON (1982) Long term culture of B lymphocytes and their precursors from murine bone marrow. Proc Natl Acad Sci 79:3608-3612.

Whitlock CA, Robertson D, Witte ON (1984) Murine B cell lymphopoiesis in long term culture. J Immunol Method 67:353-369.

Williams N, Jackson H, Sheridan APC, Murphy MJ, Elste A, Moore MAS (1978) Regulation of megakaryopoiesis in long term murine bone marrow cultures. Blood 51:245-255.

The Biology of Hematopoiesis, pages 115–122

ROLE OF STROMAL CELL FACTORS (RESTRICTINS) IN MICROORGANIZATION OF HEMOPOIETIC TISSUES

Dov Zipori, Department of Cell Biology, Weizmann Institute of Science Rehovot 76100, Israel.

INTRODUCTION

The hemopoietic system consists of a group of organs interconnected by a network of blood and lymph vessels. The vast majority of cells in the blood stream are fully mature and have a limited life span. They are continuously being replaced by maturing cells that descend from a pool of bone marrow stem cells. Pluripotent stem cells give rise to a variety of committed stem cells (progenitors) which have initially been identified by their ability to form colonies in soft agar cultures (Bradley and Metcalf, 1966; Pluznik and Sachs, 1965). They require for their in vitro growth and differentiation the presence of glycoprotein inducers termed colony stimulating factors (CSFs) (for review see Platzer, 1989). CSFs are subdivided according to the major mature cell types that they induce. For example, M-CSF and G-CSF are inducers of macrophages and granulocytes respectively. CSFs are not only required for differentiation but also sustain the survival of mature cells in culture. In view of the remarkable effects of CSFs observed in vitro it has been suggested that local production of CSF in specific sites within blood forming organs and tissues accounts for hemopoietic cell maturation and positioning. As discussed below the process of cell production and the spatial distribution of cells within the tissue is however unlikely to depend exclusively upon inducers of differentiation.

The pool of stem cells is exceedingly small. Within the bone marrow, stem cells constitute a fraction of less than one percent. The maintenance of this small population is made possible due to their potential for self renewal (Fig. 1). The mechanism that controls this process is poorly understood. It is evident from studies described below that the molecules that regulate stem cell renewal are distinct from known CSFs and that organization of hemopoietic cells into discrete patterns within hemopoietic tissues cannot be attributed to differentiation inducing molecules only.

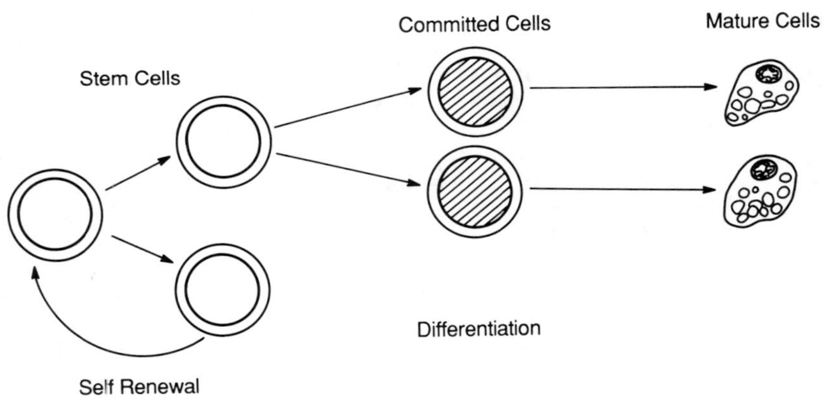

Figure 1: Alternative pathways of stem cell division: Differentiation of stem cells results in the death of the mature progeny. In order to allow the regeneration of the hemopoietic tissue, stem cells must self renew, i.e., maintain their original genotype and phenotype following division.

REGULATORS OF DIFFERENTIATION

The four major species of CSF are glycoproteins which have been purified and their genes molecularly cloned (Platzer, 1989; Metcalf, 1984). The obvious biological function of CSFs is to trigger proliferation of hemopoietic stem cells and progenitors followed by terminal differentiation.

Thus, the outcome of CSF action is the production of hundreds or thousands of mature cells from a single progenitor. Despite their designations that imply target cell specificities, their effects are not restricted to a single lineage. Interleukin-3 has the broadest target cell spectrum while M-CSF is the most restricted and affects mainly macrophages. It is however important to note that even in this latter case the macrophages which are generated due to the effect of M-CSF are secreting GM-CSF that may in turn trigger the differentiation of a variety of other cell types. This is but one example of the complex network of differentiation signals which may be elaborated by hemopoietic cells within the tissue. A further degree of complexity of the system is in the synergism among the various factors. _In situ_, cells are probably exposed simultaneously to a large number of signaling molecules and the final outcome of differentiation does not necessarily depend upon the specificity of the inducer but rather upon patterns or combination of signals. The participation of inhibitory molecules in this process is discussed below. Considered together, the various properties of CSFs strongly imply that these molecules are involved in vivo in the generation of large number of mature myeloid cells within a short time period. This is of utmost importance under conditions of stress such as those imposed by bacterial or viral infections. Indeed, we were able to demonstrate high titers of Interleukin-3 in serum of mice chronically infected with Mycobacterium lepraemurium (Resnick et al., submitted for publication).

CSFs are not only required for induction of differentiation but also for the maintenance of the mature phenotype and for activation of mature cell functions. A variety of agents which are not colony stimulating factors are nevertheless capable of facilitating differentiation by themselves or in conjunction with other molecules. Interleukin-4, Interleukin-6, 1,25 dihydroxy vitamin D_3, and prostaglandins are some examples. None of these factors including the various types of CSF can by itself, or in various combinations with the others, support long term renewal of stem cells . The only exception thus far described is IL-7 that induces proliferation of pro-B and double negative T cells, without inducing differentiation (Reviewed by Henny, 1989).

REGULATORS OF SELF RENEWAL

The abundance of differentiation inducers could potentially endanger the minute pool of stem cells. These cells which are obligatory for maintenance of intact hemopoiesis, may be drawn to terminal differentiation unless well guarded by a mechanism that does not permit excess differentiation. This mechanism seems to reside in stromal cells that form the supportive matrix (anlage) of the hemopoietic tissue. Stromal cells have been isolated in culture as cloned cell lines and were characterized as belonging to six subgroups (for review see Zipori, 1988a; Zipori, 1988b). Particular stromal cells were found to secrete a variety of cytokines including colony stimulating factors (Gimble et al., 1989). An endothelial-adipose stromal cell clone promoted long term myelopoiesis and lymphopoiesis and supported in vitro production of stem cells (Zipori and Lee, 1988). The mechanism of action of this stromal cell has not been elucidated todate. It has been clarified though that these stromal cells do not constitutively express CSF genes with the exception of CSF-1. This cytokine is also expressed by a variety of other cells devoid of any ability to promote hemopoiesis. Although it seems that CSFs do not mediate by themselves the renewal of stem cells, we examined their possible contribution to this process by transfection of endothelial-adipose stromal cells with an Interleukin-3 cDNA and selection for clones that express the gene. A comparative study of a series of such clones that differed in the expression of Interleukin-3 mRNA and Interleukin-3 bioactivity indicated that the ability of a stromal cell to express the gene does not improve its capacity to support long term hemopoiesis. In fact, clones that were producers of relatively high titer of CSF interfered with long term hemopoiesis, probably by driving the whole stem cell population to terminal differentiation (Zipori and Lee, 1988). A recent study of non cycling human stem cells indicated that these survived in culture without addition of any known cytokines (Leary et al., 1989). It is concluded that differentiation and self renewal are antagonistic processes. The function of self renewal factors from the stroma is to restrain the effect of CSFs on the stem and progenitor cell pools (Fig. 2).

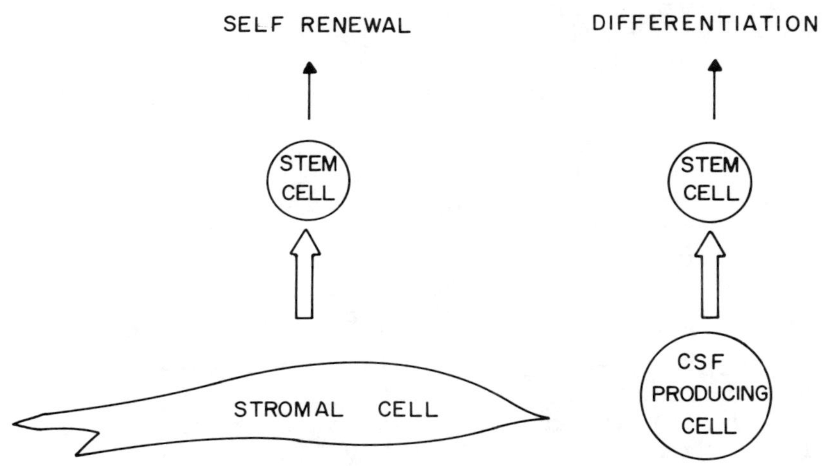

Figure 2: Stromal cell factors perform functions different from those of CSFs: Although stromal cells themselves may produce CSF they appear to influence hemopoiesis via unique molecules that support stem cell renewal rather then differentiation.

REGULATORS OF CELL ORGANIZATION

The molecules that induce differentiation and those that control stem cell renewal are sufficient to account for hemopoiesis in culture. However, the in vitro models lack one characteristic feature of the tissue, namely, the spatial organization of cells and the formation of discrete areas dominated by one cell lineage only. Although all of the hemopoietic organs are populated by cells that are descendents of a common stem cell, the cellular composition of each organ is unique and the organization of cells within the organ is highly characteristic and determines the specific functions of the tissue. It has been suggested that organ stroma dictates the pattern of cell organization. Part of this function is probably mediated by differentiation factors immobilized by components of the extracellular matrix of stromal cells (Gordon et al., 1987). Yet, due to the low target cell specificity of CSFs it is unlikely that tissue domains in which one cell type only is represented are formed solely by the local presence of the appropriate CSF. We have isolated from the surface of a stromal cell line a glycoprotein designated restrictin-P which is a specific inhibitor of plasma-like cells (Zipori et al.,1986; Zipori et al., 1988). We have obtained indirect evidence for the existence of other factors which exhibit specific inhibitory activity to other hemopoietic cell types. These findings led us to propose the theory of "restrictins" (Zipori et al., 1988, Zipori, 1989; Zipori et al., 1986).

It is assumed that stromal cells bear on their cell surfaces mosaics of inhibitory signals (restrictins) which are target cell specific. Fig. 3 demonstrates schematically that the differentiation potential of a given stem cell will only partially be expressed due to the local presence of specific restrictins. Stromal cells from the thymus, that contains an overwhelming majority of T lymphocytes are expected to harbour specific restrictins to all other hemopoietic cells. Non hemopoietic organs may either bear mosaics of specific restrictins to most hemopoietic cells or restrictins that nonspecifically inhibit any hemopoietic cell. This may explain the low occurrence of hemopoietic cells in organs such as the uterus and lung which are sources for ample amounts of CSF.

In summary, hemopoiesis is regulated on four levels. First, hemopoietic stem cells are driven by intracellular genetic program to differentiate at defined probabilities into committed progenitors. Secondly, extracellular signals originating in the stromal tissue surrounding the stem cell restrain the differentiation flow and force the stem cell to self renew. These stromal cells

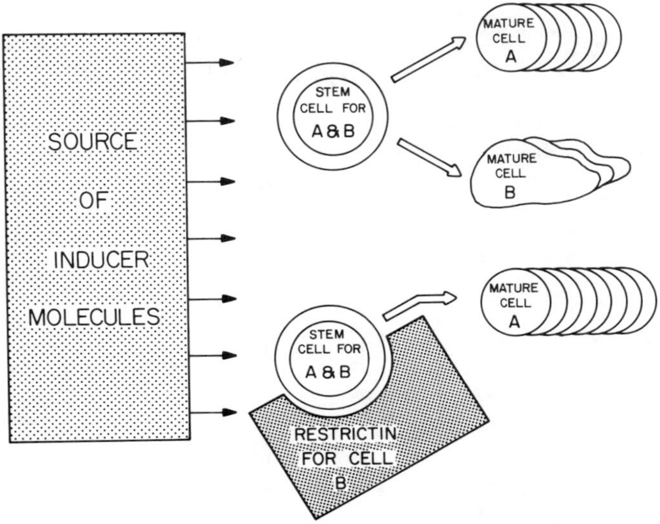

Figure 3: Putative factors termed restrictins are suggested to restrict the accumulation of specific hemopoietic cell types: The activity of lineage specific restrictins accounts for the formation of tissue sites in which only one type of hemopoietic cell is present.

antagonize the effect of the third component of the regulatory system, i.e., CSFs, the function of which is to amplify the differentiation signal and cause the production of large number of mature cells. This is achieved by their ability to induce differentiation coupled with extensive proliferation and to promote the survival and activity of the mature progeny. The fourth and final level is the organization of cells into discrete tissue specific patterns. This is proposed to be mediated by a mosaic of inhibitory signals characterized by target cell specificities that perform the "decision making" in terms of which cell population is permitted to exist at a specific site.

REFERENCES:

Bradley T.R., D. Metcalf (1966). The growth of mouse bone marrow cells in vitro. Aust. J. Exp. Biol. Med. Sci. 44:287.

Gimble J.M., C.E. Pietrangeli, A. Henley, M.A. Dorheim, J. Silver, A.E. Namen, M. Takeichi, C. Goridis, and P.W. Kincade (1989). Characterization of murine bone marrow and spleen-derived stromal cells: Analysis of leukocyte marker and growth factor mRNA transcript levels. Blood 74:303.

Gordon M.Y., G.P. Riley, S.M. Watt, M.F. Greaves (1987). Compartmentalization of a haematopoietic growth factor (GM-CSF) by glycosaminoglycans in the bone marrow microenvironment. Nature 326:403.

Henny C.S. (1989). Interleukin 7: Effects on early events in lymphopoiesis.Immunol. Today 10:170.

Leary A.G., Y. Hirai, T. Kishimoto, S.C. Clark, M. Ogawa (1989). Survival of hemopoietic progenitors in the G_0 period of the cell cycle does not require early hemopoietic regulators. Proc. Natl. Acad. Sci. USA 86:4535.

Metcalf D. (1984). The hemopoietic colony stimulating factors. Elsevier, Amsterdam.

Platzer E. (1989). Human hemopoietic growth factors. Eur. J. Haematol. 42:1.

Pluznik D.H., L. Sachs (1965). The cloning of normal "mast" cells in tissue culture. J. Cell Comp. Physiol. 66:319.

Zipori D. (1988a). Modulation of hemopoiesis by novel stromal cell factors. Leukemia, 2 (Supl. 12):9.

Zipori D., F. Lee (1988). Introduction of interleukin-3 gene into stromal cells from the bone marrow alters hemopoietic differentiation but does not modify stem cell renewal. Blood 71:586.

Zipori D. (1988b). Hemopoietic Microenvironments. In: "Hematopoiesis. Long-term effect of Chemotherapy and Radiation". N.G. Testa and R.P. Gale eds. Marcel Dekker, Inc. New York & Basel. p. 27.

Zipori D. (1989). Stromal cells from the bone marrow: Evidence for a restrictive role in regulation of hemopoiesis. Eur.J. Hematol.42:225.

Zipori D., M. Kalai, M. Tamir (1988). Restrictins: Stromal cell associated factors that control cell organization in hemopoietic tissues. Nat. Immunol. Cell Growth Regul. 7:185.

Zipori D., M. Tamir, J. Toledo and T. Oren (1986). Differentiation stage and lineage-specific inhibitor from the stroma of mouse bone marrow that restricts lymphoma cell growth. Proc. Natl. Acad. Sci. USA 83:4547.

The Biology of Hematopoiesis, pages 123–132

IN VITRO REGULATION OF HUMAN MEGAKARYOCYTE MATURATION

Alan M. Gewirtz

Departments of Medicine, Pathology, Thrombosis Research, and the Fels Cancer Research Institute, Temple University School of Medicine, Philadelphia, Pennsylvania 19140

INTRODUCTION

Megakaryocytopoiesis may be viewed as a developmental continuum which begins when an undifferentiated hematopoietic stem cell commits to maturation in the lineage of platelet producing cells (Gewirtz, 1986a; Hoffman, 1989). The commitment process results in the generation of a family of megakaryocyte progenitor cells (herein referred to as colony forming cells-megakaryocyte; CFC-Meg) which are capable of significant proliferative activity. CFC-Meg are ultimately responsible for determining the numbers of mature megakaryocytes which will populate the bone marrow. As proliferative activity declines, CFC-Meg progeny mature into precursor cells which terminally differentiate into polyploid megakaryocytes each capable of releasing several thousand platelets.

Presently, the factors responsible for controlling megakaryocyte maturation are only partially defined. Nevertheless, based on studies from a number of laboratories a general picture is beginning to emerge. The work in aggregate suggests that human megakaryocyte development is subject to a variety of regulatory influences which may be classified as effecting overall development of cells within the lineage, i.e. those of a general nature, and others which appear to control the expression of specific phenotypic properties. Data from this laboratory which support this conceptualization are presented below.

METHODS

Megakaryocyte progenitor cell assay: Depending on the experiments described, megakaryocyte colonies were grown in plasma clot cultures from progenitor cells of varying degrees of purity and with varying amounts and sources of growth factors (Gewirtz et al, 1987b, 1989).

Co-culture studies were performed in a totally autolgous system as previously described (Gewirtz et al, 1987b). A variable number of effector cells were added directly to a fixed number of target MNC ($5X10^5$/ml).

Megakaryocyte colonies were scored after identification with anti-human platelet glycoprotein antiserum in an indirect immunofluorescence assay (Gewirtz et al, 1986c, 1989). Unless otherwise stated, colony growth is reported as the mean ± S.E.M. .

Isolation of marrow immune effector cells: Monocyte-macrophages (MØ), T lymphocytes, and Natural Killer cells were isolated as described (Gewirtz et al, 1987b; Mangan et al, 1984; Timonen et al 1982; Weiner et al, 1973). NK cells of highest purity (85 ± 2% Leu 11b [+]) were obtained by immune rosetting with chromic chloride treated sheep (Indiveri et al, 1979).

Isolation and Short Term Culture of Normal Human Megakaryocytes: Megakaryocytes were enriched from the bone marrow of consenting normal donors by counterflow centrifugal elutriation (Gewirtz et al, 1987a,1989). Isolated megakaryocytes were placed into short term suspension cultures in the presence or absence of 8nM PMA (Sigma Chemical Co., St. Louis, MO) at 37°C in 5% CO_2, after which time they were fixed as described (Gewirtz et al, 1986b, 1989). Cells were deposited onto glass slides by cytocentrifugation for further analysis. Megakaryocytes were identified and staged using standard morphologic criteria (Levine, 1980). The accuracy of morphologic identification was confirmed by immunochemical identification with a mouse monoclonal antibody to platelet glycoprotein IIb/IIIa (Bennet et al, 1983).

Preparation of Human Platelet Factor 4 (PF4): Human PF4 was purified from outdated, thrombin stimulated human platelets essentially as published (Rucinski et al, 1979). Preparations gave a single band on SDS-Polyacrylamide gels, and were judged to > 95% pure.

In Situ Hybridization: In situ hybridization was carried out as described (Gewirtz et al, 1989) using purified cDNA inserts oligolabeled with biotin-11-dUTP (BRL, Gaithersburg, MD) using the method of Feinberg and Vogelstein (1984).omomycin A3

Statistical Analysis: Statistical significance of differences between groups was tested using a two-tailed Student's T Test for unpaired observations.

RESULTS

Role of immunocompentant cells in the exogenous regulation of human megakaryocytopoiesis

Since bone marrow accessory cells had been postulated to synthesize growth stimulating cytokines, we evaluated specific immune cell populations as potential sources of such growth factors. This was accomplished by determining the effect of co-culturing highly purified effector cells with partially purified marrow progenitor cells. The potential role of natural killer (NK) cells, T lymphocytes, and monocyte-macrophages was evaluated.

Patients with a proliferation of T γ lymphocytes and increased NK activity are often neutropenic, and anemic but are not commonly thrombocytopenic (Reynolds and Foon, 1984). This observation prompted us to investigate the ability of NK cells to modulate the growth of autologous CFC-Meg. A series of experiments designed to address this question were carried out, the most important aspect of which are shown in Table 1 (from Gewirtz et al, 1987).

TABLE I : Effect of Purified NK (Effector) Cells on Megakaryocyte Colony Formation by Enriched Marrow Mononuclear (Target) Cells

Exp No.	Effector (E) * Cells	Target (T)‡ Cells	T/E † 10:1	T/E 2:1
1	15 ± 1 §	41 ± 6	- - -	264 ± 40
2	- - -	30 ± 7	96 ± 29	106 ± 8
3	10 ± 3	31 ± 12	- - -	171 ± 5
mean ± SEM ¶	12 ± 2	33 ± 4	96 ± 29	182 ± 28
(n) **	(4)	(8)	(4)	(10)
df ‡‡	- - -	- - -	10	16
p value ††	- - -	- - -	.012	<.0009

* NK cells prepared by immune rosetting [purity 85 ± 2%]- number of cells plated = 5×10^5/ml

‡ adherent cell depleted, T lymphocyte depleted MNC- number plated held constant at 5×10^5/ml

† number of target cells plated kept constant at 5×10^5/ml.

§ mean ± SEM of megakaryocyte colonies enumerated in duplicate or quadruplicate culture dishes

¶ mean ± SEM of megakaryocyte colonies enumerated in all culture dishes

** total number of culture dishes scored

‡‡ degrees of freedom

The NK cells employed for these experiments were prepared by immune rosetting as described above, and were ~85% pure. In each of the three experiments a significant augmentation (p<.05, p<.001, p<.01 respectively) in megakaryocyte colony formation was noted at NK/target cell ratios of 1:2. One experiment was also performed at an NK/target cell ratio of 1:10. In contrast to results obtained with less pure effector and target cells, a three fold increase (p=.012) in colony formation, in comparison to baseline, was observed at this ratio.

NK mediated stimulation of CFU-Meg cloning efficiency could have been due to a cell contact phenomenon and/or the elaboration of a short range megakaryocyte colony stimulating activity. To distinguish these possibilities we examined the effect of centrifuging effector and target cells together (1:2 ratio), pre-incubating the cell pellet for three hours (37°C, 5% CO2) and then re-suspending the cells and plating as usual. This manipulation resulted in the loss of significant (p>.05) augmentation of megakaryocyte colony formation. Furthur, when interferon treated NK cells were utilized inhibition of CFU-Meg growth inhibition was discerned. We then assayed NK cell conditioned media (NKCM) for Meg-CSA activity. Mean colony formation per 5 x10^5 target cells in four control experiments was 34 ±7 (range 2±2 to 57±12 colonies). Addition of control medium at 5 and 10% concentration (v/v) had no effect on these numbers. In contrast, at a final NKCM concentration of 5%, 62 ±9 megakaryocyte colonies formed (p=.025). At the10% NKCM final concentration 84 ± 15 colonies were detected (p=0.009). NK cells therefore elaborate an activity with Meg-CSA. Whether this factor is IL-3 (Cuturi et al, 1989) or a unique cytokine remains to be established.

The effect of T lymphocytes (Figure 1) and monocytes on CFU-Meg cloning efficiency was also assessed. In none of the experiments performed with non-activated T lymphocytes was a statistically significant augmentation in CFU-Meg cloning efficiency observed. Similarly, when we examined the effect of Leu 3(+)helper/inducer, and Leu 2(+) suppressor/cytotoxic T cells on megakaryocyte colony formation in vitro no statistically significant effect on megakaryocyte colony formation could be demonstrated with either sub-set when cultured with target cells at target:effector ratios of 2:1, or 1:1.

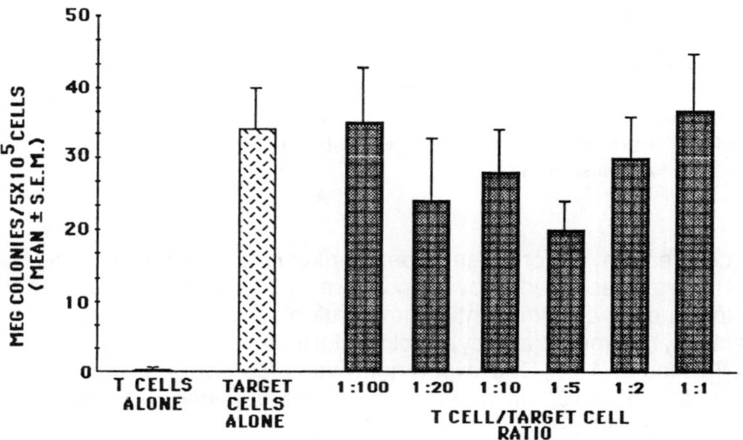

Figure 1: Effect of isolated autologous T lymphocytes on human megakaryocyte colony formation.

MØ isolated by adherence to serum coated plastic dishes also failed to increase the number of megakaryocyte colonies enumerated when co-cultured with autologous adherent cell depleted MNC. In fact, the addition of MØ to the cultures resulted in a slight, though statistically insignificant, inhibition of megakaryocyte colony formation when compared to colonies formed by target cells (adherent cell depleted MNC) alone.

Autocrine regulation

Megakaryocyte colonies are reported to develop better in the presence of platelet poor plasma than in serum (Vainchenker et al, 1982, Solberg et al, 1985). This observation suggests that platelets, or their releaseates may inhibit megakaryocyte development. A putative mediator of this effect is platelet factor 4 (PF4). We have found that highly purified human platelet factor 4 (PF4) inhibits human megakaryocytopoiesis in vitro. At $\geq$25 μg/ml, PF4 inhibited megakaryocyte colony formation ~80% in unstimulated cultures, and ~58% in cultures containing recombinant human IL-3 and GM-CSF. Since PF4 (25 μg/ml) had no effect on either myeloid or erythroid colony formation lineage specificity of this effect was suggested. A synthetic C-terminal PF4 peptide of 24, but not 13 residues, also inhibited megakaryocyte colony formation, while a synthetic 18 residue β-thromboglobulin (β-TG) peptide and native β-TG had no such effect when assayed at similar concentrations (Gewirtz, et al, 1989).

The mechanism of PF4 mediated inhibition was investigated. First, we enumerated total cell number, and examined cell maturation in control colonies (n=200), and colonies (n=100) that arose in PF4 containing cultures. Total cells per colony did not differ dramatically in the two groups (4.2±1.6 vs 6.1±3.0 respectively), but the numbers of mature "large" cells per colony was significantly decreased in the presence of PF4 when compared to controls (1.6±1.5 vs 3.9±2.3; p<.001). Second, by utilizing the human leukemia cell line HEL as a model for primitive megakaryocytic cells, we studied the effect of PF4 on cell doubling time, on the expression of both growth regulated (H3, p53, c-myc, and c-myb), and non-growth regulated (β_2-microglobulin) genes. At high concentrations of native PF4 (50μg/ml), no effect on cell doubling time, or H3, p53, or expression was discerned. In contrast, c-myc and c-myb were both upregulated.

These results suggested the PF4 inhibited colony formation by impeding cell maturation, as opposed to cell proliferation, perhaps by inducing expression of c-myc and c-myb. The ability of PF4 to inhibit a normal cell maturation function was then tested. Megakaryocytes were incubated in synthetic PF4, or β-TG peptides for eighteen hours and effect on Factor V steady state mRNA levels was determined in 600 individual cells by in situ hybridization. β-TG peptide had no effect on FV mRNA levels, while a ~60% decrease in expression of FV mRNA was found in megakaryocytes exposed to ≥100 ng/ml synthetic C-terminal PF4 peptide. Accordingly, PF4 modulates megakaryocyte maturation in vitro, and may function as a negative autocrine regulator of human megakaryocytopoiesis.

Regulation of coagulation FV expression in human megakaryocytes

The mechanisms responsible for induction of FV synthesis in megakaryocytes are unknown. To test the hypothesis that they are related to cell maturation events, we correlated FV antigen content of human megakaryocytes with cell size, morphologic stage of development, and ploidy level. Mature human megakaryocytes were isolated from normal bone marrow, deposited onto glass slides by cytocentrifugation, and fixed in methanol:acetone. Individual cells were then staged, geometric mean cell diameter (size) determined with an optical fylar, and FV antigen and nuclear DNA levels (ploidy) measured. Intrinsic megakaryocyte FV antigen levels were semi-quantified using a monoclonal antibody probe (B10) directed against the FV connecting peptide (150 kDa) (Gewirtz et al, 1986b). Cells were then reacted with Chromomycin A3 to allow for simultaneous DNA quantitation. Correlation coefficients (r) and coefficient of determination [r^2] were examined to discern potential relationships between FV expression and megakaryocyte maturation stage, size, or ploidy level (Figure 2).

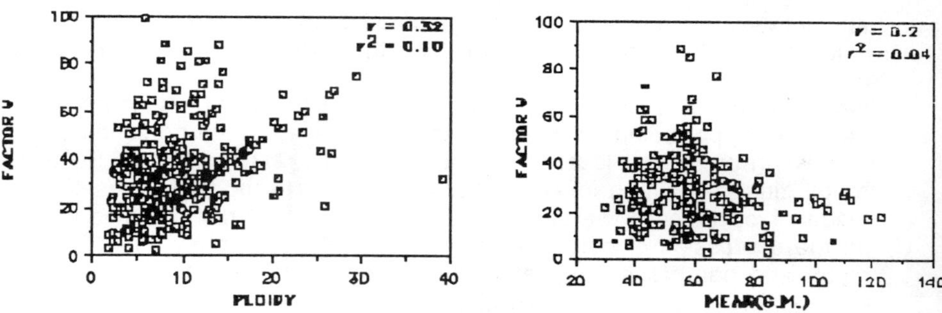

Figure 2: Megakaryocyte FV content plotted as a function of cell ploidy (left panel) or geometric mean cell diameter, an index of cell size (right panel).

A total of 1006 cells were examined, of which 12% were stage I, 8% were stage II, 35% were stage III, and 45% were stage IV. The geometric mean diameter (±SD) of cells in these stages was 48.3±11.8 μm^2, 54.9±14.4 μm^2, 61.7±20.2 μm^2, and 56.7±13.2 μm^2 respectively.

Respective ploidy values in arbitrary fluoresence units, where 2N=5%, were 28.2±18.2%, 31.4±19.3%, 54.3±26.6%, and 33.2±22.7%. Calculated r and r^2 values suggested that FV antigen levels varied independently of any of the maturation markers studied.

Subsequent experiments demonstrated that FV antigen levels could be upregulated by 24 hour exposure to 8nM phorbol myristate acetate. Analysis of FV steady state mRNA levels by in situ hybridization failed to reveal a detectable change in FV message after such treatment. We conclude that FV synthesis is neither a constitutive megakaryocyte property, nor one that is linked to the development of other cell maturation parameters. In addition, since FV protein levels are upregulated by PMA in the absence of apparent changes in the level of FV mRNA, it is likely that post-translational mechanisms regulate FV synthesis, perhaps by protein kinase C mediated protein phosphorylation.

DISCUSSION

In vitro culture systems designed to study megakaryocyte development have demonstrated the existence of several candidate, though not necessarily lineage specific, regulatory molecules. Some of these regulatory molecules promote megakaryocyte development. These include growth factors whose genes have been cloned and expressed by recombinant DNA technology such as granulocyte-macrophage colony stimulatory factor (GM-CSF)(Kaushansky et al, 1986), interleukin-3 (IL-3)(Messner et al, 1987), interleukin-6 (Ishibashi et al, 1989), and erythropoietin (Ishibashi et al, 1987). They also include proteins which have been less well characterized such as thrombopoietin (TPO)(McDonald et al, 1985; Hill and Levin, 1986), megakaryocyte stimulatory factor (MSF)(Greenberg et al, 1987), and megakaryocyte colony stimulatory factor (Meg-CSF)(Hoffman et al, 1985). The source of these factors, or factors with similar biological activites in vivo remains unclear. It is attractive to speculate however that the ancillary cells of the bone marrow are sources of these factors when appropriately stimulated (Gewirtz et al, 1987). It is also highly likely that such cells can cause clinically significant disease when their activity is inappropriately regulated (Nagasawa et al, 1986; Gewirtz et al, 1986).

Besides the stimulatory cytokines, evidence is beginning to accumulate that other molecules inhibit megakaryocyte development. Identification of these molecules was spurred by the finding of several groups that megakaryocyte colony growth is inferior in serum when compared to growth in platelet poor plasma (Vainchenker et al, 1982, Solberg et al, 1985), and by the observation that immunocytes, and their products, can cause clinically significant suppression of megakaryocyte production (Nagasawa et al, 1986; Gewirtz et al, 1986). Proteins with megakaryocyte inhibitory properties include γ interferon (Ganzer et al, 1987, transforming growth factor-β (TGF-β) (Mitjavila et al, 1988), and an incompletely characterized 12-17 kd secreted platelet glycoprotein (Dessypris et al, 1987). TGF-β and interferon can inhibit the development of cells in all hematopoietic lineages, likely by their anti-proliferative effects. The 12-17 kd glycoprotein appears to impede megakaryocyte development in a different manner by inhibiting cell maturation. Our studies suggest that a platelet specific α-granule protein, platelet factor 4 (PF4) also has inhibitory properties, and it too appears to impede cell maturation more than cell proliferation (Gewirtz et al, 1989). Since PF4, and the 12-17 kd glycoprotein are known to be synthesized by megakaryocytes they may inhibit megakaryocyte development in a truly autocrine manner.

Finally, our studies examining FV expression in mature cells suggest that the expression of specific phenotypic/functional markers may be specifically regulated, and are not necessarily linked to more generalized cell maturation and development. This finding is appealing since it provides a mechanism whereby megakaryocytes, at any given level of development may respond to acute demands for megakaryocyte derived proteins or products.

In toto, the observations discussed herein suggest what may already have been intuitively obvious. Megakaryocyte development is a complex process which appears to be the net result of stimulatory and inhibitory influences whose actions may be further modified by acute situational demands. Rapid advancements in the application of cellular and molecular techniques to this area of investigation are certain to shed even more light on this subject in the near future.

ACKNOWLEDGEMENTS: I thank my collaborators in these studies, Drs. B. Calabretta, S. Niewiarowski, and K. Mangan. The technical assistance of Nabisa Pappathi, Lu Aiquin, and Yu Min Shen, and the editorial assistance of Elizabeth R. Bien is gratefully acknowledged. Supported in part by grants from the National Cancer Institue (CA36896, and CA01324), and a Grant-In-Aid from the National Center of the American Heart Association. Dr. Gewirtz is the recipient of a Research Career Development Award from the National Cancer Institute.

REFERENCES

Bennet JS, Hoxie JA, Leitman SS, Vilaire G, and Cines DB (1983). Inhibition of fibrinogen binding to stimulated platelets by a monoclonal antibody. Proc. Natl. Acad. Sci. (USA)80:2417-2421.

Cuturi MC, Anegon I, Sherman F, Loudon R, Clark SC, Perussia B, and Trinchieri G. (1989). J. Exp. Med. 169:569-583.

Dessypris EN, Gleaton JH, Sawyer ST, Armstrong OL (1987). Suppression of maturation of megakaryocyte colony forming unit in vitro by a platelet-released glycoprotein. J Cell Physiol 130:361-368.

Feinberg AP, and Vogelstein B (1984). A technique for radiolabelling DNA restriction endonuclease fragments to high specific activity. Ann. Biochem. 137:266-267.

Ganser A, Carlo-Stella C, Greher J, Volkers B, Hoelzer D (1987). Effect of recombinant interferons alpha and gamma on human bone marrow derived megakaryocyte progenitor cells. Blood 70:1173-1179.

Gewirtz AM (1986a). Human megakaryocytopoiesis. Seminars in Hematology 23:27-42.

Gewirtz AM (1987). Recent methodologic advances in the study of human megakaryocyte development and function, in RW Colman and BJ Smith (EDS) Pharmacologic Methods for the Investigation of Coagulation and Platelets. New York, Alan R. Liss, pp.1-18.

Gewirtz AM, Calabretta B, Rucinski B, Niewiarowski S, and Xu WY (1989). Inhibition of human megakaryocytopoiesis in vitro by platelet factor 4 (PF4) and a C-terminal PF4 peptide. J. Clin. Invest. 83:1477-1486.

Gewirtz A, Keefer M, Bien R, and Barry W (1986c). Cell mediated suppression of megakaryocytopoiesis in Acquired Amegakaryocytic Thrombocytopenic Purpura. Blood 68:619-626.

Gewirtz AM, Keefer M, Doshi K, Annamali A, Chiu HC, and Colman RW (1986b). Biology of human megakaryocyte Factor V. Blood 67:1639-1648.

Gewirtz AM, Xu WY, and Mangan KF (1987). Role of Natural Killer Cells, in Comparison to T lymphocytes and Monocytes, in the Regulation of Normal Human Megakaryocytopoiesis In Vitro. J. Immunol. 139:2915-2925.

Greenberg SM, Kuter DJ, and Rosenberg RD (1987). In Vitro stimulation of megakaryocyte maturation by megakaryocyte stimulatory factor. J. Biol. Chem. 262:3269-3277.

Hill R, Levin J (1986). Partial purification of thrombopoietin using lectin chromatography. Exp Hematol 14:752-759.

Hoffman R (1989). Regulation of megakaryocytopoiesis. Blood 74:1196-1212.

Hoffman, R, Yang HH, Bruno E, Straneva J (1985). Purification and partial characterization of a megakaryocyte colony-stimulating factor from human plasma. J Clin Invest 75:1174-1182.

Ishibashi T, Kimura H, Uchida T, Kariyone S, Friese P, and Burstein SA (1989). Human interleukin-6 is a direct promotor of maturation of megakaryocytes in vitro. Proc. Natl. Acad. Sci. USA 86:5953-5957.

Ishibashi T, Koziol JA, Burstein SA (1987). Human recombinant erythropoietin promotes differentiation of murine megakaryocytes in vitro. J Clin Invest 79:286-289.

Indiveri, F., B.S. Wilson, M.A. Pellegrino, and S. Ferrrone (1979). Detection of human histocompatibility (HLA) antigens with an indirect rosette microassay. J. Immunol. Methods 29:101-109.

Kaushansky K, O'Harra RJ, Berkner K, Segal GM, Hagen FS, Adamson JW (1986). Genomic cloning, characterization and multilineage growth-promoting activity of human granulocyte-macrophage colony-stimulating factor. Proc Natl Acad Sci USA 83:3101-3105.

Levine RF (1980). Isolation and characterization of normal human megakaryocytes. Br. J. Haematol.45:487-497.

Mangan, K.F., M. Hartnett, S. A. Matis, A. Winkelstein, and T. Abo (1984). Natural Killer cells suppress human erythroid stem cell proliferation in vitro. Blood 63: 260-269.

McDonald TP, Cottrell M, Clift R, Khouri JA, Long MD: Studies on the purification of thrombopoietin from kidney cell culture media. J Lab Clin Med 106:162-174, 1985.

Messner HA, Yarnasaki K, Jamal N, Minden MM, Yang YC, Wong GG, Clark SC: Growth of human hemopoietic colonies in response to recombinant gibbon interleukin-3: comparison with human recombinant granulocyte and granulocyte-macrophage colony stimulating factor. Proc Natl Acad Sci USA 84:6765-6769, 1987.

Mitjavila MT, Vinci G, Villeval JL, Kieffer N, Henri A, Testa U, Breton-Gorius J, Vainchenker W (1988). Human platelet alpha granules contain a nonspecific inhibition of megakaryocyte colony formation: Its relationship to type B transforming growth factor (TGF-β). J Cell Physiol 134:93-100.

Nagasawa T, Sakuri T, Kashiwagi H, and Abe T (1986). Cell mediated amegakaryocytic thrombocytopenia associated with systemic lupus erythematosus. Blood 67:479-483.

Reynolds, C.W., and K.A. Foon (1984). T -lymphoproliferative disease and related disorders in humans and experimental animals: A review of the clinical, cellular, and functional characteristics. Blood 64:1146-1158.

Rucinski, B., S. Niewiarowski, P. James, D.A. Walz, and A. Budzynski. (1979). Antiheparin proteins secreted by human platelets. Purification, characterization and radioimmunoassay. Blood 53:47-62.

Solberg LA Jr, Jamal N, Messner HA (1985). Characterization of human megakaryocytic colony formation in human plasma. J Cell Physiol 124:67-74.

Timonen, T., C.W. Reynolds, J.R. Ortaldo, and R.B. Herberman (1982). Isolation of human and rat natural killer cells. J. Immunol. Methods 51:269-280.

Vainchenker W, Chapman J, Deschamps JF, Vinci G, Bouget J, Titeux M, Breton-Gorius J (1982). Normal human serum contains a factor(s) capable of inhibiting megakaryocyte colony formation. Exp Hematol 10:650-660.

Weiner, W.S., C. Bianco, V. Nussenzweig (1973). Enhanced binding of neuraminidase treated sheep erythrocytes to human T lymphocytes. Blood 42:939-946.

The Biology of Hematopoiesis, pages 133–144
Published 1990 by Wiley-Liss, Inc.

MEGAKARYOCYTE SIZE AND PLOIDY IN THROMBOCYTOPENIC OR MEGAKARYOCYTOPENIC MICE

Shirley Ebbe

Lawrence Berkeley Laboratory, University of California
Berkeley and Department of Laboratory Medicine,
University of California San Francisco

INTRODUCTION

Compensatory adjustments of megakaryocytopoiesis can be induced by perturbing the platelet count. Alterations of megakaryocyte size and ploidy are prominent, and the changes are appropriate, i.e. both are increased in response to thrombocytopenia and decreased in thrombocytosis. Sizes of megakaryocytes correlate with their ploidy (Odell et al., 1970), so when ploidy distribution within a population of cells changes, the average size of the cells also changes in the same direction. An increase in ploidy and an attendant increase in average size of megakaryocytes are prominent features of experimental thrombocytopenia (Penington and Olsen, 1970; Penington et al., 1974; Odell et al., 1976; Ebbe et al., 1988a)). However, increases in average sizes of mature megakaryocytes also occur within ploidy groups indicating that the final size of a cell may be influenced by non-ploidy dependent processes (Ebbe et al., 1988a).

It has also been found that the average sizes of mature megakaryocytes are increased when the numbers of megakaryocytes themselves are low (Ebbe and Phalen, 1979). In some cases, most notably in W/W^v and Sl/Sl^d mice, there is no attendant thrombocytopenia to explain why the megakaryocytes might have been stimulated to become larger than normal. In contrast to animals with thrombocytopenia, mature megakaryocytes of W/W^v and Sl/Sl^d mice display only a minimal trend toward higher ploidy values, the prominent macrocytosis being mediated by increases in sizes within ploidy groups (Ebbe et al., 1986 and 1989). Therefore, non-ploidy dependent mechanisms for increasing cell size appear to be important in these chronic nonthrombocytopenic megakaryocytopenias.

It is the purpose of this paper to summarize the results of measurements of megakaryocyte size and ploidy in several murine models of thrombocytopenia, megakaryocytopenia, and thrombocytosis. The aims are (1) to analyze mechanisms responsible for changes in megakaryocyte size and the extent to which they are dependent on changes in ploidy distribution, (2) to evaluate the hypothesis that a deficiency of megakaryocytes causes changes in recognizable megakaryocytes, and (3) to determine if the mechanisms responsible for macromegakaryocytosis in megakaryocytopenia differ from those that occur in thrombocytopenia.

MATERIALS AND METHODS

All methods have been described in the references throughout the text. Female CF1 mice were studied in all experiments except those involving genetically anemic mice and their +/+ controls. Fully mature (stage III) megakaryocytes were selected for measurement to ensure that DNA synthesis had been completed. The areas of cells in bone marrow smears were measured microscopically. Then the chromophore content of the nuclei of the same cells was determined by 2-wavelength microspectrophotometry after Feulgen staining. Ploidy was calculated by reference to the chromophore content of small segmented nuclei in the same marrow smears. Megakaryocyte ploidy distribution in the normal mice in all experiments was characterized by a modal value of 16N with lesser proportions of 8 and 32N and, in some cases, occasional 4 and 64N cells.

RESULTS AND DISCUSSION

Acute Immunothrombocytopenia

Acute immunothrombocytopenia was induced by a single intraperitoneal injection of guinea pig antimouse platelet serum (APS), and megakaryocytes were studied for four days thereafter (Ebbe et al., 1988a). Four hours after the APS injection, the platelet counts were about 2% of normal, and they subsequently recovered to normal. The findings in control mice and at two and four days after injection of APS illustrate the major adjustments that were observed.

On day two, there was a pronounced shift in the ploidy distribution of megakaryocytes. The proportions of 8 and 16N cells were diminished, and the proportion of 32N cells was substantially increased, but 16N remained the modal ploidy value. The failure of 32N to become the modal ploidy value contrasts with findings of Corash et al. (1987) in C57/Bl mice, Penington and Olsen (1970), Odell et al. (1976), and Jackson et al. (1984) in rats, and Martin et al. (1983) in rabbits. The difference may have been due to strain, species or other experimental variables. On day four, the ploidy distribution had reverted to normal.

The mean size of all mature megakaryocytes (average obtained from cells of all ploidy groups) was increased on day two, reflecting two abnormalities: the shift to higher ploidies and an increase in mean size of 32N cells. By day four, sizes had returned to normal.

The rate of platelet production increases about two days after induction of acute thrombocytopenia in rats (Odell et al., 1975). Kinetics of thrombocytopoiesis are similar in rats and mice (Ebbe, 1971), and rats, like the mice reported here, display marked ploidy shifts (Odell et al., 1976) and macrocytosis.(Ebbe et al., 1968a) of mature megakaryocytes on day 2 after induction of acute thrombocytopenia. These temporal associations suggest that the ploidy shift and attendant increase in megakaryocyte mass may mediate production of increased numbers of platelets.

Continuous Immunothrombocytopenia

Platelet counts were maintained at less than 10% of normal for six days by daily injections of APS; findings on days three and six were representative (Ebbe et al., 1988a).

On day three, no 8N cells were found, and the proportion of 16N was markedly reduced. At the same time there were substantial increases in proportions of 32 and 64N cells and the appearance of an occasional 128N cell; 32N became the modal ploidy class. Three days later, the ploidy shift was still prominent but less so than on day three, with the modal ploidy value returning to 16N.

Mean size of all megakaryocytes was markedly increased on both days three and six and showed little decline on day six when the ploidy distribution had reverted toward normal. On day three, 16N megakaryocytes were significantly larger than normal 16N megakaryocytes; by day six, there was substantial macrocytosis within all of the three major ploidy groups (8, 16, and 32N).

Findings in the two groups of thrombocytopenic mice reaffirm the well-known occurrence of a shift to higher ploidy values in megakaryocytes with an attendant increase in average cell size. They also indicate that the initial marked shift to higher ploidies may not be fully maintained with continued thrombocytopenia. However, the mass of megakaryocytes may be continued at a high level by an increase in average sizes within ploidy groups.

Transfusion-induced Thrombocytosis

To determine if converse changes in megakaryocyte size and ploidy would be found, mice were evaluated two and three days after a single transfusion of homologous platelets. By extrapolation from the persistently high platelet counts at those times, it was estimated that platelet counts initially were raised to about three times normal values by the transfusion.

It is known from the work of Penington et al. (1974) and Jackson et al. (1984) that a shift to lower ploidy values occurs in response to sustained thrombocytosis. Under the conditions of our experiment, little, if any, shift in ploidy distribution was demonstrable. Despite this, mean megakaryocyte sizes were significantly less than normal on both days two and three after the platelet transfusion. The reduction in overall size was mediated by reductions in mean sizes of the predominant 16N group on day two and the 32N group on both days.

These findings support the notion that megakaryocyte mass can be adjusted independently of adjustments in ploidy in response to an abrupt elevation of the platelet count.

W/W^v and Sl/Sl^d Mice

Mice of the genetically anemic strains W/W^v and Sl/Sl^d have severe megakaryocytopenia and macrocytic megakaryocytes, but no thrombocytopenia.

The ploidy distribution of W/W^v megakaryocytes was normal except for a slight increase in the proportion of 32N cells (Ebbe et al., 1989). Sl/Sl^d megakaryocytes also showed slight abnormalities which included a reduction in the proportion of 16N cells, an increase in 64N cells, and the occurrence of a small proportion of 128N cells (Ebbe, et al., 1986).

In contrast to the minimal shifts in ploidy, the megakaryocyte populations as a whole had substantially larger mean sizes in both W/W^v and Sl/Sl^d mice than in the respective controls. This was due to macrocytosis within each of the three major ploidy groups in W/W^v and within ploidy groups 16, 32, and 64N in Sl/Sl^d.

In the genetically megakaryocytopenic mice, thrombocytopenia was not a complicating factor, and ploidy shifts made only a minor contribution to megakaryocytic macrocytosis. It was mediated mainly by macrocytosis within ploidy groups, suggesting the possibility that this may be a characteristic response to megakaryocytopenia.

Post-irradiation Megakaryocytopoiesis

Sublethal irradiation (650 R, ^{60}Co) of mice produced an early severe megakaryocytopenia and thrombocytopenia which were maximal about ten days after irradiation. With the partial recovery that occurred during the second month, platelet counts could be completely normal in spite of only half normal numbers of megakaryocytes. Megakaryocytes were usually macrocytic at the same time that they were deficient in number (Ebbe and Phalen, 1979). However, almost any combination of normal or low platelet and megakaryocyte counts and normal or increased megakaryocyte sizes could occur during partial recovery from radiation. Of note, however, is the fact that megakaryocytopoiesis was never found to be completely normal during the second month after irradiation.

Most commonly, platelet and megakaryocyte numbers were decreased, platelets being disproportionately higher than megakaryocytes, and megakaryocyte sizes were increased. In that case, average sizes of all mature megakaryocytes and of 16N and 32N cells were larger than their respective controls (Ebbe et al., 1988b). There was also a modest shift in ploidy with a higher proportion of 32N cells and lower proportions of 16N and 8N cells than in unirradiated controls. These changes could have been induced by the modest deficiency of platelets, so they can not be attributed to feed-back stimulation initiated solely by the deficiency of megakaryocytes. In such animals, however, abnormalities were only partially reversed two and three days after raising the platelet count to about twice normal with a platelet transfusion.

Transfusion-induced Thrombocytosis, Post-irradiation

To evaluate the effects of an excess of platelets in megakaryocytopenia induced by irradiation, a group of mice that did not have an associated thrombocytopenia or abnormalities of megakaryocyte size or ploidy were hypertransfused with homologous platelets to platelet counts of about three times normal, and their megakaryocytes were evaluated two and three days later. By day three after platelet transfusion there was an increase in the proportion of 8N cells and a decrease in 32N. On the second day after platelet transfusion, megakaryocytes were not smaller than those of irradiated, non-transfused controls. On the third day, they were smaller due to the shift in ploidy.

Differences from the non-irradiated mice, transfused to the same extent at the same time and described above, were that appearance of micromegakaryocytosis was delayed and there were less substantive reductions in sizes within ploidy groups. These differences suggest the possibility that megakaryocytopenia may have delayed and modified the effects of transfusion-induced thrombocytosis on megakaryocytes in irradiated mice.

Hydroxyurea

Megakaryocyte numbers decline during the first three days after administration of hydroxyurea (900 mg/kg) and, at the same time, average sizes become larger than normal. Platelet counts become significantly less than normal on days four and five (Ebbe and Phalen, 1982).

Megakaryocyte sizes and ploidies were evaluated two and three days after administration of hydroxyurea (Ebbe et al., 1988b). Platelet counts did not differ from normal; megakaryocytopenia occurred on day three. The average sizes of all megakaryocytes were greater than normal on both days, as were average sizes within the 16N and 32N ploidy groups. Ploidy distribution on day two did not show changes that could have contributed to the macrocytosis, the only abnormality being a slight increase in the proportion of 8N cells. On day three there was a shift to higher ploidy with decreases in 8 and 16N cells and an increase in 32N. This ploidy shift occurred in the absence of thrombocytopenia and coincided with the onset of significant megakaryocytopenia.

Interpretation of the changes produced by a single injection of hydroxyurea requires reviewing some of the normal processes of megakaryocytopoiesis. Maturation of cells through the compartment of recognizable megakaryocytes is characterized, in part, by a progressive increase in cell size (Ebbe et al., 1968a). Based on patterns of labeling with tritiated thymidine, total maturation time can be estimated as about 68 hours (Ebbe, 1971). More than half of that time (about 36 hours) is spent within the mature stage III compartment which comprised the cells measured in the present experiments. Therefore, the most mature stage III cells would be larger than the most immature stage III cells, even though they can not be distinguished morphologically. Hydroxyurea acts mainly by depleting morphologically unrecognizable precursors (Ebbe and Phalen, 1982), and megakaryocytopenia results from diminished influx into the recognizable compartment. Two days after hydroxyurea, when the total cell number was about 80% of normal, the stage III compartment would be only partially depopulated, because about 32 hours of the elapsed 48 hours would have been required for the wave of depopulation to proceed through the less mature stages of recognizable megakaryocytes. Therefore, the age distribution of stage III cells would be shifted toward the more mature and larger cells. This disturbance in age distribution may explain the increase in average size within ploidy groups and macromegakaryocytosis that was seen on day two.

The situation on day three, when the population size was reduced to about 60% of normal, is more complex. At that time there was a persistent increase in the size/ploidy relationship that would not be explained by the same mechanism. In addition, there was a shift to higher ploidy values. The ploidy shift might occur if lower ploidy cells matured more rapidly than higher ploidy cells or if the drug affected precursors of different ploidy cells differently. However, the concurrence of the two abnormalities suggests that depopulation of the proliferating progenitor cells or their progeny may have triggered compensatory adjustments in nuclear proliferation and in rates of growth or maturation.

Size Distribution of Macrocytic Megakaryocytes

In all of the models with thrombocytopenia or megakaryocytopenia, megakaryocytes that were macrocytic for their ploidy group were observed. The size distributions of such cells were compared to the size distributions of control cells of the same ploidies. It was found that the increase in mean cell size was due to a shift to the larger sizes normally present. Of note is the fact that cells larger than any normally present in the ploidy group did not appear. The failure of sizes within ploidy groups to exceed those normally present in the same ploidy groups suggests that the amounts of nuclear DNA impose constraints on the maximum size to which the cells can grow and that those constraints are the same in normal and stimulated megakaryocytes.

Interpretation of Results

The results show that ploidy is not the only determinant of final overall megakaryocyte size, because the average size of the population of mature megakaryocytes was observed to change without attendant changes in ploidy. This phenomenon was seen two days after administration of hydroxyurea and two days after hypertransfusion of platelets in normal mice. It is also apparent that sizes within ploidy groups do not remain constant when thrombocytopoiesis is perturbed. Examples of abnormalities of average size within one or more ploidy groups were seen in all models. Therefore, this appears to be a common way by which megakaryocyte mass is adjusted.

Macrocytosis of megakaryocytes may result from different mechanisms in thrombocytopenia and megakaryocytopenia, or the mechanisms may be the same. In the following table the various models are qualitatively scored, based on whether or not certain features were absent (0), present (+), or, in contrast to simply present, were prominent (++) in an effort to decide between these choices.

Megakaryocytic Macrocytosis

	Platelets Decreased	Mega's Decreased	Ploidy Increased	Size/Ploidy Increased
Immunothrombo-cytopenia				
Acute	+ +	0	+ +	+
Sustained	+ +	0	+ +	+ +
Sl/Sl^d mice	0	+ +	+	+ +
W/W^v mice	0	+ +	+	+ +
Hydroxyurea				
2 days	0	0	0	+ +
3 days	0	+ +	+ +	+ +
Post-irradiation	+	+ +	+	+ +

In pure immunothrombocytopenia without a deficiency of megakaryocytes, shifts to higher ploidy were prominent. The size/ploidy ratio was also increased, but became prominent only with sustained stimulation.

In the pure megakaryocytopenia of genetically anemic mice, ploidy shifts were minimal, and the increased size/ploidy relationship was prominent. This suggests that the response to megakaryocytopenia may predominantly affect non-ploidy dependent mechanisms. Alternatively, it could be suggested that the pattern seen in these mice may be a characteristic of the chronically stimulated state as implied from the trend seen with prolongation of immunothrombocytopenia. After irradiation, when modest thrombocytopenia complicated megakaryocytopenia, a similar pattern of megakaryocytopoiesis prevailed.

On day two after administration of hydroxyurea the size/ploidy ratio increased without even a minimal increase in ploidy. In other megakaryocytopenic states, an increase in the size/ploidy ratio tended to predominate over ploidy shifts as a mediator of macrocytosis, but its mechanism is not known. Acceleration of megakaryocyte maturation has been demonstrated in thrombocytopenia (Ebbe et al., 1968b) and in megakaryocytopenic W/W^v mice (Ebbe et al., 1989). It may, perhaps, be a more universal phenomenon, responsible for cells growing or maturing faster and thus becoming larger, on the average, than normal for their ploidy.

An increase in ploidy was never seen without attendant evidence for an increase in the size/ploidy ratio, so in many cases the two abnormalities appeared to be linked together. One can not conclude that megakaryocytopenia and thrombocytopenia act through different pathways to induce macrocytosis, because the manifestations of thrombocytopenia and megakaryocytopenia on megakaryocyte ploidy and size overlapped. How deficiencies of either platelets or megakaryocytes are sensed by the organism is unknown. Likewise unknown is the mechanism by which the message that deficiencies exist is transmitted.

It has been proposed (Williams et al., 1982; Sparrow et al., 1987) that megakaryocytopoiesis is regulated on 2 levels: colony-forming cells by colony-stimulating factor and more mature cells by thrombopoietin or something like it, the latter affecting the phase of nuclear replication and ploidy determination. There is ample evidence for the existence of a thrombopoietin which is demonstrable in the blood of thrombocytopenic animals (McDonald, 1988; Hill and Levin, 1989), and it has been shown that thrombopoietin will induce an increase in the ploidy of megakaryocytes (Levin et al., 1982). It has also been reported that megakaryocyte colony-stimulating factor becomes demonstrable in the blood of people and animals when there is a deficiency of megakaryocytes in the marrow and that its presence is determined by a deficiency of megakaryocytes rather than of platelets (Hoffman et al., 1981; Mazur et al., 1984; Miura et al., 1988). By showing that recognizable megakaryocytes have abnormalities of ploidy and size when they are deficient in number, even in the absence of thrombocytopenia, the present results raise the possibility that megakaryocyte colony-stimulating factor may, primarily or secondarily, affect the later phases of megakarocytopoiesis. An alternative possibility is that a thrombopoietin-like mechanism may be activated by a paucity of megakaryocytes.

If megakaryocytopenia contributes to the regulation of megakaryocytopoiesis, its effects should be visible, even when there are excessive numbers of platelets. Therefore, we have asked if the effects of thrombocytosis will be modified by megakaryocytopenia. The results suggest that they will. In post-irradiation megakaryocytopenia, the reduction in megakaryocyte size that occurred in response to transfusion-induced thrombocytosis was delayed relative to that seen in unirradiated mice. Previous observations in W/W^v mice with rebound thrombocytosis (Ebbe and Phalen, 1978) and Sl/Sl^d mice with transfusion-induced thrombocytosis (Ebbe et al., 1978) showed that the sizes of the intrinsically macrocytic megakaryocytes in these mice decreased. However, the cells remained larger than those of similarly thrombocytotic +/+ control mice. These findings indicate that a high platelet count will modify the effects of megakaryocytopenia, but they suggest that the megakaryocytopenia will continue to express itself.

CONCLUSIONS

The average size of mature megakaryocytes is determined by both ploidy-dependent and nonploidy-dependent mechanisms. Homeostatic mechanisms regulating megakaryocytopoiesis are probably responsive to the number of megakaryocytes as well as to the number of platelets.

REFERENCES

Corash L, Chen HY, Levin J, Baker G, Lu H, Mok Y (1987). Regulation of thrombopoiesis: effects of the degree of thrombocytopenia on megakaryocyte ploidy and platelet volume. Blood 70:177-185.

Ebbe S (1971). The megakaryocyte: maturation and self-renewal. In Brinkhous KM, Shermer RW, Mostofi FK (eds): "The Platelet", Baltimore: Williams and Wilkins, pp 1-12.

Ebbe S, Phalen E (1978). Regulation of megakaryocytes in W/W^v mice. J Cell Physiol 96: 73-80.

Ebbe S, Phalen E (1979). Does autoregulation of megakaryocytopoiesis occur? Blood Cells 5: 123-138.

Ebbe S, Phalen E (1982). Macromegakaryocytosis after hydroxyurea. Proc Soc Exp Biol Med 171: 151-157.

Ebbe S, Stohlman F Jr, Overcash J, Donovan J, Howard D (1968a). Megakaryocyte size in thrombocytopenic and normal rats. Blood 32: 383-392.

Ebbe S, Stohlman F Jr, Donovan J, Overcash J (1968b). Megakaryocyte maturation rate in thrombocytopenic rats. Blood 32: 787-795.

Ebbe S, Phalen E, D'Amore P, Howard D (1978). Megakaryocytic responses to thrombocytopenia and thrombocytosis in Sl/Sl^d mice. Exp Hematol 6: 201-212.

Ebbe S, Bentfeld-Barker M, Adrados C, Carpenter D, Mortensen C, Yee T, Phalen E (1986). Functionally abnormal stromal cells and megakaryocyte size, ploidy, and ultrastructure in Sl/Sl^d mice. Blood Cells 12: 217-232.

Ebbe S, Yee T, Carpenter D, Phalen E (1988a). Megakaryocytes increase in size within ploidy groups in response to the stimulus of thrombocytopenia. Exp Hematol 16: 55-61.

Ebbe S, Yee T, Carpenter D, Phalen E (1988b). Megakaryocyte size and ploidy after hydroxyurea or radiation (abstract). Exp Hematol 16: 551.

Ebbe S, Carpenter D, Yee T (1989). Megakaryocytopenia in W/W^v mice is accompanied by an increase in size within ploidy groups and acceleration of maturation. Blood 74: 94-98.

Hill RJ, Levin J (1989). Regulators of thrombopoiesis: their biochemistry and physiology. Blood Cells 15: 141-166.

Hoffman R, Mazur E, Bruno E, Floyd V (1981). Assay of an activity in the serum of patients with disorders of thrombopoiesis that stimulates formation of megakaryocytic colonies. New Eng J Med 305: 533-538.

Jackson CS, Brown LK, Somerville BC, Lyles SA, Look AT (1984). Two-color flow cytometric measurement of DNA distributions of rat megakaryocytes in unfixed, unfractionated marrow cell suspensions. Blood 63: 768-778.

Levin J, Levin FC, Hull DF III, Penington DG (1982). The effects of thrombopoietin on megakaryocyte-CFC, megakaryocytes, and thrombopoiesis: with studies of ploidy and platelet size. Blood 60: 989-998.

Martin JF, Trowbridge EA, Salmon G, Plumb J (1983). The biological significance of platelet volume: its relationship to bleeding time, platelet thromboxane B_2 production and megakaryocyte nuclear DNA concentration. Thrombosis Res 32: 443-460.

Mazur EM, deAlarcon P, South K, Miceli L (1984). Human serum megakaryocyte colony-stimulating activity increases in response to intensive cytotoxic chemotherapy. Exp Hematol 12: 624-628.

McDonald TP (1988). Thrombopoietin: its biology, purification, and characterization. Exp Hematol 16: 201-205.

Miura M, Jackson CW, Steward SA (1988). Increase in circulating megakaryocyte growth-promoting activity (Meg-GPA) following sublethal irradiation is not related to decreased platelets. Exp Hematol 16: 139-144.

Odell TT Jr, Jackson CW, Friday TJ (1970). Megakaryocytopoiesis in rats with special reference to polyploidy. Blood 35: 775-782.

Odell TT, Jackson CW, Murphy JR (1975). Platelet recovery after induction of acute thrombocytopenia. Proc Soc Exp Biol Med 148: 829-833.

Odell TT, Murphy JR, Jackson CW (1976). Stimulation of megakaryocytopoiesis by acute thrombocytopenia in rats. Blood 48: 765-775.

Penington DG, Olsen TE (1970). Megakaryocytes in states of altered platelet production: cell numbers, size and DNA content. Brit J Haematol 18: 447-463.

Penington DG, Streatfield K, Weste SM (1974). Megakaryocyte ploidy and ultrastructure in stimulated thrombopoiesis. In Baldini MG, Ebbe S (eds): "Platelets: Production, Function, Transfusion and Storage", New York: Grune and Stratton, pp 115-130.
Sparrow RL, Swee-Huat O, Williams N (1987). Haemopoietic growth factors stimulating murine megakaryocytopoiesis: interleukin-3 is immunologically distinct from megakaryocyte-potentiator. Leukemia Res 11: 31-36.
Williams N, Eger RR, Jackson HM, Nelson DJ (1982). Two-factor requirement for murine megakaryocyte colony formation. J Cell Physiol 110: 101-104.

ACKNOWLEDGMENTS

Supported by the Office of Health and Environmental Research of the U.S. Department of Energy under contract no. DE-AC03-76SF00098.

The Biology of Hematopoiesis, pages 145–152

Biology and Biochemistry of the Erythropoietin Receptor

Stephen T. Sawyer
Division of Hematology
Vanderbilt University School of Medicine
Nashville, Tn 37232

Erythropoietin (EP) is the glycoprotein hormone which is the primary regulator of erythropoiesis. The binding of EP to receptor for the hormone on responsive erythroid progenitor and precursor cells apparently allows the cells to mature to erythrocytes in lieu of cell death. The development of a model erythroid cell system responsive to EP primary explanted proerythroblasts purified from the spleens of mice infected with the anemia strain of Friend virus (FVA cells) (Koury et al., 1984; Sawyer et al. 1987a) and the ability to radiolabel EP and maintain biological activity allowed the identification of the receptor for EP.

For a number of years, it was believed that iodination of EP resulted in a loss of biological activity. However, upon the availability of recombinant human EP, it has been shown in this laboratory that ^{125}I-EP can be prepared with 100% of biological activity. Tritiated EP ([^{3}H]-EP) which retained biological activity was first used to show specific binding of EP to FVA cells (Krantz and Goldwasser, 1984). Studies with ^{125}I-EP showed that the quantitative data obtained with [^{3}H]-EP was technically flawed due to the low specific activity of [^{3}H]EP. In contrast to the first report of [^{3}H]EP binding to FVA cells, ^{125}I-EP binding to the surface of FVA cells at 0°C showed a non-linear biphasic plot when the binding of increasing concentrations of EP were analyzed by the Scatchard method. This non-linearity was interpreted as the existence of two classes of EP receptors which differ in the affinity for EP. FVA cells were found to have approximately 1,000 receptors for EP of which 300 to 400 have a higher affinity for EP (Kd of 0.08 to 0.10 nM) while the remaining receptors have a lower affinity (Kd of 0.6 to 1.0nM) (Sawyer et al. 1987b,c). This biphasic Scatchard plot can also be interpreted as negative cooperativity in which the interaction of bound receptors with unbound receptors leads to the free receptors binding EP with lesser affinity. Negative cooperativity can be tested by examining the disassociation of ^{125}I-EP from occupied receptors in the presence and absence of an excess unlabeled EP. If there is negative cooperativity, ^{125}I-EP will be released faster in the presence of unlabeled EP. Experiments in this laboratory have shown that bound ^{125}I-EP is released from FVA cells at the same rate in the presence and absence of unlabeled EP indicating no negative cooperativity.

During these experiments the binding of ^{125}I-EP to Friend MEL cells, clone 745, was investigated as a control. The binding to these cells was not expected as they are totally unresponsive to EP. However, almost as many EP receptors were found on these cells as the FVA cells. These cells expressed only the lower affinity EP receptors (Kd = 0.5 to 1nM) (Sawyer et al. 1987b). Because the MEL cells which have only low affinity receptors are totally unresponsive to EP and because of the predominance of high affinity receptors occupied on FVA cells at the concentration of EP which gives the maximum biological activity, we have proposed the interaction of EP with the high affinity receptors are necessary for the full biological effect of the hormone.

In cells having only the lower affinity receptors for EP, the binding of EP to these receptors can still signal the cell to proliferate. This is also the case for FVA cells, mouse CFU-E (Landschultz et al. 1989), and human CFU-E which quickly downregulate high affinity receptors but still require EP for development when only the lower affinity receptors are expressed. The effect of EP through the lower affinity receptors is also shown in the HCD 33 and HCD 57 cells which are totally dependent on EP for survival and proliferation yet only express lower affinity receptors (Sawyer and Hankins, unpublished). Similarly in DA1, IC2, and FDCP2 cells which only have the lower affinity receptor, EP can substitute for the requirement of other hematological factors.

The number of receptors for EP on the surface of erythroid precursor cells most likely parallels the responsiveness of the cells to EP. CFU-E or cells at the proerythroblast stage of development apparently have the greatest number of receptors (approximately 1,000 receptors/cell), and the number of receptors drops substantially as the cell matures to erythroblasts and mature erythroblasts while becoming less dependent on EP at each successive stage. In the FVA cell system, the total number of receptors drops to half when the cells become basophilic erythroblasts after culture for 24h. At this stage, these basophilic FVA erythroblasts are no longer dependent on EP for maturation (Koury and Bondurant, 1988). EP receptors are rapidly lost during the next 24h of culture as the basophilic FVA erythroblast mature to reticulocytes which have no receptors. This study was carried out by measuring total receptors and grain distribution by autoradiography. These results have also been found in regenerating mouse CFU-E and human CFU-E.

When FVA cells are exposed to physiological levels of EP in culture (30 mUnits/ml) only 10% of the cells mature and 90% disintegrate during the period from 24 to 48h. Autoradiography of ^{125}I-EP bound to FVA cells at these physiological levels revealed heterogeneity of positive cells. The number of cells binding EP correlated with the percentage of cells maturing in culture. The heterogeneity in receptors explains why only a limited number of cells respond to normal EP concentrations and all the cells respond at the upper range of physiological concentrations of EP. This heterogeneity is unexplained at the molecular or cell biology level.

Binding of ^{125}I-EP to FVA cells was observed to be two-fold greater at 37°C than 0°C. Since this was typical for ligands which are internalized into the cell, the possibility that ^{125}I-EP was internalized by receptor-mediated endocytosis was pursued.

Removal of surface bound EP by a high salt, pH 2.5 wash or by digestion with proteases demonstrated endocytosis of EP within one minute. ^{125}I-EP was bound to the surface at 0°C, and the distribution of radioactivity between the cell surface, cell interior, and medium showed that upon warming, surface bound ^{125}I-EP declined as radioactivity accumulated inside the cell and then the radioactivity inside the cell declined as radioactivity was secreted into the medium. Analysis of the medium revealed that the majority of radioactivity was [^{125}I]iodotyrosine. Inhibition of lysosomal function with NH_4Cl and chloroquine greatly reduced the degradation of internalized ^{125}I-EP which suggested the degradation of EP in lysosomes after endocytosis. All of the above studies were performed in this laboratory on FVA cell (Sawyer et al., 1987b) and were repeated in human CFU-E (Sawada et al., 1988).

The fate of the receptor for EP following the receptor-mediated endocytosis into the cell is not known. By analogy to the metabolism of other growth factors and hormones, the EP receptor will probably follow one or both of two pathways within the cell. In the first pathway, the receptor and hormone are both degraded in the lysosomes following endocytosis into the cell. In the second pathway, the receptor can recycle to the surface to bind another ligand after the initial endocytosis of the receptor-ligand complex. The acidic nature of endosomes typically results in dissociation of peptide hormones and growth factors from the receptors. Since bound EP is released from the receptor at or less than pH 4.0, it is possible that the fate of EP and the receptor diverge inside the cell.

Recent experiments show evidence of EP receptor degradation as the mechanism of downregulation of the receptor in HCD 33 and HCD 57 cells exposed to EP. When these cells are taken from cultures which contain EP, they have 400 to 600 receptors for EP per cell. However, the receptor number increases five to ten-fold when EP is removed from the culture. Upon subsequent reculture in the presence of ^{125}I-EP, the receptor number is downregulated to 10-20% by 24h in culture. The recovery of EP receptors after the downregulation requires protein synthesis.

Cross-linking of ^{125}I-EP to membranes from FVA cells in this laboratory first identified two proteins of 100 kDa and 85 kDa as the receptor for EP (Sawyer et al. 1987c). Subsequent work confirmed this in normal human erythroid cells (Sawyer et al. 1989), normal murine cells (Landschultz et al. 1989) and a variety of mouse and human cell lines (Broudy et al. 1988, Hitomi et al. 1988). Digestion of the 100 and 85 kDa proteins with v8 protease resulted in very similar fragments indicating similar if not identical sequence of amino acids (Sawyer, 1989). Recently, D'Andrea et al. (1989) isolated a cDNA clone of a putative receptor for EP which encodes a 55 kDa protein by expression cloning into COS cells. Cross-linking of ^{125}I-EP to transfected COS cells revealed the presence of a 100 kDa and a 60 kDa binding proteins. D'Andrea proposed that either extensive glycosylation of the 55 kDa protein or cross-linking of two 55 kDa subunits resulted in the 100 kDa form of the EP receptor.

We investigated the possibility that the 100 kDa and 85 kDa proteins of the EP receptor identified by cross-linking differed in the extent of glycosylation of a common protein. Digestion of the solubilized cross-linked ^{125}I-EP, EP receptor complex with enzymes which hydrolyze both N-linked carbohydrate and O-linked carbohydrate showed no apparent carbohydrate on the receptor for EP. In addition, reductive alkaline hydrolysis was carried out the crosslinked receptor complex and demonstrated no O-linked carbohydrate on the EP receptor. Therefore, the difference in the 100 kDa and 85 kDa proteins cannot be carbohydrate on a protein of 55 kDa (Hosoi et al. 1988).

There is no evidence of disulfide bridging of subunits resulting in the 100 kDa and 85 kDa proteins of the EP receptor. Boiling in the cross-linked receptor in the presence of SDS and DTT or ß-mercaptoethanol and subsequent modification of free sulfhydryl groups with N-ethylmalaimide resulted in only the 100 kDa and 85 kDa proteins. These conditions are sufficient to cleave the "resistant" disulfide bridges in the insulin receptor.

EP receptors have only been analyzed structurally when cross linked to radioactive EP as purification of the receptor has not been successful to this point. Recent efforts in this laboratory have led to the ligand free labeling of EP receptors using the Denny-Jaffe reagent. The photoactivatable, cleavable, iodinated cross-linker 4[4azido-3 [^{125}I] iodophenylazo) benzoyl]-3-aminoprophlyl-N-oxy-succinimide ester was successfully conjugated to EP. The resulting conjugated, ^{125}I-Denny-Jaffe EP (^{125}I-DJ-EP), was used to label the receptor. Two bands of 140 kDa and 125 kDa labeled with this monofunctional cross-linker are identical to the bands labeled with ^{125}I-EP and homobifunctional cross-linkers. Cleavage of the cross-linked ^{125}I-DJ-EP receptor complex with dithionite resulted in the 100 kDa and 85 kDa receptor protein labeled with ^{125}I free of cross-linked EP (Hosoi et al. 1989). This experiment proved that the 100 kDa protein of the EP receptor can not be the result of simultaneously cross-linking of two 55 kDa proteins and ^{125}I-EP by bifunctional cross-linkers. These results raise the central question of the relationship of the 55 kDa protein identified by expression cloning to the 100 kDa and 85 kDa identified by cross-linking.

There appear to be three major possibilities to explain the relationship of the 55 kDa protein to the larger molecular weight forms: (1) the post-translational modification of the 55 kDa protein resulting in a 100 kDa form, (2) the 55 kDa protein is a regulatory protein which interacts with the EP binding protein which is not the 55 kDa protein, and (3) the 55 kDa protein is the binding protein for EP but has an unusual migration on SDS-PAGE. Post-translational modification other than glycosylation and disulfide bridges would be expected. Modifications might include a covalent coupling between 55 kDa subunits, or the 55 kDa protein and another protein, or addition of lipid, ubiquitin, glycosaminoglycan to the 55 kDa protein.

Covalent coupling of proteins on the cell surface except through disulfide bridges has not been described to my knowledge, although it is common in the extracellular matrix. The second possibility is that the 55 kDa protein identified as the EP receptor by expression cloning is not related to the proteins identified by cross-linking but is a regulatory protein. If the 55 kDa protein is a regulatory protein which activates the binding protein(s), these binding proteins must exist in the untransfected COS cells. An alternative hypothesis addressed by D'Andrea et al. is that the cloned cDNA encodes a protein which induces the transcription and translation of the genomic sequence for the receptor present in COS cells. This seems unlikely since the 55 kDa protein appears to be a transmembrane protein. The third possibility is that the cloned DNA encodes a 55 kDa protein which is the same binding protein identified by cross-linking; however, the protein migrates on SDS-PAGE in an anomolus fashion at 100 kDa.

REFERENCES

Broudy, V.C., Lin, N., Egrie, J., DeHaen, C., Weiss, T., Papayannopoulo, T., and Adamson, J.W., 1988, Identification of the receptor for erythropoietin on human and murine erythroleukemia cells and modulation by phorbol ester and dimethyl sulfoxide, Proc. Natl. Acad. Sci. U.S.A. 85:6513-6517.

D'Andrea, A.D., Lodish, H.F., and Wong, G., 1989, Expression cloning of the murine erythropoietin receptor. Cell. 57:277-285.

Hitomi, K., Fujita, K., Sasaki, R., Chiba, H., Okuno, Y., Ichiba, S., Takanashi, T., and Imura, H., 1988, Erythropoietin receptor of a human leukemic cell line with erythroid characteristics, Biochem. Biophys. Res. Commun. 154:902-909.

Hosoi, T., Sawyer, S.T., and Krantz, S.B., 1988, The receptor for erythropoeitin lacks detectable glycosylation, Exp. Hematol. 16:118.

Hosoi, T., Sawyer, S.T., and Krantz, S.B., 1989, Identification of erythropoietin receptor in a ligand-free form with ^{125}I-labeled, photoreactive, cleavable cross-linker (Denny-Jaffe

Reagent), Exp. Hematol. 17:224.

Koury, M.J., and Bondurant, M.C., 1988, Maintenance by erythropoietin on viability and maturation of murine erythroid precursor cells, J. Cell. Phys. 137:65-74.

Koury, M.J., Sawyer, S.T., and Bondurant, M.C., 1984, Splenic erythroblasts in anemia-inducing Friend disease: A source of cells for studies of erythropoietin-mediated differentiation, J. Cell. Physiol. 121:526-532.

Krantz, S.B., and Goldwasser, E., 1984, Specific binding of erythropoietin to spleen cells infected with the anemia strain of Friend virus, Proc. Natl. Acad. Sci. U.S.A. 81:7574-7578.

Landschultz, K.T., Noyes, A.N., Rogers, O., and Boyer, S.H. 1989, Natural history of erythropoietin binding during erythropoiesis, Blood 73:1476-1486.

Sawada, K., Krantz, S.B., Sawyer, S.T., and Civin, C.I., 1988, Quantitation of specific binding of erythropoeitin to human erythroid colony-forming cells, J. Cell. Physiol. 137:337-345.

Sawyer, S.T., 1989, The two proteins of the erythropoietin receptor are structurally similar, J. Biol. Chem. 264:13343-13347.

Sawyer, S.T., Koury, M.J., and Bondurant, M.C., 1987a, Large-scale procurement of erythropoietin-responsive erythroid cells: Assay for biological activity of erythropoietin, Methods Enzymol. 147:340-352.

Sawyer, S.T., Krantz, S.B., and Goldwasser, E., 1987b, Binding and receptor-mediated endocytosis of erythropoietin in Friend virus infected erythroid cells, J. Biol. Chem, 262:5554-5562.

Sawyer, S.T., Krantz, S.B., and Luna, J., 1987c, Identification of the receptor for erythropoietin by cross-linking to Friend virus-infected erythroid cells, Proc. Natl. Acad. Sci. U.S.A. 84:3690-3694.

Sawyer, S.T., Krantz, S.B., and Sawada, K.-I., 1989, Receptors for erythropoietin in mouse and huuman erythroid cells and placenta, Blood 74:103-109.

The Biology of Hematopoiesis, pages 153–159

STRUCTURE OF THE ERYTHROPOIETIN RECEPTOR IN STABLE FIBROBLAST TRANSFECTANTS

Alan D. D'Andrea, Gerald D. Fasman, Leonard I. Zon, Jing-Po Li, and Harvey F. Lodish

Whitehead Institute for Biomedical Research, Department of Biology, Massachusetts Institute of Technology, Cambridge, MA 02142 and The Children's Hospital, Dana-Farber Cancer Institute, Department of Pediatrics, Harvard Medical School, Boston, MA 02115.

INTRODUCTION

Erythropoietin (EPO) is a glycoprotein hormone which is the primary regulator of mammalian erythropoiesis. EPO is synthesized and released by the kidney in amounts inversely proportional to arterial oxygen content, and it circulates to the bone marrow where it stimulates resident erythroid progenitor cells via a specific receptor (EPO-R) (Erslev, 1987). To date, studies of the structure of the EPO-R have yielded conflicting results. Some investigators have demonstrated that the receptor is comprised of two noncovalent linked subunits, 100 kD and 85 kD (Sawyer et al., 1987; 1989). Others have reported that the EPO-R consists of multiple bands of lower molecular masses (Mayeux et al., 1987; Todokoro et al., 1988). Still others report that the EPO-R is a large complex of disulfide-linked subunits (McCaffery et al., 1989). Difficulty in studying the EPO-R is due, at least in part, to the small number of EPO-R per erythroblast (generally less than 1000). Also, the EPO-R has been studied only in the presence of the radiolabeled ligand, by crosslinking analyses.

The recent cloning of the mouse EPO-R cDNA (D'Andrea et al., 1989) has allowed a more detailed analysis of the EPO-R structure. Using the EPO-R cDNA we have generated stable NIH-3T3 fibroblast transfectants expressing approximately two times 10^5 receptors per cell surface. Also, we have generated polyclonal anti-peptide antibodies against predicted amino acid sequences of the EPO-R. These antisera have allowed analysis of the structure and carbohydrate processing of the EPO-R in the presence or absence of erythropoietin. These reagents will be indispensable in future analyses of the EPO-R structure and function.

RESULTS

We have generated a stable NIH-3T3 fibroblast line which expresses cell surface EPO-receptor (3T3-EPO-R). Using ^{125}I-EPO binding studies, these cells were shown to express approximately 2 x 10^5 receptors per cell surface (Figure 1). Binding studies were done at 23°C in the presence of 0.02% azide to prevent internalization, by methods modified from those published elsewhere (D'Andrea et al., 1989).

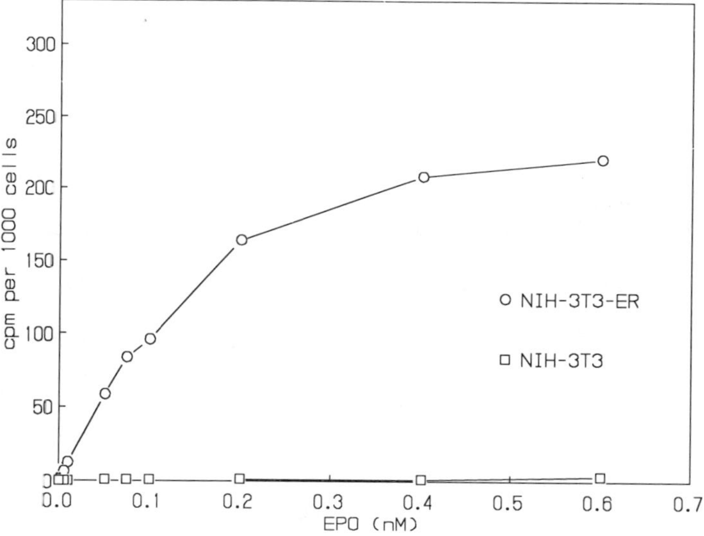

Figure 1. Binding of ^{125}I-EPO to transfected NIH-3T3 cells. The surface binding of labeled EPO was performed as described (D'Andrea et al., 1989). Each point represents the average of binding from duplicate 10 cm plates of confluent NIH-3T3 cells that synthesize EPO-R. By Scatchard plot (not shown), there are 2.1 x 10^5 EPO-R per

(Continued)

cell surface and a single affinity (K_D = 272 pM) was measured. Background binding of ^{125}I-EPO to untransfected NIH-3T3 cells was negligible (<5% of total binding to NIH-3T3-ER).

In order to generate polyclonal anti-peptide antibodies against the EPO-R, 15 amino acid synthetic peptides were prepared from the amino terminus (APSPSLPDPKFESKD) or carboxy-terminus (SLVPDSEPLHPGYVAC) of the predicted polypeptide sequence (D'Andrea et al., 1989). Peptides were coupled to KLH, and rabbits were immunized by standard techniques (Green et al., 1982). In order to screen for the presence of specific anti-peptide antibodies, we developed techniques for immunoprecipitation of the _in vitro_ translated EPO-R polypeptide. The EPO-R cDNA was transcribed with SP-6 polymerase _in vitro_ and subsequently translated with reticulocyte lysate in the presence of dog pancreatic microsomes (Mueckler and Lodish, 1986). The cell-free translated protein was a 66 kd polypeptide (Figure 2, ER). Bands depicting proteins of smaller molecular weight arise either from internal ATG translation initiation or from protease digestion of the full length 66 kD polypeptide.

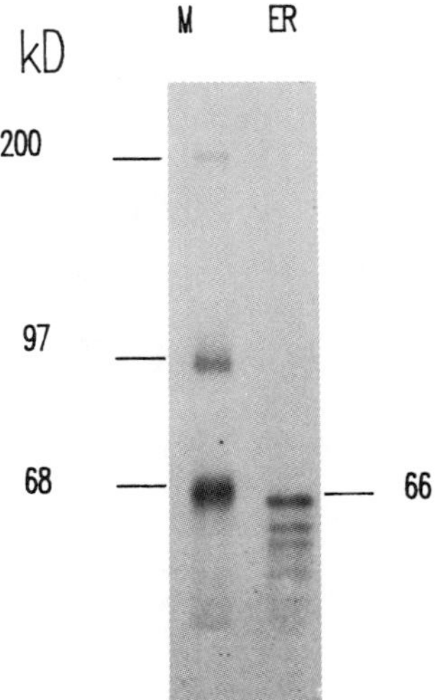

Figure 2. _In vitro_ translation of the mouse erythropoietin receptor polypeptide. Lane M contains ^{14}C marker proteins and lane ER shows the full length (66 kD) EPO-Receptor polypeptide.

Specific antisera which immunoprecipitated the in vitro translated EPO-R are demonstrated in Figure 3. An immune antiserum (I) from a rabbit immunized with the amino terminal peptide of the EPO-R immunoprecipitates the 66 kD EPO-R (lane 1), while the preimmune antiserum (P) is minimally active (lane 2). An immune antiserum from a rabbit injected with the carboxy-terminal peptide of the EPO-R also is immunoreactive with the in vitro translated protein (Figure 3, lane 3) compared to the preimmune serum (lane 4).

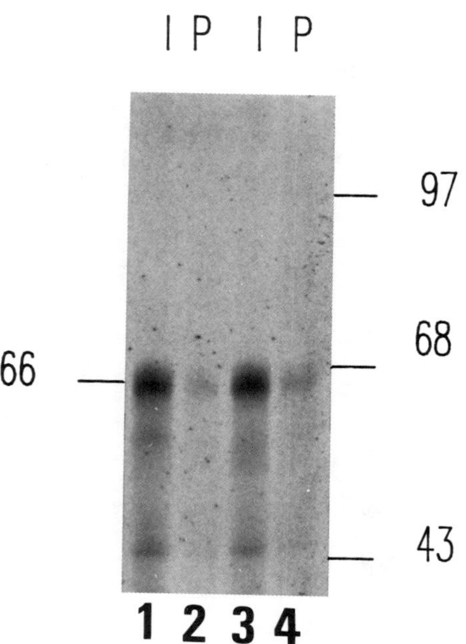

Figure 3. Immunoprecipitation of the in vitro translated EPO-Receptor polypeptide using anti-amino terminal or anti-carboxy terminal peptide antibodies.

In order to determine the size of the EPO-R polypeptide in the stable NIH-3T3 fibroblast transfectants described above in Figure 1, a Western analysis was performed using the anti-amino terminal peptide antibody

(Figure 4). Total membranes were prepared from either 3T3-ER cells (lane 1) or the non-transfected NIH-3T3 parent cells (lane 2) as described (Bischoff and Lodish, 1987). Membrane proteins were electrophoresed on a 10% polyacrylamide gel, blotted to nitrocellulose, and probed with the anti-EPO receptor antibody. Interestingly, an EPO-receptor doublet is observed at 66 kD in lane 1. These two bands are also observed on Western blots using the anti-carboxy terminal antibody (data not shown) and they presumably represent the partially processed and fully carbohydrate processed form of the EPO-Receptor polypeptide.

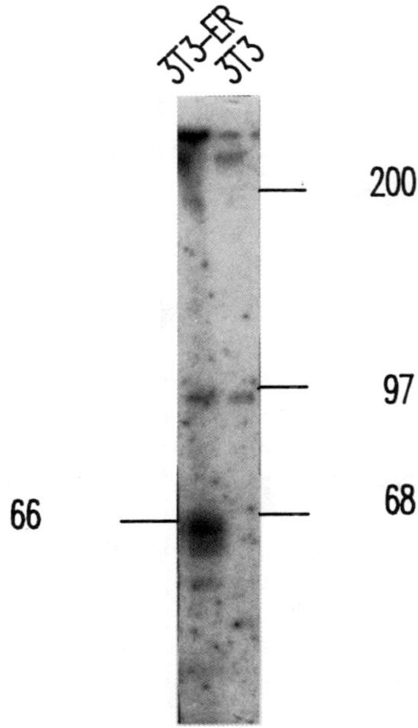

Figure 4. Western blot analysis of EPO-Receptor polypeptide expressed in stable 3T3 fibroblast transfectants. Total membranes were prepared from either NIH-3T3 cells or NIH-3T3-ER transfectants. Membranes were boiled in SDS in the presence of dithiothriotol, electrophoresed, blotted to nitrocellulose, and probed with the anti-EPO-R antisera by methods described previously (Patel and Lodish, 1987).

CONCLUSIONS

The development of a stable NIH-3T3 fibroblast transfectant expressing surface EPO-receptors should greatly facilitate the analysis of the EPO-Receptor structure. Polyclonal antisera against the amino and carboxy-terminal peptides of the EPO-R are immunoreactive with the EPO-Receptor expressed in these transfectants and will be helpful in confirming the membrane orientation of the EPO-Receptor, a putative type I membrane spanning protein by our former predictions (D'Andrea et al., 1989).

REFERENCES

Bischoff J, Lodish HF (1987). Two asialoglycoprotein receptor polypeptides in human hepatoma cells. J. Biol. Chem. 262:11825-11832.

D'Andrea A, Lodish H, Wong G (1989). Expression cloning of the murine erythropoietin receptor. Cell 57: 277-285.

Erslev A (1987). Erythropoietin coming of age. New Eng. J. Med. 316: 101-103.

Green N, Alexander H, Olson A, Alexander S, Shinnick TM, Sutcliffe, JG, Lerner RA (1982). Cell 28:477-487.

Mayeux P, Billat C, Jacquot R (1987). The erythropoietin receptor of rat erythroid progenitor cells. J. Biol. Chem. 262: 13985-13990.

McCaffery PJ, Fraser JK, Lin F, Berridge MV (1989). Subunit structure of the erythropoietin receptor. J. Biol. Chem. 264: 10507-10512.

Mueckler M, Lodish HF (1986). The human glucose transporter can insert posttranslationally into microsomes. Cell 44:629-637.

Patel VP, Lodish HF (1987). A fibronectin matrix is required for differentiation of murine erythroleukemia cells into reticulocytes. J. Cell Biol. 105: 3105-3118.

Sawyer ST, Krantz SB, Luna J (1987). Identification of the receptor for erythropoietin by crosslinking to Friend virus infected erythroid cells. Proc. Natl Acad. Sci. USA 84: 3690-3694.

Sawyer ST (1989) The two proteins of the erythropoietin receptor are structurally similar. J. Biol. Chem. 13343-13347.

Todokoro K, Kanazawa S, Amanuma H, Ikawa Y (1988). Specific binding of erythropoietin to its receptor on responsive mouse erythroleukemia cells. Proc. Natl. Acad. Sci. USA 84:4126-4130.

The Biology of Hematopoiesis, pages 161–167

DIMETHYL SULFOXIDE AMPLIFICATION OF THE ERYTHROPOIETIN RESPONSE: CLUES TO THE SIGNAL TRANSDUCTION PATHWAY

Yijuang E. Chern, Shuji Yonekura and Arthur J. Sytkowski

Laboratory for Cell and Molecular Biology,
New England Deaconess Hospital, Boston, MA 02215

INTRODUCTION

Studies of the effects of dimethyl sulfoxide on erythroleukemia cell differentiation have provided insights into the control of red blood cell development. However, relatively little information exists regarding the mode of action of the natural inducer of erythropoiesis, erythropoietin. We demonstrated previously that the biologic responses of Rauscher murine erythroleukemia cells, a transformed erythroid cell line, to erythropoietin and dimethyl sulfoxide could be segregated, suggesting dissimilar modes of action of the two inducers (Sytkowski, *et al.*, 1980). We have now examined the simultaneous effect of erythropoietin and dimethyl sulfoxide on the differentiation of clonal Rauscher lines. We have found that DMSO strongly amplifies the Epo response of these cells, indicating that the signaling pathways of these two inducers interact.

RESULTS

We used a subclone of Rauscher murine erythroleukemia, designated R28, which exhibits a relatively low response to either dimethyl sulfoxide or erythropoietin. In contrast to the use of either inducer alone, exposure of the cells to both inducers simultaneously resulted in a striking synergistic effect. After only two days, 70% of the cells were hemoglobin positive compared to less than 10% in response to either inducer alone (Figure 1).

The simultaneous presence of both inducers is not necessary for this effect. Indeed, pre-treatment of the cells with dimethyl sulfoxide followed by its removal and the addition of erythropoietin demonstrated marked amplification of the erythropoietin effect (Figure 2). We have designated pre-treatment of cells with DMSO followed by its removal prior to the addition of erythropoietin "DMSO priming".

DMSO priming is time dependent and concentration dependent. As shown in Figure 3A a slight amplification of the Epo response was seen after only 6 hours of priming, and a clear effect was observed after 12 hours with maximal amplification seen after 24-48 hours. The dose response for DMSO priming was virtually linear up to 1.5% of dimethyl sulfoxide.

There is a three-fold effect of DMSO priming on erythropoietin's biological response. Firstly, DMSO priming increases the number of Epo responsive cells (Figure 4A). Pre-treatment of R28 cells with 1% dimethyl sulfoxide for 48 hours followed by its removal and addition of erythropoietin for 48 hours resulted in 58% hemoglobin positive cells. This contrasted with only 8% hemoglobin positive cells in the absence of DMSO priming. Secondly, DMSO priming increases the rate of erythropoietin response. As seen in Figure 4B nonprimed cells exhibited a maximal erythropoietin response after 4 days of exposure to the hormone. However, DMSO primed cells required only 2 days to reach their maximum erythropoietin response. Thirdly, DMSO priming markedly increases erythropoietin sensitivity. As presented in Figure 5, there was a marked left shift of the erythropoietin dose response curve when cells were primed with dimethyl sulfoxide. The Epo activation constant (K_{act}), which was the concentration of hormone that causes 50% of the maximal response, is 0.1 U/ml and 2.0 U/ml for DMSO primed and unprimed cells respectively, representing a 20-fold increase in erythropoietin sensitivity.

These multiple effects of DMSO priming on the Epo biologic response are all consistent with an amplification of the Epo signal transduction pathway by the chemical inducer. One effect of DMSO on Epo signal transduction pathway is shown in Figure 6. In this study, the erythropoietin receptor density on Rauscher cells was measured by ^{125}I-erythropoietin binding. Unprimed cells contain approximately 3,000 erythropoietin receptors per cell. However, after 24 hours of DMSO priming the erythropoietin receptor density is markedly up-regulated. Saturation curves have demonstrated a density greater than 15,000 per cell. These results suggest that receptor up-regulation is at least part of a mechanism by which DMSO priming amplifies the erythropoietin signal pathway.

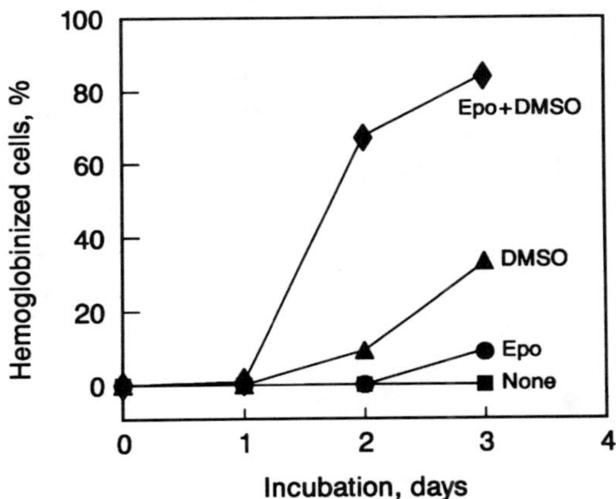

Figure 1. Synergistic effect of erythropoietin and DMSO on differentiation of Rauscher erythroleukemia cells. Cells were treated with 10 U/ml Epo (●), 1% DMSO (▲), Epo plus DMSO (♦) or no addition (■). The percentage of Hb^+ cells was assessed every day under each condition.

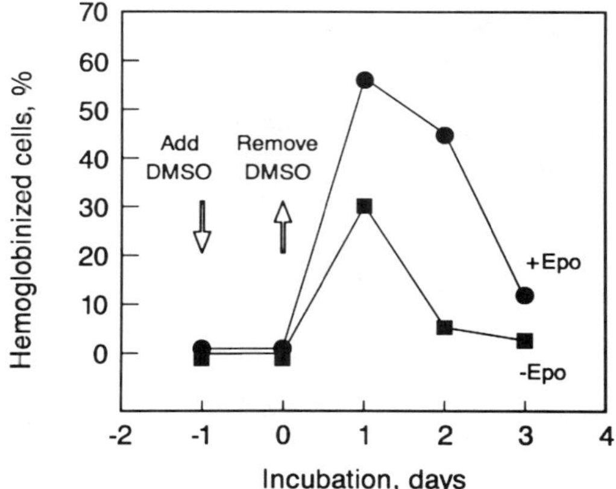

Figure 2. DMSO "priming" amplifies erythropoietin induction of Rauscher cells. Cells were pre-treated with 1% DMSO for 24 hours, washed twice with 3% FBS/DMEM and resuspended in fresh medium in the presence (●) or absence (■) of 10 U Epo/ml at day 0. The percentage of Hb^{+} cells was assessed every day under each condition. Note the Epo-specific response after only 1 day of exposure to the hormone.

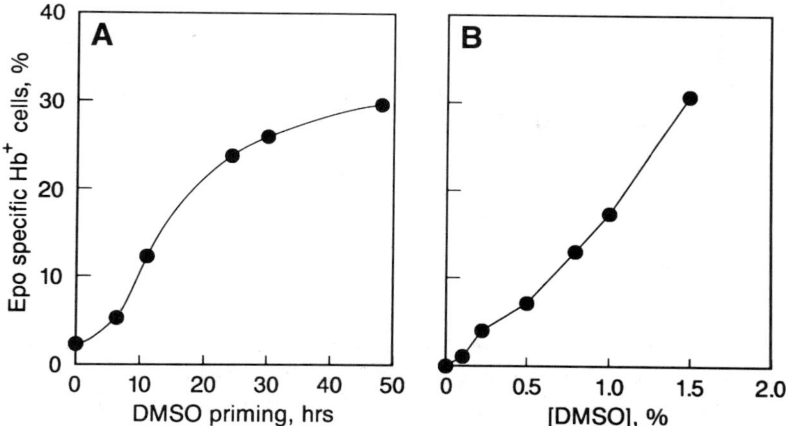

Figure 3. DMSO priming of the Epo-response is time-dependent (A) and concentration dependent (B). Panel A: Cells were grown in 1% DMSO for the times indicated. Cells were washed twice with 3% FBS/DMEM to remove DMSO and replaced with in fresh medium containing Epo (10 U/ml). Panel B: Cells were pre-treated with DMSO at the indicated concentrations for 24 hours, washed twice with 3% FBS/DMEM to remove DMSO and replated in fresh medium with Epo (10 U/ml). The percentage of Hb^{+} cells was measured after 24 hours of treatment with Epo.

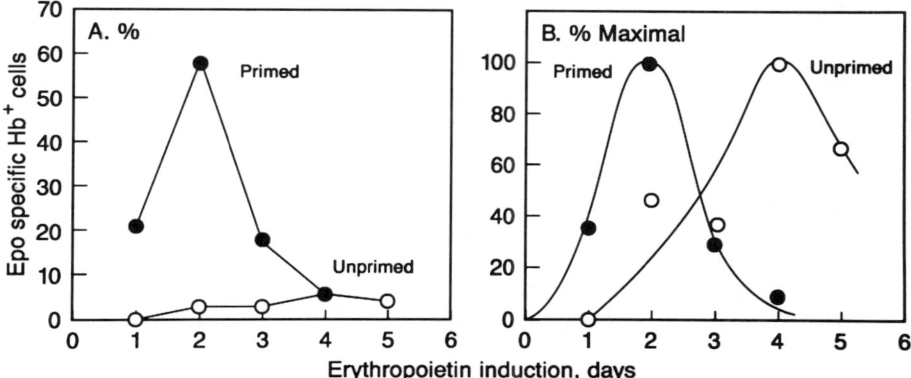

Figure 4. DMSO priming increases number of Epo-responsive cells (A) and rate of Epo response (B). Panel A: Cells were grown in the absence (○) or presence (●) of 1% DMSO for 48 hours, washed twice with 3% FBS/DMEM and exposed to Epo (40 U/ml) beginning on day 0. Net Epo specific Hb^+ response was obtained by subtracting the basal Hb^+ cell number at the times indicated. Panel B: The same set of data in (A) was normalized to percent of maximal Hb^+ response.

DISCUSSION

A modification of the erythropoietin response by DMSO has been reported in another murine erythroleukemia cell line (Mishina and Obinatu, 1985). Addition of DMSO to TSA8 cells allows the cells to form erythropoietin dependent colonies, suggesting that these cells are converted into a more CFU-E-like stage of differentiation. In this regard the amplified biologic responses exhibited by DMSO primed Rauscher cells, especially the 2 day maximal response rate and the dose response curve, are also remarkedly similar to the normal murine CFU-E. However, up-regulation of the Epo receptor was not found in TSA8 cells in contrast to the marked increase in receptor density reported here.

Three other hematopoietic growth factors, IL-3, GM-CSF and BPA have been reported to effect the erythropoietin response (Clark and Kamen, 1987; Feldman, et al., 1987). In this regard DMSO may be thought to mimic the functions of these other growth factors in triggering the maturation of red blood cells. Thus, it will be important to analyze DMSO's action further with regard to the modes of action of these natural inducers. Such comparisons may be fruitful in efforts toward the design of therapeutic agents that may be used in conjunction with recombinant growth factors. Moreover, DMSO and other chemical agents may be considered as convenient probes of Epo's signal transduction pathway.

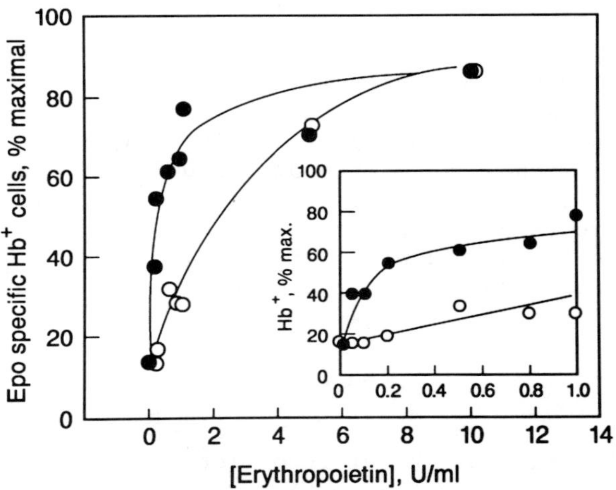

Figure 5. DMSO priming markedly increases Epo-sensitivity of Rauscher cells. Cells were grown in the absence (○) or presence (●) 1% DMSO for 48 hours, washed twice with 3% FBS/DMEM and replated in the presence of specific concentration of Epo for 24 hours. Net Epo response was obtained by subtracting the basal Hb^+ cell number (no addition of Epo) from the total Hb^+ cell number at various Epo concentrations. Data were normalized using the percent of maximal Epo-specific response (obtained at 10 U/ml). The percentage of Hb^+ cells induced by Epo at 10 U/ml was 10% and 41% for unprimed cells and primed cells respectively. Inset: Horizontal scale enlarged to facilitate comparison at low Epo concentrations.

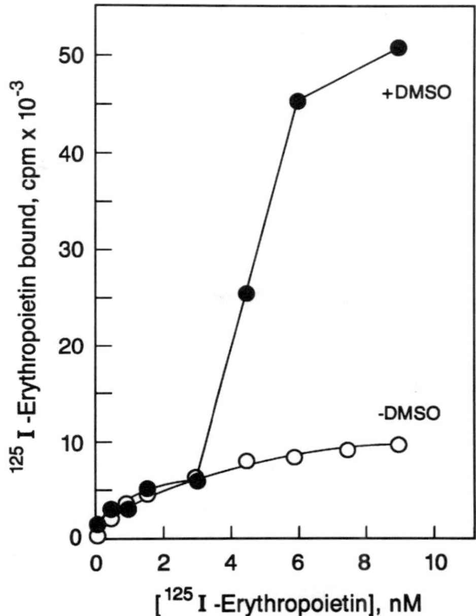

Figure 6. DMSO treatment increases the number of Epo receptor in Rauscher cells. Cells were grown in the absence (○) or presence (●) of 1% DMSO for 24 hours.

REFERENCES

Sytkowski AJ, McIntyre CJ, Perrine SP, Salvado AJ (1980). The biochemistry of erythropoietin: An approach to its mode of action. Exp. Hematol. 8:52-64.

Mishina Y, Obinata M (1985). Induction of commitment of murine erythroleukemia cells (TSA8) to CFU-E with DMSO. Exp. Cell Res. 162:319.

Clark SC, Kamen R (1987). The human hematopoietic colony-stimulating factors. Science 238:1229.

Feldman L, Cohen CM, Riordan MA, Dainiak N (1987). Purification of a membrane-derived human erythroid growth factor. Proc. Natl. Acad. Sci. USA 84:6775-6779.

The Biology of Hematopoiesis, pages 169–178

THE MECHANISM OF ACTION OF MURINE INTERLEUKIN-3: CURRENT STATUS

Alice L-F Mui, Sudish C. Murthy, Poul H.B. Sorensen, Gerald Krystal

Department of Pathology, University of British Columbia, and the Terry Fox Laboratory, Vancouver, Canada

INTRODUCTION

Murine interleukin-3 (mIL-3) is a potent hemopoietic growth factor that is produced by activated T lymphocytes and stimulates the proliferation and differentiation of pluripotent stem cells and committed myeloid and early lymphoid progenitors (Schrader, 1986). Although its role in maintaining steady-state hemopoiesis is still uncertain, it is thought to be a key immune system regulator of hemopoiesis. Studies into the mechanism of action of mIL-3 in our laboratory as well as others have used, almost exclusively, immortalized mIL-3 dependent cell lines. This has been necessitated by difficulties in acquiring adequate numbers of homogeneous, mIL-3 responsive, normal progenitor cells for biochemical analysis. Thus, although much data has been generated using these non-differentiating cell lines, the results obtained, and presented here, may not accurately reflect the message transduction pathways utilized by normal hemopoietic target cells. With this caveat in mind we will attempt to summarize the information gathered to date on the mechanism of action of mIL-3.

PROPERTIES OF MURINE INTERLEUKIN-3

Murine IL-3 is produced physiologically by antigen-activated T lymphocytes and perhaps, as well, by astrocytes and glioma cells in the brain (Farrar et al., 1989; Frei et al., 1986) and by mast cells in response to IgE receptor-mediated activation (Wodnar-Filipowicz et al., 1989). It has been purified to homogeneity from WEHI-3 cell conditioned medium (Ihle et al., 1982; Clark-Lewis et al., 1984) and from pokeweed mitogen stimulated mouse spleen cell conditioned medium (Cutler et al., 1985; Murthy et al., 1989). Complementary DNA and genomic DNA clones that encode the protein have been isolated (Fung et al., 1984; Yokota et al., 1984; Miyatake et al., 1985) and the predicted full length protein contains 140 amino acid residues. However, a shorter form lacking the first 6 amino acids has also been purified (Ihle et al., 1983). The protein sequence indicates a M.wt. of 15,102 with 4 potential N-glycosylation sites, which results in purified mIL-3 preparations varying from 16 to 32 kd (Cutler et al., 1985; Murthy et al., 1989; Ziltener et al., 1988). There is also some recent evidence for a low level of 0-linked glycosylation (Murthy et al., 1989). The entire 140 amino acid species of mIL-3, as well as a number of mIL-3 analogs, have been chemically synthesized and assays of the various products have shown that, 1) glycosylation is not essential for biological activity, 2) a disulfide bridge between cysteines 17 and 80 is required for full biological activity, 3) the difference of 6 amino acids between the two isolated forms does not affect its activity and 4) an amino terminal fragment (1 to 79) is partially active (Clark-Lewis, 1986).

PROPERTIES OF THE MURINE INTERLEUKIN-3 RECEPTOR

Scatchard analyses using ^{125}I-mIL-3 and various mIL-3 dependent cell lines are consistent with a single affinity class of cell surface receptors with an apparent K_D of ~1 nM (Murthy et al., 1989). The fact that the biological response to mIL-3 occurs two orders of magnitude below this concentration (Murthy et al., 1989) suggests, in the absence of any evidence for additional affinity classes, that very few bound ligand molecules are required to elicit a biological response. However, even though there appears to be only one affinity class, crosslinking studies using ^{125}I-mIL-3 and disuccinimidyl suberate (DSS) reveal two radiolabeled species with apparent M.wts. of 140 kd (p140) and 70 kd (p70) (Murthy et al., 1989). The p70/p140 ratio is not altered by incubating cells with very low concentrations of mIL-3, confirming the presence of only one affinity class, although there is a slight increase in this ratio if cells are incubated for longer times at 4°C, before crosslinking (Murthy et al., 1989). Interestingly, if the concentration of crosslinker is increased, more p70 is observed, a finding not consistent with p140 being a dimer of p70. More importantly, as we (Murthy et al., 1989) and Isfort et al. (1988) have shown, if intact mIL-3 dependent cells are shifted up to 37°C after ^{125}I-mIL-3 binding and crosslinking at 4°C, a dramatic increase in the relative intensity of p70 is observed. This can be prevented by first boiling the sample for 1 min in SDS sample buffer (Murthy et al., 1989). These and other data suggest that p140 is the bonafide mIL-3 receptor and is cleaved to p70 by a closely associated protease that is activated by mIL-3 binding and chemical crosslinking. Furthermore, this putative protease is released from inhibitory restraints when plasma membranes are prepared (i.e., only p70 is typically seen when crosslinking studies are carried out with plasma membranes (Murthy et al., 1989)). In addition, characterization studies involving N-glycanase treatment of the two crosslinked species suggest that the mIL-3 receptor contains 2 N-linked carbohydrate moieties with M.wts. of 3 and 8 kd (Murthy et al., 1989).

In order to assess the role of the mIL-3 receptor in the mechanism of action of mIL-3 we have developed assays capable of detecting detergent solubilized mIL-3 binding activity (Mui et al., 1989) and used these to devise a simple 2 step purification procedure for the receptor (Mui et al., 1989). This protocol involves incubating intact B6SUtA$_1$ cells, which possess approximately 100,000 mIL-3 receptors under conditions of mIL-3 starvation (Murthy et al., 1989), with biotin labeled mIL-3. Following detergent solubilization of the cells, advantage is taken of the fact that the mIL-3 receptor is tyrosine phosphorylated after mIL-3 binding (see below) by incubating supernatants with bead bound antiphosphotyrosine antibodies. The phenyl phosphate eluates are then chromatographed through streptavidin agarose. Low pH elution of bound material yields an apparently homogeneous mIL-3 binding protein with a M.wts. of 140 kd (Mui et al., 1989). This protein has a similar mobility in the presence and absence of reducing agents on SDS-PAGE (as does DSS crosslinked receptor), suggesting that disulfide bridges, if present, do not significantly restrain this polypeptide from assuming a random coil conformation in the presence of SDS (Mui et al., 1989). Moreover, from N-glycanase studies it appears that the purified receptor possesses approximately 10 kd of N-linked sugar (Mui et al., 1989), confirming reports with DSS crosslinked material (Murthy et al., 1989).

CHANGES IN THE mIL-3 RECEPTOR AS A CONSEQUENCE OF mIL-3 BINDING

Within 2 minutes of adding mIL-3 to B6SUtA$_1$ cells, two membrane associated proteins, p140 and p68, become tyrosine phosphorylated (Sorensen et al., 1989). Experiments involving DSS crosslinking of ^{125}I-mIL-3 to these cells, SDS dissociation of potential mIL-3 receptor complexes and precipitation of individual tyrosine phosphorylated proteins with antiphosphotyrosine antibodies reveal that the tyrosine phosphorylated p140 corresponds to the intact mIL-3 receptor (Sorensen et al., 1989). However, the tyrosine phosphorylated p68 does not appear to be the same protein as the mIL-3 binding fragment, p70. One possibility is that it represents the other cleaved product of p140. Interestingly, the phosphorylated p140 can be shown by highly resolving SDS-PAGE to consist of two species and these might represent different degrees of phosphorylation or precursor product forms of an initial cleavage event.

Experiments using partially purified mIL-3 receptor preparations and the ATP analog, 5-p-fluorosulfonylbenzoyl [8-^{14}C] adenosine, which becomes covalently bound to ATP binding sites on protein kinases, suggest that the mIL-3 receptor may possess an endogenous tyrosine kinase activity (Mui et al., 1989). Studies are in progress using purified receptor preparations and liposomes to confirm these findings. Also of interest is our recent finding that there might be a cytosolic inhibitor of tyrosine specific mIL-3 receptor phosphorylation (Table 1). In these studies,

TABLE 1

Tyrosine phosphorylation of the mIL-3R in plasma membranes

Sample	mIL-3	cpm associated with beads
B6SUtA$_1$ pm	+	11 076
	-	10 292
B6SUtA$_1$ cytosol	+	5 982
	-	4 004
B6SUtA$_1$ pm + cytosol	+	9 148
	-	3 422

$B6SUtA_1$ plasma membranes in the presence and absence of their cytosols have been incubated with ^{32}P-γ-ATP. Antiphosphotyrosine antibody precipitation of detergent solubilized tyrosine phosphorylated proteins reveal that cytosols inhibit the tyrosine phosphorylation (or enhance dephosphorylation) of membranes and that this is reversed to a significant extent by mIL-3. Also of interest is our recent finding that the protease activity associated with the receptor in intact cells, membrane and crude membrane lysates (Murthy et al., 1989) is still present in apparently homogeneous preparations of mIL-3 receptor. Specifically, upon storage of the purified p140 at 4°C there is a slow conversion of this protein to a 70 kd species and this is markedly accelerated by the presence of DSS suggesting that crosslinking alters the conformation of the receptor to make it more susceptible to cleavage (Mui et al., 1989). The presence of protease activity in apparently pure receptor preparations suggests that either the preparation is contaminated with a leupeptin, aprotinin and PMSF resistant protease or, more intriguingly, that the receptor itself possesses an intrinsic protease activity. However, there is no evidence as yet that this does indeed occur under physiological conditions. Nonetheless, there is growing evidence that proteases may play a role in message transduction. For example, Downing et al (1989) recently showed that protein kinase C (PKC) down modulates CSF-1 receptors by activating a protease that cleaves the 150 kd receptor. Proteases have also been implicated in the mechanism of action of the epidermal growth factor receptor (Seger et al., 1988) the insulin receptor (Shoelson et al., 1988) and the IL-2 receptor (Loughnan et al., 1988).

EARLY EVENTS FOLLOWING mIL-3 BINDING TO ITS CELL SURFACE RECEPTOR

Murine IL-3 binds rapidly to its receptor on mIL-3 dependent cells at 37°C, reaching saturation binding within 30 min (Murthy et al., 1989). Internalization of surface bound complexes is >90% complete by 60 min at 37°C and, starting 2 hrs later, mIL-3 is degraded within lysosomes in a sequential fashion, first releasing a 1 kd and then a 3 kd fragment before being totally digested to TCA soluble material (Murthy et al., 1989). An examination of mIL-3 receptor re-expression following down regulation by saturating levels of mIL-3, indicates that in the presence of cycloheximide, these receptors are capable of recycling back to the cell surface. Alternatively, these results are consistent with there being a large intracellular pool of mIL-3 receptors that is not exhausted during the 6 hr exposure to cycloheximide used in this study (Murthy et al., 1989). If the receptors are indeed recycled it suggests that cleavage of p140 to p70 does not occur to any significant extent, although, even as an infrequent event, it may still constitute an important step in mitogenesis.

In investigating early events, many investigators have focussed in on protein phosphorylation changes that occur following addition of mIL-3 to cells (Sorensen et al., 1989; Isfort et al., 1988; Morla et al., 1988; Koyasu et al., 1987; Evans et al., 1987). This was initially prompted, in part, by studies showing that oncogenes encoding tyrosine kinases could abrogate mIL-3 dependence (Pierce et al., 1985) and that mIL-3 dependent cell lines could proliferate to a limited extent in the presence of sodium orthovanadate or TPA (Sorensen et al., 1989). In B6SUtA$_1$ cells, aside from the tyrosine specific phosphorylations of membrane bound p140 and p68 described above, a number of cytosolic proteins have been shown to become tyrosine phosphorylated, i.e., p40, p55 and p90 (Sorensen et al., 1989). Similar results have been reported with other mIL-3 dependent cell lines, although the M.wts. of the phosphorylated proteins may vary somewhat with the cell line used (Morla et al., 1988).

Another early event that has been reported is the translocation and activation of PKC (Farrar et al., 1985), although this does not appear to be achieved by increased hydrolysis of inositol phospholipids or by increases in intracellular calcium levels (Whetton et al., 1988). To complicate matters further, there is some controversy concerning the role of PKC in the mechanism of action of mIL-3 since the phorbol ester TPA, which can substitute for diacylglycerol in binding and activating PKC, is synergistic with mIL-3 in stimulating the proliferation of some mIL-3 dependent cell lines but markedly inhibits mIL-3 induced proliferation in others. Nonetheless, early mIL-3 induced events that appear to be mediated by PKC activation, at least in some mIL-3 dependent cell lines, include activation of the Na^+/H^+ antiport, resulting in intracellular alkalinization (Whetton et al., 1988) and activation of the glucose transporter, leading to increased intracellular ATP (Whetton et al., 1986). Murine IL-3 may also cause a very rapid change in plasma membrane organization but studies with TPA suggest that this is probably not mediated by PKC (Laskay et al., 1988). This does not rule out that ser/thr specific protein phosphorylations may play a role in this event, however, since two other ser/thr specific kinases have recently been shown to be activated by mIL-3, i.e., protein kinase P (Klemm and Elias, 1987) and c-raf-1 (Carroll et al., 1989).

LATE EVENTS

Murine IL-3, like other hemopoietic growth factors, is not only a proliferation inducer but a survival factor as well. Elegant work from Dexter's laboratory suggests that it may carry out this latter function, at least in part, by maintaining high intracellular ATP levels through activation of the glucose transporter (Whetton et al., 1986).

A comparison of rapid tyrosine phosphorylation events induced by mIL-3 and mGM-CSF in B6SUtA$_1$ cells (which proliferate equally well with either of these two growth factors) suggest that only one cytosolic protein, p90, is phosphorylated in response to both (Sorensen et al., 1989). Thus, phosphorylated p90 may be a common later-acting intermediate involved in transmitting the mitogenic signal in these cells. Similarly, pp68, a cytosolic protein rapidly phosphorylated on serine residues when mIL-2, mIL-3 or mGM-CSF responsive cells are administered their appropriate growth factor (Evans et al., 1987) may play an important role in carrying the signal transduction message to the nucleus. There is also recent evidence that activated PKC migrates into the nucleus of mIL-3 dependent cells in response to mIL-3 and ser/thr phosphorylates nuclear proteins (Adunyah and Elias, 1988).

Lastly, mIL-3 has been shown to alter the expression of specific genes. For example, increases in the levels of the mIL-2 receptor (p55) (Birchenall-Sparks et al., 1986; Ihle et al., 1988) and the γ T cell receptor (Ihle et al., 1988) have been demonstrated. More importantly, both c-myc and c-fos (Rapp et al., 1985) mRNA have been reported to be elevated in response to mIL-3. This is especially interesting in view of data showing that mIL-3 dependance is abrogated by v-myc (Rapp et al., 1985) and that abrogation of mIL-3 dependence by oncogenes encoding protein tyrosine kinases, such as abl, src, fms and trk, result in the constitutive expression of c-myc (Ihle et al., 1988). A summary of the early and late events mentioned above are depicted in Fig. 1.

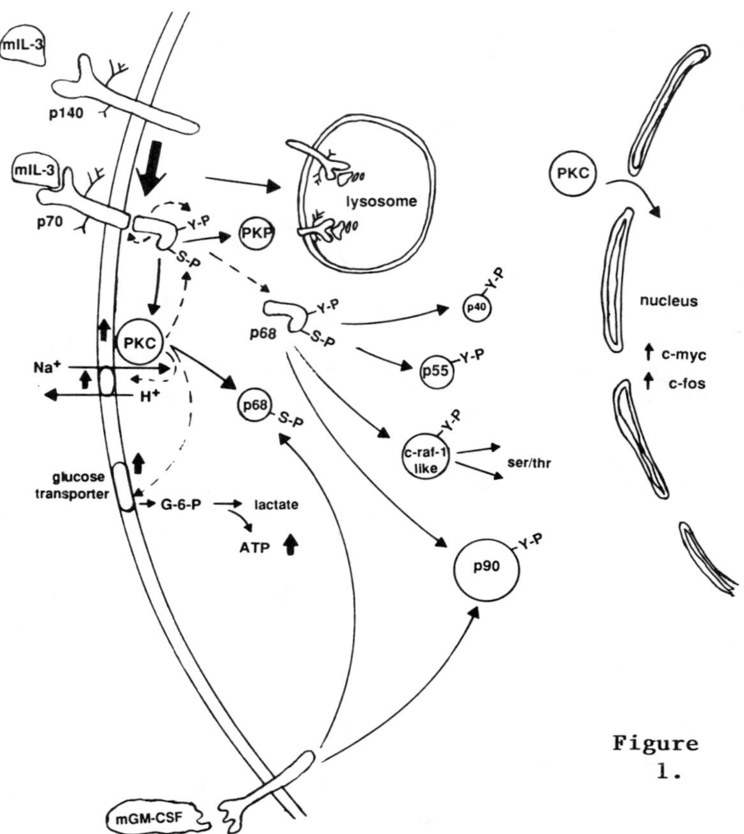

Figure 1.

REFERENCES

1. Adunyah SE, Elias L (1988). Il-3 induced intranuclear redistribution of protein kinase C and phorbol 12,13 dibutyrate binding activities in DA-1 leukemic cells. FASEB J 2: #4, Abstr #313.
2. Birchenall-Sparks MC, Farrar WL, Rennick D, Kilian PL, Ruscetti FW (1986). Regulation of expression of the interleukin-2 receptor on hematopoietic cells by interleukin-3. Science 233: 455-458.
3. Carroll MC, Clark-Lewis I, Rapp UR, May WS (1989). The multipotential hematopoietic growth factor IL-3 induces rapid phosphorylation of a c-raf-1-like protein in FDC-P1 cells. Exp Hematol 17: #6, Abstr #353.
4. Clark-Lewis I, Aebersold R, Ziltener H, Schrader JW, Hood LE, Kent SBH (1986). Automated chemical synthesis of a protein growth factor for hemopoietic cells, interleukin-3. Science 231: 134-139.

5. Clark-Lewis I, Kent SBH, Schrader JW (1984). Purification to apparent homogeneity of a factor stimulating the growth of multiple lineages of hemopoietic cells. J Biol Chem 259: 7488-7494.
6. Cutler RL, Metcalf D, Nicola NA, Johnson GR (1985). Purification of a multipotential colony-stimulating factor from pokeweed mitogen-stimulated mouse spleen cell conditioned medium. J Biol Chem 260: 657-6587.
7. Downing JR, Roussel MF, Scherr CJ (1989). Ligand and protein kinase C downmodulate the colony-stimulating factor 1 receptor by independent mechanisms. Mol Cell Biol 9: 2890-2896.
8. Evans SW, Rennick D, Farrar WL (1987). Identification of a signal-transduction pathway shared by haematopoietic growth factors with diverse biological specificity. Biochem J 244: 683-691.
9. Farrar WL, Thomas TP, Anderson WB (1985). Altered cytosol/membrane enzyme redistribution on interleukin-3 activation of protein kinase C. Nature 315: 235-237.
10. Farrar WL, Vinocour M, Hill JM (1989). In situ hybridization histochemistry localization of interleukin-3 mRNA in mouse brain. Blood 73: 137-140.
11. Frei K, Bodmer S, Schwerdel C, Fontana A (1986). Astrocyte-derived interleukin-3 as a growth factor for microglia cells and peritoneal macrophages. J Immunol 137: 3521-3527.
12. Fung MC, Hapel AJ, Ymer S, Cohen DR, Johnson RM, Campbell HD, Young IG (1984). Molecular cloning of cDNA for murine interleukin-3. Nature 307: 233-237.
13. Ihle JN, Isfort R, Cleveland JL, Weinstein Y (1988). Mechanisms in interleukin-3 mediated growth regulation of early myeloid cells. J Cell Biochem Suppl 12A, Abstr #C025.
14. Ihle JN, Keller J, Henderson L, Klein F, Palaszynski E (1982). Procedures for the purification of interleukin-3 to homogeneity. J Immunol 129: 2431-2436.
15. Ihle JN, Keller J, Oroszlan S, Henderson LE, Copeland TD, Fitch F, Prystowsky MB, Goldwasser E, Schrader JW, Palaszynski E, Dy M, Lebel B (1983). Biologic properties of homogeneous interleukin 3. J Immunol 131: 282-287.
16. Isfort R, Huhn RD, Frackelton AR Jr., Ihle JN (1988). Stimulation of factor-dependent myeloid cell lines with Interleukin 3 induces tyrosine phosphorylation of several cellular substrates. J Biol Chem 263: 19203-19209.
17. Isfort RJ, Stevens D, May WS, Ihle JN (1988). Interleukin 3 binds to a 140-kDa phosphotyrosine-containing cell surface protein. Proc Natl Acad Sci USA 85: 7982-7986.
18. Klemm DJ, Elias L (1987). A distinctive phospholipid-stimulated protein kinase of normal and malignant murine hemopoietic cells. J Biol Chem 262: 7580-7585.
19. Koyasu S, Tojo A, Miyajima A, Akijama T, Kasuga M, Urabe A, Schreurs J, Arai K, Takaku F, Yahara I (1987). Interleukin 3-specific tyrosine phosphorylation of a membrane glycoprotein of Mbr 150 000 in multi-factor-dependent myeloid cell lines. EMBO J 6: 3979-3984.
20. Laskay G, Dale RE, Jelinek J, Spooncer E, Dexter TM (1988). Interleukin-3-specific modification of cell membrane "fluidity" of haemopoietic cells. Growth Factors 1: 67-73.
21. Loughnan MS, Sanderson CJ, Nossal GJV (1988). Soluble interleukin-2 receptors are released from the cell surface of normal murine B lymphocytes stimulated with interleukin 5. Proc Natl Acad Sci USA 85: 3115-3119.
22. Miyatake S, Yokota T, Lee F, Arai K (1985). Structure of the chromosomal gene for murine interleukin-3. Proc Natl Acad Sci USA 82: 316-320.

23. Morla AO, Schreurs J, Miyajima A, Wang JYJ (1988). Hematopoietic growth factors activate the tyrosine phosphorylation of distinct sets of proteins in interleukin-3-dependent murine cell lines. Mol Cell Biol 8: 2214-2218.
24. Mui ALF, Sorensen PHB, Kay RJ, Krystal G (1989). Purification and characterization of the murine interleukin-3 receptor, in Redding C (ed): Hematopoiesis, vol 120. New York, Alan R Liss, Inc (in press).
25. Mui ALF, Sorensen PHB, Murthy SC, Krystal G (1989). Properties of the murine interleukin-3 receptor. Exp Hematol Today - 1989 (in press).
26. Murthy SC, Eaves CJ, Krystal G (1989). A simple three-step purification procedure for Interleukin 3 involving absorption to fixed cells. Exp Hematol 17: 997-1003.
27. Murthy SC, Mui ALF, Krystal G (1989). Characterization of the Interleukin-3 receptor. Exp Hematol (in press)
28. Murthy SC, Sorensen PHB, Mui ALF, Krystal G (1989). Interleukin-3 down-regulates its own receptor. Blood 73: 1180-1187.
29. Pierce JH, Di Fiore PP, Aaronson SA, Polter YM, Pumphrey J, Scott A, Ihle JN (1985). Neoplastic transformation of mast cells by Abelson-MuLV: Abrogation of IL-3 dependence by a nonautocrine mechanism. Cell 41: 685-693.
30. Rapp UR, Cleveland JL, Brightman K, Scott A, Ihle JN (1985). Abrogation of IL-3 and IL-2 dependence by recombinant murine retrovirus expressing v-myc oncogenes. Nature 317: 434-438.
31. Schrader JW (1986). The panspecific hemopoietin of activated T lymphocytes (interleukin-3). Annu Rev Immunol 4: 205-230.
32. Seger R, Yarden Y, Kashles O, Goldblatt D, Schlessinger J, Shaltiel S (1988). The epidermal growth factor receptor as a substrate for a kinase-splitting membrane proteinase. J Biol Chem 263: 3496-3500.
33. Shoelson SE, White MF, Kahn CR (1988). Tryptic activation of the insulin receptor. J Biol Chem 263: 4852-4860.
34. Sorensen P, Mui ALF, Krystal G (1989). Interleukin-3 stimulates the tyrosine phosphorylation of the 140 kilodalton interleukin-3 receptor. J Biol Chem (in press).
35. Sorensen PHB, Mui ALF, Murthy SC, Krystal G (1989). Interleukin-3, GM-CSF and TPA induce distinct phosphorylation events in an IL-3 dependent multipotential cell line. Blood 73: 406-418.
36. Whetton AD, Heyworth CM, Dexter TM (1986). Phorbol esters activate protein kinase C and glucose transport and can replace the requirement for growth factor in interleukin-3-dependent multipotent stem cells. J Cell Sci 84: 93-104.
37. Whetton AD, Monk PN, Consalvey SD, Huang SJ, Dexter TM, Downes CP (1988). Interleukin 3 stimulates proliferation via protein kinase C activation without increasing inositol lipid turnover. Proc Natl Acad Sci USA 85: 3284-3288.
38. Whetton AD, Vallance SJ, Monk PN, Cragoe EJ, Dexter TM, Heyworth CM (1988). Interleukin-3-stimulated haemopoietic stem cell proliferation. Biochem J 256: 586-592.
39. Wodnar-Filipowicz A, Heusser CH, Moroni C (1989). Production of the hemopoietic growth factors GM-CSF and interleukin-3 by mast cells in response to IgE receptor-mediated activation. Nature 339: 150-152.
40. Yokota T, Lee F, Rennick D, Hall C, Arai N, Mosmann T, Nabel G, Cantor H, Arai K (1984). Isolation and characterization of a mouse cDNA clone that expresses mast-cell growth-factor activity in monkey cells. Proc Natl Acad Sci USA 81: 1070-1074.
41. Ziltener HJ, Fazekas de St Groth B, Leslie KB, Schrader JW (1988). Multiple glycosylated forms of T cell-derived interleukin-3 (IL-3). J Biol Chem 263: 14511-14517.

The Biology of Hematopoiesis, pages 179–187
Published 1990 by Wiley-Liss, Inc.

STRUCTURE AND FUNCTION OF INTERLEUKIN-2 RECEPTORS

Warren J. Leonard, Michael Sharon, and James R. Gnarra

Cell Biology and Metabolism Branch, National Institute of Child Health and Human Development, National Institutes of Health, Bethesda, MD 20892

Introduction

The interaction of interleukin-2 (IL-2) and IL-2 receptors serves a critical regulatory control mechanism in the T-cell immune response (reviewed in Leonard *et al.*, 1989; Leonard and Sharon, in press). Following antigen activation, the 15.5 kD polypeptide hormone IL-2 is produced, principally by the CD4 positive population of T lymphocytes. Concomitantly, subpopulations of both CD4-positive and CD8-positive T cells express high affinity IL-2 receptors. The interaction of IL-2 with these high affinity receptors results in proliferation and expansion of specialized effector T cells, capable of mediating helper, suppressor, and cytotoxic T cell functions. In the absence of continued antigen presentation, IL-2 production and high affinity IL-2 receptor expression diminish, with a concomitant decrease in the antigen induced response. Thus, although the specificity of the response is determined by antigen, it is the quantity of IL-2 produced, the level of IL-2 receptors expressed, and the time course of these events which serve to control the magnitude and duration of the T cell response. High dose IL-2 can also stimulate proliferation of resting T cells in the absence of antigen stimulation.

Three classes of IL-2 receptors: existence of IL-2Rα and IL-2Rß.

In addition to the high affinity IL-2 receptors referred to above, IL-2 receptors are now known to also include low and intermediate affinity classes of receptors (reviewed in Leonard *et al.*, 1989; Leonard and Sharon, in press). These three classes of receptors result from different combinations of two binding proteins, IL-2Rα and IL-2Rß. Low affinity sites contain the α chain but not the ß chain, intermediate affinity sites contain the ß chain but not the α chain, and high affinity sites contain both α and ß chains. The IL-2 receptor system is therefore a unique situation in receptor biology-- it is one in which there are two proteins each of which can independently bind ligand, and which in addition can associate with each other to form a receptor of even higher affinity.

Data proving the existence of both α and ß chains came from affinity labeling studies (Sharon *et al.*, 1986; Tsudo *et al.*, 1986; Teshigawara *et al.*, 1987). In these experiments, ^{125}I-IL-2 was bound and covalently cross-linked to cells expressing different classes of IL-2 receptors, cellular extracts prepared and samples analyzed on SDS polyacrylamide gels. In addition to free IL-2 at the dye front, two cross-linked complexes of 68-72 kD and 85-92 kD were identified (Sharon *et al.*, 1986). These corresponded to IL-2 cross-linked to IL-2Rα (also known as p55 or Tac antigen, a protein known since 1982 to represent an IL-2 binding protein, originally named as the protein recognized by anti-Tac monoclonal antibody) and to IL-2Rß (p70), respectively.

Resting cells express predominantly IL-2Rß:

IL-2Rß can be detected on resting T cells, although the percent of cells expressing this protein may be low (Siegel *et al.*, 1987; Dukovich *et al.*, 1987; Sharon *et al.*, 1988a). Based on affinity labeling studies, both CD4 positive and CD8 positive populations of T cells have been reported to contain cells expressing this protein (Sharon *et al.*, 1988a). However, in flow cytometric studies, only the CD8 positive cells have a subpopulation which clearly stain with antibodies directed against IL-2Rß (Tsudo *et al.*, 1989). Assuming that both the affinity labeling data and flow cytometric data are valid, it is possible that the CD8 positive population contains a small number of cells that express modest levels of the ß chain (as detected by flow cytometry), whereas the CD4 positive cells perhaps more uniformly express a small number of ß chains. This could result in the identification of receptor by affinity labeling but without a significant shift noted in fluroescent intensity in flow cytometric studies.

The resting cells most enriched for IL-2Rß expression are the large granular lymphocytes (LGLs)(Siegel *et al.*, 1987), which are the cells possessing the most potent natural killer (NK) activity. When either LGLs or resting T cells are are cultured in high dose IL-2, the cells respond with proliferation and the evolution of lymphokine activated killer (LAK) activity. Interestingly, the culturing of cells in high dose IL-2 results in the upregulation of the ß chain and the *de novo* high level expression of the α chain, yielding high affinity IL-2 receptors (Siegel *et al.*, 1987). The IL-2 induced responses of these cells can therefore be divided into two phases: the first requires high concentrations of IL-2, sufficient to saturate intermediate affinity receptors; the second only requires low concentrations of IL-2, sufficient to saturate high affinity receptors (Siegel *et al.*, 1987).

As noted, IL-2Rα is not expressed on unstimulated T cells and LGLs but rather is only detected following cellular activation. With activation, the induction of IL-2Rα is so profound that on the activated cells it exceeds IL-2Rß expression by 10 to 20 fold (see Leonard *et al.*, 1989; Leonard and Sharon, in press). Only low and high affinity receptors are generally detected on the activated cells, suggesting that all or nearly all the ß chains are associated with α chains.

Structure of the α and ß chains:

cDNAs encoding both the α and ß chains have been identified and characterized (Leonard et al., 1984; Hatakeyama et al., 1989). Based on deduced amino acid sequences (see Figure 1), both have similarly sized extracellular domains (219 and 214 amino acids, respectively). However, the cytoplasmic domains are extremely different in size. The α chain has a very short intracellular domain of only 13 amino acids. This domain is very positively charged, suggesting that it can serve a cytoplasmic anchoring function; however, it certainly is unlikely to contain an enzymatic activity such as a kinase. In contrast, the ß chain has a cytoplasmic domain of 286 amino acids, consistent with its having a greater role in IL-2 mediated signal transduction. However, there is no clear consensus for a kinase domain. Nevertheless, even if no enzymatic activity is encoded, such a large domain makes it possible that this chain might be able to link to a signal transduction mechanism within the cell.

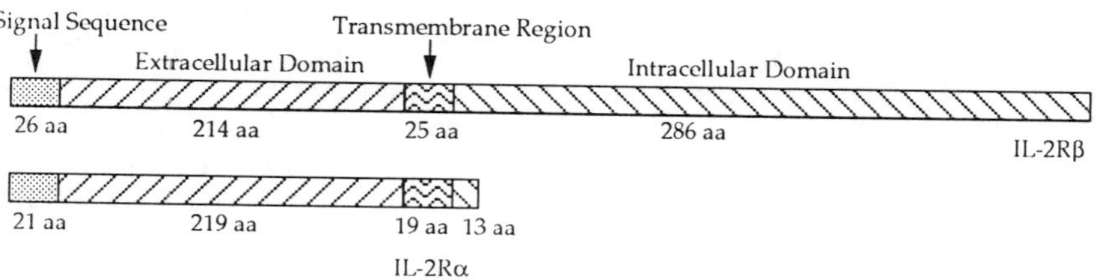

Figure 1: Schematic comparison of the deduced amino acid sequences of the α and ß chains of the human IL-2 receptor. Shown are the signal peptide, extracellular domain, transmembrane domain, and intracellular domain.

The ß chain on YT and HUT-102B2 cells is tyrosine phosphorylated:

In order to try to elucidate the mechanism(s)

of IL-2 mediated signal transduction, we investigated whether the ß chain was phosphorylated. On two leukemic cell lines studied (YT and HUT-102B2 cells), we have established that the ß chain is a phosphoprotein (Sharon _et al._, 1989a). This conclusion is based in part on a shift in the migration of the affinity labeled IL-2/IL-2Rß complex on SDS gels following incubation with alkaline phosphatase. A combination of immunoprecipitation and immunoblotting experiments with anti-phosphotyrosine antibodies strongly suggested that this phosphorylation was at least in part on tyrosine residues (Sharon _et al._, 1989a). Experiments designed to evaluate _in vitro_ kinase activity suggest that the ß chain is not a kinase. Because these experiments were performed on leukemic cells not responsive to IL-2, we were unable to determine whether the observed phosphorylation was induced by IL-2.

A 100 kD protein is associated with the murine IL-2 receptor:

In order to try to evaluate the inducibility of the phosphorylation, we began to study the murine CTLL-2 cell line, a cell line which is extremely responsive to IL-2. In so doing, we confirmed a more complex pattern of IL-2 affinity labeling, and therefore became involved in definitively identifying a 100 kD protein that is a component of the murine IL-2 receptor (Sharon _et al._, 1989b).

When IL-2 was bound and cross-linked to murine CTLL-2 cells, in addition to bands corresponding to the α and ß chains, an additional band of 115 kD was detected. Although this type of finding had been previously observed (Saragovi and Malek, 1987), it had never been resolved whether this band resulted from IL-2 being bound to a new 100 kD protein, whether two IL-2 molecules were bound to a single ß chain, whether one IL-2 plus another protein of approximately 25 kD were cross-linked together with a single ß chain, etc. Importantly, when we affinity labeled resting splenocytes and splenocytes activated with concanavalin A (Con A), we detected on resting cells only the band corresponding to the ß chain, whereas the pattern seen on Con A activated cells recapitulated the pattern detected on CTLL-2 cells (Sharon <u>et al.</u>, 1989b). Thus, the phenomenon was not unique to a leukemic cell line, but was also found on physiologically activated cells. In order to elucidate the composition of the band, we biosynthetically labeled CTLL-2 cells with ^{35}S-methionine, bound unlabeled IL-2, cross-linked with the thio cleavable cross-linker dithiobissuccinimidyl propionate (DSP), immunoprecipitated the samples with anti-IL-2 antibodies, and then analyzed these immunoprecipitates on two dimensional non-reducing/reducing diagonal gels. In this experiment, the cross-linker was cleaved in the second dimension, allowing proteins to which IL-2 had been cross-linked to fall from the diagonal. We were able to directly identify a 100 kD protein falling from the diagonal from an M_r of 115 kD prior to reduction, most consistent with the cleavage of s single IL-2 molecule. We were also able to cross-link this identical 100 kD protein (as proven by peptide mapping) to the α and/or ß chain(s) of the murine IL-2 receptor in the absence of IL-2. Thus, we have definitively established the existence of 100 kD associated protein (p100). The potential role(s) played by this protein in IL-2 binding and in signal transduction remain to be elucidated. p100 can be identified in association with high affinity IL-2 receptors; it remains an open question as to whether it can associate with low and intermediate IL-2 receptors. Because transfection experiments with the α and ß chains of the IL-2 receptor suggest that an additional chain may be needed both for high affinity binding and for function, it is reasonable to consider p100 as one such candidate.

<u>Other proteins associated with the IL-2 receptor</u>:

Reports have been published noting two other IL-2 receptor associated proteins. First, the OKT27 antigen (intercellular adhesion molecule-1, ICAM-1) has been reported to be associated with the IL-2 receptor based on fluorescent energy transfer experiments (Szollosi et al., 1987). Second, HLA class I is also associated, based on the ability to directly cross-link ^{125}I-IL-2 to class I molecules (Sharon et al., 1988b). This cross-linking event requires the binding of IL-2 to IL-2 receptors. There is no reason to suspect that HLA class I molecules directly bind IL-2; rather it appears that IL-2 binds to its receptors and then cross-links to adjacent class I molecules. Thus, there are data in support of several proteins that may associate with α and/or ß chains. The IL-2 receptor therefore indeed may turn out to be a very complex structural/functional unit which needs much additional investigation to elucidate the mechanisms of IL-2 mediated signal transduction.

References:

Dukovich, M., Wano, Y., Bich Thuy, L.-t., Katz, P., Cullen, B.R., Kehrl, J.H., and Greene, W.C. (1987). A second human interleukin-2 binding protein that may be a component of high-affinity interleukin-2 receptors.

Hatakeyama, M., Tsudo, M., Minamoto, S., Kono, T., Doi, T., Miyata, T., Miyasaka, M., and Taniguchi, T. (1989). Interleukin-2 receptor ß chain gene: generation of three forms by cloned α and ß chain cDNAs. Science 244:551-556.

Leonard, W.J, Depper, J.M., Crabtree, G.R., Rudikoff, S., Pumphrey, J., Robb, R.J., Kronke, M., Svetlik, P.B., Peffer, N.J., Waldmann, T.A., and Greene, W.C. (1984). Molecular cloning and expression of cDNAs for the human interleukin-2 receptor. Nature (London) 312:626-631.

Leonard, W.J., Sharon, M. and Cross, S.L. (1989). The human interleukin-2 receptor: structure and molecular regulation. In The Year in Immunology 1988 (edited by J. Cruse and R.E. Lewis, Jr.) vol 5, pp. 46-58, S. Karger AG Medical and Scientific Publishers, Basel, Switzerland).

Leonard, W.J. and Sharon, M. (in press). Growth factors and receptors. In Molecular

Genetics of Cancer (edited by J. Cossman), Elsevier Press, New York).

Saragovi, H. and Malek, T.R. (1987). The murine interleukin 2 receptor. Irreversible cross-linking of radiolabeled interleukin 2 to high affinity interleukin 2 receptors reveals a noncovalently associated subunit. J. Immunol. 139:1918-1926.

Sharon, M. Klausner, R.D., Cullen, B.R.. Chizzonite, R. and Leonard, W.J. (1986). Novel interleukin-2 receptor subunit detected by cross-linking under high-affinity conditions. Science 234:859-863.

Sharon, M., Siegel, J.P., Tosato, G., Yodoi, J., Gerrard, T.L., and Leonard, W.J. (1988a). The human interleukin-2 receptor beta chain (p70): Direct identification, partial purification, and patterns of expression on peripheral blood mononuclear cells. J. Exp. Med. 167:1265-1270.

Sharon, M., Gnarra, J.R., Baniyash, M., and Leonard, W.J. (1988b). Possible association between IL-2 receptors and class I HLA molecules on T cells. J. Immunol. 141:3512-3515.

Sharon, M., Gnarra, J.R., and Leonard, W.J. (1989a). The beta chain of the IL-2 receptor (p70) is tyrosine phosphorylated on YT and HUT-102B2 cells. J. Immunol. 143:2530-2533.

Sharon, M., Gnarra, J.R., and Leonard, W.J. (1989b). Identification of a distinct 100 kDa protein that interacts with the murine IL-2 receptor. Clin. Res. vol 37.

Siegel, J.P., Sharon, M., Smith, P.L., and Leonard, W.J. (1987). The IL-2 receptor beta chain (p70): Role in mediating signals for LAK, NK, and proliferative activities. Science 238: 75-78.

Szollosi, J., Damjanovich, S., Goldman, C.K., Fulwyler, M.J., Aszalos, A.A., Goldstein, G., Rao, P., Taller, M.A., and Waldmann, T.A. (1987). Flow cytometric resonance energy transfer measurements support the association of a 95-kDa peptide termed T27 with the 55-kDa Tac peptide. Proc. Natl.

Acad. Sci. USA 84: 7246-7250.

Teshigawara, K., Wang, J.-M., Kato, D., and Smith, K.A. (1987). Interleukin 2 high affinity receptor expression requires two distinct binding proteins. J. Exp. Med. 165:223-238.

Tsudo, M., Kozak, R.W., Goldman, C.K., and Waldmann, T.A. (1986). Demonstration of a non-Tac peptide that binds interleukin-2: A potential participant in a multichain interleukin 2 receptor complex. Proc. Natl. Acad. Sci. USA 83:9694-9698.

Tsudo, M. Kitamura, F., and Miyasaka, M. (1989). Characterization of the interleukin 2 receptor ß chain using three distinct monoclonal antibodies. Proc. Natl. Acad. Sci. USA 86:1982-1986.

The Biology of Hematopoiesis, pages 189–196

CHARACTERIZATION OF HEMATOPOIETIC GROWTH FACTOR RECEPTORS

Linda S. Park and Steven Gillis

Immunex Corporation, Seattle, WA 98101

INTRODUCTION

The hematopoietic process is governed by a complex network of regulatory factors, most of which are popularly referred to as cytokines. The colony stimulating factors are the classical group of factors which have been shown to be involved in regulating the survival, proliferation and differentiation of hematopoietic progenitor cells, where G-CSF and CSF-1 are relatively specific for end stage progenitors of the granulocytic and monocytic lineages respectively, and GM-CSF and IL-3 act on earlier multi-potential hematopoietic progenitors. More recently, the picture of growth factor control has become increasingly complex with demonstrations that a number of other cytokines are capable of acting on hematopoietic precursors, in some cases alone, and in some cases in synergy with other cytokines.

This paper will discuss what is known about the receptors for the classical colony stimulating factors GM-CSF, IL-3 and G-CSF, as well as some new aspects of the receptors for other hematopoietic regulatory factors, particularly those which illustrate ways in which receptors may be involved in regulating biological responses to cytokines. Discussion will focus on the following topics: (1) Recent findings that show that while most cytokines bind specifically to a single receptor, human GM-CSF and IL-3 are capable of binding to a common receptor species on both normal cells and blasts from patients with acute nonlymphocytic leukemia; (2) The receptor for IL-7, which appears to play an important role in the regulation of events early in lymphopoiesis; (3) The discovery that in addition to classical membrane bound receptors, at least some cytokine receptors may have natural soluble forms which are secreted from cells and can efficiently bind a cytokine in solution. The IL-4 receptor will be used as an illustration; and (4) A comparison of the structure of recently cloned cytokine receptors which places several of these receptors in a new cytokine receptor family.

RESULTS AND DISCUSSION

To begin a discussion of the receptors for the colony stimulating factors it is useful to consider an overview of their distribution on human cells in comparison to the expression of receptors for two of the other factors involved in hematopoiesis, IL-4 and IL-1 (Park et al., 1990a). First, one of the general trademarks of the receptors for cytokines is that they are expressed at extremely low levels on the cell surface, most frequently at less than 1000 receptors/cell. This is quite different than the expression of receptors for the more classical peptide growth factors such as insulin, EGF and PDGF, which are expressed at much higher levels. Second, the receptor expression for some of the cytokines is considerably more restricted than the expression for others. Expression of the IL-4 receptor, for instance, is basically ubiquitous. While this helps explain why IL-4 exhibits such a diversity of biological activities, it raises a major question of how these biological activities may be regulated *in vivo.* The IL-1 receptor is similar. While not quite so widely expressed as the IL-4 receptor, it is none-the-less found on most cell lineages. Initially it appeared that receptors for GM-CSF and G-CSF were restricted to hematopoietic cells of the myelomonocytic lineage, including mature neutrophils and monocytes. However, receptors for both have now been found to be expressed on some cells of non-hematopoietic lineage, such as small cell carcinoma and adenocarcinoma (Berdel et al., 1989). Whether the receptors for GM-CSF and G-CSF found on non-hematopoietic cells are the same as those found on hematopoietic cells is not yet clear. Receptors for interleukin-3, in addition to being present on monocytes and some cell lines of myelomonocytic origin, are also expressed on cells of early or pre-B cell phenotypes (Park et al., 1989a). Expression of IL-3 receptors on pre-B cells raises the question of whether IL-3 may play a role in lymphopoiesis. The answer to this is not yet known.

With regard to IL-3 receptor, some very interesting observations have fallen out of research on this receptor, specifically that GM-CSF and IL-3 appear to interact via binding to a common receptor species. During studies of the human IL-3 receptor, we initially compared the binding characteristics of IL-3 with both purified human monocytes and JM-1 cells, a human pre-B cell line. Equilibrium binding studies generated linear Scatchard plots, indicative of a single class of receptors for IL-3. On both cells, the IL-3 receptor was expressed at very low levels (<200 receptors/cell), and had a binding affinity of about 1 x 10^{10} M^{-1}. However, when specificity of ^{125}I-IL-3 binding to these two cell types was examined an interesting difference was found. Binding of ^{125}I-IL-3 to the JM-1 cell line could only be inhibited by an excess of unlabeled IL-3, and not by an excess of a number of other cytokines or growth factors. This indicates that on JM-1 cells, IL-3 binds to a specific receptor to which no other cytokines bind. This result has been typical for the other cytokines studied to date which bind to a specific receptor that binds no other cytokines. However, with human monocytes we found that human GM-CSF consistently produced a small, but reproducible, inhibition of IL-3 binding.

Besides human monocytes, the only cell line available that bound both IL-3 and GM-CSF was the myelogenous leukemia cell line KG-1. Binding of ^{125}I-IL-3 to these cells was also found to be effectively inhibited by GM-CSF. GM-CSF was able to compete radiolabeled IL-3 binding with basically the same capacity on a molar basis as IL-3 itself. Even at a very large molar excess this inhibition was only partial however. Similarly, unlabeled IL-3 could compete GM-CSF binding, but again only partially. G-CSF and CSF-1 were ineffective in competing for binding of either IL-3 or GM-CSF. It should be stressed that this inhibition occurred at 4°C where internalization of receptors cannot occur, as well as at 37°C showing that it is not due to transmodulation where binding of one cytokine is capable of down regulating the receptor for another. This inhibition of binding appears instead to be due to direct competition for binding at the cell surface. Further characterization of the temperature dependence of this phenomenon showed that the ability of either unlabeled IL-3 or unlabeled GM-CSF to inhibit ^{125}I-IL-3 binding was very similar at both 4°C and 37°C. Another interesting aspect to this cross-competition was that different variants of the KG-1 cell line stably displayed different capacities for cross-competition, ranging from 40% to 80%. In addition, equilibrium binding data showed that binding of both radiolabeled IL-3 and GM-CSF to KG-1 produced curvilinear Scatchard plots, indicative of receptor heterogeneity on these cells. This is in contrast to what was obtained by equilibrium binding of GM-CSF to HL-60 cells (which do not bind IL-3) and IL-3 to JM-1 cells (which do not bind GM-CSF), where linear Scatchard plots were obtained.

It therefore appears there is more than one kind of receptor for IL-3 and GM-CSF. HL-60 cells have receptors that only bind GM-CSF, JM-1 cells have receptors that only bind IL-3, and KG-1 cells are capable of binding both. On these cells, GM-CSF and IL-3 are able to partially compete for each others binding suggesting that at least part of the binding is to some common receptor species. How is this cross-competition mediated at the molecular level? This is not yet known. One obvious hypothesis is that there is actually a unique protein capable of binding both GM-CSF and IL-3 that is present on some cells, such as KG-1. A second is that the dual GM-CSF/IL-3 receptor is actually a complex made up of subunits that can bind only IL-3 or GM-CSF, but which are closely enough associated that these ligands are capable of interfering with each other's binding, perhaps by steric hindrance or conformational change. Although we have carried out a number of affinity crosslinking experiments on cells that bind only IL-3, only GM-CSF, or both, our results do not clearly support either model.

What does this receptor heterogeneity mean in terms of biological activities exhibited by GM-CSF and IL-3? While the answer to this is not yet known either, we do know that this receptor heterogeneity is seen not only on normal primary cells, but also on blasts from patients with acute nonlymphocytic leukemia. A large number of labs over the last few years have looked at the ability of ANL blasts to respond to colony stimulating factors and other cytokines, both in terms of proliferation and differentiation. The most common theme that has emerged from this research is that the pattern of responsiveness of ANL cells from different patients shows striking variability and it has been essentially impossible to draw any definitive correlations between cytokine responsiveness and leukemic subtype. More recently we and others have begun to look at the distribution of receptors for the colony stimulating factors on ANL cells and whether receptor expression might be correlated with responsiveness to CSFs (Park et al., 1989b). What has been found is that in general ANL cells of various subclasses express low levels of receptors for all three of these CSFs. Furthermore, the expression of receptors is not an indicator of whether ANL cells will respond to a particular CSF or how well they will respond. Perhaps the most definitive statement that can be made is that the expression of receptors for all three CSFs on ANL blasts renders them theoretically capable of responding to all these factors, even if no response is measured in a particular assay system. Like KG-1 cells, we found that ANL blasts exhibit heterogeneity in the receptors for IL-3 and GM-CSF that they express. Equilibrium binding to most ANL blasts produces curvilinear Scatchard plots with both ^{125}I-GM-CSF and ^{125}I-IL-3. Furthermore, when the ability of IL-3 and GM-CSF to cross-compete for binding at 4°C was examined on ANL blasts from several patients it was found that GM-CSF could partially compete radiolabeled IL-3 binding and IL-3 could partially compete radiolabeled GM-CSF binding with considerable patient to patient variation. It therefore appears that ANL cells display considerable heterogeneity in the receptors they express for IL-3 and

GM-CSF. An understanding of how these cells respond to these CSFs may very well require a better understanding of the biological significance of this receptor heterogeneity.

I now want to leave the pathway of myelopoiesis and move to a brief discussion of an important new regulator of lymphopoiesis - interleukin 7. Although a number of factors have been characterized which operate during myelopoiesis, very little has been known until recently about factors involved in the regulation of early lymphopoiesis. IL-7 was originally identified, purified and cloned on the basis of its ability to stimulate growth of B-cell precursors. It has now been shown to be involved in T-lymphopoiesis and recent experiments showing *in vivo* administration of IL-7 results in an increase in platelets suggest it may also be involved in some way in myelopoiesis. What do we know about the receptor for this cytokine? Equilibrium binding of murine IL-7 to a pre-B cell line called IxN/2b that is absolutely dependent on IL-7 for survival and proliferation generates curvilinear Scatchard plots with both a high and low affinity region (Park et al., 1990b). This characteristic, which is seen at both 4°C and 37°C, indicates possible receptor heterogeneity. A variety of murine cell types were examined for expression of IL-7 receptors and all cells expressing IL-7 receptors were found to exhibit both high and low affinity binding sites. All pre-B cell lines tested had IL-7 receptors, while in contrast mature B cell lines did not. Receptors could also not be detected on purified primary B cells, which could explain why no effects of IL-7 on mature B cells have been observed. In the T cell lineage, IL-7 receptors were variably expressed on T-cell lines, thymocytes, and purified mature T cells. From affinity crosslinking studies it appears the receptor is a protein of about 75 kDa which may be capable of dimerization.

Another receptor system from which we have learned a great deal is the receptor for IL-4. IL-4 is a molecule which has a broad range of effects including activities on B cells, T cells and hematopoietic progenitors. The receptor for IL-4 has recently been cloned (Mosley et al., 1989) as briefly summarized below. Using the cytotoxic T cell line CTLL, which expresses about 2000 receptors/cell, we selected a cell line expressing approximately 1 million receptors per cell by sequential rounds of fluorescence activated cell sorting using a fluorescein derivative of IL-4. Using this high expressing cell line and the low expressing parent line from which it was derived, a cDNA probe relatively specific for the IL-4 receptor was generated by a hybrid subtraction method which was then used to clone an IL-4 receptor cDNA. Two classes of cDNA were obtained. One coded for a membrane bound form of the IL-4 receptor and one encoded a form representing a possible secreted form of the IL-4 receptor. The membrane bound form of the receptor binds IL-4 and has an expressed molecular weight which is identical to that demonstrated for the natural IL-4 receptor. It has a typical structure for a membrane bound receptor with an extracellular domain of 208aa, a 24 aa transmembrane domain and a 553aa cytoplasmic domain.

In contrast, the cDNA isolated for the soluble form of the receptor encoded a protein containing essentially the entire extracellular domain but missing the transmembrane and cytoplasmic domains. Isolation of this natural soluble form raised the possibility that while cytokines normally bind to cell surface receptors to elicit a biological response, secretion of a soluble receptor form could interrupt this process by preventing binding to its surface bound receptor. Secretion of soluble receptors could therefore represent a new regulatory pathway for shutting off cellular responses to cytokines. When cDNA clones which coded for a soluble receptor were transiently expressed in COS-7 cells and supernatants tested, we found that the soluble IL-4 receptor was in fact capable of completely inhibiting ^{125}I-IL-4 binding to its receptor on CTLL cells. Furthermore, we found that COS cell supernatants containing the soluble IL-4 receptor were able to effectively inhibit the ability of CTLL cells to proliferate in response to IL-4, but not IL-2.

In addition to discovery of a soluble form, we have also learned from the IL-4 receptor how some of the cytokine receptors may be related. When the sequence of the cloned IL-4 receptor was searched against the Genbank DNA and NBRF protein databases it was found to be unique. However, when we compared the IL-4 receptor sequence to those of several cytokine receptors which have very recently been cloned, we found significant homology between the extracellular domains of the receptors for IL-4, IL-6, erythropoietin and the β subunit of the IL-2 receptor (Idzerda et al., 1990). Distinguishing features include four conserved cysteines and a Trp-Ser-X-Trp-Ser motif near the transmembrane domain.

Figure 1 shows a schematic representation of these four receptors as well as the receptors for CSF-1 and IL-1 (drawn to scale). The extracellular domains of the receptors for IL-6, EPO, IL-2β and IL-4 are shown with the position of the four invariant cysteine residues and the WSXWS motif indicated. The CSF-1 and IL-1 receptors are known to belong to the immunoglobulin gene superfamily where CSF-1R contains five immunoglobulin like domains and the IL-1R contains three. The IL-6 receptor is an interesting hybrid between these two families containing a single immunoglobulin domain at the N-terminus followed by the domain characteristic of what we are calling the hematopoietin receptor family (Idzerda et al., 1990).

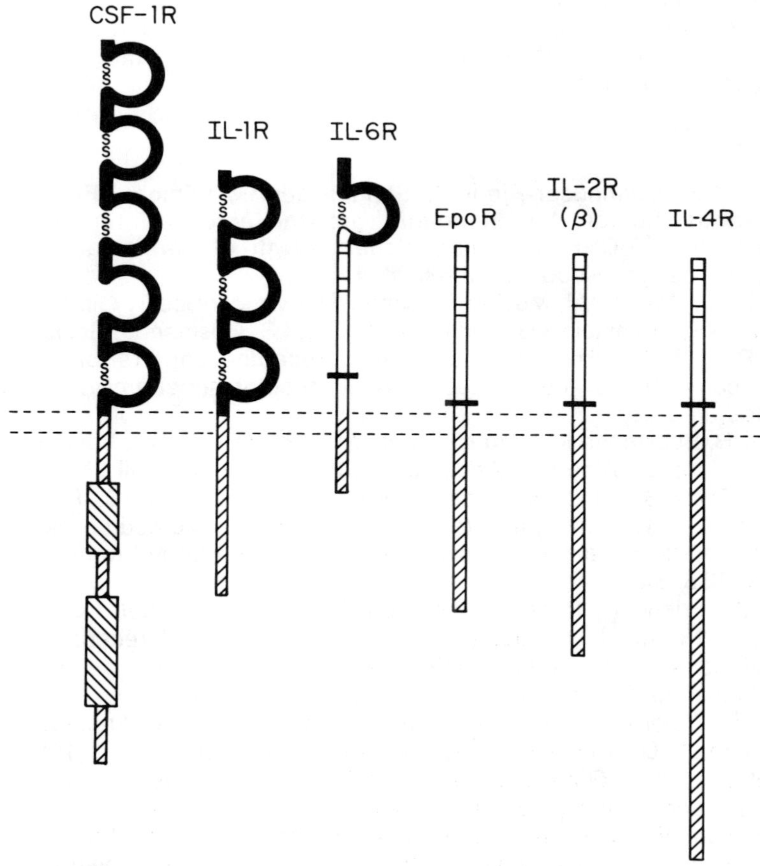

Figure 1. Cytokine receptor families. Horizontal dashed lines show transmembrane domain, hatched boxes show cytoplasmic domain, open or solid boxes show extracellular domain. Horizontal lines in open boxes show position of conserved cysteine residues and the solid black bar shows position of the WSXWS motif.

Compared to the homology in the extracellular domain, the other important point to note is the lack of similarity in the cytoplasmic domains. Not only are differences in size obvious, but alignment programs fail to find significant sequence homology between them. The CSF-1R is the only one of these six which has tyrosine kinase activity, where the split tyrosine kinase domains are indicated. How these other receptors may function to transmit a biological signal is largely unknown, and represents one of the new frontiers in unraveling the interactions of the complex network of cytokines and cytokine receptors that regulate hematopoiesis.

REFERENCES

Berdel WE, Danhauser-Riedl S, Steinhauser G, Winton EF (1989). Various human hematopoietic growth factors (Interleukin-3, GM-CSF, G-CSF) stimulate clonal growth of nonhematopoietic tumor cells. Blood 73:80-83.

Idzerda RL, March CJ, Mosley B, Lyman SD, VandenBos T, Gimpel SD, Din WS, Grabstein KH, Widmer MB, Park LS, Cosman D, Beckmann MP (1990). Human interleukin-4 receptor confers biological responsiveness and defines a novel receptor superfamily. J Exp Med, in press.

Mosley B, Beckmann MP, March CJ, Idzerda RL, Gimpel SD, VandenBos T, Friend D, Alpert A, Anderson D, Jackson J, Wignall JM, Smith C, Gallis B, Sims JE, Urdal D, Widmer MB, Cosman D, Park LS (1989). The murine interleukin-4 receptor: Molecular cloning and characterization of secreted and membrane bound forms. Cell 59:335-348.

Park LS, Friend D, Price V, Anderson D, Singer J, Prickett KS, Urdal DL (1989a). Heterogeneity in human interleukin-3 receptors. A subclass that binds human granulocyte/macrophage colony stimulating factor. J Biol Chem 264:5420-5427.

Park LS, Waldron PE, Friend D, Sassenfeld HM, Price V, Anderson D, Cosman D, Andrews RG, Bernstein ID, Urdal DL (1989b). Interleukin-3, GM-CSF, and G-CSF receptor expression on cell lines and primary leukemia cells: Receptor heterogeneity and relationship to growth factor responsiveness. Blood 74:56-65.

Park LS, Gillis S, Urdal DL (1990a). Hematopoietic growth-factor receptors. In: *Colony-Stimulating Factors - Molecular and Cellular Biology.* Marcel Dekker, Inc., NY, pp. 39-75.

Park LS, Friend DJ, Schmierer AE, Dower SK, Namen AE (1990b). Murine interleukin-7 receptor: Characterization on an IL-7-dependent cell line. J Exp Med, in press.

The Biology of Hematopoiesis, pages 197–204

CONTROL OF LYMPHOKINE PRODUCTION BY PROTEIN KINASE C

Julianne J. Sando, E. Chris Homan and David E. Jensen

Department of Pharmacology and Cancer Center
Univ. of Virginia, Charlottesville, VA 22908

INTRODUCTION

Lymphokine production by T cells is normally stimulated by antigen and the macrophage product Interleukin 1 (IL1). Replacement of these stimuli with tumor-promoting phorbol esters (PEs) and Ca^{2+} ionophores implicated Protein Kinase C (PKC) and Ca^{2+} in this pathway. PEs replace a diacylglycerol requirement for activation of PKC, a Ca^{2+}- and phospholipid-dependent kinase which can also be activated by a Ca^{2+}-dependent protease to generate a cofactor-independent kinase (for review, see Nishizuka, 1988). In an attempt to focus on just the PKC component of lymphocyte activation, we have used the EL4 mouse thymoma cell line which produces large amounts of several lymphokines including Interleukin 2 (IL2), Interleukin 3 (IL3) and Granulocyte/Macrophage-Colony Stimulating Factor (GM-CSF) in response to PEs alone. Resistant lines of EL4 cells exist which fail to exhibit any of the responses of the sensitive cells to PEs.

PKC ACTIVATION IN SENSITIVE AND RESISTANT EL4 CELLS

In early studies we found that stimulation of EL4 cells with PE caused a loss of PKC from cytosol in both sensitive (S-EL4) and resistant (R-EL4) lines (Kraft et al, 1982). Previous studies had failed to detect any differences in number or affinity of PE receptors in S-EL4 vs R-EL4 cells (reviewed in Sando et al, 1989) thus suggesting that the defect in R-EL4 cells was not at the level of PKC. However the defect in these cells is early in the pathway since R-EL4 cells even fail to exhibit the substrate adherence response which occurs during the first 30 min of PE treatment.

The subsequent identification of at least 7 isozymes of PKC (Nishizuka, 1988) raised the possibility that S-EL4 and R-EL4 cells might differ in isozyme content. Northern analysis has revealed that both lines contain mRNA for alpha (type III) and beta (type II) PKC but not gamma (type I) (not shown). Expression of types II and III PKC protein in both lines was verified by purification and Western blotting with isozyme-specific antibodies (Table 1).

Table 1: PKC Isozymes in Sensitive and Resistant EL4 Cells

	PKC activity (cpm/90 ul)*	Antibody Reactivity**		
		MC5	beta	beta 2
S-EL4				
HA1	7,000	-	+	++
HA2	5,000	+	-	-
R-EL4				
HA1	29,000	-	+	++
HA2	20,000	+	-	-

*Cytosolic extracts from S-EL4 or R-EL4 cells were chromatographed over DE52 followed by hydroxyapatite. Phospholipid-dependent PKC activity in the two hydroxyapatite peaks, HA1 nd HA2, was assayed as in Walker and Sando (1988).
**Samples of the peak fractions were probed on a Western blot with MC5 antibody (Amersham) or beta-specific antibodies which were a generous gift from Drs. Kikkawa and Nishizuka.

Immunologic (Berry et al, 1989) and RNA expression (Koretzky et al, 1989) data for the existence of types II and III PKC in other lymphocytes has also been presented. Two cell lines lacking PKC beta RNA still responded to antigen stimulation with production of IL2, arguing that type III PKC is sufficient for this response (Koretzky et al, 1989). Whether type II PKC can also stimulate lymphokine production is unknown. It is interesting to note that type III PKC may be more dependent on Ca^{2+} than is type II (Nishizuka, 1988). Studies of PKC activation in different lipid systems suggest that both isozymes may require Ca^{2+} for association with membrane phospholipids but that type III has an additional Ca^{2+} requirement that is unrelated to membrane binding (Walker and Sando, submitted). The failure of R-EL4 to respond to PE might, then, be due to lesser activation of type III PKC, possibly due to inadequate Ca^{2+} concentrations. Pilot experiments demonstrated a resting Ca^{2+} of ~100 nM in R-EL4 cells and ~200 nM in S-EL4 cells. Although this difference might lead to differential activation of type III PKC in the two cells, we were unable to stimulate IL2 production from resistant cells by addition of Ca^{2+} ionophore with PE.

While no qualitative differences in PKC isozyme content were found in S-EL4 vs R-EL4, purification of PKC from R-EL4 cells resulted in consistently greater recovery of activity in both isozyme fractions (Table 1). Huang et al have reported (1988) that the PKC half life is much longer in R-EL4 cells. Such an effect could be due to a difference in PKC itself or, perhaps, in the availability of a protease or other inactivating enzyme in sensitive vs. resistant cells. The increased recovery of both isozymes in R-EL4 cells may tend to favor a defect in those cells at the level of an inactivating enzyme rather than in PKC itself. The decreased recovery of S-EL4 PKC may suggest that generation of a catalytic fragment of PKC or perhaps rapid inactivation of PKC is important for lymphokine production. Although no direct evidence to support such a mechanism exists, the above-mentioned difference in intracellular Ca^{2+} could contribute to differential PKC proteolysis.

NUCLEAR EFFECTS OF PKC

Since lymphokine production is dependent on transcription and protein synthesis, the signal initiated by PKC activation must eventually reach the nucleus. In EL4 cells, PE-stimulated production of IL2 (Harrison et al, 1987), IL3 and GM-CSF mRNA (not shown) is blocked by addition of protein synthesis inhibitors between 1 and 2 hours after addition of PE. This may indicate that PKC activation first stimulates production of an intermediate factor that is required for lymphokine transcription. An alternative interpretation is that a protein not affected by PKC but with a short half life is required for lymphokine transcription. Nuclear effects of PKC activation could be directed at the hypothetical intermediate transcriptional event and/or more directly at transcription of the lymphokines.

Genes for many PE-induced proteins have been found to contain a PE responsive element (TRE) in the 5' flanking DNA.

Angel et al (1987) identified a protein, AP1, which binds to this region and more recent work has shown homology of this protein with the product of the jun oncogene (Bohmann et al, 1987; Angel et al, 1988). Jun-jun homodimers can stimulate transcription from TRE-containing genes but heterodimers of jun and the fos oncogene product bind DNA with higher affinity (Chiu et al, 1988; Gentz et al, 1989). Since PEs cause rapid induction of fos and jun in some cells, and the IL2 gene contains a TRE consensus sequence, fos and jun are candidates for intermediates in PE-induced IL2 transcription.

The observation that the regulatory domain of PKC contains a cysteine-rich region much like many DNA binding transcription factors raised the question of whether PKC might affect transcription via a direct interaction of this domain with DNA. Hata et al (1989) have recently shown that transfection of a catalytic fragment of PKC stimulates transcription of a reporter gene containing a TRE, indicating that transcriptional responses do not require the PKC regulatory domain. This result suggests that kinase activity and thus one or more substrates of PKC may be required for the transcriptional effects of PEs. Whether transcription-regulatory phosphorylation events occur in the nucleus or elsewhere in the cell has not been determined. We did not find intact PKC in nuclei of EL4 cells before or after PE treatment, but existence of the catalytic fragment in nuclei could not be ruled out (Jensen and Sando, 1987).

IDENTIFICATION OF PKC SUBSTRATES

Accumulating evidence indicates that phosphorylation/ dephosphorylation may control the activity of a number of transcription factors. Fig. 1 shows that nuclei do contain potential PKC substrates but these were only phosphorylated after addition of exogenous PKC to the nuclear preparation in vitro. It is possible that PKC substrates or more distal proteins in the PKC pathway translocate to the nucleus after phosphorylation events elsewhere. The transcription factor NFkB has been shown to translocate from cytosol to membrane upon stimulation of lymphocytes (Baeuerle and Baltimore, 1988).

Earlier in vitro studies revealed the existence of a number of potential PKC substrates in cytosol from EL4 cells (Kramer and Sando, 1986). Since PKC is usually activated at a membrane surface, the potential significance of cytosolic substrates has been questioned. We found, however, that most of the cytosolic substrates bound phosphatidylserine in a Ca^{2+}-dependent manner. Thus cytosolic proteins may become phosphorylated upon their reversible association with membranes where active PKC is known to exist. One ~45 kDa protein, found in S-EL4 but not R-EL4 cells, is a candidate for involvement in PE-stimulated lymphokine production.

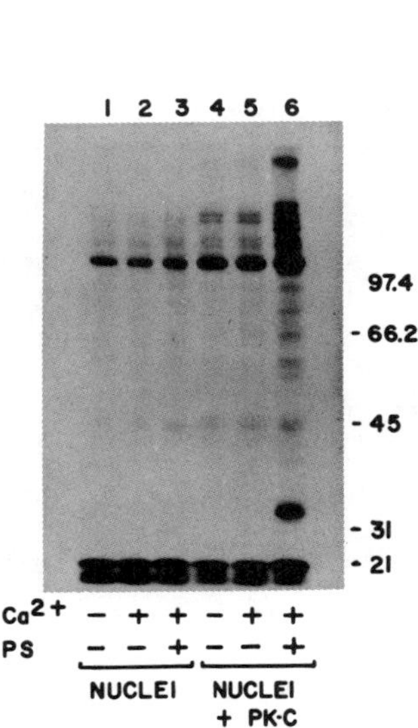

Fig. 1. Nuclear PKC Substrates. Nuclei were isolated as in Jensen & Sando, lysed, and incubated with ^{32}P-ATP + Ca^{2+}, lipid, and/or PKC purified as in Walker & Sando 1988. Resolved proteins were detected by autoradiography.

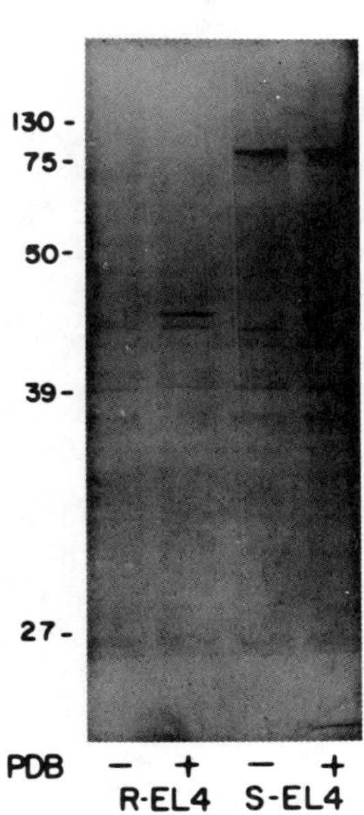

Fig. 2. Tyr-Phosphorylated Proteins in S-EL4 and R-EL4. Cells were incubated with or without PE for 10 min. Blots of resolved proteins were probed with anti-P-tyr antibody generously provided by Drs. Payne and Weber.

Many membrane proteins have been identified as PKC substrates. A number of these are receptors with associated tyrosine protein kinase activity which is diminished after PKC-mediated phosphorylation. In T cells, several components of the CD3/antigen receptor complex are phosphorylated in response to PE (Cantrel et al 1985), and CD3 or PE stimulation of Jurkat cells results in serine phosphorylation of the src tyrosine kinase (Ledbetter et al, 1987). Another membrane-associated tyrosine kinase, $p56^{lck}$, is also phosphorylated in response to PE treatment of lymphocytes (Casnellie and Lamberts, 1986). This kinase is associated with the CD4 and CD8 surface antigens in lymphocytes and dissociates from CD4 (not CD8) after PE treatment, possibly due to PKC-mediated phosphorylation and internalization of CD4 (Hurley et al, 1989). PE-stimulated phosphorylation of a MAP2 serine kinase has also been observed in lymphocytes (Hanekom et al, 1989). Thus the involvement of PKC in a phosphorylation cascade involving a number of additional serine/threonine as well as tyrosine kinases and phosphatases is likely.

To identify effects of PE on tyrosine phosphorylation, we probed Western blots of control and PE-treated S-EL4 and R-EL4 cells with an anti-phosphotyrosine antibody. Fig. 2 shows that PE induced tyr phosphorylation of a 45 kDa protein in both cell lines. A less prominent protein of slightly smaller size was induced by PE in S-EL4 only. Also indicated in this figure is the constitutive phosphorylation of a protein of ~80 kDa in S-EL4 only. The identity of these proteins is under investigation as is their subcellular localization and the mechanism by which PKC leads to their increased phosphorylation on tyr.

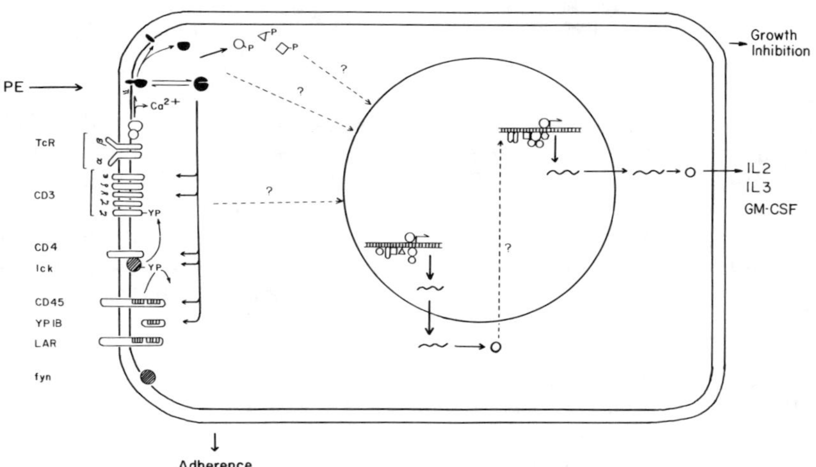

Fig. 3. Potential steps in lymphokine production.

SUMMARY

As illustrated in Fig. 3, our understanding of lymphokine production is incomplete. Nuclear effects of PKC are probably mediated by phosphorylated substrates. Some of the substrates are themselves being identified as kinases and phosphatases, adding more complexity to the pathway. Use of resistant cell lines is one of the approaches that may help link early phosphorylation events with later transcriptional responses.

Supported by grants GM31184, DK40031 (NIH) & FRA-306 (ACS).

REFERENCES

Angel P, Imagawa M, Chiu R, Stein B, Imbra RJ, Rahmsdorf HJ, Jonat C, Herrlich P, Karin M (1987) Phorbol ester-inducible genes contain a common cis element recognized by a TPA -modulated trans-acting factor. Cell 49:729-739.

Angel P, Allegretto EA, Okino ST, Hattori K, Boyle WJ, Hunter T, Karin M (1988) Oncogene jun encodes a sequence-specific trans-activator similar to AP-1. Nature 332:166-171.

Baeuerle PA, Baltimore D (1988) Activation of DNA-binding activity in an apparently cytoplasmic precursor of the NFkB transcription factor. Cell 53:211-217.

Berry N, Ase K, Kikkawa U, Kishimoto A, Nishizuka Y (1989) Human T cell activation by phorbol esters and diacylglycerol analogues. J Immunol 143:1407-1413.

Bohmann D, Bos TJ, Admon A, Nishimura T, Vogt PK, Tjian R (1987) Human proto-oncogene c-jun encodes a DNA binding protein with structural and functional properties of transcription factor AP-1. Science 238:1386-1392.

Cantrell DA, Davies AA, Crumpton MJ (1985). Activators of protein kinase C down-regulate and phosphorylate the T3/T -cell antigen receptor complex of human T lymphocytes. Proc Natl Acad Sci 82:8158-8162.

Casnellie JE, Lamberts RJ (1986). Tumor promoters cause changes in the state of phosphorylation and apparent molecular weight of a tyrosine protein kinase in T lymphocytes. J Biol Chem 261:4921-4925.

Chiu R, Boyle WJ, Meek J, Smeal T, Hunter T, Karin M (1988) The c-fos protein interacts with c-jun/AP-1 to stimulate transcription of AP-1 responsive genes. Cell 54:541-552.

Gentz R, Rauscher FJ III, Abate C, Curran T (1989) Parallel association of fos and jun leucine zippers juxtaposes DNA binding domains. Science 243:1695-1699.

Hanekom C, Nel A, Gittinger C, Rheeder A, Landreth G (1989)

Complexing the CD-3 subunit by a monoclonal antibody activates a microtubule-associated protein 2 (MAP-2) serine kinase in Jurkat cells. Biochem J 262:449-456.
Harrison JMR, Lynch KR, Sando JJ (1987). Phorbol esters induce Interleukin 2 mRNA in sensitive but not in resistant EL4 cells. J Biol Chem 262:234-238.
Hata A, Akita Y, Konno Y, Suzuki K, Ohno S (1989) Direct evidence that the kinase activity of protein kinase C is involved in transcriptional activation through a TPA -responsive element. FEBS Lett 252:144-146.
Huang FL, Arora PK, Hanna EE, Huang KP (1988) Proteolytic degradation of protein kinase C in the phorbol ester -induced interleukin-2 secreting thymoma cells. Arch Biochem Biophys 267:503-514.
Hurley TR, Luo K, Sefton BM (1989) Activators of protein kinase C induce dissociation of CD4, but not CD8, from $p56^{lck}$. Science 245:407-409.
Jensen DE, Sando, JJ (1987). Absence of protein kinase C in nuclei of EL4 mouse thymoma cells. Cancer Res 47:4830-4834.
Koretzky GA, Wahi M, Newton ME, Weiss A (1989). Heterogeneity of protein kinase C isozyme gene expression in human T cell lines. Protein kinase C-beta is not required for several T cell functions. J Immunol 143:1692-1695.
Kramer CM, Sando JJ (1986). Substrates for protein kinase C in cytosol of EL4 mouse thymoma cells. Cancer Res 46:3040 -3045.
Kraft AS, Anderson WB, Cooper HL, Sando JJ (1982). Decrease in Cytosolic Calcium/Phospholipid-dependent protein kinase activity following phorbol ester treatment of EL4 thymoma cells. J Biol Chem 257:13193-13196.
Ledbetter JA, Gentry LE, June CH, Rabinovitch PS, Purchio AF (1987) Stimulation of T cells through the CD3/T-cell receptor complex: Role of cytoplasmic calcium, protein kinase C translocation, and phosphorylation of $pp60^{src}$ in the activation pathway. Mol Cel Biol 7:650-656.
Nishizuka Y (1988). The molecular heterogeneity of protein kinase C and its implications for cellular regulation. Nature 334:661-665.
Sando JJ, Kramer CM, Harrison JR, Jensen DE (1989). Role of protein kinase C in stimulation of Interleukin 2 production. In Colburn NH (ed): "Genes and Signal Transduction in Multistage Carcinogenesis" Marcel Dekker, pp 279-308.
Walker JM, Sando JJ (1988). Activation of Protein kinase C by short chain phosphatidylcholines. J Biol Chem 263:4537-4540
Walker JM, Sando JJ (1989). Differential activation of protein kinase C isozymes. submitted.

The Biology of Hematopoiesis, pages 205–213
Published 1990 by Wiley-Liss, Inc.

PHORBOL ESTERS, LIPOPOLYSACCHARIDES AND COLONY STIMULATING FACTOR PRODUCTION

Dov H. Pluznik and Matthias Bickel

Division of Cytokine Biology, HFB-800,
Center for Biologics, Evaluation and Research,
Food and Drug Administration, Bethesda, MD 20892

INTRODUCTION

Colony stimulating factors (CSFs) are glycoproteins that regulate the proliferation and differentiation of hemopoietic stem cells into mature granulocytes and macrophages. Four different subclasses of CSF have been identified: Granulocyte Macrophage-CSF (GM-CSF), Multi-CSF, also known as Interleukin 3 (IL3), Macrophage-CSF and Granulocyte-CSF. All four subclasses have been biochemically purified and their genes cloned and expressed in various prokaryotic and eukaryotic cells (Metcalf, 1986). The different subclasses of CSF can be obtained from various organs, tissue extracts and cell lines. Lymphoid cells are a particularly good source for CSFs. T cells, when stimulated with antigens, mitogens or phorbol esters such as 12-*O*-tetradecanoyl-phorbol-13-acetate (TPA), secrete GM-CSF and IL3 as well as other lymphokines such as interleukin 2 (IL2) and interferon γ (Mosmann and Cossman, 1987). Certain B cell lines when stimulated with lipopolysaccharides (LPS) secrete GM-CSF (Bickel et al.,1987a). B cells present in bone marrow, when stimulated with a combination of LPS and TPA, also secrete GM-CSF (Pluznik and Mergenhagen, 1986).

The molecular pathways leading to the activation of genes which are responsible for secretion of bioactive molecules such as GM-CSF are largely unknown. In general they involve the stimulation of cell surface receptors, followed by a signal transduction in the form of second messengers such as diacylglycerol and inositol-1,4,5-triphosphate. Diacylglycerol stimulates protein kinase C whereas inositol-1,4,5-triphosphate releases calcium from intracellular stores. These processes lead finally to the expression of specific genes that are responsible for the production of the bioactive molecules. To study such pathways in the case of GM-CSF, research in our laboratory has been focused on the production of this CSF in B and T cell lines representing homogeneous lymphocyte populations.

INDUCTION OF GM-CSF IN B CELLS AND THE EFFECT OF Ca^{2+} ANTAGONISTS

Two B cell lines, B-lymphoma M12.4.1 (Kim et al., 1979) and B-hybridoma TH2.2 (Hamano et al., 1982) were used to study the release of GM-CSF after stimulation with LPS. TH2.2 cells have IgM receptors on their surface and thus are also capable of responding to exposure with anti IgM antibodies by producing GM-CSF (Bickel et al., 1987a). Cells in serum-free medium were stimulated with LPS-W from *Salmonella abortus equi*. Production of CSF depends on the amount of LPS added to the cell cultures. Fifty µg/ml of LPS induced optimal amounts of CSF as determined by bioassays of cell supernatants on the GM-CSF and IL3 dependent cell line PT-18 (Pluznik et al., 1984). Highest GM-CSF levels in the culture supernatants were reached 24 hours after addition of LPS. Since no cell line has been characterized that depends on GM-CSF only, rabbit anti-murine recombinant GM-CSF antibodies (10 µg/ml) (Mochizuki et al., 1986) were used to confirm the identity of the secreted CSF. These antibodies completely neutralized the biological activity of the CSF released by the B cell lines (Bickel et al., 1987a). The same antibodies had no effect on known sources of IL3 activity when assayed either on the PT-18 or on the IL3 dependent cell line, DA-1 (Ythier et al., 1985). These data demonstrate that the CSF activity released by LPS-stimulated B cell lines was GM-CSF.

Conflicting reports exist regarding the nature of interaction of LPS with its target cells. It is unclear whether LPS binds to specific cell surface receptors and whether such binding is followed by stimulation of the cells (Coutinho et al., 1978, Lei and Morrison, 1988). Since Ca^{2+} release from intracellular stores occurs when cells are stimulated, we tested the possible involvement of Ca^{2+} in the pathway of events leading to secretion of GM-CSF. TH2.2 cells were stimulated with 50 µg/ml LPS in the presence of two Ca^{2+} antagonists: 8-(N,N-diethylamino)-octyl

3,4,5-trimethoxybenzoate hydrochloride (TMB-8), which blocks the Ca^{2+} release from intracellular bound stores (Malagodi and Chiou, 1974) or with the synthetic compound n-(6-aminohexyl)-5-chloro-1-naphthalenesulfonamide (W-7), an antagonist to the Ca-binding protein calmodulin (Fujii et al., 1985). Regardless of the amounts of TMB-8 up to 10 µM and W-7 up to 16.7 µM no change in GM-CSF activity could be detected in the supernatants. (These antagonists also had no effect on the indicator cell line PT-18). These experiments suggested that GM-CSF expression does not depend on the release of cytosolic free ($[Ca^{2+}]i$) or on calmodulin. To further analyze this observation we measured directly whether the stimulation of TH2.2 cells with LPS will induce the intracellular release of $[Ca^{2+}]i$. Cells were loaded with the indicator acetomethoxy quin-2, a membrane- permeable derivative of the Ca-sensitive fluorescent probe quin-2 (Tsien, 1980). Increase in fluorescence intensity is directly proportional to increase in $[Ca^{2+}]i$. TH2.2 cells were stimulated with LPS and fluorescence intensity measured in real time. No increase of the emitted fluorescent signal was observed within 5 minutes after LPS stimulation. However, when anti IgM antibodies were subsequently added to the same cells a rapid increase in fluorescence intensity was detected. This data further support the hypothesis stated above that production of GM-CSF after treatment of these B cells with LPS is independent of release of $[Ca^{2+}]i$. As for the generation of GM-CSF with anti IgM antibodies in these cells, either its production is via a different pathway which is Ca^{2+} dependent, or the Ca^{2+} signal which is observed in these cells after stimulation with anti IgM antibodies is not related to CSF production.

INDUCTION OF GM-CSF IN T CELLS

Two T cell lines of independent origin, the thymoma EL-4 (Farrar et al., 1980) and the hybridoma 2B4 (Samelson and Schwartz, 1983), were used in experiments to study GM-CSF production upon stimulation with TPA. Similar to what we observed in LPS treated B cells, highest GM-CSF levels in serum-free culture supernatants were reached 24 hours after the addition of optimal amounts of TPA (20nM) (Bickel et al., 1988). TPA-stimulated T cells also produce IL2 and IL3 in addition to GM-CSF. Since PT-18 cells respond to both CSFs (GM-CSF and IL3) we took advantage of earlier observations that the immunosuppressive drug cyclosporin A (CsA) inhibits IL3 production but not that of GM-CSF

(Palacios, 1985, Bickel et al., 1987b). We had reported that doses of CsA up to 0.5 µg/ml inhibited the production of IL3 in EL-4 and 2B4 cells. Under these treatment conditions (20 nM TPA and 0.5 µg/ml CsA), activity released by these cells and assayed on PT-18 cells reflects the effect of GM-CSF exclusively. Confirmation of this fact was obtained by utilizing rabbit anti-murine recombinant GM-CSF antibodies to neutralize the biological activity in supernatants from TPA stimulated cells that were exposed to CsA. These antibodies completely neutralized this activity (Bickel et al., 1987b).

The observation that GM-CSF activity is resistant to CsA treatment might also provide additional support for the hypothesis that GM-CSF production is independent of intracellular Ca^{2+} fluxes, since CsA has been shown to interfere with calmodulin (Colombini et al., 1985). The findings that TPA proved to be a very potent inducer of GM-CSF activity in these cells points to a possible involvement of protein kinase C in the pathway leading to GM-CSF release since TPA interacts directly with this enzyme (Castagna et al., 1982).

CONTROL OF GM-CSF PRODUCTION ON THE GENE LEVEL IN B AND T CELLS

To further study the pathways that lead to GM-CSF release in LPS-treated B cells and in TPA-stimulated T cells, we analyzed whether the inducible appearance of biological activities is reflected in the mRNA levels. RNA was isolated and analyzed by Northern blotting as described elsewhere (Bickel et al., 1987a, 1987b). ^{32}P-labelled cDNA probes for GM-CSF were used to detect specific mRNA. The data obtained in these analyses matched the data obtained by bioassays: mRNA can only be detected in cells that have been exposed to LPS or TPA. Highest levels were detected 5 8 hours after treatment. RNA levels rise transiently, disappearing after 12 hours. The kinetics of mRNA production might help to explain why biological activity in supernatants peaks at 20 to 24 hours after stimulation and does not increase further thereafter.

We had reported earlier that CsA does not inhibit GM-CSF production in T cells, both at the level of detection of biological activity and mRNA. In studies on IL2 production in T cells evidence was presented that CsA blocks cytokine synthesis at a transcriptional level (Krönke et al., 1984). Why would IL2 and GM-CSF differ in their sensitivity to CsA? Comparison of steady-state levels of IL2 and GM-CSF mRNA after TPA treatment show both transcripts are induced in EL-4 and 2B4 cells. High levels of mRNA obviously can be reached by various mechanisms in the cells, e.g. increase in the rate of transcription or stabilization of mature transcripts. The effects of CsA suggested that the induction of GM-CSF and IL2 transcripts are possibly reached through different pathways.

In a first approach to analyze such possibilities we used the drug 5,6-dichloro-1-β-D-ribofuranosylbenzimidazole (DRB) an inhibitor of transcription initiation (Efrat and Kaempfer, 1984), to ask whether this drug also differentiates between GM-CSF and IL2 production in T cells. Results obtained from experiments with TPA and DRB treated cells were very similar to those obtained with CsA. GM-CSF production was not affected by DRB, whereas IL2 was completely inhibited (Bickel et al., 1990). Data obtained for biological activity of GM-CSF and IL2 could also be reproduced at the level of Northern analyses. GM-CSF transcript levels were not significantly reduced by DRB whereas IL2 levels were sharply diminished.

We next assessed transcriptional activity directly by performing nuclear run-on analyses in TH2.2 and EL-4 cells (Bickel et al., 1989, Pluznik et al., 1989). As anticipated, we found that the GM-CSF gene was transcribed in untreated TH2.2 and EL-4 cells and did not change significantly when cells were treated with LPS or TPA, respectively. In addition, CsA did not have a significant effect on GM-CSF transcription in EL-4 cells. On the other hand, there was no IL2 transcription in untreated EL-4 cells and TPA-induced IL2 transcription was clearly inhibited by CsA and DRB.

These data together suggest that the GM-CSF gene is in fact transcribed by transcriptional complexes which are somehow resistant to the effect of DRB or CsA. But why could we not detect the effects of these transcripts in Northern analysis in unstimulated cells? One possibility could be due to limited sensitivity of this type of analysis. To increase sensitivity, we took advantage of a method that has been used to detect low copy number of double-stranded viral RNAs (Robertson and Hunter, 1975). Solution hybridization of large amounts of total RNA to cRNA probes, followed by chromatographic separation of double-stranded from single-stranded RNA on CF-11 cellulose, allowed us to detect these low abundance GM-CSF transcripts in unstimulated EL-4 cells.

Since we now were able to detect low amounts of GM-CSF mRNA in unstimulated cells, we next asked the question whether cycloheximide (Chx), a protein synthesis inhibitor, also would allow the detection of these transcripts, based on its known effect to stabilize certain mRNAs (Friedman et al., 1984, Reed et al., 1987). Our data showed that Chx induced GM-CSF mRNA in unstimulated cells while under the same experimental conditions no IL2 mRNA was detected (Bickel et al., 1989).

All these observations suggest that GM-CSF transcripts in unstimulated cells might be rapidly decaying, whereas transcripts are rendered stable upon LPS or TPA addition. To answer this question we measured the half-life of the GM-CSF mRNA in unstimulated and TPA-stimulated T cells. EL-4 cells were stimulated with TPA or left untreated for 6 hours after which the cells were incubated with actinomycin D (10 mg/ml) and at various time intervals RNA was isolated and the amount of GM-CSF mRNA analyzed. With improved methods for Northern analyses, which included the use of high specific activity cRNA probes, cross-linking of RNA to nylon membranes by exposure to UV light, optimizing signal to noise ratios by lowering background, and prolonged autoradiographic exposures of the blots, we could detect GM-CSF mRNA in unstimulated cells. These methods allowed the direct comparative measurement of GM-CSF half-lives in TPA-stimulated vs unstimulated cells. Our results clearly showed a highly significant increase of GM-CSF mRNA half-life after TPA induction (Bickel et al., 1990). Does LPS act in a similar fashion on B cells? Studies by Thorens et al. (1987) on macrophages stimulated with LPS allowed the inference that LPS also prolongs the half-life of GM-CSF mRNA.

The mechanism of stabilization of the GM-CSF mRNA with TPA is unclear. GM-CSF mRNA contains an AU-rich region in the 3' untranslated portion of its message. These elements have been shown to destabilize normally stable messages such as globin when they are placed at the 3' end (Shaw and Kamen, 1986). Thus, degradation of GM-CSF mRNA before stimulation with TPA may be due to cytoplasmic proteins which interact with this AU rich region of the mRNA and direct its destruction (Malter, 1989). These proteins may be rapidly turned over and hence be highly susceptible to inhibition of protein synthesis. Support but not proof for such a possibility was obtained from our experiments in which cycloheximide was shown to stabilize the GM-CSF mRNA in unstimulated cells.

REFERENCES

Bickel M, Amstad P, Tsuda H, Sulis C, Asofsky R, Mergenhagen SE, Pluznik DH (1987a). Induction of granulocyte-macrophage colony-stimulating factor by lipopolysaccharide and anti-immunoglobulin M-stimulated murine B cell lines. J Immunol 139:2984-2988.

Bickel M, Tsuda H, Amstad P, Evequoz V, Mergenhagen SE, Wahl SM, Pluznik DH (1987b). Differential regulation of colony stimulating factors and interleukin 2 production by cyclosporin A. Proc Natl Acad Sci (USA) 84:3274-3277.

Bickel M, Wahl S, Mergenhagen SE , Pluznik DH (1988). Granulocyte-macrophage colony-stimulating factor regulation in murine T cells and its relation to cyclosporin A. Exp Hematol 16:691-695.

Bickel M, Mergenhagem SE, Pluznik DH (1989). Regulation of granulocyte-macrophage colony-stimulating factor in murine lymphocytes. In Baum SJ, Dicke KA, Lotzova E, Pluznik DH (eds): "Experimental Hematology Today-1988", New York, Springer Verlag, pp 62-67.

Bickel M, Cohen RB, Pluznik DH (1990). Post-transcriptional regulation of granulocyte-macrophage colony stimulating factor synthesis in murine T cells. (submitted).

Castagna M, Takai Y, Kaibushi K, Sano K, Kikkawa V, Nishizuka Y (1982). Direct activation of calcium-activated, phospholipid-dependent protein kinase by tumor-promoting phorbol esters. J Biol Chem 257:7847-7851.

Colombani PM, Robb A, Hess AD (1985). Cyclosporin A binding to calmodulin: a possible site of action on T lymphocytes. Science 228:337-339.

Coutinho A, Forni L, Watanabe T (1978). Genetic and functional characterization of an antiserum to the lipid A-specific triggering receptor on murine B lymphocytes. Eur J Immunol 8:63-67.

Efrat S, Kaempfer R (1984). Control of biologically active interleukin 2 messenger RNA formation in induced human lymphocytes. Proc Natl Acad Sci (USA) 81:2601-2605.

Farrar JJ, Fuller-Farrar J, Simon pl, Hilfiker ML, Stadler BM, Farrar WL (1980). Thymoma production of T cell growth factor (interleukin 2). J Immunol 125:2555-2561.

Friedman AP, Manly SP, McMahon M, Kerr IM, Stark GR (1984). Transcriptional and posttranscriptional regulation of interferon-induced gene expression in human cells. Cell 38:745-755.

Fujii Y, Ohno S, Hidaka H (1985). Quantitative radioautographic study of intracellular localization of calmodulin antagonost, W-7, in chinese-hamster ovary cells. Histochemistry 82:75-80.

Hamano T, Kim KJ, Leiserson WM, Asofsky R (1982). Establishment of B cell hybridomas with B cell surface antigens. J Immunol 129:1403-1406.

Kim KJ, Kanellopoulos-Langevin C, Mervin RM, Sachs DH, Asofsky R (1979). Establishment and characterization of Balb/c lymphoma lines with B cell properties. J Immunol 122:549-554.

Krönke M, Leonard WJ, Depper JM, Arya SK, Wong-Staal F, Gallo RC, Waldman TA, Greene WC (1984). Cyclosporin A inhibits T cell growth factor gene expression at the level of mRNA transcription. Proc Natl Acad Sci (USA) 81:5214-5218.

Lei MG, Morrison DC (1988). Specific endotoxic lipopolysaccharide-binding proteins on murine splenocytes. J Immunol 141:996-1005.

Malagodi MH, Chiou CY (1974). Pharmacological evaluation of a new Ca^{2+} antagonist, TMB-8: Studies in smooth muscles. Eur J Pharmac 27:25-33.

Malter JS (1989). Identification of an AUUUA-specific messenger RNA binding protein. Science 246:664-666.

Metcalf D (1986). The molecular biology and functions of granulocyte-macrophage colony stimulating factors. Blood 67:257-267.

Mochizuki DY, Eisenman JR, Conlon PJ, Park SL, Urdal LD (1986). Development and characterization of antiserum to murine granulocyte-macrophage colony stimulating factor. J Immunol 136:3709-3712.

Mosmann TR, Cossman RL (1987). Two types of mouse helper T-cell clone. Implications for immune regulation. Immunol Today 8:223-227.

Palacios R (1985). Cyclosporin A inhibits antigen-and lectin-induced but not constitutive production of interleukin 3. Eur J Immunol 15:204-206.

Pluznik DH, Cunnigham RE, Noguchi PD (1984). Colony stimulating factor (CSF) controls proliferation of CSF-dependent cells by acting during G1 phase of the cell cycle. Proc Natl Acad Sci (USA) 81:7451-7455.

Pluznik DH, Mergenhagen SE (1986). Synergistic action of lipopolysaccharide and tumor promoting phorbol esters: A two-signal requirement for colony stimulating factor production by murine bone marrow cells. Exp Hematol 14:1029-1036.

Pluznik DH, Bickel M, Mergenhagen SE (1989). B lymphocyte derived hematopoietic growth factors. Immunol Invest 18:103-116.

Reed JC, Alpers JD, Nowell PC (1987). Expression of *c-myc* proto-oncogen in normal human lymphocytes. Regulation by transcriptional and posttranscriptional mechanisms. J Clin Invest 80:101-106.

Robertson HD, Hunter T (1975). A sensitive method for the detection and characterization of double helical ribonucleic acid. J Biol Chem 250:418- 425. Samelson LE,

Schwartz RH (1983). T cell clone-specific alloantisera that inhibit or stimulate antigen-induced T cell activation. J Immunol 131:2645-2661.

Shaw G, Kamen R (1986). A conserved AU sequence from the 3' untranslated region of GM-CSF mRNA mediates selective mRNA degradation. Cell 46:659-667.

Thornes B, Mermod JJ, Vassalli P (1987). Phagocytosis and inflammatory stimuli induce GM-CSF mRNA in macrophage through posttranscriptional regulation. Cell 48:671-679.

Tsien RY (1980). New calcium indicators and buffers with high selectivity against magnesium and protons: design, synthesis, and properties of prototype structures. Biochemistry 19:2396-2404.

Ythier AA, Abud-Filho M, Williams JM, Loertscher R, Schuster MW, Nowill A, Hansen JA, Maltezos D, Storm TB (1985). Interleukin 2-dependent release of interleukin 3 activity by T4+ human T cell clones. Proc Natl Acad Sci (USA) 82:7020-7024.

The Biology of Hematopoiesis, pages 215–223

SYNERGISTIC INTERACTIONS BETWEEN TWO SIGNAL TRANSDUCTION PATHWAYS DURING MEGAKARYOCYTE PROLIFERATION

Michael W. Long
Division of Hematology/Oncology, Department of Pediatrics, University of Michigan, Ann Arbor, MI 48109

Both clinical and laboratory studies indicate that there are at least two levels of regulation within the megakaryocytic lineage: expansion of the progenitor cells (i.e. proliferation) versus differentiation. The earliest clinical study, by Harker and Finch, elegantly demonstrated that patients with megakaryocyte-platelet dyscrasia must have separate controls exerted over expansion of the lineage versus megakaryocyte size (maturation) (Harker, and Finch, 1969). Subsequently, Williams, Long, and others demonstrated the need for multiple factors during *in vitro* murine megakaryocyte development (Williams *et al.* 1982; Long *et al.* 1982b; Long *et al.* 1982a; Long *et al.* 1985; Long *et al.* 1984; Long *et al.* 1988; Straneva *et al.* 1986; Bruno *et al.* 1989; Gewirtz *et al.* 1983).

The *in vitro* proliferation of both human and murine megakaryocyte progenitor cells thus requires the obligate presence of a megakaryocyte colony stimulating activity (Hoffman *et al.* 1985; Williams *et al.* 1986; Long *et al.* 1988). This ability to support megakaryocyte colony formation *in vitro* is a function of both the recombinant interleukin-3 or GM-CSF molecules (Quesenberry *et al.* 1985; Hoffman *et al.* 1985; Long *et al.* 1988). Under the influence of these hematopoietic growth factors, megakaryocyte progenitor cells *in vitro* generate heterogeneous colonies of pure megakaryocytes as well as mixed-phenotype colonies which contain megakaryocytes. Examination of pure megakaryocyte colonies reveals that the maturational development is limited, with the majority of the cells being immature. These early-acting factors thus seem to regulate proliferation and expansion of the lineage while bringing about limited degrees of maturation (Hoffman *et al.* 1985; Long *et al.* 1988).

Optimal megakaryocyte development *in vitro* (for both murine and human cells) requires both the presence of either IL-3 or GM-CSF, as well as a late-acting auxiliary factor(s) which by itself lacks the sole ability to stimulate megakaryocyte colony development, but synergizes with colony stimulating factors to augment megakaryocyte proliferation and differentiation (Williams *et al.* 1986; Long *et al.* 1988). In the human system, these distal-acting activities stimulate increases in colony frequency, cytoplasmic content, antigenic expression, DNA content, and shift the morphological distribution from immature to mature cells (Long *et al.* 1988). Finally, administration of crudely purified preparations of CM containing this activity to murine recipients results in an increase in the rate of platelet production as well as circulating platelet count (Williams *et al.* 1990). Thus, the *in vitro* actions of these synergistic co-regulators mimic *in vitro* all of the known actions of thrombopoietin-enriched preparations when administered *in vivo* (Long *et al.* 1988).

To understand the cytoplasmic events occuring during factor-mediated megakaryocyte development requires large numbers (10^7 - 10^8) of purified target cells (i.e. megakaryocyte progenitor cells or immature megakaryocytes). The low frequency of mature megakaryocytes in the bone marrow (Rabellino *et al.* 1979; Long, and Heffner, 1988), coupled with the even lower frequency of the factor-dependent target cells precludes direct studies on the cellular biochemistry occurring during megakaryocyte proliferation and/or differentiation. However, use of the murine system allows direct detection of megakaryocyte colonies (based on their expression of a lineage-specific cytochemical marker, acetylcholinesterase (Jackson, 1973; Long, and Williams, 1981)). As well, pharmacological probes of cellular activation such as tumor-promoting phorbol diesters for calcium-mediated, protein kinase C related events, or cholera toxin for adenylate cyclase, are known to stimulate these signal transduction systems in other cell systems. By analogy, it is possible to probe megakaryocyte signal transduction events utilizing known pharmacological activators of these systems and directly assess lineage-specific responses by culturing progenitor cells of each lineage.

We hypothesized that if two synergistic co-regulators are required for megakaryocyte development, then it should be possible to implicate two signal transduction systems in this process and these systems should show synergistic interactions. We report that megakaryocyte proliferation requires co-activation of the protein kinase C - calcium mobilization system as well as the adenylate cyclase complex. Finally, synergistic interactions occur between the calcium-protein kinase C system and the adenylate cyclase complex. These observations thus document the biochemical basis of multifactoral regulation of megakaryocytopoiesis.

ACTIVATION OF PROTEIN KINASE C-MEDIATED SIGNAL TRANSDUCTION EVENTS DURING MEGAKARYOCYTE PROLIFERATION AND MATURATION.

We previously described the role of synergistic co-regulators found in conditioned medium prepared from murine pulmonary cells (Williams *et al.* 1982; Long *et al.* 1982b; Long *et al.* 1982a). Such conditioned media (CM) alone failed to support megakaryocyte colony formation and are devoid of detectable levels of colony-stimulating activity, but are a biological source of activities capable of stimulating the later phases of megakaryocyte development. We observed that phorbol myristate acetate, the most powerful of the tumor promoting phorbol diesters, was capable of substituting for this biological source of megakaryocyte potentiating activity, generating a three-fold increase in megakaryocyte colony formations over a range of 10^{-10} - 10^{-6} M (Long *et al.* 1984). This phorbol diester (or its vehicle, DMSO), alone, does not stimulate megakaryocyte colony formation, nor synergize with sources of lung CM, demonstrating that PMA is not a megakaryocyte colony stimulating activity (Long *et al.* 1984). Moreover, megakaryocyte progenitor cells respond equivalently to phorbol diesters under serum-free conditions (Long *et al.* 1986; Long *et al.* 1984; Long *et al.* 1988). The role of accessory cells in phorbol diester-mediated colony development was ruled out using two alternative procedures. Firstly, bone marrow cells exhaustively depleted of adherent cell populations also show a three-fold augmentation of IL-3 dependent colony formation observed when unfractionated populations of bone marrow cells were used as targets (Long *et al.* 1984). Moreover, adherent cells fail to augment IL-3 driven megakaryocyte colony formation when stimulated with high concentrations of phorbol dibutyrate (an active tumor promoting phorbol diester which is more readily washed out of the cell membrane) (Long *et al.* 1984). Finally, phorbol diesters also show synergistic interactions with IL-3 in cultures of highly purified progenitor cell populations (Long *et al.* 1988) It is felt, therefore, that effects of phorbol diesters were not mediated by a population of auxiliary cells producing megakaryocyte synergistic activities.

Examination of the structure:activity relationship between various phorbol diesters and augmentation of megakaryocyte colony development indicated that the two tumor promoting compounds, PMA and phorbol dibutyrate, were able to substitute for the biological co-regulator in megakaryocyte colony forming assays. In contrast, both phorbol 12, 13-diacetate and the parent alcohol phorbol, itself, were inactive either alone or in combination with IL-3, consistent with their lack of an *in vivo* effect in skin tumor promotion (Slaga *et al.* 1980). Interestingly, mezerein, a plant derived ester of 12-hydroxydaphentoxin, which is a competitive analog of phorbol acetate at low concentrations (10^{-12} - 10^{-9} M) (Solanki *et al.* 1981), was capable of inhibiting both PMA-driven colony formation as well as the functional effects of the biological source of synergistic co-regulator. This observation showed that PMA and the biologically synergistic, co-regulator, must share a final common denominator for the induction of differentiation. Given that tumor promoting phorbol diesters are highly lipophilic, they do not function via a membrane receptor but instead bypass the receptor and activate a novel protein kinase (protein kinase C) which plays a role in mediating membrane signal transduction events (Niedel *et al.* 1983; Nishizuka, 1984). This suggests that protein kinase C is the cellular site at which PMA and the biologically derived synergistic co-regulator share a final common signal transduction pathway.

The use of phorbol diesters as probes of megakaryocyte developments also allowed the detection of a previously unrecognized population of megakaryocyte progenitor cells which morphologically resembled erythroid bursts. These megakaryocyte burst colonies contained large numbers of megakaryocytes and were comprised of 2-8 subcolonies (Long *et al.* 1985). Thus, a megakaryocyte burst forming cells are early hematopoietic progenitor cells restricted to megakaryocyte development and characterized by a higher proliferative potential and more mature colony forming megakaryocyte progenitor cells. Additionally, these cells show distinctly different rates of colony development *in vitro*, were separable from the colony forming cell by their physical-chemical characteristics, and demonstrated *in vitro* responsiveness to hematopoietic growth factors (Long *et al.* 1986; Long *et al.* 1985). For example, purified IL-3 alone was capable of stimulating development of the colony forming cells, generating maximal colony numbers between 10 and 40 ng/ml. Nonetheless, PMA augmented colony formation (numbers) at all concentrations of IL-3 tested, demonstrating that IL-3, while obligate, is not sufficient for optimal colony formation (Long *et al.* 1986; Long *et al.* 1985). In contrast to its effects on colony-forming cells IL-3, alone, failed to support the development of the burst forming colonies. Thus, megakaryocyte bursts were only observed in the presence of both types of megakaryocyte regulator: IL-3 and the synergistic co-regulator (or its substitute, phorbol myristatecetate). The above studies show that both classes of murine progenitor cells (i.e. the CFC-Mk and BFC-Mk) respond to two regulatory activities but only at the level of the burst forming cell is the requirement for both absolute. We conclude, then, that a progenitor:progeny relationship exists between the high proliferative (BFC-Mk) and low proliferative potential colony-forming megakaryocyte progenitor cells (CFC-Mk).

THE ROLE OF ADENYLATE CYCLASE IN MEGAKARYOCYTE PROLIFERATION.

The hormone-sensitive adenylate cyclase system consists of the central catalytic unit and two heteromeric protein complexes, all intercollated with the lipids of the plasma membrane (Gilman, 1984a; Gilman, 1984b). This protein complex mediates both positive and negative signals from several types of receptors and ultimately stimulates or inhibits adenylate cyclase catalytic activity. Usually, the receptors for adenylate cyclase mediated stimulatory factors interact with a pair of homologous guanine nucleotide binding regulatory proteins (GNBP) which mediate the stimulation (G_S) or inhibition (G_I) of the catalytic unit of adenylate cyclase. Stimulation of these two types of regulatory GNBP yields an integrated response, eventually resulting in an elevated or decreased cellular concentration of cyclic AMP, thus effectively modulating subsequent protein phosphorylation events (for review see (Gilman, 1984a; Gilman, 1984b)). There are a number of pharmacological probes of adenylate cyclase system: cholera toxin, which stimulates the G_S subunit of the adenylate cyclase complex (Gilman, 1984a; Gilman, 1984b); forskolin, which directly stimulates the catalytic unit of adenylate cyclase (Stenstrom *et al.* 1985); NECA, (5-[N]-ethyl-carboxyamidoadenosine) which is a analog of adenosine and thus is a ligand for the adenosine receptor (Marone *et al.* 1985) and, finally, dibutyryl-cyclic AMP which is a non-hydrolysable analog of cAMP.

Examination of megakaryocyte colony formation stimulated by IL-3 and cholera toxin demonstrated that cholera toxin did not augment IL-3 driven megakaryocyte colony formation (Long *et al.* 1988). As well, cholera toxin alone had no effect. However, cholera toxin further amplified the synergistic interaction observed between IL-3 and tumor promoting phorbol diesters (PMA). The addition of as little as 10 ng/ml cholera toxin results in a detectable increase in PMA-stimulated megakaryocyte colony frequency generating six times as many colonies as observed with IL-3 alone. Interestingly, cholera toxin also caused a similar elevation in the burst forming progenitor cells, markedly enhancing the cellularity and size of these colonies. Moreover, the presence of cholera toxin, IL-3 and PMA allowed observation of a population of megakaryocyte progenitor cells which are analogous to the high proliferative potential colony forming cells (HPP-CFC) observed in the granulocytic lineage, generating megakaryocyte colonies measuring 1-2 mm in diameter (Long *et al.* 1988).

The mechanism by which cholera toxin augments megakaryocyte colony proliferation seems to be one of increasing the absolute number of megakaryocyte colonies as well as changing the sensitivity of the megakaryocyte progenitor cells to PMA. For example, in the presence of cholera toxin, the 50% maximal effect of (EC_{50}) concentration of PMA is reduced by one log for the more mature colony forming cells and for two logs for the burst forming cells (Long *et al.* 1988). It should be noted that the amplification in megakaryocyte colony formation observed with cholera toxin, as well as phorbol diesters is lineage specific as the addition of cholera toxin to IL-3 driven granulocyte or erythroid colony formation either inhibits or has no effect (respectively) on these hematopoietic progenitor cells (Long *et al.* 1988).

Further studies addressing the intracellular activation of adenylate cyclase utilized other probes to substitute for cholera toxin. Thus, forskolin, NECA, and dibutyryl cyclic AMP all show similar augmentation of the synergistic interactions between IL-3 and phorbol diester (Mazur *et al.* 1988; Long, 1989). Each probe of the adenylate cyclase complex acts on a separate region of the complex and all results in a 2-3 fold amplification of IL-3, PMA-driven megakaryocyte colony formation: stimulation of adenylate cyclase agonist receptor with NECA, stimulation of the G_S subunit of the GNBP, forskolin stimulation of the catalytic unit itself, and finally substitution of dibutyryl cyclic AMP for its naturally occurring analog. The above data clearly demonstrate that adenylate cylcase activation strongly augments megakaryocyte proliferation, and further suggest that megakaryocyte proliferation is directly coupled to cyclase mediated signal transduction events.

Our observations indicate that the cellular processes effecting megakaryocyte progenitor cell proliferation are influenced by alterations in both the protein kinase C and adenylate cyclase systems. While the adenylate cyclase system and protein kinase C (and/or calcium calmodulin) are observed synergistically interact during megakaryocyte development, the final effect of these interactions is that megakaryocyte progenitor cell response to activation of second messenger systems must depend on the effector of these transductions systems: differences in phosphoproteins. These remain to be elucidated.

REFERENCES

Bruno E, Miller ME, and Hoffman R (1989) Interacting cytokines regulate *in vitro* human megakaryocytopoiesis. Blood 73:671-677.

Gewirtz AM, Bruno E, Elwell J, and Hoffman R (1983) *In vitro* studies of megakaryocytopoiesis in thrombocytotic disorders of man. Blood 61:384-389.

Gilman AG (1984a) G proteins and dual control of adenylate cyclase. Cell 36:577-579.

Gilman AG (1984b) Guanine nucleotide-binding regulatory proteins and dual control of adenylate cyclase. J Clin Invest 73:1-4.

Harker LA, and Finch CA (1969) Thrombokinetics in man. J Clin Invest 48:963-974.

Hoffman R, Yang HH, Bruno E, and Straneva, JE (1985) Purification and partial characterization of a megakaryocyte colony-stimulating factor from human plasma. J Clin Invest 75:1174-1182.

Jackson CW (1973) Cholinesterase as a possible marker for early cells of the megakaryocytic series. Blood 42:413-421.

Long MW, Williams N, and Ebbe S (1982a) Immature megakaryocytes in the mouse: physical characteristics, cell cycle status, and in vitro responsiveness to thrombopoietic stimulatory factor. Blood 59:569-575.

Long MW, Williams N, and McDonald TP (1982b) Immature megakaryocytes in the mouse: in vitro relationship to megakaryocyte progenitor cells and mature megakaryocytes. J Cell Physiol 112:339-344.

Long MW, Smolen JE, Szczepanski P, and Boxer, LA (1984) Role of phorbol diesters in *in vitro* murine megakaryocyte colony formation. J Clin Invest 74:1686-1692.

Long MW, Gragowski LL, Heffner CH, and Boxer LA (1985) Phorbol diesters stimulate the development of an early murine progenitor cell. The burst-forming unit-megakaryocyte. J Clin Invest 67:431-438.

Long MW, Heffner CH, and Gragowski LL (1986) In vitro differences in responsiveness of early (BFU-Mk) and late (CFU-Mk) murine megakaryocyte progenitor cells. Prog Clin Biol Res 215:179-186.

Long MW, and Heffner CH (1988) Detection of human megakaryocyte antigens by solid-phase radioimmunoassay. Exp Hematol 16:62-70.

Long MW, Hutchinson RJ, Gragowski LL, Heffner CH, and Emerson SG (1988) Synergistic regulation of human megakaryocyte development. J Clin Invest 82:1779-1786.

Long MW, and Williams N (1981) Immature megakaryocytes in the mouse: Morphology and quantitation acetylcholinersterase staining. Blood 58:1032-1039.

Long MW, Heffner CH, and Gragowski LL (1988) Cholera toxin and phorbol diesters synergistically modulate murine hematopoietic progenitor cell proliferation. Exp Hematol 16:195-200.

Long MW (1989) Signal transduction events in *In Vitro* megakaryocytopoiesis. Blood Cells 15:205-235.

Marone G, Petracca R, and Vigorita S (1985) Adenosine receptors on human inflammatory cells. Int Archs Allergy Appl Immunol 77:259-263.

Mazur EM, Cohen JL, and Bogart L (1988) Growth characteristics of circulating hematopoietic progenitor cells from patients with esssential thrombocythemia. Blood 71:1544-1550.

Niedel JE, Kuhn LJ, and Vandenbark GR (1983) Phorbol diester receptor copurifies with protein kinase C. Proc Natl Acad Sci USA 80:36-40.

Nishizuka Y (1984) The role of protein kinase C in cell surface signal transduction and tumour promotion. Nature 308:693-698.

Quesenberry PJ, Ihle JN, and McGrath E (1985) The effect of interleukin 3 and GM-CSA-2 on megakaryocyte and myeloid clonal colony formation. Blood 65:214-217.

Rabellino EM, Nachman RL, Williams N, Winchester RJ, and Ross GD (1979) Human megakaryocytes. I. Characterization of the membrane and cytoplasmic components of isolated marrow megakaryocytes. J Exp Med 149:1273-1287.

Slaga J, Fischer SM, Nelson K, and Gleason GL (1980) Studies on the mechanism of skin tumor promotion: Evidence for several stages in promotion. Proc Natl Acad Sci USA 77:3659-3663.

Solanki V, Slaga TJ, Callaham M, and Huberman, E (1981) Down regulation of specific binding of [20-3H]phorbol 12,13-dibutyrate and phorbol ester-induced differentiation of human promyelocytic leukemia cells. Proc Natl Acad Sci USA 78:1722-1725.

Stenstrom S, Seppala M, Pfenning M, and Richelson E (1985) Inhibition by ethanol of forskolin-stimulated adenyolate cyclase in a murine neuroblastoma clone (N1E-115). Biochem Pharmacol 34:3655-3659.

Straneva JE, Goheen MP, Hui SL, Bruno E, and Hoffman R (1986) Terminal cytoplasmic maturation of human megakaryocytes *in vitro*. Exp Hematol 14:919-929.

Williams JL, Heffner CH, and Long MW (1990) Regulation of *in vitro* human megakaryocyte maturation. In: "Megakaryocytes: Molecular and Cellular Biology," New York: Alan Liss, in press.

Williams N, Eger RR, Jackson HM, and Nelson DJ (1982) Two-factor requirement for murine megakaryocyte colony formation. J Cell Physiol 110:101-104.

Williams N, Oon SH, Jackson H, and Lim R (1986) Studies on megakaryocyte potentiator: its production and some biochemical characteristics. Prog Clin Biol Res 215:91-103.

The Biology of Hematopoiesis, pages 225–226

REGULATION OF ERYTHROPOIETIN GENE EXPRESSION

Eugene Goldwasser and Nega Beru

Department of Biochemistry and Molecular Biology and Department of Medicine, Section of Hematology/ Oncology, The University of Chicago

A line of mouse spleen cells (IW32) transformed by a helper-independent ecotropic, murine leukemia virus, expresses erythropoietin (epo) constitutively. There are both a normal and a rearranged epo gene in these cells with the rearranged gene being amplified about six-fold. Dnase-1 hypersensitivity expriments indicate that the normal gene is not expressed and that the rearranged gene is. We have shown that there are no viral sequences within 4.5 kb upstream and 9.5 kb downstream of the epo gene, suggesting that expression is not due to viral LTR sequences. We have analyzed the upstream sequence of the rearranged epo gene and found, on the complementary strand, 2 CAAT boxes, a TATA box, a ribosome binding site, 2 SP-1 binding sites and an open reading frame encoding 25 amino acids. This "new" gene is expressed in these cells, in two other similarly transformed cells, in mouse bone marrow but not in the liver, brain, kidney or spleen. We suggest that constitutive expression of the epo gene in these hemopoietic cells is a consequence of the adventitious rearrangement of the epo gene to the proximity of the "new" gene which is expressed in these cells. To date, we have found no homology in the data banks with the "new" gene, either at the nucleotide or at the amino acid level.

The regulation of the normal renal epo gene has been studied by the mobility shift assay. Computer matching has shown a segment of the upstream region from 30 to 60 bp upstream of the start site that is identical in the mouse and human genes. Using a synthetic 31 base oligonucleotide we found that the 5' 17 base segment of this sequence specifically binds a component extracted from the nuclei of mouse kidney. This component has an apparent molecular size of 24 kd on a SDS gel. This factor is decreased about 10 fold when the nuclei are taken from kidney of hypoxic mice. Additonal evidence suggests that the specific binding component of the nuclei is a ribonucleoprotein. It would appear then, that the renal epo gene is regulated, in part, by a negative trans-acting factor, the loss of which permits the gene to be switched on.

The Biology of Hematopoiesis, pages 227–232

ERYTHROPOIETIN STRUCTURE-FUNCTION RELATIONSHIPS

Jean-Paul Boissel and H. Franklin Bunn

Division of Hematology and Department of Medicine, Brigham and Women's Hospital, Harvard Medical School, Boston, Massachusetts, 02115

INTRODUCTION

The glycoprotein hormone erythropoietin (Epo) is the primary regulator of erythropoiesis in man and other mammals (Goldwasser, 1984; Golde and Gasson, 1988). The molecular cloning of the Epo genes of man (Jacobs et al, 1985; Lin et al, 1985), monkey (Lin et al, 1986) and mouse (Shoemaker et al, 1986) has greatly enhanced studies on the molecular events responsible for Epo production as well as its mechanism of action. The hormone is produced in the fetal liver and adult kidney in response to hypoxic stimulus. As the hormone circulates in plasma, it is available for binding to receptors on the surface of erythroid precursor cells in the bone marrow, inducing proliferation and terminal maturation.

The human erythropoietin gene codes for a 193 aa protein. Following cleavage of a 27 aa leader sequence, the mature protein has a calculated molecular weight of 18,490. Post-translational glycosylation is clearly required for in vivo function. Human Epo contains 39% carbohydrate giving it an Mr of 30,400 when measured accurately by sedimentation equilibrium (Davis et al, 1987). Complex N-linked glycosylation (85% tetra-antennary) takes place on three asparagine residues (Residues 24, 38 and 83) (Lai et al, 1986). When the formation of complex polysaccharides is blocked by the inhibitor 1-deoxymannojirimycin, the Epo product contains approximately 50% less carbohydrate but retains full biological activity (Wojchowski et al, 1987). Likewise, when glycosylation is attenuated by expression in insect cells, the Epo product contains only around 30% of its normal complement of carbohydrate but is fully active (Wojchowski et al, 1987). Site-directed mutagenesis (Asn→Glu) at position 24 did not affect biosynthesis whereas at 38 and 83, there was no detectable protein in the cell extract or medium despite normal levels of mRNA (Dube et al, 1987). Human and monkey Epo have one O-linked glycosylation site at Ser126 (Sasaki et al, 1987). All of the N-linked glycosylation sites are preserved in monkey and mouse Epo while in mouse Ser126 is replaced by Pro. It is not known whether mouse Epo has any alternative O-linked glycosylation sites. Surprisingly, abolition of O-linked glycosylation by the site directed mutation 126 Ser→Gly causes human

Epo to lose all of its biological activity (Dube et al, 1987). Thorough structural analyses show that recombinant Epo expressed in mammalian cells [Chinese hamster ovary cells (CHO)] is nearly identical in carbohydrate sequence to the native protein (Sasaki et al, 1987; Takeuchi et al, 1988). Desialated Epo (Goldwasser et al, 1974) has normal or even enhanced (Mufson and Gesner, 1987) biologic function in vitro but has no activity when assayed in vivo.

Human and monkey Epo contains two disulphide bonds, Cys29-Cys33 and Cys7-Cys161 (Sitkowsky, 1980; Wang et al, 1985). Both appear to be essential for the function of the molecule. Reduction of both disulfide bonds results in loss of biological activity. Mouse Epo lacks the former disulfide bond because of replacement of Cys by Pro at position 33. In contrast, site directed mutagenesis of 33 Cys→Pro in human Epo results in complete loss of biological activity (Lin, 1987). As with O-linked glycosylation mentioned above, the limited data from site-directed mutagenesis are in apparent conflict with inter-species comparisons of primary structure.

One approach to delineate the functional domains of a protein is to develop monospecific antibodies that recognize limited epitopes on the surface of the molecule. Sytkowski and his colleagues (1985, 1987) have raised antibodies to peptides (9-19 residues) corresponding to seven non-overlapping putative hydrophilic stretches on human Epo. Although all but one of the 7 antibodies bound tightly to Epo, only anti-peptides 99-118 and 111-129 blocked Epo's biological activity. This result makes region 99-129 a candidate for the domain that interacts with the Epo receptor. However steric factors, owing to the large size of the antibody, as well as the likely contribution of non-contiguous residues in a globular protein make this experiment difficult to interpret.

Another powerful approach for delineating structure-function relationships of a protein is to study a series of scanning mutants in which the entire coding region has been sequentially and systematically altered. In this brief report we describe preliminary results on deletion mutants of human Epo.

RESULTS AND DISCUSSION

The method of Kunkel et al (1987) was employed for the preparation of mutants of Epo. This strategy entails placing the gene to be mutated into an M13 vector and transforming the E Coli strain CJ236 (dut- ung-) which is deficient in two enzymes: dUTPase (dut) and uracil N-glycolase (ung). Deficiency of the former results in elevated levels of dUTP, thereby competing with dTTP for incorporation into DNA. Deficiency of uracil N-glycosylase prevents the removal of uracil that has been incorporated into DNA. The uracil containing single strand template is isolated and hybridized with the complementary mutated primer and filled in by the addition of dNTPs and Klenow. This heteroduplex vector is then used to transform E Coli MV1190, which contains normal levels of the two enzymes. Thus the parental (non-mutated, uracil containing) strand is not replicated. This strategy enables highly efficient selection of the newly synthesized mutant strand. In the mutant Epo's that we have prepared to date, the per cent positive plaques, as determined by DNA sequencing, ranged between 40 and 85 %.

In deciding on a logical and sequential choice of Epo mutants to test structure-function relationships, we have relied heavily on current information on Epo structure: the primary sequences of human, monkey and mouse Epo's, and schematized in the Figure below, as well as the sites for disulfide bonds and carbohydrate attachment. Stretches of primary structure that are homologous are more likely to represent functionally important domains. The figure below depicts both conservative and non-conservative amino acid replacements. The primary structure also permits a crude prediction of secondary structure. Chou-Fasman rules (1978) when applied to human Epo predict stretches of α helix and β sheet as depicted below. This result agrees reasonably well with the measured α helical content of 50% in human Epo (Davis et al. 1987; Lai et al. 1986). As in certain other globular proteins, the Chou-Fasman algorithm overpredicts β-pleated sheet in Epo. Also shown in this figure is the prediction of a computer algorithm of the surface residues of human Epo according to Emini et al (1985).

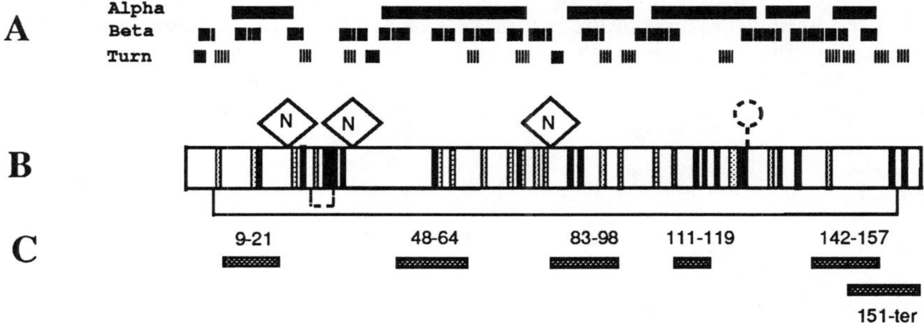

Figure 1 Scheme depicting the structural features of Epo and the deletion mutants tested to date.

A. Predictions of α helix, β pleated sheet and non-helical turns according to Chou-Fasman rules.

B. Homologies in primary sequence between human, monkey and mouse Epo's. Conservative amino acid replacements are shown by shading, non-conservative by black spaces. The remaining white spaces show sequence identity. The two disulfides bonds in primate Epo's are shown below. Mouse Epo lacks the one in dashed lines. The N-linked glycosylation sites are shown by diamonds and the O-linked (lacking in mouse Epo) by the dashed circle.

C. Deletion mutants that were prepared and tested (see Table 1).

As a starting point in choosing a set of informative Epo mutants, deletion mutants have been prepared corresponding to each of the seven predicted stretches of surface residues. These correspond reasonably well to stretches of conserved primary structure. The boundaries of these deletions (depicted in the above figure and shown in detail in the Appendix) are as follows: Δ9-21 (i.e. residues 9 through 21 deleted), Δ48-64, Δ83-98, Δ111-119, Δ142-150, Δ151-157 and Δ151-term. The first six were prepared by using mutant primers that loop out the deleted segment and the last employed a mutation to a termination codon at position 150.

Expression of normal and mutant Epo's For expression in mammalian cells we have used the RK1-4MA expression vector, kindly supplied by Dr. Randy Kauffman at Genetics Institute. In this vector, the Epo cDNA insert is driven by a strong adenovirus promoter. The addition of non-coding DHFR sequence at the 3' end of the Epo mRNA imparts added stability to the message. With the use of the RK1-4MA vector, normal Epo and the 7 deletion mutants have been expressed transiently in the Cos7 monkey kidney cell line. These deletions preserve the reading frame and therefore do not alter the amino acid sequence 3' to the deletion. The Epo radioimmune assay and the ex vivo bioassay of Krystal (1983) were used to measure Epo in the medium. Cell lysates were prepared in the presence of inhibitors of proteolysis. Northern blot analysis showed that all mutants produced about the same amount of mRNA as that of the wild type. Epo levels after 48 hours incubation are shown in the Table below:

Table 1. Expression and Production of Normal and Mutant Epo's in Cos7 Cells

Mutant	Epo mRNA	Cytosolic Epo RIA mU/ml	Secreted Epo RIA mU/ml	Secreted Epo Bioassay mU/ml
Wild type	+	415	9900	8700
Δ9-21	+	<0.5	<0.5	<1.0
Δ48-64	+	<0.5	<0.5	<1.0
Δ83-98	+	<0.5	<0.5	<1.0
Δ111-119	+	350	9200	7500
Δ142-150	+	<0.5	<0.5	<1.0
Δ151-157	+	<0.5	<0.5	<1.0
Δ151-term	+	<0.5	<0.5	<1.0

The wild type Epo cDNA produces and exports a large quantity of immunologically reactive and biologically active Epo in Cos7 cells. One deletion mutant, Δ111-119, produced and exported nearly as much Epo as the wild type. This mutant Epo appears to have full biological activity. Thus the site on Epo responsible for receptor binding and/or internalization is very unlikely be include residues 111-119. Moreover the efficient export of this mutant can probably be explained by the fact that the deleted residues do not include any of the glycosylation sites and should not affect disulfide bond formation. In contrast, no

Epo was detected in the media or cytosol following transfection with any of the other deletion mutants. Experiments are currently underway to determine whether these mutants have blocked processing or export.

The results presented here on scanning deletion mutants of Epo are in excellent agreement with a preliminary computer generated model of the three dimensional structure of Epo, developed recently by Dr. Fred Cohen at the University of California, San Francisco. The constraints of primary structure and the known disulfide bonds indicate a possible globular structure composed of two antiparallel pairs of alpha helical bundles. All deletions that we made within each of these 4 helical domains resulted in an unstable Epo product with no detectable biologic activity. In contrast the one deletion mutant (Δ111-119) which lies well outside the predicted alpha helical bundles was stable with full retention of biologic activity. Examination of linker scanning mutants should enable a rigorous test of this structural model and should also provide information on the biologically important domains of the molecule, particularly the receptor binding site.

ACKNOWLEDGEMENT

This work was supported by Grant RO1 HL42949-01 from the National Heart, Lung and Blood Institute of the National Institutes of Health.

REFERENCES

Chou PY, Fasman GD (1978). Empirical predictions of protein conformation. Ann Rev Biochem 47:251-276.

Davis JM, Arakawa T, Strickland TW, Yphantis DA (1987). Characterization of recombinant human erythropoietin produced in Chines hamster ovary cells. Biochemistry 26:2633-2638.

Dube S, Lin N, Manger R, Fisher JW, Powell JS (1987). Erythropoietin (EP) requires specific addition of carbohydrate (CHO) side chains for intracellular processing and secretion. Blood 70:170a.

Emini EA, Hughes JV, Perlow DS, Boger J (1985). Induction of hepatitis A virus-neutralizing antibody by a virus-specific synthetic peptide. J Virol 55:836-839.

Golde DW, Gasson JC (1988). Hormones that stimulate the growth of blood cells. Scientific American, July:62-68.

Goldwasser E, Kung CK-H, Eliason J (1974). On the mechanism of erythropoietin-induced differentiation. XIII. The role of sialic acid in erythropoietin action. J Biol Chem 249:4202-4206.

Goldwasser E (1984). Erythropoietin and its mode of action. Blood Cells 10:147-162.

Jacobs K, Shoemaker C, Rudersdorf R, Neill SD, Kaufman RJ, Mufson A, Seehra J, Jones SS, Hewick R, Fritsch EF, Kawakita M, Shimizu T, Miyake T (1985). Isolation and characterization of genomic and cDNA clones of human erythropoietin. Nature 313:806-810.

Krystal G (1983). A simple microassay for erythropoietin based on ^{3}H-thymidine incorporation into spleen cells from phenylhydrazine treated mice. Exp Hematol 11:649-660.

Kunkel TA, Roberts JD, Zakour RA (1987). Rapid and efficient site-specific mutagenesis without phenotypic selector. Meth Enzymol 154:367-382.

Lai P-H, Everett R, Wang F-F, Arakawa T, Goldwasser E (1986). Structural characterization of human erythropoietin. J Biol Chem 261:3116-3121.

Lin F-K, Suggs S, Lin C-H, Browne JK, Smalling R, Egrie JC, Chen KK, Fox GM, Martin F, Stabinsky Z, Badrawi SM, Lai P-H, Goldwasser E (1985). Cloning and expression of the human erythropoietin gene. Proc Natl Acad Sci USA 82:7580-7585.

Lin F-K, Lin C-H, Lai P-H, Browne JK, Egrie JC, Smalling R, Fox GM, Chen KK, Castro M, Suggs S (1986). Monkey erythropoietin gene: cloning, expression and comparison with the human erythropoietin gene. Gene 44:201-209.

Lin F-K (1987). The molecular biology of erythropoietin. NATO ASI Series H8:23-36.

Mufson RA, Gesner TG (1987). Binding and internalization of recombinant human erythropoietin in murine erythroid precursor cells. Blood 69:1485-1490.

Sasaki H, Bothner B, Dell A, Fukuda M (1987). Carbohydrate structure of erythropoietin expressed in Chinese hamster ovary cells by a human erythropoietin cDNA. J Biol Chem 262:12059-12076.

Shoemaker CB, Mitsock LD (1986). Murine erythropoietin gene: cloning, expression, and human gene homology. Mol & Cell Biol 6:849-858.

Sytkowski AJ (1980). Denaturation and renaturation of human erythropoietin. Biochem Biophys Res Commun 96:143-149.

Sytkowski AJ, Fisher JW (1985). Isolation and characterization of an anti-peptide monoclonal antibody to human erythropoietin. J Biol Chem 260:14727- 14731.

Sytkowski AJ, Donahue KA (1987). Immunochemical studies of human erythropoietin using site-specific anti-peptide antibodies. J Biol Chem 262:1161-1165.

Takeuchi M, Takasaki S, Miyazaki H, Kato T, Hoshi S, Kochibe N, Kobata A (1988). Comparative study of the asparagine-linked sugar chains of human erythropoietins purified from urine and the culture medium of recombinant Chinese hamster ovary cells. J Biol Chem 263:3657-3663.

Wang FF, Kung CK-H, Goldwasser E (1985). Some chemical properties of human erythropoietin. Endocrinology 116:2286-2292.

Wojchowski DM, Orkin SH, Sytkowski AJ (1987). Active human erythropoietin expressed in insect cells using a baculovirus vector: a role for N-linked oligosaccharide. Biochim Biophys Acta 910:224-232.

The Biology of Hematopoiesis, pages 233–239

INTERLEUKIN-1 STIMULATION STABILIZES GM-CSF mRNA IN HUMAN VASCULAR ENDOTHELIAL CELLS: PRELIMINARY STUDIES ON THE ROLE OF THE 3' AU RICH MOTIF

G.C. Bagby, G. Shaw, M.C. Heinrich,
S. Hefeneider, M.A. Brown, T.G. DeLoughery,
G.M. Segal, and L. Band

Molecular Hematology (G.C.B., M.C.H., L.B.) and Immunology Research (S.H.) Laboratories, V.A. Medical Center; Division of Hematology and M. Oncology (G.C.B., M.C.H., M.A.B., T.G.D., G.M.S.), Oregon Health Sciences University, Portland, OR 97201, and Genetics Institute (G.S.), Cambridge, MA 02140

The hematopoietic activity of IL-1 is mediated indirectly and derives from its ability to induce the expression of other interleukin and CSF genes which themselves function as direct-acting effector molecules (Sieff et al., 1988; Bagby, 1989a). Because vascular endothelial cells (EC) abound in hematopoietic tissues and respond to IL-1 by producing IL-6, GM-CSF, G-CSF, ELAM-1, and IL-1 (Warner et al., 1987; Sironi et al., 1989; Bagby et al., 1989b; Segal and Bagby, 1988; Zsebo et al., 1988; Bevilacqua et al., 1989) these cells play a vital role in regulating hematopoietic cellular growth and differentiation.

The complexity of the interleukin/CSF network is enormous. Indeed, it is now clear that any two or more of these hematopoietic microenvironmental cells are capable of forming a complex intercellular communication network involving many cytokines each of which has heterogeneous biological activities. In this network abound hierarchies (Bagby, 1989a; Sieff et al., 1988), synergistic bioactivities (Hoang et al., 1988; Williams and Broxmeyer, 1988; Ikebuchi et al., 1988), autocrine amplification mechanisms (Tartakovsky et al., 1988; Dalton et al., 1989; Cozzolino et al., 1989), and paracrine amplification loops (Lindemann et al., 1989; Sisson and Dinarello, 1988). Although the surface of this CSF/ interleukin network has been merely scratched, it is clear that paracrine abnormalities may also account for certain pathophysiological attributes of hematopoietic neoplasms (Griffin et al., 1987; Bagby et al., 1988; Oster et al., 1989; Kawano et al., 1989).

The role of EC in the IL-1/CSF network has been a focus of our group for a number of years (Bagby et al., 1983). One of our current objectives is to elucidate the exact molecular mechanisms by which IL-1 induces expression by of hematopoietic growth factors and interleukins. First, we and others determined that IL-1 induces GM-CSF mRNA accumulation in ECs (Broudy et al., 1987; Sieff et al., 1987; Zsebo et al., 1988). In our laboratory similar results were found using IL-6, G-CSF, and IL-1β cDNAs as probes.

TRANSCRIPTIONAL CONTROL OF GM-CSF EXPRESSION

We tested the notion that IL-1 induces transcription of the cytokine genes by using nuclear runoff analysis, DNase I hypersensitivity site analyses and promoter-reporter analysis. None of these studies demonstrated a transcriptional effect (not shown). Based on these observations reasoned that IL-1's inductive effect is entirely post-transcriptional, a notion congruent with that recently reported by Gasson's group in promoter-reporter analysis of GM-CSF gene expression in fibroblasts (Nimer et al., 1989).

GM-CSF GENE TRANSCRIPT METABOLISM

GM-CSF and G-CSF mRNA molecules are very short lived in uninduced cells (Shaw and Kamen, 1986; Ernst et al., 1989). Shaw and Kamen (Shaw and Kamen, 1986) have demonstrated that an AU rich motif in the 3' untranslated region of the GM-CSF gene mediates transcript instability. This motif is shared by a variety of IL-1 inducible cytokines, including G-CSF, TNF-α, IL-6 (Shaw and Kamen, 1986), IL-8 (Mukaida et al., 1989), ELAM-1 (Bevilacqua et al., 1989), and IL-1 (Shaw and Kamen, 1986). Although the ribonucleases which account for the degradation of cytokine mRNA have not been identified, that these cytokines have intrinsically short half lives suggested to us that IL-1 might increase transcript levels by slowing the rate of mRNA decay.

We employed Actinomycin-D chase (Bagby et al., 1989b) experiments to test this notion. While the half life of GM-CSF mRNA in unstimulated EC was less than 2 hours, GM-CSF mRNA in IL-1-stimulated cells was completely stable for more than 6 hours of Actinomycin D exposure (Bagby et al., 1989b).

THE AU-RICH 3′ UT, mRNA DECAY AND TRANSLATION

The AU rich 3′ untranslated regions of certain transcripts for cytokines and nuclear proto-oncogenes clearly play a role in the function and metabolism of gene transcripts. In addition to the evidence (cited above) from Shaw and Kamen (Shaw and Kamen, 1986), Wreschner and Rechavi have determined that transcripts with AU rich 3′ untranslated regions are unstable in a crude cell free system (Wreschner and Rechavi, 1988). They propose that there exists an inverse correlation between RNA stability and content of 3′ UT $(U)_nA$ sequences.

Others have recently reported that AU rich 3′UT of mRNAs inhibit translation. Kruys and her colleagues have found that translation of *in vitro* transcripts in Xenopus oocytes is inhibited by the AU rich 3′ untranslated regions of β-interferon (Kruys et al., 1988), c-fos, and GM-CSF (Kruys et al., 1989). While this model does clearly show that cytoplasmic factors can identify unique structural elements of the 3′ UT, the dearth of ribonucleases in oocytes (the AU rich mRNAs are quite stable in oocytes [Kruys et al., 1989]) and the short half-life of wild-type transcripts in cells of higher eukaryotes suggest that this model may not be wholly relevant to cytokine gene control. Translational control, while obviously important, will be difficult to analyze in stromal cells without first defining the differential kinetics of mRNA decay and the role of the AU rich element in the IL-1 mRNA-degradation response. Therefore, we have chosen to focus on the role of the AU rich region on differential mRNA metabolism in whole cells. Accordingly we sought to transfect cells with reporter genes attached to AU rich 3′ regions or mutants thereof to: 1) confirm that the AU rich element is a decay element, and 2) to test the notion that IL-1 treatment of the transfected cell would stabilize the reporter transcript.

PROMOTER-REPORTER DECAY EXPERIMENTS WITH L CELLS

After having determined that murine L cells possessed high affinity receptors for recombinant human IL-1α (not shown), we transfected murine L cells with the promoter reporter decay plasmids originally described by Shaw and Kamen (Shaw and Kamen, 1986). In these constructions the 3′ untranslated region of the rabbit β-globin gene was mutated by insertion of either the AU rich element of GM-CSF, or a mutant element in which every ATTTA sequence was disrupted by one or more point mutations (Fig. 1). L cells were transformed by calcium phosphate precipitation (Rosenthal, 1989) and selected in G418. After selection, confluent cells were exposed to either control medium or to recombinant human IL-1α (3 ng/ml) overnight and RNA was extracted (MacDonald et al., 1987) for Northern blot analysis (Fig. 2). The AU rich region did function as an instability element, but apparently not as an IL-1 response element in these cells.

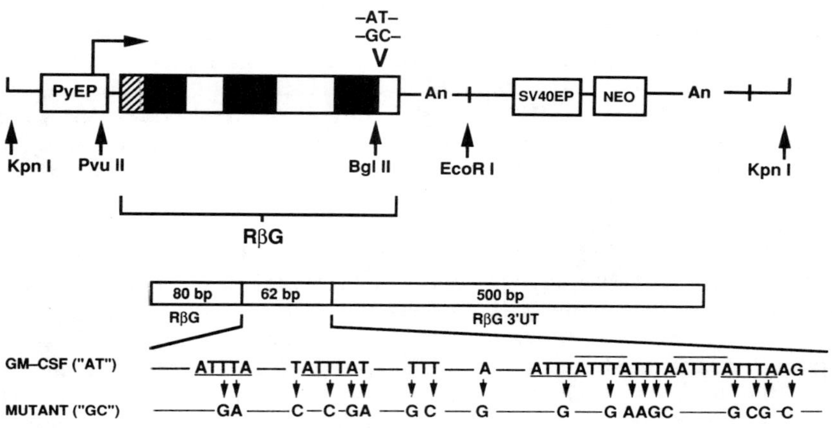

Figure 1. Two plasmids were used for L-cell transfection. TOP: Each contained polyoma early promoter upstream of rabbit β-globin and SV40 promoted neo gene for selection. The 3′ untranslated region of the rabbit β-globin gene was mutated by insertion of one of two 62 base pair elements; AT or GC. BOTTOM: The structure of the AT and GC inserts. Note that in GC the reiterated ATTTA sequences are each disrupted by from one to four point mutations (arrows).

These observations could be explained in two equally plausible ways. First, the 3′ UT is not an IL-1 response element in these or in any other cell. Alternatively, unique second messenger systems required to couple the IL-1 stimulus with the GM-CSF mRNA response in human ECs might not exist in L-cells. We carried out studies designed to prove that L cells could respond to IL-1. We stimulated L cells with human IL-1 alpha (kindly supplied by Peter Lomedico) overnight then tested the supernatant medium for GM-CSA using normal murine marrow cells as targets. IL-1 failed to induce GM-CSF or G-CSF expression in these cells. Similarly, L cells transfected with a human genomic GM-CSF clone,GM-CSFpUC-18, (kindly provided by Dr. Judy Gasson) did express GM-colony stimulating activity for human marrow cells, but GM-CSF expression did not increase in IL-1-stimulated cells. Consequently, we have concluded that while L cells might be appropriate cellular models for studies on constitutive RNA decay, they are not appropriate prototypes for studies on the mechanisms by which IL-1 stabilizes AU rich transcripts.

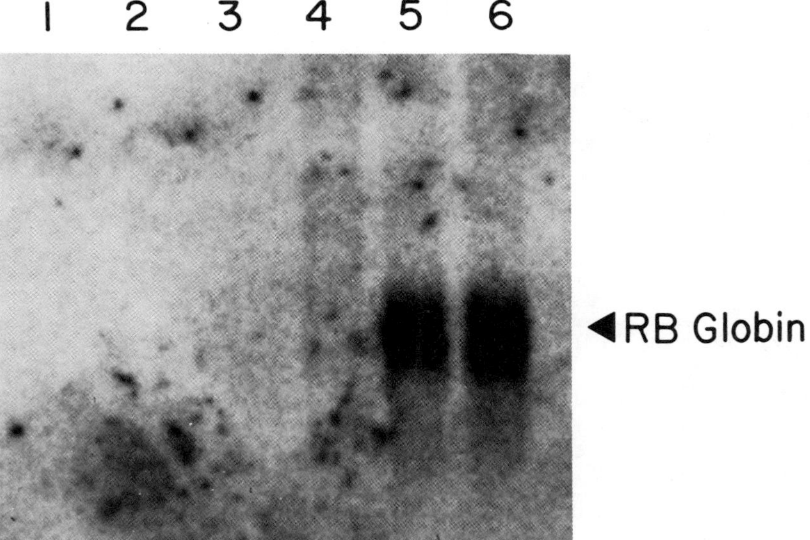

Figure 2. Rabbit β-globin RNA from untransformed L cells treated with medium or IL-1 are shown in lanes 1 and 2 respectively. In lanes 3 and 4 is RNA from the 3′ AU

(Continued)

(Fig. 2 Continued)

transfectants. Lane three RNA is from cells treated with medium alone, lane four is RNA from cells treated with human IL-1 alpha. In neither case was RNA detectable. In lanes four and five, rabbit β-globin RNA from the GC mutants is readily detectable, but no effect of IL-1 treatment (lane 6) is seen.

SUMMARY

To date, the notion that the AU rich motif in the 3′ UT of GM-CSF mRNA can function as an IL-1 response element has not been adequately examined. We suspect that it must play some role because virtually all IL-1 inducible genes have AU rich 3′ untranslated regions. Thus, we will continue to address these technical problems so that the hypothesis can be more clearly tested. Nonetheless, we can state with reasonable certainty that: 1) IL-1 induces expression of GM-CSF in EC by inducing accumulation of mRNA, 2) the GM-CSF gene is constitutively transcribed but the half life of the mRNA is short, 3) IL-1 induced mRNA accumulation results from stabilization of the transcript, 4) although most IL-1 responsive genes have AU-rich domains in their 3′ untranslated regions, it is not yet clear that these AU-rich regions are sufficient to function as an IL-1 response element, and 5) murine L cells cannot be used for studies on the molecular biology of cytokine induction by IL-1.

REFERENCES

Bagby GC, McCall E, Bergstrom KA, Burger D (1983). *Blood* 62:663-668.

Bagby GC, Dinarello CA, Neerhout RC, Ridgway D, McCall E, (1988). *J Clin Invest* 82:1430-1436.

Bagby GC (1989a). *Blood Rev* 3:152-161.

Bagby GC, Shaw G, Segal GM (1989b). *J Invest Derm* 93:48S-52S.

Bevilacqua MP, Stengelin S, Gimbrone MA, Seed B (1989) *Science* 243:1160-1165.

Broudy VC, Kaushansky K, Harlan JM, Adamson JW (1987). *J Immunol* 139:464-468.

Cozzolino F, Rubartelli A, Aldinucci D, Sitia R, Torcia M, Shaw A, Di Guglielmo R (1989). *Proc Natl Acad Sci USA* 86:2369-2373.

Dalton BJ, Connor JR, Johnson WJ (1989). *Arthritis Rheum* 32: 279-287.

Ernst TJ, Ritchie AR, O'Rourke R, Griffin JD (1989). *Leukemia* 3:620–625.

Griffin JD, Rambaldi A, Vellenga E, Young DC, Ostapovicz D, Cannistra SA (1987). *Blood* 70:1218–1221.

Hoang T, Haman A, Goncalves O, Letendre F, Mathieu M, Wong GG, Clark SC (1988). *J Exp Med* 168:463–474.

Ikebuchi K, Ihle JN, Hirai Y, Wong GG, Clark SC, Ogawa M (1988). *Blood* 72:2007–2014.

Kawano M, Tanaka H, Ishikawa H, Nobuyoshi M, Iwato K, Asaoku H, Tanabe O, Kuramoto A (1989). *Blood* 73:2145–2148.

Kruys V, Marinx O, Shaw G, Deschamps J, Huez G (1989). *Science* 245:852–855.

Kruys VI, Wathelet MG, Huez GA (1988). *Gene* 72:191–200.

Lindemann A, Riedel D, Oster W, Ziegler-Heitbrock HWL, Mertelsmann R, Herrmann F (1989). *J Clin Invest* 83:1308–1312.

MacDonald RJ, Swift GH, Przybyla AE, Chirgwin JM (1987). *Methods Enzymol* 152:219–227.

Mukaida N, Shairoo M, Matsushima K (1989) *J Immunol* 143: 1366–1371.

Nimer SD, Gates MJ, Koeffler HP, Gasson JC (1989). *J Immunol* 143:2374–2377.

Oster W, Cicco NA, Klein H, Hirano T, Kishimoto T, Lindemann A, Mertelsmann RH, Herrmann F (1989). *J Clin Invest* 84:451–457.

Rosenthal N (1989). In Berger SL and Kimmel AR (eds): *Methods in Enzymology*, New York: Alan R. Liss, pp 704–720.

Segal GM, Bagby GC (1988). *Int J Cell Cloning* 6:306–312.

Shaw G, Kamen R (1986). *Cell* 46:659–667.

Sieff CA, Tsai S, Faller DV (1987). *J Clin Invest* 79:48–51.

Sieff CA, Niemeyer CM, Mentzer SJ, Faller DV (1988). *Blood* 72: 1316–1323.

Sironi M, Breviario F, Proserpio P, Biondi A, Vecchi A, Van Damme J, Dejana E, Mantovani A (1989). *J Immunol* 142:549–553.

Sisson SD, Dinarello CA (1988). *Blood* 72:1368–1374.

Tartakovsky B, Finnegan A, Muegge K, Brody DT, Kovacs EJ, Smith MR, Berzofsky JA, Young HA, Durum SK (1988) *J Immunol* 141:3863–3867.

Warner SJC, Auger KR, Libby P (1987) *J Immunol* 139:1911–1917.

Williams DE, Broxmeyer HE (1988). *Blood* 72:1608–1615.

Wreschner DH, Rechavi G (1988). *Eur J Biochem* 172:333–340.

Zsebo KM, Yuschenkoff V, Schulter S, Chong D, McCall E, Dinarello CA, Altrock B, Bagby GC (1988). *Blood* 71:99–103.

The Biology of Hematopoiesis, pages 241–248

ACTIVATOR PROTEINS WHICH REGULATE IMMUNOGLOBULIN HEAVY CHAIN GENE TRANSCRIPTION IN B LYMPHOCYTES

Christopher Roman, Karen Riggs, Kevin Merrell and Kathryn Calame
Department of Microbiology, Columbia University College of Physicians and Surgeons, New York, N.Y. 10032

INTRODUCTION

We wish to understand the molecular mechanisms in B lymphocytes which regulate the cell-specific and developmental stage-specific transcription of immunoglobulin heavy chain (IgH) genes. IgH transcription has provided a paradigm for mechanisms which operate on highly regulated eukaryotic genes (reviewed in Calame, 1989). Two DNA elements, a promoter, located within 250 base pairs (bp) of the cap site, and an enhancer, located in the first intron approximately 2.0 kb 3' to the cap site, are known to be important for regulated transcription from heavy chain variable region (V_H) transcription initiation sites.

Fig. 1 illustrates multiple positive activator proteins which are known to bind to a V_H promoter and the IgH enhancer and to be important for their function. (The figure minimizes the number of proteins involved because less well characterized proteins are not included.)

Our current understanding of the cell-type distribution of these proteins does not fully explain the B-cell specific expression of IgH genes. One of the two proteins which binds at the octamer (8) site, Oct-2, is present in B cells and a few other lineages including macrophages and neurons (L. Staudt, personal communication). The others all have a ubiquitous tissue distribution when assayed for DNA binding activity (Sen and Baltimore, 1986; Peterson and Calame, 1987). Thus more subtle differences in the relative amounts or transcriptional activity of some of these proteins may determine B-cell specificity.

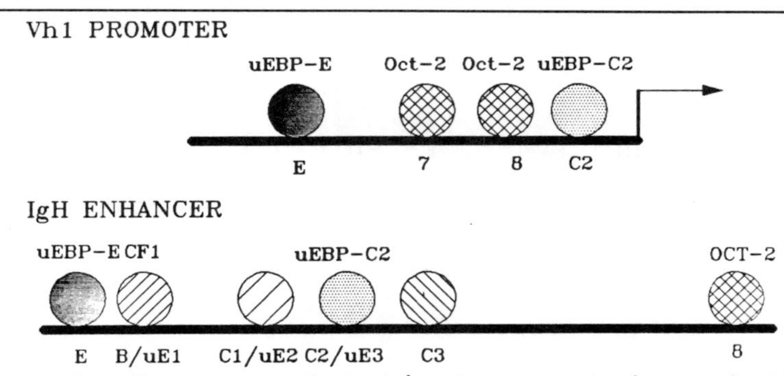

Fig. 1. Summary of Activator Proteins Binding to the Immunoglobulin Heavy Chain Enhancer and V_{H1} Promoter. The relative locations of proteins (above circles) and binding sites (below circles)are indicated but not drawn to scale.

A striking observation is that three of the proteins which bind to the enhancer (at sites E, C2 and octamer or 8) also bind to the V_{H1} promoter (Peterson et al 1988; Peterson and Calame, 1989). This suggests that the enhancer may function by providing proteins to the transcription initiation region. Further, it may be that the low, enhancer-independent transcription of unrearranged V_H promoters observed in early B cells (Yancopoulos and Alt,1985) may occur because some of these factors have increased activities. A suggested mechanism for how enhancers may provide transcription factors to distant promoters involves the formation of intrastrand DNA loops mediated by protein-protein interactions between proteins bound at the enhancer and promoter (Ptashne, 1986). Our recent results provide specific evidence consistent with this model.

Here we describe further studies on three IgH enhancer-binding proteins: uEBP-E, uEBP-C2 and uEBP-B, which we suggest should be renamed CF1.

uEBP-E IS A MEMBER OF THE FOS-JUN FAMILY

A Southwestern screen of a lambdaGT11 expression library (Singh, et al 1987) using a multimerized E site olignucleotide as a probe identified a cDNA clone encoding a polypeptide which could bind specifically to E sites in both the IgH enhancer and promoter. A fusion protein which contains the expressed cDNA yields a chemical-endonuclease footprint on the enhancer which is indistinguishable from that of the native uEBP-E protein. Northern analysis using the cDNA demonstrates that the mRNA, like the native protein, is present ubiquitously at low levels.

Derived amino-acid sequence from the partial uEBP-E cDNA has revealed a number of interesting characteristics (Fig.2A). uEBP-E is a member of a family of DNA binding proteins which includes c-fos, c-jun, CREB, C/EBP, and GCN4 which is characterized by a motif comprising a stretch of basic amino-acids followed by a several heptad repeats of leucine residues. The basic region is believed to bind directly to the DNA molecule. The sequence of leucine repeats are believed to form an amphipathic alpha-helix whose hydrophobic face mediates dimerization between two polypeptides thereby juxtaposing two basic regions to form one functional DNA binding domain (Landshulz, et al 1988a).

uEBP-E shares the highest degree of homology in the basic region with the CCAAT/Enhancer Binding Protein (C/EBP) (Landshulz et al, 1988b). This similarity is reflected in the high degree of homology between their respective known DNA binding sites;indeed, a C/EBP fusion protein is capable of binding to E sites _in vitro_. In addition, the homology extends through the leucine repeat, particularly at amino-acids which would contribute to the putative dimerization interface. We are currently examining the possibility that uEBP-E and C/EBP form heteromers by _in vitro_ co-expression of both polypeptides.

A PROTEIN BINDING TO uE3/C2 IS A MEMBER OF THE "MYC HOMOLOGY" FAMILY OF DNA-BINDING PROTEINS

We have cloned a cDNA for a protein which binds specifically to site C2/uE3 of the heavy-chain enhancer by Southwestern screening of a lambdaGT11 cDNA expression library. The protein produced from the cDNA _in vitro_ yields footprints on known DNA binding sites for uEBP-C2 on the IgH enhancer and V_{H1} promoter indistinguishable from the native protein.

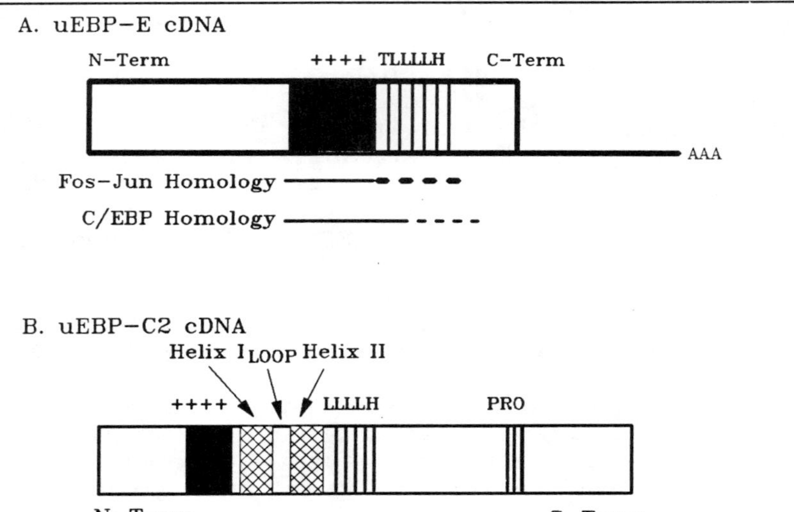

Fig. 2 Diagrams of IgH Transcription Factor cDNAs. A. The uEBP-E clone has 283 bp of 3' untranslated and 170 amino acids of coding; the clone does not contain the N terminus. The "zipper" region is shown (HLLLLT) as is the basic region (+++). B. The uEBP-C2 clone has 1.23 kb of 3' untranslated and 290 amino acids of coding; the clone contains neither the poly A site nor the N terminus.

Expression of this mRNA analyzed by Northern blotting revealed low levels in most murine adult tissues and cell lines, including spleen and two plasmacytoma lines P3X and M603. This is consistent with the ubiquitous distribution of C2/uE3 binding activity we have detected *in vitro*. However there is approximately 5-10 fold higher levels of steady-state uEBP-C2 mRNA in adult brain compared to other adult tissues and cell lines. We are currently performing *in situ* hybridizations on rat fetal sections to determine if uEBP-C2 is differentially expressed during embryogenesis.

The sequence of the uEBP-C2 protein shows that

share a motif known as the "myc homology region" (MHR)(Murre, et.al 1988) (Fig. 2B). These factors include a number of other proteins known to be important for developmental programming and/or transcriptional regulation, N-myc, L-myc, c-myc, MyoD1, daughterless, USF, and lyl-1. The MHR comprises a basic cluster of amino-acids, followed by two putative amphipathic helices separated by a variable loop. The basic region is believed to interact directly with the DNA molecule, whereas the amphipathic helices are believed to mediate dimerization between two polypeptides in order to juxtapose two basic regions to form one DNA binding domain (Murre, et.al 1988). In addition, uEBP-C2 contains a series of heptad leucine repeats immediately following the MHR. This "leucine zipper" represents a second putative dimerization motif in uEBP-C2. Following the leucine repeats is a sequence rich in prolines; such a region is characteristic of the transcriptional transactivation domain of CTF/NF-1 (Mermod et al 1989).

The presence of two dimerization motifs in uEBP-C2 is consistent with the possibility that this protein can form higher order multimers, namely dimers and tetramers, characteristic of native uEBP-C2 (Peterson and Calame, 1989). A tetrameric complex of uEBP-C2 would also comprise two DNA binding domains, and would thus be consistent with a model whereby a tetramer of uEBP-C2 could bind simultaneously to two binding sites, namely in the IgH promoter and enhancer, thereby juxtaposing these elements to potentiate transcription.

COMMON FACTOR 1 IS AN ACTIVATOR WHICH BINDS TO BOTH THE c-MYC PROMOTER AND THE IgH ENHANCER

We have previously described a repressor of c-myc transcription called plasmacytoma repressor factor (PRF) which binds 280 base pairs 5' of the P1 start site of transcription (Kakkis, et al. 1989). PRF has only been found in plasmacytomas. A second protein factor has been identified which interacts with PRF and may be directly involved in the mechanism of repression. This protein is ubiquitous in its distribution and has been designated CF1 (common factor 1).

Due to its ubiquitous distribution, we suspected that CF1 might be a positive factor. This was tested by cloning five copies of the CF1 recognition sequence upstream of the partial tk promoter present in the reporter plasmid pBLCAT2 (Luckow and Schutz, 1987) to form a construct designated pBL(CF1-5)CAT2 (Fig. 3B). When pBL(CF1-5)CAT2 was transiently transfected into L-cells, the amount of CAT activity present in the harvested cell extracts was four times the activity present in control cells transfected with pBLCAT2. Transient transfection of the plasmacytoma cell line P3X showed a 2.5 fold increase in CAT production from pBL(CF1-5)CAT2 over pBLCAT2. These experiments show that CF1 is able to act as an activator of transcription.

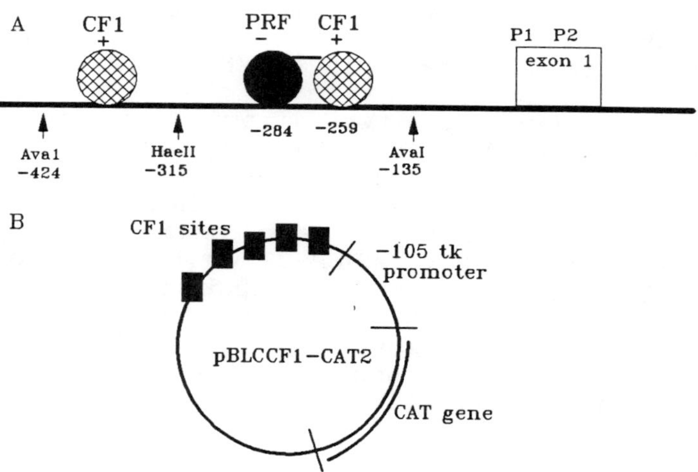

Fig. 3. c-Myc Regulatory Elements. A. The locations of CF1 and PRF binding sites relative to the first transcription start are indicated. The 5' CF1 site is only approximately mapped. B. Construct containing CF1 sites used for transfection studies.

Using an oligonucleotide multimer of the IgH enhancer B site as a competitor in gel mobility shift assays, we noted that it competed for binding to the CF1 site in the c-myc promoter. Results from a number of further experiments strongly support the notion that CF1 is identical with the IgH enhancer protein uEBP-B. First, oligonucleotides corresponding to both sites cross compete on c-myc and IgH enhancer probes for binding to these sites. Comparison of the two binding sites shows an 8 out of 11 sequence similarity. Secondly, both proteins are ubiquitous in their distribution. Third, both have been shown to have rapid off-rates (less than 30 sec.)(Kakkis et al, 1989; Peterson and Calame, 1987). Finally, when proteins in a plasmacytoma nuclear extract are separated by their electrostatic properties on an FPLC Mono Q column, binding to the IgH B site and c-myc CF1 site appear to co-purify. Thus we believe that uEBP-B and CF1 are the same protein. Because the name CF1 has greater generality, CF1 has been retained as the designation for this protein.

SUMMARY

While our results do not completely explain the B-cell specificity or other regulated aspects of IgH transcription, they show that IgH transcriptional factors belong to several different DNA-binding families which are capable of dimerization. It may be that formation of heteromultimers provides an additional level of regulation which might confer functional tissue specificity. Our results also suggest that enhancers and promoters may interact through protein-protein interactions, looping out the intervening DNA. Finally, we have shown that the same protein may regulate several genes including IgH and c-myc, indicating that transcriptional regulatory mechanisms for different genes are both complex and interconnected.

REFERENCES

Calame, K. (1989) Immunoglobulin Gene Transcription: Molecular Mechanisms, Trends in Genetics, in press.

Kakkis, E., Riggs, K., Gillespie, W. and Calame, K. (1989) A Repressor of c-Myc Transcription,

Nature 339, 712-14

Lanshulz, W., Johnson, P. and McKnight, S. (1988a) The Leucine Zipper, a Hypothetical Structure Common to a New Class of DNA Binding Proteins" Sci. 240, 1759-64

Landshulz, W., Johnson, P., Adashi, E., Graves, B. and McKnight, S. (1988b) Isolation of a Recombinant Copy of the Gene Encoding C/EBP, Genes and Dev. 2, 786-800

Lucknow, B. and Schutz, G.(1987) CAT Constructions with Multiple Unique Restriction Sites for the Functional Analysis of Eukaryotic Promoters and Regulatory Elements, Nuc. Acids Res. 15, 5490-94

Mermod, N., O'Neill, E., Kelly, T., Tjian, R. (1989) The Proline-Rich Transcriptional Activator of CTF/NF1 is Distinct from the Replication and DNA Binding Domain, Cell 58, 741-753.

Murre, C., McCaw, P. and Baltimore, D. (1989) A New DNA Binding and Dimerization Motif in Immunoglobulin Enhancer Binding, daughterless, Myo D and myc Proteins, Cell 56, 777-783

Peterson, C. and Calame, K. (1987) Complex Protein Binding within the Mouse Immunoglobulin Heavy-Chain Enhancer, Mol. Cell. Biol. 7, 4194-4203

Peterson, C. and Calame, K. (1989) Proteins Binding to Site C2 (uE3) in the Immunoglobulin Heavy-Chain Enhancer Exist in Multiple Oligomeric Forms, Mol. Cell. Biol. 9, 776-786

Peterson, C., Eaton, S. and Calame, K. (1988) Purified uEBP-E Binds to Immunoglobulin Enhancers and Promoters, Mol. Cell. Biol. 8, 4972-4980

Ptashne, M. (1986) Gene Regulation by Proteins Acting Nearby and at a Distance, Nature 322, 697-701

Singh, H., LeBowitz, J, Baldwin, A. and Sharp, P. (1988) Molecular Cloning of an Enhancer Binding Protein: Isolation by Screening of an Expression Library with a Recognition Site DNA, Cell 52, 415-423

Yancopoulos, G. and Alt, F. (1985) Developmental Control and Tissue Specific Expression of Unrearranged V_H Gene Segments, Cell 40:271-281

The Biology of Hematopoiesis, pages 249–256

TOPOISOMERASE INHIBITORS SUPPRESS RELEASE OF GLOBIN SEQUENCES INTO SMALL SOLUBLE DNA IN ERYTHROBLASTS

Phyllis R. Strauss*

Department of Biology, Northeastern University, Boston Massachusetts 02115

INTRODUCTION

Topoisomerases are enzymes that alter the topology of DNA by permitting one strand or helix of the nucleic acid to pass through another(Wang, 1985; Yanagida and Wang, 1987). Type II topoisomerases are able to catenate and decatenate DNA and to relax supercoiled DNA through staggered breaks. Type I topoisomerase is able to relax supercoiled DNA via single strand nicks. The type II enzyme is clearly required during cell division for the final stages in separation of sister chromatids(Holm et al., 1989). While the type I enzyme is apparently not required for cell viability, it is often preferentially associated with regions of the genome undergoing active transcription(Gilmour and Elgin, 1987). Inhibition of topoisomerase II in a topoisomerase I minus strain of yeast, however, results in rapid loss of cell viability(Brill et al., 1987; Brill and Sternglanz, 1988).

A variety of anti-tumour agents which result in DNA strand breaks in dividing cells act via their ability to stabilize the topoisomerase-DNA intermediate(Liu, 1989; Drilica and Franco, 1988). For example, VM26(teniposide) stabilizes a covalent DNA-topoisomerase II intermediate, while camptothecin stabilizes the covalent DNA-topoisomerase I complex. The covalent complexes have been studied by filter binding assays(Pommier et al., 1985) and by sequence analysis(Udvardy et al., 1985).

We recently showed that inhibitors of

topoisomerases affect the formation of hematopoietic colonies by cultured human bone marrow cells(Dainiak et al., 1989). Not only was colony formation altered but also hemoglobinization was delayed even in colonies where hemoglobin biosynthesis normally occurs. Inhibition of both topoisomerase classes together produced the most profound effects.

One indication of both active transcription and DNA replication is chromatin lability as reflected in both DNase I hypersensitive sites in actively transcribed genes(Weintraub and Groudine, 1976; Elgin, 1988) and also the release of small soluble DNA(sm-sol) DNA(Strauss et al., 1984). Release of sm-sol DNA is cell cycle dependent(Bai and Strauss, 1988; Strauss, 1989) and requires functional topoisomerases(Zhang et al., 1986). The DNA which is released is enriched in transcriptionally active sequences(Strauss, 1988). In this report we present further data showing that sm-sol DNA from murine erythroblasts is enriched in globin sequences compared with sm-sol DNA obtained from lymphoblasts. After treatment of cells with inhibitors of topoisomerases, the amount of released DNA is altered and sequence enrichment no longer occurs.

METHODS AND MATERIALS

Erythroblasts were obtained from the spleens of anemic mice(Obinata and Ikawa,1978); lymphoblasts were obtained from the spleens of mice immunologically stimulated with concanavalin A (Strauss et al., 1977). DNA was obtained from soluble fractions of cells lysed either with 0.5% Nonidet P40(Strauss et al., 1984) at 4oC or with 0.5% sodium dodecyl sulfate(SDS)(Strauss, 1989) at room temperature. Dot blots were prepared as described by Maniatis et al.(1982), hybridized at 42oC in 47% formamide and washed at 60oC in 2XSSC containing 0.1% SDS. Mouse beta globin cDNA was obtained from Edgell(Rochaix et al., 1978); the globin 3' 450 bp untranslated region was obtained from Benezra(1986); while the kappa epsilon probe was obtained from Garrard(Xu et al., 1986). Autoradiograms were scanned by means of a Shimadzu CS-930 chromatoscanner to obtain relative amounts of a given sequence for several DNA concentrations from each fraction.

RESULTS AND DISCUSSION

Table I shows the effects of treatment of

erythroblasts with an inhibitor of topoisomerase II (100 ug/ml VM26 for 30 min at 37oC), of topoisomerase I(125 ug/ml camptothecin for 30 min at 37oC), or with the two inhibitors together. Exposure of erythroblasts to VM26 reduces release of sm-sol DNA somewhat, while exposure to camptothecin enhances release slightly. However, as in the case of effects of topoisomerase inhibitors on lymphoblasts(Zhang et al., 1986), the presence of both inhibitors together results in considerable inhibition of release.In this case, maximal inhibition was 50% of the controls treated with DMSO.

TABLE 1. Effects of Topoisomerases Inhibitors on Release of Small Soluble DNA by Erythroblasts

TREATMENT	SMALL SOLUBLE DNA (ug/10^8 cells)*
DMSO	17.6±2.1(SE, 4)
VM26	14.1±2.1(SE, 4)
CAMPT	22.0±3.3(SE, 4)
VM26+CAMPT	9.4±1.0(SE, 4)

*Mean±S.E.

Since topoisomerase inhibitors alter the release of DNA into the soluble fraction, it was of interest to determine their effects on sequence content of released and insoluble DNA. First, however, the sequence content of sm-sol and insoluble DNA from erythroblasts from anemic mice and lymphoblasts from immunologically stimulated mice was compared. The probes selected were globin cDNA for a sequence that is both heavily transcribed and translated in erythroblasts but neither transcribed nor translated in lymphoblasts; the 450 bp 3' untranslated region of globin which is translated but not transcribed by erythroblasts; and the kappa (epsilon) region of the murine immunoglobulin light chain, which is the transcription termination region for both cell types(Figure 1). Dot blot analysis(Table 2 and Figure 2) reveals that erythroblast sm-sol DNA is enriched four-fold over lymphoblast sm-sol DNA in globin coding sequencing, enriched two fold over lymphoblast DNA in globin translated but untranscribed regions and not enriched at all in a sequence which is not transcribed by either cell type.

Figure 2 also shows that treatment with the topoisomerase inhibitors, particulary VM 26, reduces the sequence content of the globin coding region released into the soluble fraction. Table 3 presents the data for the effects of the drugs alone and together on the sequence content of all three loci examined in this study. The most pronounced effects are on the globin coding region where release is inhibited by 75%. The degree of inhibition for the

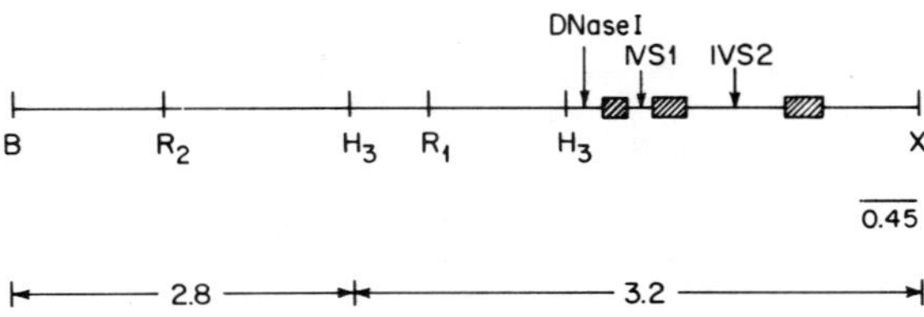

Figure 1. Restriction Map of a 6.0 Kilobase Xba/Bam H1 Fragment Containing the Mouse Beta Major Globin Gene(Benezra et al., 1986). The globin cDNA probe contains the three globin exons, while the 450 bp 3' untranslated region contains the 0.45 kbp fragment 3' to the third exon.

Table 2. Enrichment of Actively Transcribed Sequences in Small-soluble DNA of Erythroblasts*

SEQUENCE	SEQUENCE CONTENT PER 10^8 CELLS (sm-sol/insol)		
	ERYTHROBLASTS	LYMPHOBLASTS	E:L
BETA GLOBIN	13.4	3.3	4.0
BETA GLOBIN 450 UT	19.0	9.0	2.1
KAPPA(E)	3.7	3.5	1.0

*Total area units of each sequence in sm-sol DNA are divided by total area units in recovered insoluble DNA average of 3 04 4 determinations.

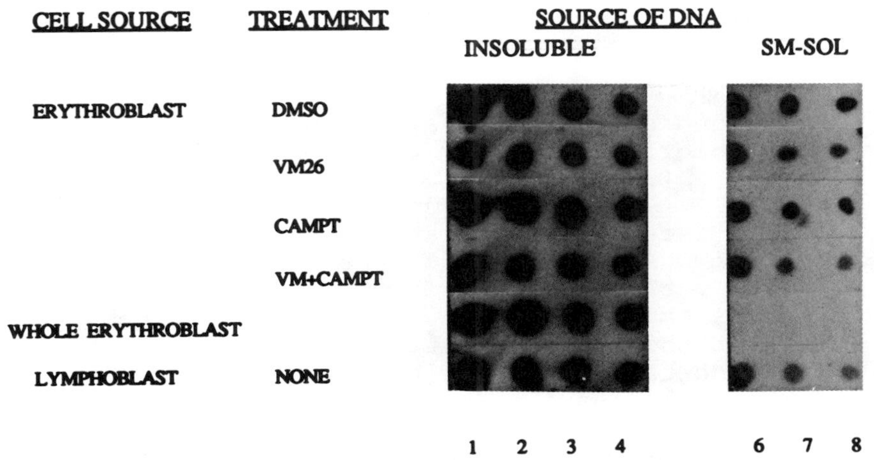

CELL SOURCE | TREATMENT | SOURCE OF DNA: INSOLUBLE | SM-SOL

ERYTHROBLAST DMSO

VM26

CAMPT

VM+CAMPT

WHOLE ERYTHROBLAST

LYMPHOBLAST NONE

1 2 3 4 6 7 8

Figure 2 Distribution of Globin Coding Sequences between Small-soluble and Insoluble DNA of Erythroblasts and Lymphoblasts--Effects of Topoisomerase Inhibitors Cells were treated with dimethyl sulfoxide(DMSO), the solvent for the inhibitors, VM26 (tenposide, 100 ug/ml), campt(camptothecin, 125 ug/ml) or the two inhibitors together. The dot blot was constructed so that the insoluble DNA from 6.4, 4.8, 3.2 and $1.6X10^{6}$ cells was applied in columns 1, 2, 3 and 4 respect-ively, while the sm-sol DNA from 2, 1, and $0.8X10^{7}$ cells was applied in columns 5, 6 and 7.

Table 3. Effects of Anti-topoisomerase Agents on the Release of Selected Sequences in Small-soluble DNA

CELL TYPE	SEQUENCE	TREATMENT	SEQUENCE CONTENT OF SM-SOL DNA (PERCENTAGE OF CONTROL)
ERYTHRO- BLAST	GLOBIN	DMSO	100
		VM26	26
		CAMPT	79
		VM+CAMPT	26
	GLOBIN 450 UT	DMSO	100
		VM26	50
		CAMPT	100
		VM+CAMPT	52
	KAPPA(E)	DMSO	100
		VM26	68
		CAMPT	108
		VM+CAMPT	50

Each percentage is the mean of three or four experiments in which total area units released into the soluble fraction from cells treated as indicated

(Continued)

(Table 3 Continued)
was divided by the total areas units released into the soluble fraction from cells treated with DMSO.

<u>sequence</u> exceeds considerably the inhibition on the <u>amount</u> of DNA released into the soluble fraction. Therefore, the effect is far more pronounced on some sequences than on others. This is born out by the fact that the release of the globin 3' untranslated region and the kappa(epsilon) region are progressively less inhibited.

These results directly confirm an effect of the topoisomerase inhibitors on the chromatin structure of erythroblasts. Thus, the observation that the inhibitors prevent colony formation and delay hemoglobinization in bone marrow cultures may result from altered chromatin structure preventing normal gene expression.

REFERENCES

Bai, X.-H. and Strauss, P. R. 1988 Release of detergent soluble DNA in Chinese hamster ovary(CHO) cells is cell cycle dependent J. Cell Biol. 107, 77a

Benezra, R., Cantor, C. R. and Axel, R. 1986 Nucleosomes are phased along the mouse beta-major globin gene in erythroid and non-erythroid cells Cell 44, 697-704

Brill, S. J. and Sternglanz, R. 1988 Transcription-dependent DNA supercoiling in yeast DNA topoisomerase mutants Cell 54, 403-411

Brill, S. J., DiNardo, S., Voelkel-Meiman, K. and Sternglanz, R. 1987 Need for DNA topoisomerase activity as a swivel for DNA replication and for transcription of ribosomal RNA Nature(London) 326, 414-416

Dainiak, N., Kreczko, S., Hanspal, M. and Strauss, P. R. 1989 DNA topoisomerase inhibitors block erythropoiesis and delay hemoglobinization in vitro J. Cellul. Physiol. 138, 87-96

Drilica, K. and Franco, R. J. 1988 Inhibitors of DNA topoisomerases Biochemistry(Wash.) 27, 2253-2259

Elgin, S. C. R. 1988 The formation and function of DNase I hypersensitive sites in the process of gene activation J. Biol. Chem. 263, 19259-19262

Gilmour, D. S. and Elgin, S. C. 1987 Localization of specific topoisomerase I interactions within the transcribed region of active heat shock genes by usung the inhibitor camptothecin Mol. Cell. Biol. 7, 141-148

Holm, C., Stearns, T. and Botstein, D. 1989 DNA topoisomerase II must act at mitosis to prevent nondisjunction and chromosome breakage Mol. Cell. Biol. 9, 159-168

Liu, L. F. 1989 DNA topoisomerase poisons as antitumor drugs Annu. Rev. Biochem. 58, 351-375

Maniatis, T., Fritsch, E. F. and Sambrook, J. 1982 Molecular Cloning, A Laboratory Manual Cold Spring Harbor Laboratory, Cold Spring Harbor NY

Obinata, M. and Ikawa, Y. 1978 Change in message sequences during erythroid differentiation Nucleic Acids Res. 8, 4271-4282

Pommier, Y., Minford, J. K., Schwartz, R. E., Zwelling, L. A., and Kohn, K. W. 1985 Effects of the DNA intercalators 4'-(9-acridinylamino)methanesulfon-m-anisidide and 2-methyl-hydroellipticinium on topoisomerase II mediated DNA strand cleavage and strand passage Biochemistry(Wash.) 24, 6410-6416

Rochaix, J. D., Rougeon, F. and Mach, B. 1978 Electron microscope analysis of mouse and rabbit globin and immunoglobulin gene sequences Gene 3, 9-16

Strauss, P. R. 1989 Dynamic heirarchies of chromatin organization and small soluble DNA--An overview In: The Eukaryotic Nucleus: Molecular Biochemistry and Macromolecular Assemblies Ed. P. R. Strauss and S. Wilson, Telford Press Caldwell NJ In press

Strauss, P. R., Andrutis, A. T., Leong, S. R., Nickeson, S. and Supple, E. 1984 Characterizationm of rapidly labeled detergent-soluble DNA in murine splenocytes Biochemistry(Wash.) 23, 915-921

Strauss, P. R., Sheehan, J. F. and Kashket, E. R. 1977 Membrane transport by murine spleen cells. II. Nucleoside uptake and transport after in vivo mitogen stimulation J. Immunol. 118, 1328-1334

Udvardy, A., Schedl, P., Sander, M. and Hsieh, T.-s.

Drosophila topoisomerase II Cell 40, 933-941

Wang, J. C. 1985 DNA topoisomerases Annu. Rev. Biochem. 54, 665-697

Weintraub, H. and Groudine, M. 1976 Chromosomal subunits in active genes have an altered conformation Science 193, 848-856

Wu, H.-Y., Shyy, S., Wang, J. C. and Liu, L. F. 1988 Transcription generates positively and negatively supercoiled domains in the template Cell 53, 433-440

Xu, M., T.-C., Bernard, M. B., Rose, S. M., Cockerill, P. N., Huang, S.-Y. and Garrard, W. T. 1986 Transcription termination and chromatin structure of the active immunoglobulin kappa gene locus J. Biol. Chem. 261, 3838-3845

Yanagida,, M. and Wang, J. C. 1987 Yeast topoisomerases and their structural genes In: Nucleic acids and molecular biology vol. 1(F. Eckstein and D. M. J. Lilley, eds.) Springer-Verlag, Berlin Heidelberg pp. 196-209

Zhang, L.-H., Mui, S. C., Todt, J. T. and Strauss, P. R. 1986 Role for topoisomerases in the release of DNA into the detergent-soluble fraction of eukaryotic cells Proc. Natl. Acad. Sci.(USA) 83, 5871-5874

*Supported by funds from the Research Corporation and from Northeastern University

The Biology of Hematopoiesis, pages 257–267

CONTROL OF HEMATOPOIETIC GROWTH FACTORS

Makoto Akashi, H. Phillip Koeffler

Division of Hematology/Oncology, UCLA School of Medicine, Los Angeles, California

INTRODUCTION

Life span of mature blood cells is ephemeral, requiring hematopoiesis throughout life. A complex network of hematopoietic progenitor cells and cytokines maintain an enormous daily production of granulocytes, monocytes, erythrocytes, platelets, and lymphocytes. This population of hematopoietic cells must be able to respond rapidly to changing needs such as bleeding, infections, cancer, or exposure to cytotoxic agents. Hematopoietic growth factors, many of which are known as colony stimulating factors (CSFs), are a family of glycoproteins that promote growth and differentiation of hematopoietic progenitor cells and enhance the function of the mature blood cells. Numerous studies _in vitro_ suggest that proliferation of hematopoietic progenitor cells require the continuous presence of these factors. A variety of tissues are capable of producing many of the hematopoietic growth factors.

MESENCHYMAL CELLS

Mesenchymal cells originate from either mesoderm or ectoderm. Three of the major cells that compose the mesenchymal cells include fibroblasts, vascular endothelial, and smooth muscle cells. Pluznik and Sachs originally showed that fibroblasts could produce CSF (Pluznik and Sachs, 1965); somewhat more recently endothelial cells and smooth muscles were found to be capable of stimulating granulopoiesis. Sustained myelopoiesis in long term culture of bone marrow cells requires the presence of stromal cells composed of a complex network of cell types including fibroblasts and endothelial cells. These cells produce low levels of hematopoietic growth factors.

Bagby and co-workers initially noted that macrophages exposed to lipopolysaccharide produced factors that stimulated both endothelial cells (Bagby et al, 1983a) and fibroblasts (Bagby et al, 1983b) to produce CSFs. Several years later, we (Munker et al, 1986) found that tumor necrosis factor (TNF) was able to stimulate fibroblasts, endothelial cells, and smooth muscle cells to produce CSFs. We showed that both TNF (Munker et al, 1986) and interleukin-1 (IL-1) (Koeffler et al, 1987) were able to stimulate mesenchymal cells to produce both granulocyte(G)-and granulocyte-macrophage (GM)-CSF. Similar findings have been made by others (Bagby et al, 1986; Zucali et al, 1986). Further studies have shown that mesenchymal cells cultured with either TNF, IL-1 or lymphotoxin produced macrophage (M)-CSF (Kaushansky et al, 1988; Akashi et al, in press), as well as IL-1 (Yamato et al, 1989b; Nawroth et al, 1986), and IL-6 (Kohase et al, 1986; Akashi et al, submitted) (Figure 1). We have noted that mRNA for each of these growth factors is produced in a coordinate fashion after mesenchymal cells are cultured with either TNF or IL-1. M-CSF mRNA levels increase the least after stimulation of the cells. Also, lymphotoxin has 30% amino acid homology with TNF alpha and perhaps uses the same cellular receptors as TNF alpha. Nevertheless, potency of lymphotoxin to produce CSF appears to be less than TNF (Akashi et al, in press) (Figure 1).

Mesenchymal cells have detectable levels of CSF mRNA within 30-60 minutes of exposure to TNF (Koeffler et al, 1988). Peak levels occur at about 4 hours and then decrease, returning to near baseline at 24 hours (Koeffler et al, 1988). Levels of CSF mRNA can be increased by TNF in the absence of protein synthesis (Koeffler et al, 1988). TNF slightly increases the rate of transcription of CSF but it more markedly increases the stability of the mRNAs coding for G- and GM-CSF (Koeffler et al, 1988). Protein kinase C (PKC) stimulators also increase the accumulations of CSF mRNA (Figure 2). Promoter-reporter gene constructs of GM-CSF transfected into fibroblasts and stimulated with either TNF or IL-1 showed no enhancement of reporter-gene activity. In contrast, a PKC stimulator markedly increased levels of the reporter-gene (Nimer et al, 1989). These results are consistent with our notion that TNF and IL-1 do not have a major effect on transcription of CSF but modulate levels of CSFs post-transcriptionally. PKC stimulators such as 12-Otetradeconylphorbol 13-acetate and teleocidin appear to stimulate transcription and enhance stability of these CSF mRNAs (Koeffler et al, 1988; Akashi et al, in press).

Further studies by us show that TNF causes rapid alkalination of mesenchymal cell; this probably occurs through stimulation of the Na^+/H^+ antiporter (Yamato et al, submitted). Amiloride blocks this alkalinization, but does not block accumulation of GM-CSF mRNA. Further studies show that TNF enhances levels of CSF mRNA even after activity of PKC was blocked (Yamato et al, 1989). These experiments in concert with our promoter-reporter gene studies provide strong evidence that TNF does not mediate its action through either PKC or Na/H^+ antiporter.

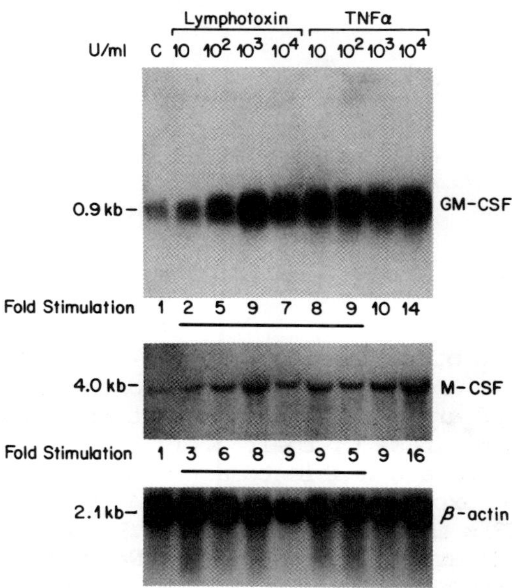

Figure 1: Dose-dependent effect of lymphotoxin and TNF alpha on levels of GM-CSF, M-CSF and IL-6 mRNA in human lung fibroblasts. Fibroblasts were cultured with either lymphotoxin or TNF alpha for 8 hrs. Cytoplasmic RNA was analyzed by electrophoresis and trans-ferred to a nylon-membrane. Fold stimulation of levels of mRNA as compared to levels in untreated cells was equalized for levels of beta-actin.

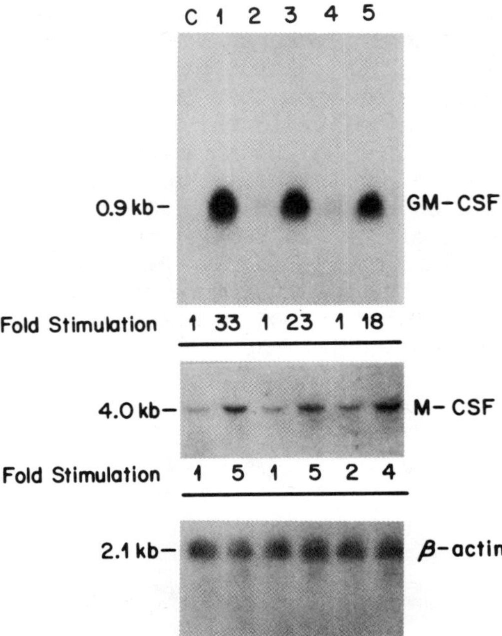

Figure 2: Effect of various derivatives of phorbol ester on expression of GM- and M-CSF studied by Northern analysis. TPA, PDD, and PDB are phorbol esters that are potent activators of protein kinase C; their derivatives, 4-O-methyl TPA and 4-alpha-PDD are unable to activate protein kinase C. Fibroblasts were exposed to each compound (50nM) for 2 hrs and levels of CSFs mRNA measured. The 0.9 and 4.0 kb hybridizing bands are consistent with mRNA coding for GM-CSF and M-CSF, respectively. Fold stimulation of levels of CSFs mRNA as compared to levels in untreated cells was calculated as described in Figure 1. Abbreviations: TPA, 12-O-tetradecanoylphorbol 13-acetate; PDD, phorbol 12,13-decanoate; PDB, phorbol 12,13-dibutyrate.

Using an array of agonist and antagonist, we find that those agents that increase levels of intracellular Ca^{++} and K^{+} also increase levels of CSF mRNA (Yamato _et al_, 1989a). Increase of K^{+} levels may stimulate the Ca^{++}/K^{+} pump causing increased levels of cytosolic Ca^{++}. In addition we find that NaF in the presence of Al^{+++} is a potent stimulator of levels of CSF mRNA (Yamato et al, 1989a). This stimulation cannot be blocked by pertussis toxin suggesting that NaF/Al^{+++} may be enhancing the activity of G-binding proteins that are insensitive to the action of pertussis toxin. This observation is consistent with preliminary data suggesting that transformation of mesenchymal cells by transfection of activated H-ras can lead to their increased expression of GM-CSF mRNA.

Some tumors are able to synthesize CSF constitutively and patients with these tumors often have peripheral blood leukocytosis. We examined cell lines from tumors that produced CSFs; these tumors were associated with leukocytosis in the patients (Ross and Koeffler, manuscript in preparation). Cells of each expressed high levels of GM-, G-, M-CSF mRNA as well as IL-1 and IL-6 mRNA. Furthermore, the stability of mRNA coding for each of these growth factors was 10-20 fold greater than that in non-transformed cells. The tumors have well-defined oncogene alterations that may be closely associated with inappropriate stability of normally transiently expressed genes.

MONOCYTES/MACROPHAGES

Macrophages are pivotal in inflammation and immunity. In the 1970's, monocytes/macrophages were found to produce CSF (Golde and Cline, 1972; Chervenick and LoBuglio, 1972). Further studies have found that human monocytes/macrophages from many tissues produce predominantly G- and M-CSF, as well as IL-1, IL-6 and TNF, but synthesize very little GM-CSF. However, other studies found that murine macro-phages accumulate GM-CSF when exposed to LPS, fetal calf serum, or thioglycolate or when the cells phagocytose and adhere in the presence of fibronectin (Thorens et al, 1987). Resting macrophages produce little CSFs, but their synthesis of CSFs markedly increase with activation after exposure to a variety of physiologically relevant agents including TNF, interferon-gamma (IFN-gamma), GM-CSF, IL-3, IL-1, and endotoxin. Besides producing M-CSF, IL-1 and TNF, these cells have receptors for these cytokines suggesting that under certain circumstances these cells might develop an autocrine stimulation which might foster inflammation. This inflammation may be either salutary (e.g., bacterial infections) or detrimental (e.g., rheumatoid arthritis). Nuclear run-on transcription assay and half-life studies showed that the induction of G- and M-CSF genes is due to mRNA stabilization (Earnest et al, 1989).

TNF and IL-1B are made in abundant amounts by activated macrophages; lymphotoxin is mostly synthesized by activated lymphocytes. A number of conditions including bacterial invasion are known to stimulate these cells to synthesize TNF, IL-1 and lymphotoxin which can enhance CSF production by mesenchymal cells. This inter-communication of cells results in a cascade of synthesis of cytokines in regions of inflammation such as sites of bacterial and viral infections, rheumatoid arthritis and some collagen vascular disorders (Figure 3). Steady-state hematopoiesis in the bone marrow perhaps is in part regulated by the constant, short-range production of cytokines synthesized by mesenchymal cells, macrophages and lymphocytes.

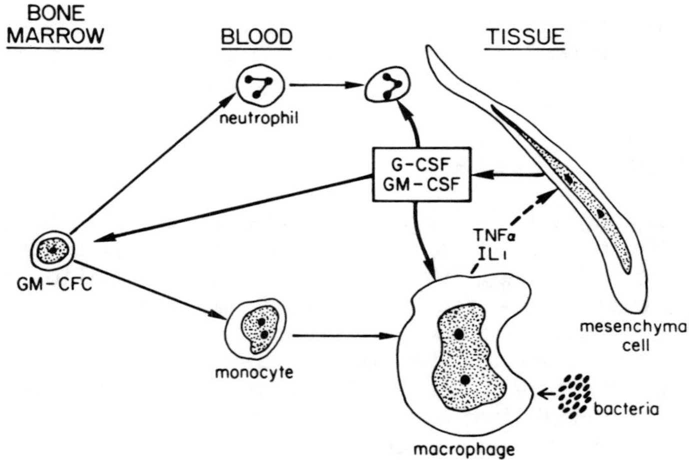

Figure 3: Possible role of TNF in host defenses. Bacteria stimulate macrophages to synthesize TNF and IL-1, as well as G- and M-CSF. The TNF and IL-1 stimulate mesenchymal cells to produce G-, GM- and M-CSF. These cytokines enhance the activity of granulocytes and macrophages as well as to stimulate hematopoiesis.

LYMPHOCYTES

Cline and Golde first showed that human lymphocytes *in vitro* produce significant CSF (Cline and Golde, 1974); these cells especially synthesize large amounts when stimulated with lectin or antigenic stimulation. CSF can be synthesized by both $CD4^+$ and $CD8^+$ lymphocytes; the former are the most potent producers of cytokines. T-lymphocytes can produce all the interleukins and GM-CSF. The cells lack the ability to secrete G- and M-CSF suggesting that trans-regulatory proteins may be different in mesenchymal cells and T-lymphocytes, and those that regulate G- and M-CSF production possibly are different from those that control GM-CSF. A recent study showed that mRNA for M-CSF can accumulate in natural killer cells stimulated with IL-2 and CD16 ligands. Only T-lymphocytes secrete IL-3.

COMPARISONS OF PRODUCTION OF CSF BY MESENCHYMAL CELLS, T-LYMPHOCYTES, MACROPHAGES

In the resting state, both mesenchymal cells and macrophages transcribe cytokines, but do not accumulate these mRNAs (Table 1). With stimulation, cytokine mRNA accumulates in macrophages and mesenchymal cells as well as T-lymphocytes. Maximal mRNA accumulation occurs after 2-8 hrs. of stimulation in all three cell types. The constellation of cytokines produced by each of these cells differs. For example, G- and M-CSF mRNA can be synthesized by mesenchymal cells and macrophages, but not by T-lymphocytes; GM-CSF mRNA is produced predominately by T-lymphocytes and mesenchymal cells, but very little is synthesized by human macrophages. Many of the same signals of CSF production are operative in two or three of the cell types including IL-1, TNF, agents that increase intracellular calcium levels, endotoxin and stimulators of protein kinase C. T-lymphocytes are unique for several reasons. Studies suggest that they require two signals for CSF-production instead of one; only one is probably required for macrophages and mesenchymal cells. T-lymphocytes can be stimulated by specific antigens to produce CSFs.

Stabilization of the shortlived mRNAs play a pivotal role in the accumulation of cytokines in each of the cell types. Stabilization occurs after the cells are exposed to most stimulators listed in Table 1. This may occur in part through AU-rich sequences present in the 3' untranslated

TABLE 1: REGULATION OF CSF

Variables	Mesenchymal Cells	T-Lymphocytes	Macrophages
CSF produced in activated state:	G-, M-, GM-CSF, IL-1, IL-6	GM-CSF, All Interleukins	G- and M-CSF IL-1, IL-6
CSF-Produced in resting state:	Transcription, little accumulation	No transcription	Transcription, little accumulation
Maximal level of CSF mRNA after activation:	4-8 hrs.	4-8 hrs.	2-8 hrs.
Mechanism of enhanced accumulation of CSF mRNA:			
Stimulator:			
GM-CSF, IL-3	-	-	stabilization
TNF, IL-1	stabilization	-	stabilization
PKC stimulator	increased stability and increased transcription		
GM-CSF mRNA T1/2:			
Resting:	<.25 hrs	-	?
Activated (TNF or Mitogen):	0.6 hrs	0.6 hrs	?
TPA or CHX:	>4 hrs	> 2 hrs	?
Signal Pathway for CSF Synthesis:	one signal	two signals	?
Signals include:	TNF, IL-1 PKC Ca^{++} NaF	IL-1 PKC Ca^{++} Specific Antigens	TNF, IL-1 PKC
Critical region for GM-CSF Expression:	DNA Sequences from -53 to +1		

regions of most of the genes coding for these cytokines (Shaw and Kamen, 1986). In contrast, protein kinase C activators stimulate both transcription as well as stabilization of these CSF mRNAs in each of the cell types. These activators require promoter sequences encompassed by -53 to the start site of transcription of the GM-CSF gene in mesenchymal cells and lymphocytes (Chan et al, 1986).

CONCLUSION

Hematopoietic cells are produced and destroyed continuously under precise control. Regulation of induction of hematopoietic growth factors reflects an integrated network of bioregulator molecules. Some act directly on the hematopoietic progenitor cells; others affect accessory cells; and some have both direct and indirect affects on the hematopoietic cells. Many hematopoietic growth factor genes have been cloned and their products have been expressed in mammalian cells. Use of these clones has provided the opportunity to evaluate the regulation of expression of CSFs and the evaluation of their affects on the target cells.

REFERENCES

Akashi M, Loussaraian AH, Adelman DC, Saito M, Koeffler HP. Role of lymphotoxin in expression of IL-6 in human fibroblasts: stimulation and regulation (submitted).

Akashi M, Saito M, Koeffler HP. Lymphotoxin: Stimulation and regulation of colony-stimulating factors in fibroblasts. Blood (in press).

Bagby GC, McCall E, Bergstrom KA, Burger D (1983). A monokine regulates colony-stimulating activity production by vascular endothelial cells. Blood 62:663.

Bagby GC, McCall E, Layman DL (1983). Regulation of colony-stimulating activity production: Interactions of fibroblasts, mononuclear phagocytes and lactoferrin. J Clin Invest 71:340.

Bagby GC, Diarello CA, Wallace P, Wagner C, Hefeneider S, McCall E (1986). Interleukin-1 stimulates granulocyte macrophage colony-stimulating activity release by endothelial cells. J Clin Invest 78:1316.

Chan JY, Slamon DJ, Nimer SD, Golde DW, Gasson JC (1986). Regulation of expression of human granulocyte-macrophage colony-stimualing. Proc Natl Acad Sci USA 83:8669.

Chervenick PA, LoBuglio AF (1972). Human blood monocytes, stimulators of granulocyte and mononuclear colony formation in vitro. Science 178:164.

Cline MJ, Golde DW (1974) Production of colony-stimulating activity by lymphocytes. Nature 248:703.

Earnest TJ, Ritchie AR, Demetri GD, Griffin JD (1989). Regulation of granuloctye- and monocyte-colony-stimulating factor mRNA levels in human blood monocytes is mediated primarily at a post-transcriptional level. J Biol Chem 264:5700.

Golde DW, Cline MJ (1972). Identification of colony-stimulating cells in human peripheral blood. J Clin Invest 51:2981.

Kaushansky K, Broudy VC, Marlan JM, Adamson JW (1988) Tumor necrosis factor-alpha and tumor necrosis factor-beta (lymphotoxin) stimulate the production of granulocyte-macrophage colony-stimulating factor, macrophage colony-stimulating factor, and IL-1 in vivo. J Immunol 141:3410.

Koeffler HP, Gasson J, Ranyard J, Souza L, Shephard M, Munker R (1987). Recombinant human TNFa stimulates production of granulocyte colony-stimulating factor. Blood 70:55.

Koeffler HP, Gasson J, Tobler A (1988). Transcriptional and posttranscriptional modulation of colony-stimulating factor expression by tumor necrosis factor and other agents. Mol Cell Biol 8:3423.

Kohase M, Henriksen-DeStefano D, May Lt, Vilcek J, Sehgal PB (1986). Induction of beta2-interferon by tumor necrosis factor: A homeostatic mechanism in the control of cell proliferation. Cell 45:659.

Munker R, Gasson J, Ogawa M, Koeffler HP (1986). Recombinant human TNF induces production of granulocyte-monocyte colony-stimulating factor. Nature 323:79.

Nawroth PP, Bank I, Handley D, Cassimeris J, Chess L, Stem D (1986). Tumor necrosis factor/cachectin interacts with endothelial cell receptors to induce release of interleukin-1. J Exp Med 163:1363.

Nimer S, Gates MJ, Koeffler HP, Gasson JC (1989). Multiple mechanisms control the expression of granulocytes-macrophage colony-stimulating factors by human fibroblasts. J Immunol 143:2374-2377.

Pluznik DH, Sachs L (1965). Cells in tissue culture. J Cell Comp Physiol 66:319.

Ross HJ, Koeffler HP (manuscript in preparation).

Shaw G, Kamen R (1986). A conserved AU sequence from 3' untranslated region of GM-CSF mRNA mediates selective mRNA degradation. Cell 46:659.

Thorens B, Mermod JJ, Vassalli P (1987). Phagocytosis and inflammatory stimuli induce GM-CSF mRNA in macrophages through posttranscriptional regulation. Cell 48:671.

Yamato K, El-Hajjaoui Z, Kuo JF, Koeffler HP (1989a) Granulocyte-Macrophage Colony-Stimulating Factor: Signals for its mRNA accumulation. Blood 74:1314-1320.

Yamato K, El-Hajjaoui Z, Koeffler HP (1989b). Regulation of levels of IL-1 mRNA in human fibroblasts. J Cell Physiol 139:610-616.

Yamato K, Kurtz I, El-Hajjaoui Z, Koeffler HP. Tumor necrosis factor stimulates Na^+/H^+ antiporter in human fibroblasts: Dissociation between intracellular alkalinization and cytokine mRNA accumulation (submitted).

Zucali JR, Diarello CA, Oblon DJ, Gross MA, Anderson L, Weiner RS (1986). Interleukin-1 stimulates fibroblasts to produce granulocyte-macrophage colony-stimulating activity and prostoglandin E_2. J Clin Invest 77:1857.

ACKNOWLEDGEMENTS

This grant is supported in part by NIH grants and the 4E Leukemia Fund in memory of Marilyn Levine and Irvin Epstein. We would like to thank Elisa Weiss for excellent secretarial help.

The Biology of Hematopoiesis, pages 269–276

LYMPHOHEMATOPOIETIC FACTORS AND BIOLOGICAL CONTROL MECHANISMS

William L. Farrar and Diana Linnekin

Laboratory of Molecular Immunoregulation, National Cancer Institute, Frederick Cancer Research Facility, Frederick, MD 21701-1013

INTRODUCTION

Lymphohematopoietic cell growth, differentiation and functional activation is regulated by both cellular contact as well as by soluble mediators referred to collectively as cytokines. Though not functioning through previously characterized second messenger pathways, cytokine stimulation of both serine/threonine (Evans et al., 1986, 1987) and tyrosine kinases (Farrar and Ferris, 1989, Ferris et al., 1988, 1989) has been demonstrated in previous work from our laboratory.

Recent studies in our laboratory have sought to address the relationship of serine/threonine and tyrosine kinase activation in stimulation of human lymphoid and myeloid cells. Previous models of study have focused primarily on murine cell lines to address cytokine signal transduction. The objective of this work was to identify kinase substrates of potential importance in transduction of the proliferative signal in human lymphoid and myeloid cells and to determine the relationship between activation of serine and tyrosine phosphotransferase systems in response to IL 2, IL 3 and GM-CSF.

RESULTS

The human myeloid leukemic cell line, AML 193 has been shown to proliferate in response to GM-CSF and IL 3 (Santoli et al., 1987). Previous work from this laboratory demonstrated IL 3 and G-CSF induced phosphorylation of a 68 kDa protein in NSF60.8 cells, a murine myeloid cell line responsive to multiple growth factors (Evans et al., 1986, 1987). We were therefore interested if this response was conserved in human hematopoietic cells. Factor deprived AML 193 cells were labeled with ^{32}P-orthophosphate and stimulated with concentrations of human GM-CSF and IL 3 corresponding to those producing optimal proliferation. Phosphoproteins were resolved using high resolution 2 dimensional gel electrophoresis. Radiolabeled proteins were visualized using autoradiography. Figure 1 demonstrates the increase in phosphorylation of a protein of approximately 68 kDa in response to IL 3 and GM-CSF.

Figure 1

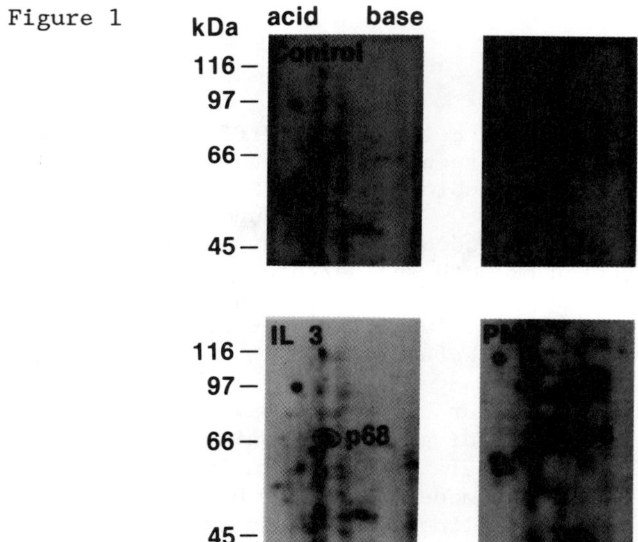

The kinetics of p68 phosphorylation after treatment with either IL 3 or GM-CSF were identical. Maximum increases in phosphate incorporation occurred after a 10′ stimulation with GM-CSF or IL 3 and were 302% and 497% greater than the control, respectively. Phosphoamino acid analysis of acid hydrolyzed p68 demonstrated all phosphorylation to occur on serine residues (data not shown). Radiolabeled cell lysates from cytokine stimulated AML 193 cells were compared to NSF60.8 cells treated with IL 3, GM-CSF and G-CSF. The protein identified as a major phosphosubstrate in AML 193 cells migrated with an identical charge-mass ratio as that phosphorylated in factor stimulated NSF60.8 cells (data not shown). In addition, as reported for the cloned murine T lymphocyte line CT6, p68 is phosphorylated in response to IL 2 stimulation. These data provide strong evidence for remarkable conservation in phosphosubstrates for a serine/threonine kinase activated by lymphohematopoietic growth factors.

Stimulation of AML 193 cells and human T lymphocytes with phorbol myristate acetate resulted in serine phosphorylation of a 68 kDa protein with identical pI (4.8-5.2) as the substrate phosphorylated in response to IL 2, IL 3 and GM-CSF. The convergence of growth factors and a pharmacological activator of PKC on an identical substrate suggests a possible role for PKC or a serine kinase with similar substrate specificity in signaling by these cytokines. The objective of the next study was to determine if PKC and the cytokine activated serine kinases shared the same phosphorylation sites. Preliminary data suggest that limited proteolysis of p68 from PMA, GM-CSF or IL 3 treated cell produced identical peptide maps (data not shown). However, to further address this question, work is in progress to resolve the peptide fragments from complete proteolysis of p68 using 2 dimensional high voltage thin layer chromatography. This will eliminate potential ambiguity inherent in a 1 dimensional system for peptide resolution.

Activation of tyrosine kinases has previously been associated with cellular proliferation. We have observed tyrosine phosphorylation in response to IL 2 in several cell lines as well as in human T lymphocytes (Farrar and Ferris, 1989, Ferris et al., 1989). In addition, we have reported IL 3 induced activation of tyrosine phosphorylation in the murine myeloid cell line FDC-P1 (Ferris et al., 1988). The objective of the next series of studies was to determine if either IL 3 or GM-CSF activated tyrosine kinase(s) in a human myeloid cell line. We now report the phosphorylation of a 140 kDa protein after stimulation of AML 193 cells with either factor. Quiescent AML-193 cells were radiolabeled with ^{32}P-orthophosphate, stimulated with either GM-CSF or IL 3 for the appropriate time period and lysed with extraction buffer. Lysates were clarified with high speed centrifugation and immunoprecipitated with a monoclonal antibody directed against phosphotyrosine. Using one dimensional SDS-PAGE for resolution of proteins, GM-CSF and IL 3 produced phosphorylation of the 140 kDa protein (Fig. 2, lanes 1-4). The p140 protein was not phosphorylated after PMA stimulation. The kinetics of p140 stimulation in response to either factor were identical. Increases in phosphate incorporation of 249% and 795% over control were observed as early as 0.5′ after stimulation with IL 3 and GM-CSF respectively. Maximum phosphorylation of p140 occurred 2.5′ post factor treatment and responses returned to control values between 20 and 30′ later (data not shown). These data indicate that the phosphorylation of p140 occurs rapidly after cytokine stimulation and stand is support of the hypothesis that this protein has an important role in cytokine signal transduction. Two dimensional electrophoresis using IEF in the first dimension indicated that the pI of the GM-CSF and IL 3 stimulated phosphotyrosylprotein was 4.6 to 4.8. Interestingly, stimulation of NSF60.8 cells with GM-CSF, IL 3 or G-CSF also resulted in phosphorylation of a protein of approximately 140 kDa (data not shown). Studies characterizing the murine and human p140 proteins are currently being conducted in our laboratory.

Figure 2

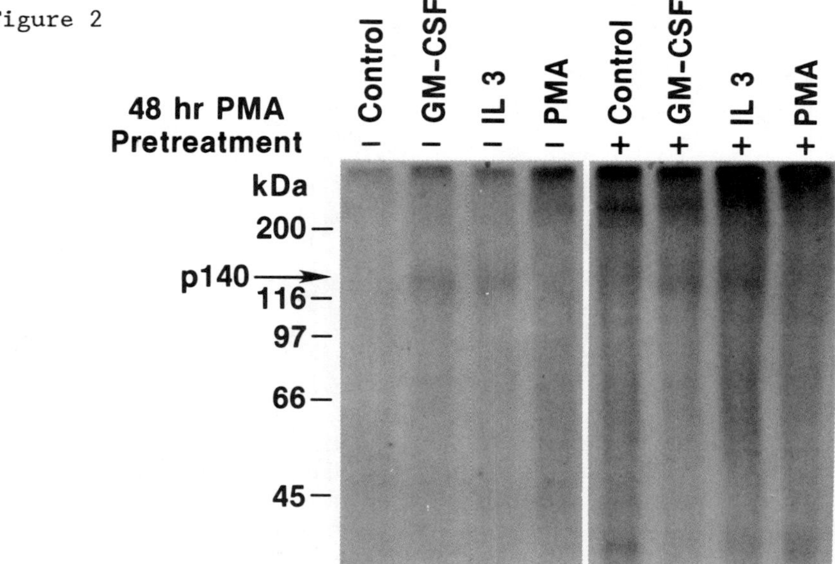

The role of PKC in the transduction of the tyrosine kinase signal was tested by prolonged treatment of target cells with high concentrations of PMA. This procedure has been shown to deplete cells of PKC isozymes through acceleration of PKC degradation (Young et al., 1987). AML 193 cells were cultured with 500 ng/ml PMA for 48 hours and then compared with control cells for capacity to phosphorylate the 140 kDa protein in response to GM-CSF or IL 3. Phosphorylation of p140 after GM-CSF or IL 3 stimulation was identical in control and PKC depleted cells (Figure 2, lanes 1-3 compared to lanes 5-7). These data indicate that activation of the tyrosine kinase associated with the receptor, is independent of the PKC isozyme family.

The effects of PKC depletion on cytokine activation of serine/threonine kinase(s) were also examined. In contrast to tyrosine kinase substrates, phosphorylation of p68 did not increase in cytokine stimulated AML 193 cells pretreated with PMA (data not shown). However, the basal level of p68 phosphorylation in PKC depleted cells is 351% greater than in untreated controls. This degree of phosphorylation probably represents close to maximum levels since PMA stimulation of normal AML 193 cells produces an increase in p68 phosphate incorporation of 433%. Therefore, this method of eliminating PKC does inhibit cytokine or PMA induced increases in p68 phosphorylation but through the elevation of basal levels of serine phosphorylation rather than inhibition of stimulus induced increases.

DISCUSSION

These studies demonstrate the coactivation of a serine/threonine kinase (Fig. 1) and a tyrosine kinase(s) (Fig. 2) in the human myeloid cell line, AML 193 in response to cytokines. Phosphorylation of p68 is a response conserved between species (human and mouse), common to a number of growth factors (IL 2, IL 3 and GM-CSF) as well as hematopoietic cell lineages (myeloid and lymphoid). This degree of conservation suggests an important role for this protein in cytokine signal transduction. Ongoing work in our laboratory is directed at the sequencing and identification of this phosphosubstrate.

The characterization of the serine/threonine kinase activated by IL 2, IL 3 and GM-CSF is crucial to elucidating the mechanism of action of these molecules. Efforts to evaluate the role of PKC in IL 3 and GM-CSF induced p68 phosphorylation were confounded by the high levels of basal phosphorylation in cells pretreated with high concentrations of PMA. Glazer et al. have reported the liberation of the Ca^{++} and lipid independent catalytic domain of PKC, termed PKM, in HL-60 cells after pretreatment with high concentrations of PMA (Aquino et al., 1988). Unregulated phosphorylation by PKM could explain the high backgrounds observed in AML 193 cells depleted of PKC through these means.

Limited proteolysis of p68 with V8 protease was performed as another approach in determining the role of PKC in GM-CSF and IL 3 induced phosphorylation of p68. One dimensional analysis of peptide maps from cytokine and PMA stimulated p68 phosphoproteins suggests that phosphorylation occurs at similar sites. These data support the role of PKC or a serine kinase with similar substrate preference in cytokine elicited kinase activation. However, 2 dimensional separation of peptide fragments will be necessary to more rigorously support this interpretation.

An exciting finding of these studies is the tyrosine phosphorylation of a protein of approximately 140 kDa by both human GM-CSF and IL 3. Previous reports have identified a 140 kDa protein phosphorylated in murine cells in response to IL 3, however no work to date has shown this response shared with GM-CSF (Isfort et al., 1988, Sorenson, 1989). The identification of a tyrosine kinase substrate phosphorylated within seconds of factor addition and conserved as a substrate among hematopoietic growth factors as well as between mouse and human myeloid cells indicates this protein may be key to signal transduction of these factors. The cytokine induced tyrosine kinase(s) is independent of PKC based on the capacity of PKC depleted AML 193 cells to phosphorylate p140 after treatment with GM-CSF or IL 3.

The identification and characterization of the kinases associated with and activated by the receptors for lymphohematopoietic factors will be crucial to understanding the mechanisms of action of these molecules.

Evidence to date indicates that these receptors will probably form a new class of binding proteins capable of associating with tyrosine kinases not encoded in the receptor itself. Recent work has demonstrated several means of receptor effector coupling previously unappreciated. The receptor for atrial natriuretic peptide contains the enzyme guanyl cyclase, the receptor for insulin-like growth factor 2 binds two ligands at different sites on the extracellular domain, and the formyl peptide receptor of the PMN couples to a tyrosine kinase through a G protein inhibited by pertussis toxin (Chinkers et al., 1989, MacDonald, et al., 1988 and Huang et al., 1988). Thus, perhaps other unidentified coupling mechanisms could explain some of the intriguing observations made regarding IL 2, IL 3 and GM-CSF binding and signal transduction. Examples of these are activation of tyrosine kinase(s) through receptors seemingly devoid of intrinsic tyrosine kinase enzyme, GM-CSF stimulated guanyl cyclase activity and the competition between GM-CSF and IL 3 for binding protein on some cells (Coffey et al., 1987, Gesner et al, 1988).

REFERENCES

Aquino, A., Hartman, K.D., Knode, M.C., Grant, S., Huang, K., Niu, C. and Glazer, R.I. (1988). Role of PKC in Phosphorylation of Vinculin in Adriamycin-resistant HL-60 Leukemia Cells. Canc. Res. 34:3324-3330.

Chinkers, M., Garbers, D.L., Chang, M., Lowe, D., Chin, H., Goeddel, D. and Schulz, S. (1989). A Membrane Form of Guanylate Cyclase is an Atrial Natriuretic Peptide Receptor. Nature 338:78-81.

Coffey, R.G., Davis, J.S. and Djeu, J.Y. (1988). Stimulation of Guanylate Cyclase Activity and Reduction of Adenylate Cyclase Activity by GM-CSF in Human Blood Neutrophils. J. Immunol. 40:2695-2701.

Evans, S.W., Rennick, D. and Farrar, W.L. (1986). Multilineage Hematopoietic Growth Factor IL 3 and Direct Activators of Protein Kinase C Stimulate Phosphorylation of Common Substrates. Blood 68:906-913.

Evans, S.W., Rennick, D. and Farrar, W.L. (1987). Identification of a Signal-Transduction Pathway Shared by Haematopoietic Growth Factors with Diverse Biological Specificity. Biochem. J. 244:683-691.

Farrar, W.L. and Ferris, D.K. (1989). Two-dimensional Analysis of IL 2-Regulated Tyrosine Kinase Activation Mediated by the p70-75 Subunit of the IL 2 Receptor. J. Biol. Chem. 264:12562-12568.

Ferris, D.K., Willette-Brown, J., Martensen, T. and Farrar, W.L. (1988). Interleukin 3 Stimulation of Tyrosine Kinase Activity in FDC-P1 Cells. Biochem. Biophys. Res. Commun. 154:991-996.

Ferris, D.K., Willette-Brown, J., Ortaldo, J. and Farrar, W.L. (1989). IL-2 Regulation of Tyrosine Kinase Activity is Mediated Through the p70-75 Subunit of the IL-2 Receptor. J. Immunol. 143:870-877.

Gesner, T., Mufson, R., Norton, C., Turner, K., Yang, Y. and Clark, S. (1988). Specific Binding, Internalization, and Degradation of Human Recombinant IL-3 by Cells of the Acute Myelogenous, Leukemia Line, KG-1. J. Cell. Phys. 136:493-501.

Huang, C., Laramee, G.R., and Casnellie, J.E. (1988). Chemotactic factor Induced Tyrosine Phosphorylation of Membrate Associated Proteins in Rabbit Peritoneal Neutrophils. Biochem. Biophys. Res. Commun. 151:794-801.

Isfort, R., Huhn, R.D., Frackelton, R. and Ihle, J.N. (1988). Stimulation of Factor-dependent Myeloid Cell Lines with IL 3 Induces Tyrosine Phosphorylation of Several Cellular Substrates. J. Biol. Chem. 263:19203-19209.

MacDonald, R., Pfeffer, S., Coussens, L., Tepper, M., Brocklebank, C., Mole, J., Anderson, J., Chen, E., Czech, M. and Ullrich, A. (1988). A Single Receptor Binds Both Insulin-Like Growth Factor II and Mannose-6-Phosphate. Science 239:1134-1138.

Santoli, D., Yang, Y., Clark, S.C., Kreider, B.L., Caracciolo, D. and Rovera, G. (1987). Synergistic and Antagonistic Effects of Recombinant Human IL 3, IL-1, G-CSF and M-CSF on the Growth of GM-CSF Dependent Leukemic Cell Lines. J. Immunol. 139:3348-3354.

Sorenson, P.H.B., Mui, A., Murthy, S. and Krystal, G. (1989). IL 3, GM-CSF and TPA Induce Distinct Phosphorylation Events in an IL 3 Dependent Multipoteintial Cell Line. Blood. 13:406-418.

Young, S., Parker, P.J., Ullrich, A and Stabel, S. (1987). Down-regulation of Protein Kinase C is Due to an Increased Rate of Degradation. Biochem. J. 244:775-779.

The Biology of Hematopoiesis, pages 277–285

CYTOGENETIC AND MOLECULAR ANALYSIS OF THE DELETIONS OF CHROMOSOME 5 IN MYELOID DISORDERS

Michelle M. Le Beau

Section of Hematology/Oncology, Department of Medicine, University of Chicago, Chicago, Illinois, 60637

INTRODUCTION

Recurring chromosomal rearrangements are characteristic of human malignant diseases, particularly the leukemias and lymphomas (Le Beau and Rowley, 1986). During the past few years, the genes that are located at the breakpoints of a number of the recurring abnormalities have been identified. Molecular analysis has revealed that alterations in expression of these genes or in the properties of the encoded proteins resulting from the rearrangement play an integral role in the process of malignant transformation. Perhaps the best examples are Burkitt's lymphoma and chronic myelogenous leukemia in which _MYC_ and immunoglobulin sequences [t(8;14)] or _ABL_ and _BCR_ sequences [t(9;22)] are juxtaposed. In the former disease, the expression of _MYC_ is altered by the immunoglobulin genes, and in the latter disease, the size and properties of the _ABL_ protein are altered.

To date, the major emphasis of the molecular analysis of the chromosomal abnormalities in human leukemias and lymphomas has involved the recurring translocations, in which two gene sequences are juxtaposed, resulting in the activation of an oncogene in a dominant fashion. However, another aspect of molecular-cytogenetic analysis that has recently received considerable attention is the loss of genetic material. Such a loss may result from chromosomal loss or deletion as well as by other genetic mechanisms such as mitotic recombination. The consequences of these abnormalities is the development of homozygosity or hemizygosity resulting in a gene dosage effect or in the unmasking of a recessive allele on the structurally "normal" homologue

(Hansen and Cavenee, 1988; Klein, 1988).

Retinoblastoma is the prototypic model for the study of recessive oncogenes or tumor suppressor genes. Knudson proposed that this malignant tumor is the result of two distinct genetic changes, each causing loss of function of one of the two homologous alleles at a single genetic locus, termed the RB1 locus. Mutations affecting this locus may be inherited from a parent, may arise during gametogenesis, or they may occur somatically. The RB1 gene encodes a 105 kd nuclear phosphoprotein that has DNA-binding activity. This protein forms complexes with the adenovirus E1A and the SV40 large T oncoproteins. Mutations in the E1A gene that prevent this interaction lead to loss of tumorigenicity.

Tumor suppressor genes have been implicated in the pathogenesis of a number of tumors for which loss of heterozygosity has been demonstrated. These tumors include Wilms' tumor, rhabdomyosarcoma and hepatoblastoma (11p), ductal breast carcinoma (13q), small cell lung carcinoma and renal carcinoma (3p), meningioma (22q), colon carcinoma (5q), and acute lymphoblastic leukemia (9p). The affected genes have not yet been identified in these disorders. The high frequency of loss of genetic material in acute myeloid leukemia (AML) suggests that, as for a number of solid tumors, recessive mutations and loss of function of a tumor suppressor locus may be involved in the pathogenesis of some malignant myeloid disorders.

CHROMOSOMAL ABNORMALITIES IN THERAPY-RELATED AML (t-AML)

The occurrence of a myelodysplastic syndrome (MDS) or AML has been recognized as a late complication of cytotoxic therapy (either radiation and/or chemotherapy) used in the treatment of both malignant and non-malignant diseases (t-MDS/t-AML) (Koeffler and Rowley, 1985). The association of abnormalities of chromosome 5 and/or 7 with these diseases was first noted by Rowley et al. who observed loss of an entire chromosome 5 or 7 or a deletion of the long arm of these chromosomes [del(5q)/del(7q)] in cells from 23 of 26 patients (88%) examined. This association has been confirmed by other investigators, and in our analysis of 122 consecutive patients with t-MDS/t-AML, 113 (93%) of whom had a clonal chromosomal abnormality (Le Beau et al., 1986a and unpublished data). This can be compared with our series of

329 patients with AML de novo who were studied during the same period (1970-1989), of whom 67% had an abnormal karyotype. Consistent clonal abnormalities leading to the loss or deletion of chromosome 5 and/or 7 were observed in 94 of the 113 patients (83%) with abnormal karyotypes (77% of all patients). Among these 94 patients, 20 patients had a -5, 26 patients had a del(5q), 8 patients had loss of 5q following unbalanced translocations, 50 patients had a -7, 10 patients had a del(7q), and 11 patients had loss of 7q as a result of an unbalanced translocation. Thirty-one patients had abnormalities of both chromosomes 5 and 7. A del(5q) was the most common structural aberration in our series. In contrast, only 58 of 329 patients (18%) with AML de novo had a similar aberration of one or both of these chromosomes [9% had a -5 or del(5q)]. In t-AML, one seldom finds the specific rearrangements that are closely associated with the distinct morphologic subsets of AML de novo, such as the t(15;17) in acute promyelocytic leukemia (Fourth International Workshop, 1984; Le Beau et al., 1986a).

ABNORMALITIES OF CHROMOSOME 5 IN OTHER MYELOID DISORDERS

In addition to t-AML, a -5/del(5q) has also been observed in the malignant cells of ~10% of patients with AML de novo (Nimer and Golde, 1987). These patients frequently have had significant occupational exposure to potential environmental carcinogens, leading to the suggestion that these abnormalities may be a marker of mutagen-induced leukemia. A distinct clinical syndrome associated with a del(5q) is also seen in older patients, especially in females (Van den Berghe et al., 1985). Morphologically, this disorder, termed the "5q- syndrome", is characterized by refractory macrocytic anemia (RA) and the presence of abnormal megakaryocytes with mono- or bilobulated nuclei in the bone marrow. These patients have a del(5q) as their sole cytogenetic abnormality, and tend to have a relatively mild course that usually does not progress to acute leukemia, whereas in patients with AML, the del(5q) is usually accompanied by additional abnormalities (Van den Berghe et al., 1985).

IDENTIFICATION OF THE CRITICAL REGION OF CHROMOSOME 5

To determine the location of genes on 5q that may be involved in myeloid leukemogenesis, we previously examined the breakpoints and the extent of the deletions in patients with the RA 5q- syndrome, t-MDS/t-AML, or AML de novo. Our analysis revealed that these deletions were interstitial; that is, two breaks occurred in the long arm with loss of the intermediate segment. Moreover, the deletions were relatively similar, with a proximal breakpoint commonly in q13 to q15 and a distal breakpoint in q33 to q35. By comparing the breakpoints in 17 patients with t-MDS/t-AML, we previously identified a region consisting of bands q23 and q31 that was deleted in each patient (Le Beau et al., 1986a). This segment has been termed the critical region.

To refine the critical region of 5q, we have recently examined the breakpoints of the deletions in an expanded series of 93 patients, all of whom had a del(5q). This analysis included 29 patients who had t-MDS/t-AML, 50 patients who had de novo MDS or AML, and 14 patients who had the RA 5q- syndrome (Fig. 1). Sixty-four patients had a distal breakpoint in 5q33.3; distal breakpoints in 5q31-32 or in 5q34-35 were observed in 7 and 22 patients, respectively. For patients with t-MDS/t-AML or de novo MDS/AML, the identification of patients who had a _proximal_ breakpoint in q31 and of other patients who had a _distal_ breakpoint in this band, allowed us to refine the critical region of 5q to q31. We have also identified 4 patients who have balanced rearrangements involving 5q31, providing further support that the critical region of 5q may actually be limited to q31. Thus, it is likely that loss of a gene(s) located within this band is involved in the pathogenesis of myeloid disorders characterized by a del(5q).

IDENTIFICATION OF GENES IN THE CRITICAL REGION OF 5Q

A number of genes encoding growth factors and growth factor receptors have been mapped to the critical region of 5q (Fig. 2). Four of these genes encode hematopoietic growth factors, two of which are colony-stimulating factors (CSFs) that are required for the growth and maturation of myeloid progenitor cells _in vivo_. By using _in situ_ hybridization and the analysis of somatic cell hybrids, we previously localized the interleukin-3 (_IL3_, 5q23-31), granulocyte-macrophage CSF (_GMCSF_, 5q23-31), macrophage-CSF (_CSF1_, 5q33.1), and _FMS_ (5q33) genes to chromosome 5 (Fig. 2) (Huebner et al., 1985; Le Beau et al., 1986b, 1987). Other genes that have been mapped to the critical region of 5q

CRITICAL REGION ON CHROMOSOME 5

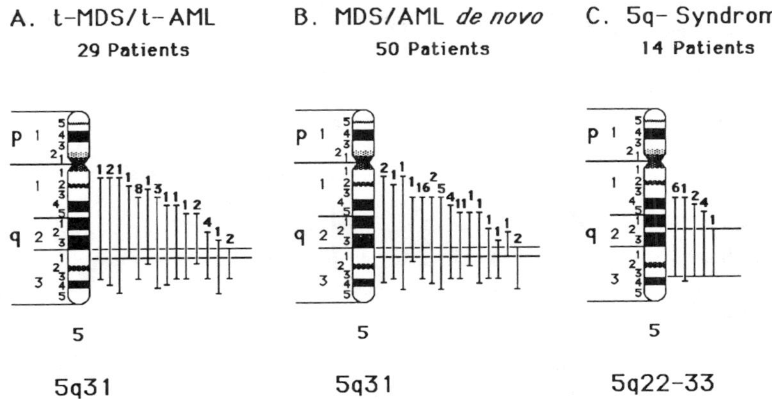

Figure 1. Diagram of the banding pattern of chromosome 5 illustrating the breakpoints and deletions in 93 patients with (A) t-MDS/t-AML (29 patients); (B) MDS/AML de novo (50 patients); and (C) the RA 5q- syndrome (14 patients). Each vertical bar represents the region that was deleted; the numbers above the lines indicate the number of patients with this deletion. The dashed horizontal lines indicate the critical region that was deleted in each patient.

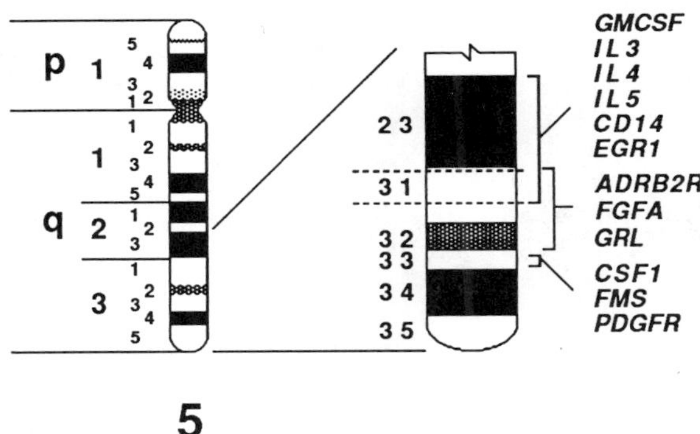

Figure 2. Diagram of the banding pattern of chromosome 5 illustrating the localization of the GMCSF, IL3, IL4, IL5, CD14, EGR1, ADRB2R, FGFA, glucocorticoid receptor (GRL), CSF1, FMS, and platelet derived growth factor receptor (PDGFR) genes. The critical region of 5q is indicated by dashed horizontal lines (band q31).

include the genes encoding the β_2-adrenergic receptor (ADRB2R, 5q31-32), endothelial cell growth factor (FGFA, 5q31-32), and the CD14 antigen (5q23-31), a myeloid-specific differentiation-associated antigen (Wasmuth and Ferrell, 1989). In situ hybridization of probes for these genes to metaphase cells from bone marrow aspirates of AML patients with a del(5q) revealed that, with the exception of the CSF1 and FMS genes, each of these genes was deleted in the 5q- chromosome of all patients examined (Le Beau, 1987).

More recently, we have localized the genes encoding two other hematopoietic growth factors, namely IL4 (B-cell stimulatory factor-1) and IL5 (eosinophil-differentiation factor) to chromosome 5, at bands q23-31 (Le Beau et al., 1989b). Hybridization of the IL4 and IL5 probes to metaphase cells obtained from bone marrow aspirates revealed that both genes were deleted in the 5q- chromosome of two patients with RA or t-AML who had a del(5)(q14q33.3), in one patient with RA who had a similar distal breakpoint [del(5)(q14q33.3)], and in that of a fourth patient, with t-MDS, who had a del(5)(q23q35) (Le Beau et al., 1989b).

The EGR1 gene encodes a 533 amino acid protein, which contains three DNA-binding zinc fingers (Sukhatme et al., 1988). Proteins containing "zinc fingers" have received considerable attention, as this motif is characteristic of one class of proteins that bind to DNA and regulate gene expression. The properties of the EGR1 gene and protein suggest that this gene may function as a transcriptional regulator in diverse biological processes. By using in situ hybridization, we localized this gene to 5q23-31, the same bands to which the GMCSF, IL3, IL4, and IL5 genes are localized, and demonstrated loss of EGR1 as a result of a del(5q) (Sukhatme et al., 1988, and unpublished results).

PHYSICAL LINKAGE OF GENES IN THE CRITICAL REGION OF 5Q

The identification of a functional family of genes on the long arm of chromosome 5 that regulate the growth of hematopoietic cells is intriguing, and raises questions regarding the evolution and regulation of these genes. In this regard, it is notable that the IL4 and IL5 genes have biological and structural similarities to the genes encoding IL3 and GMCSF. Long-range mapping using pulsed field gel electrophoresis (PFGE) revealed that the IL3 and GMCSF genes were physically linked within 9 kb (Yang et al., 1988). By using similar techniques, we confirmed these results and demonstrated that the _IL4_ and _IL5_ genes were linked within 310 kb. Moreover, we found that the _IL4_/_IL5_ and _GMCSF_/_IL3_ probes do not co-hybridize to the same PFGE restriction fragments and are separated by at least two _Not_I sites, suggesting that these two linkage groups are not closely linked to each other (Chandrasekharappa et al., 1989).

ANALYSIS OF GENES IN THE CRITICAL REGION OF 5Q

By analogy to retinoblastoma, it is possible that structural rearrangements of a leukemia-related gene may be present on the cytogenetically "normal" chromosome 5 homologue. To examine whether rearrangements of genes in the critical region of 5q had occurred, we have begun an analysis of DNA from leukemia cells with a del(5q) (3 patients) or a rearrangement that involved 5q31 (1 patient). Southern blot analysis using PFGE and probes for the _GMCSF_, _IL4_, _IL5_, _EGR1_, _CD14_, and _FGFA_ genes did not reveal the presence of rearrangements (Le Beau et al., 1989a).

DISCUSSION

The genetic consequences of a deletion may be a reduction in the level of a gene product, or in the loss of a wild type allele. In the latter case, loss of function of both alleles may occur, in one instance through a detectable chromosomal deletion and in the other, as the result of a mutation. The identification of a cluster of genes encoding hematopoietic growth factors in the critical region of 5q suggests a role for these genes in the autocrine growth of leukemia cells characterized by a del(5q). Recent studies demonstrate that some myeloid leukemia cells have the capacity for autocrine growth (Young and Griffin, 1986). Nonetheless, autocrine growth of leukemia cells with a del(5q) as a result of aberrant expression of a growth factor gene located on 5q has not yet been documented.

The high frequency of loss of genetic material in AML suggests that loss of function of a tumor suppressor locus may be involved in the pathogenesis of some malignant myeloid disorders. The properties of the _EGR1_ gene and encoded protein suggest that this gene may be a more suitable candidate than those encoding growth factors or receptors for playing a role in the malignant transformation of myeloid cells with a del(5q). That is, the EGR1 protein is a DNA-binding protein with transcriptional regulatory activity; thus, the EGR1 gene may function as a tumor suppressor locus whose absence or loss of function could lead to deregulated cell growth. In this regard, the RB1 protein has also been demonstrated to have DNA-binding properties. To determine the role of the various genes located in the critical region of chromosome 5 in the pathogenesis of MDS and AML in patients with del(5q), a detailed molecular characterization of these loci and their encoded products in myeloid leukemia cells is necessary.

ACKNOWLEDGMENTS

We thank Susan Jarman for secretarial assistance.

REFERENCES

Chandrasekharappa SC, Rebelsky MS, Firak TA, Le Beau MM, Westbrook CA (1989). A long-range restriction map of the interleukin 4 and interleukin 5 linkage group on chromosome 5. Genomics, in press.

Fourth International Workshop on Chromosomes in Leukemia (1984). Cancer Genet Cytogenet 11:249-360.

Hansen MF, Cavenee WK (1988). Tumor suppressors: Recessive mutations that lead to cancer. Cell 53:172-173.

Huebner KM, Isobe M, Croce CM, Golde DW, Kaufman SE, Gasson JC (1985). The gene encoding GM-CSF is at 5q21-q32, the chromosome region deleted in the 5q- anomaly. Science 230:1282-1285.

Klein G (1988). The approaching era of the tumor suppressor genes. Science 238:1539-1545.

Koeffler HP, Rowley JD (1985). Therapy-related acute nonlymphocytic leukemia. In Wernick PH, Canellos GP, Kyle RA, Schiffer CA (eds): "Neoplastic Diseases of the Blood", vol. 1, New York: Churchill Livingstone, pp 357-381.

Le Beau MM (1987). Cytogenetic and molecular analysis of the del(5q) in myeloid disorders: Evidence for the involvement of colony-stimulating factor and FMS genes. In Gale RP, Golde DW (eds): "Recent Advances in Leukemia and Lymphoma", UCLA Symposium on Molecular and Cellular

Biology, New Series, vol. 61, New York: Alan R. Liss, pp 71-81.

Le Beau MM, Albain KS, Larson RA, Vardiman JW, Davis EM, Blough RR, Golomb HM, Rowley JD (1986a). Clinical and cytogenetic correlations in 63 patients with therapy-related myelodysplastic syndromes and acute nonlymphocytic leukemia: Further evidence for characteristic abnormalities of chromosomes 5 and 7. J Clin Oncol 4: 325-345.

Le Beau MM, Chandrasekharappa SC, Lemons RS, Schwartz JL, Larson RA, Arai N, Westbrook CA (1989a). Molecular and cytogenetic analysis of chromosome 5 abnormalities in myeloid disorders: Chromosomal localization and physical mapping of IL-4 and IL-5. Cancer Cells 7:53-58.

Le Beau MM, Epstein ND, O'Brien SJ, Nienhuis AW, Yang YC, Clark SC, Rowley JD (1987). IL-3 maps to human chromosome 5 and is deleted in myeloid leukemias with a del(5q). Proc Natl Acad Sci USA 84:5913-5917.

Le Beau MM, Pettenati MJ, Lemons RS, Diaz MO, Westbrook CA, Larson RA, Sherr CJ, Rowley JD (1986b). Assignment of the GM-CSF, CSF-1, and FMS genes to human chromosome 5 provides evidence for linkage of a family of genes regulating hematopoiesis and for their involvement in the deletion 5q in myeloid disorders. Cold Spr Harb Symp Quant Biol 51:899-909.

Le Beau MM, Rowley JD (1986). Chromosomal abnormalities in leukemia and lymphoma. Adv Hum Gen 15:1-54.

Nimer SD, Golde DW (1987). The 5q- abnormality. Blood 70:1705-1712.

Sukhatme VP, Cao X, Chang LD, Tsai-Morris CH, Stamenkovich D, Ferreira PCP, Cohen DR, Edwards SA, Shows TB, Curran T, Le Beau MM, Adamson ED (1988). A zinc finger-encoding gene coregulated with c-fos during growth and differentiation and after cellular depolarization. Cell 53:37-43.

Van den Berghe H, Vermaelen C, Mecucci C, Barbieri D, Tricot G (1985). The 5q- anomaly. Cancer Genet Cytogenet 17: 189-255.

Wasmuth JJ and Ferrell R (1989). Report of the committee on the genetic constitution of chromosome 5. Human Gene Mapping 10. Cytogenet Cell Genet, in press.

Yang Y-C, Kovacic S, Kriz R, Wolf S, Clark SC, Wellems TE, Nienhuis A, Epstein N (1988). The human genes for GM-CSF and IL-3 are closely linked in tandem on chromosome 5. Blood 71:958-961.

Young DC, Griffin JD (1988). Autocrine secretion of GM-CSF in acute myeloblastic leukemia. Blood 68:1178-1181.

The Biology of Hematopoiesis, pages 287–299

The Combination of Il-3 and Il-6 Enhances Retrovirus Mediated Gene Transfer into Hematopoietic Stem Cells

David M. Bodine*, Nancy Seidel*, Stefan Karlsson#, and Arthur W. Nienhuis*

*Clinical Hematology Branch, NHLBI, and #Developmental and Metabloic Neurology Branch, NINDS, Bldg. 10, 7C103, NIH, Bethesda MD USA 20892

Introduction

All cells in the peripheral circulation are descendents of a pluripotent hematopoietic stem cell (PHSC). This cell has the capacity to self-renew or become committed to the myeloid or lymphoid lineages (for review see reference 1). Retroviral mediated gene transfer into PHSC has a number of attractive applications. The introduction of new genetic material into the uncommitted stem cell provides genetic markers to study the differentiation of various cell lineages (2,3). In addition, perfection of this technology may allow gene replacement therapy for certain genetic disorders affecting the hematopoietic system (4). Retroviral mediated gene transfer has been used to transfer several genes into murine bone marrow cells, including the genes for human β globin (5,6,7), human adenosine deaminase (ADA) (8), murine Interleukin-3 (9), murine Granulocyte Macrophage Colony Stimulating Factor (10), murine dihydrofolate reductase (11), and bacterial neomycin resistance (neo^r; 2,3,12,13).

Retroviral infection of PHSC is a rare event. Previous studies have shown that cellular DNA replication is required for integration of murine leukemia virus DNA into the host genome of mammalian cells (14,15). However, 97% of purified mouse stem cells are in the G_0 or G_1 phases of the cell cycle (16). Lack of stem cell DNA replication may explain the low frequency of infection of these cells in gene transfer experiments. Pretreatment of the donor marrow with 5-fluorouracil (5FU), which increases both stem cell cycling (17,18) and the relative number of stem cells (19), has been shown to facilitate retroviral gene transfer (3).

Several hematopoietic growth factors, including Interleukin-3 (IL-3) and Interleukin-6 (IL-6), have been proposed to affect PHSC (for review see ref. 20). Il-3 is required for the formation of multilineage blast cell colonies that are believed to be derived from very primitive progenitor cells (21). The combination of IL-3 and IL-6 shortens the time interval between plating and the appearance of blast colonies. The authors have proposed that combination of IL-3 and IL-6 shortens the G_0 period of the blast cell colony progenitor cells and promotes entry into the cell cycle (22). Lemischka et al. (3) have shown that retroviral gene transfer to Spleen Colony Forming Units (CFU-S) is greatly enhanced in the presence of IL-3, although the frequency of stem cell infection appeared to be less than 10%. Because we have recently reported that IL-3 and IL-6 synergize to increase both CFU-S number and competitive repopulating ability of stem cells in culture (28), we have tested the effects of these growth factors on retroviral mediated gene transfer into these cells.

Methods

Cells and Viruses. The $\psi\beta$S1 producer line has has a titer of $2x10^6$ neo^r cfu/ml (6). Helper virus was assayed as described previously (6). No helper virus was detected in supernatent from the producer cells at the time of infection or in serum from mice 5 months post transplantation.

Growth Factors. Recombinant E. coli derived human IL-6 (rhuIL-6, ref. 23) was provided by Steve Clark of Genetics Institute. The plasmids pCDIL-3 (24), and pCDIL-6 (25) were provided by Frank Lee of DNAX. These plasmids were transfected into COS cells and growth factor containing supernatent collected 72 hours post transfection. The biological activities of murine IL-3 and IL-6 were assayed on 32D (26) and T1165 (27) cells respectively using known standards as controls.

Mice. WBB6F1-W/W^v recipients for long term gene transfer experiments, and female C57BL/6J (donors for

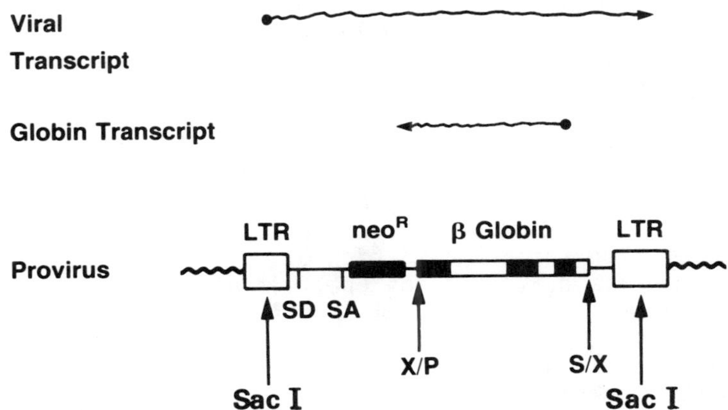

Fig. 1 Diagram of the human β globin provirus (below) it's transcripts and their directions (above). The dark boxes represent the coding regions of the neo^r and the human β globin genes; open boxes, the intervening sequences of the human β globin gene. Restriction sites indicated are: the Sac I (Sst I) sites in the long terminal repeats, the Ssp I (S) site and the Pst I (P) site at the 5′ and 3′ ends respectively of the human β globin gene, both were converted to Xho I sites for cloning into the virus.

all experiments) were all purchased from The Jackson Laboratory. Young (4-6 weeks old) donor mice were treated with 150 mg/kg 5-fluorouracil (5FU; Fluka) intravenously 48 hours before bone marrow harvest.
<u>Gene Transfer Protocol</u>. Marrow cells were harvested as above, and resuspended at a concentration of 5 X 10^5/ml in DMEM with 15% FCS and 15% WEHI-3D cell conditioned medium. Additional growth factors (200 U/ml rhuIl-6; 15% 5637 cell conditioned medium) were added as indicated. Ten ml of this cell suspension was plated on Sarstedt plates and incubated at 37° C, 5% CO_2 for 48 hours (28;29). The cells were recovered by centrifugation, counted, and resuspended in medium containing the same growth factors and 6 μg/ml

polybreen (Sigma). A total of 3 X 10^6 cells were added to 10 cm plates of ψβS1 producer cells split 1:5 24 hours previously. Following 48 hours of co-cultivation, the cells were recovered by centrifugation, washed, counted, and resuspended in PBS for injection into WBB6F1-$\underline{W}/\underline{W}^v$ recipients. Each mouse was injected with 1 X 10^6 cells. Three months post transplantation, and at three month intervals thereafter, individual mice were injected interperitineally with .5 mg phenylhydrazine daily for 5 days to destroy existing red blood cells. RNA was extracted from reticulocyte rich blood two days post treatment. Immunoflourescent analysis of red blood cells was performed 10 days later. Analysis of mouse hemoglobins, immunoflourescent analysis of human β globin chains, DNA analysis, and RNase protection assays were carried out as described previously (6).

Results

The retrovirus produced by the ψβS1 producer cell line is described in reference 6 and is shown in Figure 1. The human β globin gene is inserted in the antisense orientation to prevent splicing of the introns during retroviral RNA synthesis and packaging.

The Combination of IL-3 and IL-6 Increases the Frequency of Retroviral Gene Transfer to Stem Cells.

We compared the effects of Il-3, 5637 conditioned medium, and Il-6 on stem cell infection. RNase protection analysis of RNA extracted from reticulocyte rich peripheral blood from these animals demonstrated that 11 were expressing human human β globin mRNA at six months post transplantation (Figure 2). Table 1 shows that the combination of IL-3 and IL-6 augmented stem cell infection. The use of IL-3 alone or the addition of 5637 conditioned medium to IL-3 and IL-6 gave a lower level of stem cell infection. In fact, treatment of cells with 5637 conditioned medium in the presence of IL-3 plus IL-6 inhibited the repopulating potential of bone marrow cells in a competitive repopulation assay (30,28). We have also compared several variations of the original gene transfer protocol described by Dick et al. (2). Of 14 animals reconstituted with bone marrow cells cocultured for 48 hours in the presence of IL-3 and IL-6, no animals were DNA positive at three months

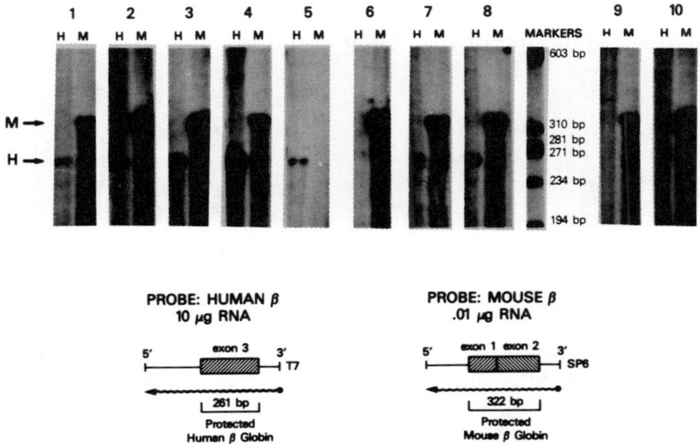

Fig. 2 RNase protection analysis of mice expressing the transduced human β globin gene 6 months post transplantation. Eight positive (1-8) and two negative (9-10) animals are shown. Mice were treated with phenylhydrazine prior to extraction of RNA from reticulocyte rich blood. Ten μg and 0.01 μg of RNA respectively was hybridized to the human and mouse probes shown below the figure.

post transplantation. In contrast, pre-incubation (29) of the same bone marrow cells in IL-3 and IL-6 for 48 or 96 hours prior to the 48 hour cocultivation yielded 4/10 and 4/9 DNA positive animals at three months post transplantation, respectively (Table 1).

Transduced Human β Globin Genes are Expressed in Long Term Reconstituted Mice.

Southern blot analysis of peripheral blood DNA showed that 18 of the 19 mice described above contained approximately 0.1 copy of the human β globin provirus per genome. No proviral sequences were detected in 10 mice that did not express human β globin mRNA. These results indicate that RNA

Table I. Frequency of Infection of PHSC Cocultured in the Presence of Combinations of Growth Factors.

Expt.[a]	Growth Factor/s[b]			Mice positive 6 mo. Post Transplant
	Il-3	5637[c]	Il-6[d]	#+/total (%)
1.	+	-	-	2/17 (12)[e]
2.	+	+	-	1/14 (7)[e]
3.	+	+	+	2/10 (20)[e]
4.	+	-	+	6/11 (55)[e]
5.	+	-	+	4/10 (40)
6.[f]	+	-	+	4/9 (44)

All experiments used 2 day post 5FU bone marrow cells prestimulated in the presence of the indicated growth factors for 48 hours prior to a 48 hour coculture with producer cells. ND= not analyzed.a) Experiments 1-4, 5,6 used the same pools of donor bone marrow cells and were infected with the $\psi\beta$S1 virus (titer: $2x10^6$ neo^r cfu/ml).b) Experiments 1-4 used 15% WEHI conditioned medium as a source of IL-3; experiments 5,6 200U/ml COS cell derived IL-3. c) Experiments 2 and 3 used 15% 5637 conditioned medium as a source of several growth factors including IL-1α and G-CSF. d) Experiments 3 and 4 used 200U/ml recombinant human IL-6; experiments 5,6 used 200U/ml COS cell derived murine IL-6 e) Experiment 4 vs. Experiment 1: $\chi^2 = 4.3$; $p < 0.05$; Experiment 4 vs. Experiment 1, 2, and 3: $\chi^2 = 7.8$; $p < 0.05$; Experiments 4 and 5 vs. Experiment 1: $\chi^2 = 4.07$; $p < 0.05$; Experiments 4 and 5 vs. Experiments 1, 2, and 3: $\chi^2 = 7.1$; $p < 0.05$. f) 96 hour prestimulation; 48 hour coculture.

expression is sufficient to identify positive animals. The average level of expression of human β globin mRNA in these animals was approximately 0.15% that of the mouse β globin genes (Figure 2), although there was considerable variation about that number. Immunoflourescent staining of peripheral red blood cells with a monoclonal antibody against human β globin showed that between 5% and 15% of the red cells contained human β globin chains, consistent with the gene copy number we observed. Peripheral blood DNA from one animal contained approximately 1 copy of the human β globin provirus per genome. Figure 3 shows that there was only one proviral insertion site in the

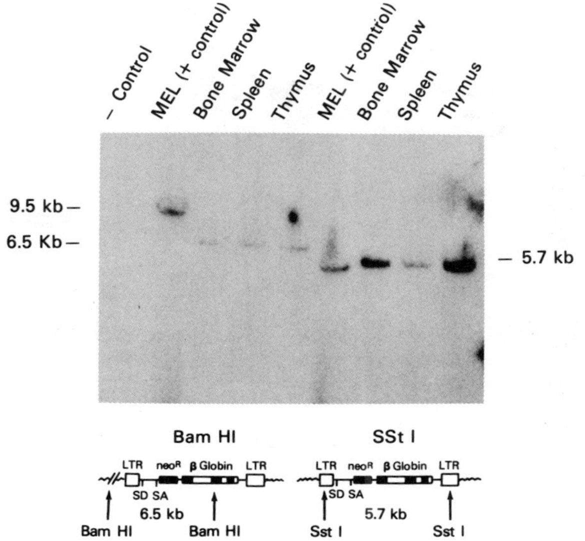

Fig. 3 Southern blot analysis of Mouse B5. DNA was isolated from bone marrow, spleen, and thymus, and digested with Bam H1 to detect insertion sites, or Sst I to estimate copy number.

bone marrow, thymus and spleen of this animal, indicating reconstitution by a single or very limited number of stem cells. Immunoflourescent staining of peripheral red blood cells with a monoclonal antibody against human β globin showed that over 60% of the red cells contained human β globin chains. The amount of human β globin mRNA in this animal was approximately 1.0% that of the mouse β globin genes. This data together with our previous studies and those of others (5,6) demonstrates the transduced human β globin gene is expressing 1-2% the amount of mRNA as the endogenous mouse β globin genes per gene copy.

One animal was sacrificed 10 months post transplantation, and RNA extracted from peripheral blood mononuclear cells, bone marrow, spleen, thymus, and liver was analyzed for the presence of the transduced neo^r and human β globin mRNAs, as well as endogenous mouse β globin mRNA. Figure 4 shows that human and mouse β globin mRNA were detected only in RNA from bone marrow and the spleen, and not in RNA

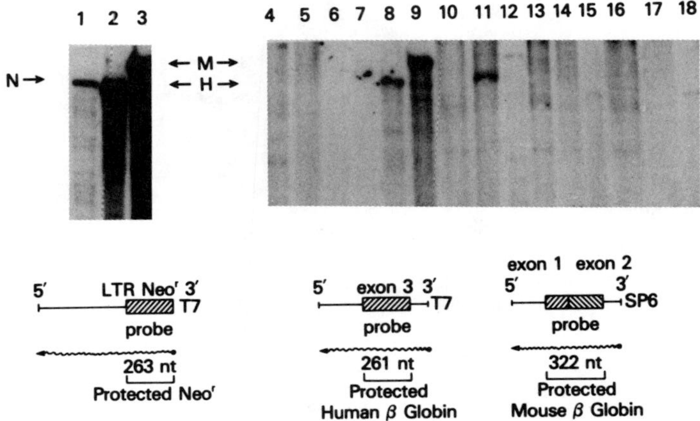

Fig. 4 RNase protection of neo^r (10 μg of RNA; lanes 1,4,7,10,13, 16), human β globin (10 μg of RNA; lanes 2,5,8,11,14,17), or mouse β globin (0.01 μg RNA; lanes 3,6,9,12,15,18) transcripts in RNA isolated from infected MEL cells (lanes 1-3), peripheral blood mononuclear cells (lanes 4-6), spleen (lanes 7-9), bone marrow (lanes 10-12), thymus (13-15), and liver (16-18).

from peripheral blood mononuclear cells or thymus. No neo^r transcripts were detected in RNA from any tissue. Thus the transduced human β globin gene shows an erythroid specific pattern of expression.

The Transduced Human β Globin Gene is Expressed in Repopulated Secondary Recipients

Two animals were sacrificed 12 months post transplantation and 10^7 bone marrow cells from these mice used to repopulate secondary <u>W</u>/<u>W</u>^{v} recipients. Three months post transplantation these mice were fully reconstituted with marrow carrying the "single" hemoglobin marker of the original C57BL/6J donor. Analysis of RNA from these secondary animals revealed the presence of human β globin mRNA in 4 of 5 animals examined (Figure 5).

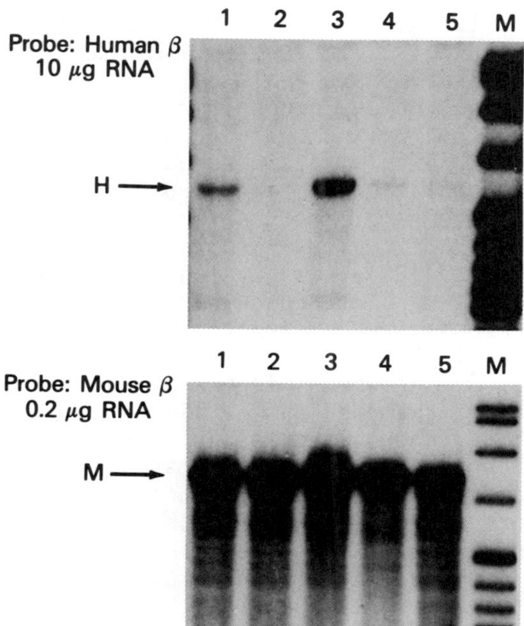

Fig. 5 Identification of human β globin mRNA in secondary mice transplanted with cells from long term gene transfer animals. RNA was extracted from phenylhydrazine treated secondary recipients three months post transplant. A. 10 μg of reticulocyte RNA from 5 secondary transplant mice (lanes 1-5) was probed with the human β globin probe described below the figure. B. 0.2 μg of reticulocyte RNA from 5 secondary transplant mice (lanes 1-5) were probed with the mouse β globin probe described below the figure. The markers in the lanes marked M are from top to bottom: 622, 527, 407, 309, 242/238, 217, 201, 190, and 180 base pairs in length. Panels A and B were not exposed for the same length of time.

Discussion

We have previously shown that the combination of IL-3 and IL-6 increases the number of CFU-S and repopulating potential of bone marrow cells in liquid culture (28). These results are consistent with the observations that IL-3 maintains multipotent colony forming cells in serum free medium and in long term bone marrow culture without inducing commitment (31,32). The synergistic effects of IL-3 and IL-6 on CFU-S that we observed are analogous to those described on blast colony progenitors (22) and multipotent colony forming cells in serum free medium (33). Because our experiments were not done with a purified cell population, we cannot prove that the effects we observed are direct effects of the added growth factors. However, our results are analogous to those of others (21,22), who have shown that IL-3 and IL-6 act directly on blast colony progenitor cells. In addition we demonstrated a direct correlation between the percentage of CFU-S in the cell cycle and the percent of CFU-S that were infected by retroviruses (28). We have not examined the cycling status of PHSC in a competitive repopulation assay, but based on the increased susceptibility of PHSC treated with IL-3 and IL-6 to retroviral infection demonstrated here, we infer that some of these cells are in cycle.

Treatment with IL-3 and IL-6 increased the frequency of stem cell infection 5 fold over that seen with IL-3 alone. Two previous studies have examined retroviral mediated transfer of human β globin genes to murine PHSC. Dzierzak et al. (5) reported that 8 of 108 mice (7.4%) expressed the human β globin gene, and that approximately 10% of the PHSC in those mice carried the β globin provirus. The bone marrow cells were infected in the presence of IL-3 only, using a virus with a titer of ~ $2x10^5$ neo^r cfu/ml. A second study had a much higher frequency of long term mice that expressed the human β globin gene (7). In this experiment the bone marrow cells were infected with a virus with a titer of $4x10^6$ neo^r cfu/ml and selected in G418 to select for stem cells that had incorporated the proviral genome. At least 3 X 10^7 bone marrow cells were utilized to reconstitute each mouse. This is equivalent to 1.5 X 10^9 cells per kilogram, far more than the number of marrow cells available for reconstitution of a large experimental animal or man. We conclude that the preselection protocol as currently applied is an impractical approach to human gene therapy.

Although infection in the presence of IL-3 plus IL-6 increases the frequency of gene transfer, the fact remains that most stem cells are not infected. Other studies have shown that using an extremely high titer retrovirus containing the human ADA gene, approximately 50% of the reconstituted animals expressed the ADA gene for 6 months (8). As in all animals reconstituted without _in vitro_ selection to date, approximately 10% of the stem cells in these animals were infected. Perhaps infection in the presence of IL-3 plus IL-6 with a very high titer virus would lead to a greater efficiency of gene transfer.

The expression of the transduced human β globin gene in mouse erythroid cells is very low. Recent experiments have shown that relatively small segments of the locus activating region for the human β globin gene cluster (35) can increase the level of expression of human β globin genes in transgenic mice to near that of the endogenous mouse β globin genes (36, 37). We are attempting to incorporate these sequences into a retrovirus to increase the level of expression of the transduced human β globin gene following gene transfer with the long term goal of somatic gene therapy for human hemoglobinopathies.

Acknowledgements
The authors would like to thank Thalia Papayannopoulou for the gift of the monoclonal antibody against human β globin and for help with the assays. We would also like thank Steve Clark for the gift of rhuIL-6, Frank Lee for the pCDIL-3 and pCDIL-6 plasmids, Rick Nordan for the T1165 cell line, and Jane Barker and David Williams for advice and discussions.

References

1. Ogawa, M., Porter, P.N., and Nakahata, T. (1983) Blood 61, 823-829.
2. Dick, J.E., Magli, M.C., Huzar, D., Phillips, R.A., and Bernstein, A. (1985) Cell 42, 71-79.
3. Lemischka, I.R., Raulet, D.H., and Mulligan, R.C. (1986) Cell 45, 917-927.
4. Anderson, W.F. (1984) Science 226, 401-409.
5. Dzierzak, E.A., Papayannopoulou, Th. and Mulligan, R.C. (1988) Nature (London) 331, 35-41.
6. Karlsson, S., Bodine, D.M., Perry, L., Papayannopoulou, Th., and Nienhuis, A.W. (1988) Proc. Natl. Acad. Sci. (USA) 85, 6062-6066.

7. Bender, M.A., Gelinas, R.E., and Miller, A.D. (1989) Mol. Cell. Biol. 9, 1426-1434.
8. Belmont, J.W., MacGregor, G.R., Wagner-Smith, K., Fletcher, F.A., Moore, K.A., Hawkins, D., Villalon, D., Chang, S.M-U., and Caskey, C.T. (1988) Mol. Cell. Biol. 8, 5116-5125.
9. Wong, P.M.C., Chung, S.W., Dunbar, C.E., Bodine, D.M., Ruscetti, S., and Nienhuis, A.W. (1989) Mol. Cell. Biol. 9, 798-808.
10. Johnson, G.R., Gonda, T.J., Metcalf, D., Hariharan, I., and Cory, S. (1989) EMBO 8, 441-448.
11. Williams, D.A., Lemischka, I.R., Nathan, D.G., and Mulligan, R.C. (1984) Nature (London) 310, 476-480.
12. Keller, G., Paige, C., Gilboa, E., and Wagner, E.F. (1985) Nature (London) 318, 149-154.
13. Eglitis, M.A., Kantoff, P., Gilboa, E., and Anderson, W.F. (1985) Science 230, 1395-1398.
14. Harel, J., Rassart, E., and Jolicoeur, P. (1981) Virology 110, 202-207.
15. Richter, A., Ozer, H.L., Des Groseillers, L., and Jolicoeur, P. (1984) Mol. Cell. Biol. 4, 151-159.
16. Spangrude, G.J., Heimfeld, S., and Weissman, I.L. (1988) Science 241, 58-62.
17. Hodgson, G.S., and Bradley, T.R. (1979) Nature (London) 281, 381-382
18. Van Zant, G. (1984) J. Exp. Med. 159, 679-690.
19. Nakano, T., Waki, N., Asai, H. and Kitamura, Y. (1989) Blood 73, 425-430.
20. Metcalf, D. (1989) Nature (London) 339, 27-30.
21. Suda, T., Suda, J., Ogawa, M., and Ihle, J.N. (1985) J. Cell. Physiol. 124, 182-190.
22. Ikebuchi, K., Wong, G.G., Clark, S.C., Ihle, J.N., Hirai, Y, and Ogawa, M. (1987) Proc. Natl. Acad. Sci. (USA) 84, 9035-9039.
23. Wong, G.G., Witek-Giannotti, J.S., Temple, P.A., Kriz, R., Ferenz, C., Hewick, R.M., Clark, S.C., Ikebuchi, K., and Ogawa, M. (1988) J. Immunol. 140, 3040-3044.
24. Yokota, T., Lee, F., Rennick, D., Hall, C., Arai, N., Mossmann, T., Nabel, G., Cantor, H., and Arai, K. (1984) Proc. Natl. Acad. Sci. (USA) 81, 1070-1074.
25. Chiu, C.P., Moulds, C., Coffman, R.L., Rennick, D., and Lee, F. (1988) Proc. Natl. Acad. Sci. (USA) 85, 7099-7103.

26. Greenberger, J.S., Sakakeeny, M.A., Humphries, R.K., Eaves, C.J., and Eckner, R.J. (1983) Proc. Natl. Acad. Sci. (USA) 80, 2931-2935.
27. Nordan, R.P., and Potter, M. (1986) Science 233, 566-569.
28. Bodine, D.M., Karlsson, S., and Nienhuis, A.W. (1989) Proc. Nat. Acad. Sci. USA 86, in press.
29. Lim, B., Apperly, J., Orkin, S.H., and Williams, D.A. (1989) Proc. Nat. Acad. Sci. USA 86, in press.
30. Harrison, D.E. (1980) Blood 55, 77-81.
31. Sonoda, Y., Yang, Y-C., Wong, G.G., Clark, S.C., Ogawa, M. (1988) Proc. Natl. Acad. Sci (USA) 85, 4360-4364.
32. Kobayashi, M., Van Leeuwen, B.H., Elsbury, S., Martinson, M.E., Young, I.G., and Hapel, A.J. (1989) Blood 1836-1841.
33. Rennick, D., Jackson, J., Yang, G., Wideman, J., Lee, F., and Hudak, S. (1989) Blood 73, 1828-1835.
34. Mueller-Sieburg, C.E., Townsend, K., Weissman, I.L., and Rennick, D. (1988) J. Exp. Med. 167, 1825-1840.
35. Forrester, W.C., Takegawa, S., Papayannopoulou, Th., Stamatoyannopoulos, G., and Groudine, M. (1987) Nucl. Acids Res. 15, 10159-10177.
36. Grosveld, F., Van Assendelft, G.B., Greaves, D.R., and Kollias, G. (1987) Cell 51, 75-85.
37. Ryan, T.M., Behringer, R.R., Martin, N.C., Townes, T.M., Palmiter, R.D., and Brinster, R.L. (1989) Genes Develop. 3, 314-323.

The Biology of Hematopoiesis, pages 301–311

RETROVIRAL GENE TRANSFER: APPLICATIONS TO HUMAN THERAPY

Eli Gilboa

Memorial Sloan-Kettering Cancer Center,
Program in Molecular Biology, 1275 York Avenue,
New York, New York 10021

The concept of "gene therapy" was formulated long before the technical basis for its application was even conceivable, to describe a proposed treatment of patients suffering from genetic disorders to replace a defective gene with a functional counterpart. The technical basis of gene therapy is the ability to introduce genes with high efficiency into the somatic cells of live individuals. Now, with the advent of increasingly efficient gene transfer techniques, gene therapy may soon become a reality, as evidenced by an increasing number of laboratories which are exploring this new avenue to human therapy. In recent years it also became apparent that gene therapy, as defined for the treatment of genetic disorders, represents the tip of the iceberg of the potential of this new technology. This hidden and yet poorly appreciated potential of gene therapy will be the overall theme of this short review, and Table I lists several areas in which it may have usefull applications in human therapy.

Drug resistance genes introduced into hemopoietic cells can serve as selectable markers in vivo to enrich for hemopoietic cells carrying the drug resistant gene, and any gene which is physically linked to it.

Table I. **In vivo gene transfer - Applications to human therapy.**

1. Genetic disorders - gene therapy
2. Drug resistance - In vivo selection
3. Immunization - Cellular immune responses
4. Targetted delivery of cytokines - Tumor destruction

Methotrexate (MTX) resistant DHFR genes which can be selected with MTX, or the **mdr** gene which can be selected with vinblastine or other agents are possible candidates for in vivo selection. Introduction of selectable markers into hemopoietic cells may be exploited to improve the success of bone marrow transplantations, because the introduction of a selectable gene into the donor marrow may be used to confer growth advantage to the normal donor-derived hemopoietic cells in the transplanted patient.

Perhaps the major impact of in vivo gene transfer capabilities will be experienced in the field of immunology and immunotherapy because this technology will provide an extremely powerfull tool to manipulate the immune system in the live individual. For example, in vivo gene transfer may be used to develop alternative immunization protocols designed to elicit **cellular** immune responses, as opposed to currently employed immunization protocols which elicit primarily a **humoral** immune response. Several lines of evidence suggest that medical intervention designed to boost the cellular arm of the immune response will be beneficial to patients suffering from diseases such as AIDS, immunocompromised individuals at risk from CMV infection, or cancer patients. It was recently realized that while a humoral response is generated when antigen is presented directly to the immune system, a cellular response is elicited primarily when the foreign antigen is expressed de novo from within the antigen presenting cell. The basis of this immunization strategy is therefore that introduction of genes encoding a foreign antigen into the antigen presenting cells of the individual will elicit primarily a cellular immune response. Histocompatibility restrictions will necessitate the use of very efficient gene transfer systems to deliver genes with high efficiency into autologous cells of the patient.

Another potentially important use of effective gene transfer techniques is the delivery of cytokines to their appropriate targets in the body. It has been shown that in vivo administration of cytokines can be used to manipulate the immune system for the benefit of the patient. The most celebrated case is IL-2 which was shown in some cases to potentiate the immune system of cancer patients, and contribute to tumor regression. The short half life of cytokines in the serum requires the administration of very high doses of lymphokine which can lead to intolerable toxicities limiting their usefulness. This is not surprising since secretion of cytokines in vivo is highly localized, mediated by a limited number of specialized cells, reaching high and effective concentrations only at the appropriate site of the body, for example at the site of the tumor. Using gene transfer it may be possible to mimick the physiological state of lymphokine secretion by introducing the corresponding gene into antigen specific T-cells, which will then act as vehicles to transport the lymhokine gene to the appropriate region of the body, resulting in its localized and continuous secretion. Since a weak, though ineffective, T-cell response is induced by many tumor types which may be further amplified in vitro, and since the tumor specific T-cells will be used as vehicles for lymphokine delivery and not as effector cells, this approach may be applied to a wide range of tumor systems.

Finally, methodologies mediated via gene transfer may be used for the treatment of infectious diseases. As an example of the growing potential of gene therapy beyond its original definition for the treatment of genetic disorders,

I will further expand on this topic.

Retroviral gene transfer

Retroviral based gene transfer is one of several techniques that can be considered for the introduction of genes into the somatic cells of live individuals. The suitability of these viruses as vehicles for gene transfer, i.e. vectors, stems from their mode of replication. An obligatory step in the replication of retroviruses involves the integration of the viral genes into the cell chromosome, a process which does not affect the viability the infected cell, the integrated viral DNA serving as the template for the expression of the viral genes and the systhesis of progreny viral RNA. In the laboratory it is possible to experimentally exchange the viral genes with the gene of interest to create a hybrid virus which will deliver the foreign gene into the target cell. Retroviral gene transfer is not only an efficient technique for stable gene transfer with a wide host range but most importantly, it is also an experimentally controllable gene transfer system since in contrast to vaccinia or Adenovirus based systems, it employs replication defective viruses which do not spread beyond the primary target cell. (see Gilboa, 1986 for a review).

Gene inhibition mediated via gene transfer

The term "gene inhibition" is used here to describe a method in which a cell is genetically altered via gene transfer to result in the functional inactivation of a particular gene. A DNA template designed to inhibit the expression of an essential viral gene will result in the inhibition of viral replication, and if introduced into the cell prior to infection with the virus, it will render the cell resistant to viral infection. The term "intracellular immunization" was proposed to describe gene inhibition strategies designed to "protect" cells from viral replication (Baltimore, 1988).

Antisense RNA inhibition is one of several experimental strategies that can be used to inhibit gene expression, by constructing DNA templates which upon introduction into the cell will express RNA complementary to the target RNA, (i.e. antisense RNA) and bring about the functional inactivation of the corresponding gene. The feasibility of using antisense RNA inhibition to stably inhibit the function of specific genes was demonstrated in various studies (for a review see van der Krol, 1988) and it was also shown to inhibit the replication of HTLV-I in human T-lymphoid cells (Ruden and Gilboa, 1989). Although antisense RNA inhibition is a very attractive strategy, (availability of a partial sequence of a gene may suffice for its inactivation) the experience of many investigators in using this technique was somewhat dissapointing. The limiting factor in the successfull application of this experimental tool appears to be the synthesis of effective levels of antisense RNA in the target cell which are required in considerable excess over the target RNA to effect inhibition of gene function.

So the primary objective in developing effective antisense RNA inhibition methodologies has to be the design of DNA templates which will generate high levels of corresponding RNA. Although much attention is given to the identification of a "strong" promoter, the improtance of this factor is not clear. Our experience using retroviral gene transfer cannot confirm the existence of consistently "strong" or "weak" promoters. It may be that the importance of post-transcriptional processing events in generating high levels of RNA transcripts has been overlooked. Various studies have shown that events such as splicing, polyadenylation/termination or even translation may determine the nuclear transport and accumulation of the RNA in the cell. Finally, in a gene transfer setting, the vector also may inadvertantly affect the expression of transduced genes.

Retroviral vectors represent an interesting example in which the vector design may have an unwelcome influence on the expression of the transduced gene. The negative influence of the retroviral transcriptional unit i. e. the viral LTR, is mainly responsible for the poor expression of transduced genes, and vector design strategies have been explored to "separate" between the viral transcriptional unit and that of the transduced gene. Retroviral vectors carrying deletions of the promoter and enhancer region in the 3'LTR (self-inactivating vectors) have not gained much popularity because other parameters of vector function were compromised in the process, i.e. viral titer. (Yu, et.al., 1986).

Fig 1: The principle of double copy (DC) vectors.

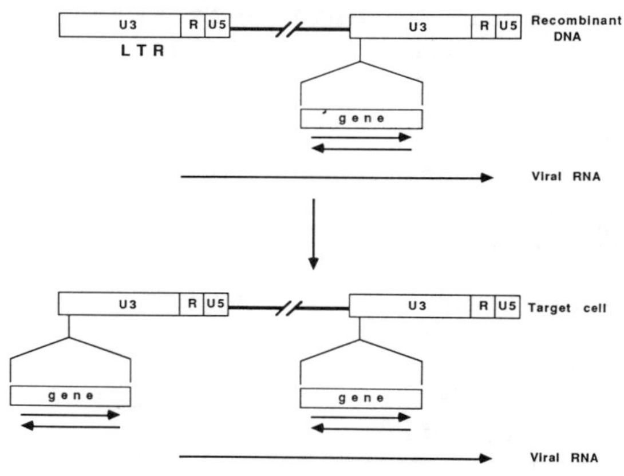

Another approach to limit the influence of the viral transcriptional unit on the expression of the transduced gene was recently described (Hantzopoulos et.al, 1989), and is shown in Fig 1. The unique feature of this type of retroviral vector is that the foreign gene is inserted into the U3 region of the 3'LTR. It is the consequence of the mechanism of replication of retroviruses that in the infected cell the gene will be duplicated and will appear also in the 5'LTR, hence the name of this type of vector, **double copy (DC) vector.** The important result is that in its new position, in the 5'LTR, the gene is placed outside the viral transcriptional unit, eliminating or at least reducing the negative effects of the retroviral transcriptional unit.

In the course of our studies we have explored a variety of promoters to express genes and antisense templates in the context of retroviral vectors and we were not successfull in identifying consistently "strong" promoters. In fact, the activity of promoters such as early SV40, immediate early CMV, human actin, HSV TK and others promoters was not reproducible, adding to our suspicion that factors other then promoter function (vector design, post-transcriptional events) play an important role in the accumulation of RNA in the cell.

The common denominator of most if not all promoters that have been used to express stably transduced genes, via retroviral vectors or other gene transfer methods, is that they are recognized by RNA polymerase II. The difficulties encountered in using these promoters recommends for consideration the use of alternative transcriptional units, in particular for the synthesis of non-coding RNA transcripts i.e. antisense RNA: A procarytic expression system based on the T7 RNA polymerase was shown to be very effective in a vaccinia based vector (Fuerst et.al. 1986) and may be used in a stable gene transfer setting as well. The potential problems with this approach is that the T7 generated transcripts may be unstable in the mammalian nucleous and the added complexity of this system which requires also the introduction of a functional T7 RNA polymerase gene into the target cell may limit the usefulness of this approach. **SnRNA** which are expressed very efficently from a modified RNA polymerase II system represent another option. **RNA polymerase III** transcriptional units are particularly attractive candidates since they represent a highly active transcriptional unit. It is estimated that, on a molar basis, the amount of steady state t-RNA transcribed from a t-RNA gene equals, within an order of magnitude, the total amount of mRNA content of a mammalian cell. Preliminary studies from our laboratory indicate that t-RNA-antisense fusion templates delivered into cells via retroviral vectors express high levels of antisense RNA, and the constitutive expression of antisense RNA renders cells partially resistant to replication of M-MuLV, or HIV.

Table II. **Strategies for gene inhibition mediated via stable gene transfer.**

1. Antisense RNA
2. Dominant negative mutants
3. Ribozymes
4. RNA binding decoys
5. False primers

Antisense RNA inhibition represents one of several strategies that can be employed for gene inhibition and Table II lists additional strategies that can be considered for this purpose. The use of **dominant negative mutants** was proposed on theoretical grounds by Herskowitz (1987) and used by Friedman et.al (1988) to inhibit the replication of HSV. The attractiveness of this approach is that it may not require the generation of large excess of the dominant mutant product to obtain significant inhibition. However, at best it is laborious and may not be universally applicable. Haseloff and Gerlach (1988) have shown that **ribozymes**, RNA molecules that catalyse endonucleolytic cleavage of RNA, can be used to cleave RNA molecules with experimentally determined sequence specificity. This approach would represent an attractive alternative to antisense RNA since ribozymes will inactivate the target RNA irreversibly (antisense

RNA though may do the same) and they can function catalytically. Another approach, involving the use of **RNA binding decoys** is applicable to genes which are positively regulated by factors which bind to RNA. The synthesis of excess RNA molecules encoding the recognition sequence of the RNA binding factor will then act as a decoy and lead to gene inhibition. HIV gene expression is particularly suitable for inhibition via such decoys since its expression is positively regulated by two RNA binding activators, the **tat** and **rev** gene products. Finally, **false primers** may be used to inhibit the replication of retroviruses. This strategy is based on unique features of the replication cycle of retroviruses which involve the primer dependent initiation of reverse transcription and an associated RNase H activity which degrades the template RNA. False priming would consist of the synthesis of RNA molecules that can act as primers for reverse transcription placed along the retroviral genome and leading to the degradation of the viral RNA. The caveat of this approach is that it requires that the 3'end of the primer RNA be complementary to the RNA template. Pol III transcriptional units can be engineered to generate such primers.

Applications to human therapy

Gene inhibition methodologies which render the cell resistant to viral replication may be usefull in the treatment of infectious diseases, provided an efficient in vivo gene transfer system exists to introduce the DNA template into the appropriate cells of the individual. AIDS may be a suitable disease candidate for such treatment which would consists of an autologous bone marrow transplantation protocol in which hemopoietic stem cells contained within the bone marrow are transduced ex-vivo with an antisense vector and then reinfused into the cytoblated patient to reconstitute the hemopoietic system with cells which are now resistant to HIV replication. If, as one may expect, the virus resistant hemopoietic cells in the transplanted patient will have a growth advantage over the HIV infected cells (which are destined to die), a relatively low efficiency of gene transfer may suffice to repopulate the hemopoietic system with HIV resistant T-lymphoid cells and restore immune functions. However, major caveats exists which must be considered first. Foremost, is the availability of an adequate gene transfer technology to deliver the antisense templates into the hemopoietic stem cells. Second, is the issue of whether HIV infection is directly or indirectly responsible for $CD4^+$ T-cell depletion. If the primary effect of HIV is indirect, a gene inhibition protocol as discussed here may not be effective. Furthermore, macrophages which constitute an important if not major reservoir of HIV are not eliminated in a cytoblation protocol and therefore will persist in the transplanted patient for a considerable period.

On a final note, although emphasis here was an theraputic applications, it will be very difficult to overemphasize the importance of developing gene inhibition methods for basic research. This is so because eucaryotic cells were so far refractile to extensive genetic manipulations as we were accustomed in the procaryotic system. The reason, of course, is that eucaryotic cells are diploid, a fact which prevented the derivation of a large collection of usefull mutants. The use of gene inhibition procedures discussed here will circumvent this limitation since they generate phenotypic though genetically stable mutations in diploid or polyploid cells and consequently may open the eucaryatic and mammalian cell to extensive genetic manipulation.

REFERENCES

Baltimore, D. (1988). Gene therapy intracellular immunization. Nature, 335, 395-396.

Friedman, A.D., Triezenberg, S.J. and Mcknight, S.L. (1988). Expression of a truncated viral transactivator selectively impedes lytic infection by its cognate virus. Nature, 335, 452-454.

Fuerst, T.R., Niles, E.G., Studier, F.W., and Moss, B. (1986). Eukaryotic transient-expression system based on reconbinant vaccinia virus that synthesizes bacteriophage T7 RNA polymerase. Proc. Natl. Acad. Sci. USA, 83, 8122-8126.

Gilboa, E. (1986). Retrovirus vectors and their uses in molecular biology. BioEssay 5, 252-258.

Hantzopoulos P.A., Sullenger, B.A., Ungers, G., and Gilboa, E. (1989). Improved gene expression upon transfer of the adenosine deaminase minigene outside the transcriptional unit of a retroviral vector. Proc. Natl. Acad. Sci. USA, 86, 3519-3523.

Haseloff, J. and Gerlach W.L. (1988). Simple RNA enzymes with new and highly specific endoribonuclease activities. Nature, 334, 585-591.

Herskowitz, I. (1987). Functional inactivation of genes by dominant negative mutations. Nature, 329, 219-222.

von Ruden, T. and Gilboa, E. (1989). Inhibition of human T-cell leukemia virus type I replication in primary human T cells that express antisense RNA. J. Virol. 63, 677-682.

van der Krol, A.R., Mol, J. N. M. and Stuitje A.R. (1988). Modulation of eukaryotic gene expression by complementary RNA or DNA sequences. Biotechniques, 6, 958-976.

Yu, S. -F., Ruden, T.V., Kantoff, P.W., Garber, C., Seiberg, M., Ruther, U., Anderson, W.F., Wagner, E.F., and Gilboa, E., (1986). Self-inactivating retroviral vectors designed for transfer of whole genes into mammalian cells. Proc. Natl. Acad. Sci. USA, 83, 3194-3198.

The Biology of Hematopoiesis, pages 313–322

DEVELOPMENTAL CONTROL OF HUMAN GLOBIN GENE EXPRESSION

Bernard G. Forget, M.D.

Department of Internal Medicine,
Yale University School of Medicine,
333 Cedar Street, New Haven, CT 06510

INTRODUCTION

During normal human development, there is a perinatal switch from the synthesis of fetal hemoglobin or HbF ($\alpha_2\gamma_2$) to adult hemoglobin or HbA ($\alpha_2\beta_2$). The study of various naturally occurring mutations associated with elevated HbF levels in adult life has provided numerous insights into mechanisms that can potentially regulate the fetal to adult hemoglobin switch. Such mutations constitute a heterogeneous group of disorders termed hereditary persistence of fetal hemoglobin or HPFH (for reviews see Bunn and Forget, 1986; Stamatoyannopoulos and Nienhuis, 1987; and Weatherall and Clegg, 1981).

The nondeletion forms of HPFH are particularly noteworthy. In contrast to most other syndromes of persistent HbF production where both linked $^G\gamma$ and $^A\gamma$ genes are overexpressed, only one or the other γ gene is overexpressed in the usual nondeletion types of HPFH. These can therefore be subdivided into two types: $^G\gamma$ HPFH and $^A\gamma$ HPFH. Because of this restricted pattern of expression, it was assumed that the mutations in these syndromes must be located near the affected gene and initial molecular studies focused initially on the DNA sequence analysis of the promoter regions of the overexpressed γ genes in nondeletion HPFH.

RESULTS

Mutations Associated with Nondeletion HPFH

The results of structural analyses revealed a number of different point mutations in the promoter region of the overexpressed γ gene in different individuals with different types of nondeletion HPFH. These point mutations have clustered in three distinct regions of the 5' flanking DNA of the affected γ globin genes (Figure 1). A number of different mutations have been identified in the region approximately 200 base pairs from the "cap site" or site of transcription initiation, specifically at positions -202 (Collins et al 1984; Gilman et al 1988), -198 (Tate et al, 1986), and -196 (Giglioni et al, 1984; Ottolenghi et al, 1987; Gelinas et al, 1986). This region of DNA which was not previously suspected of playing a role in the regulation of gene expression is very G-C rich and its sequence bears homology to that of known control elements of other genes such as the 21 bp repeat of the SV40 virus promoter and the distal element of the thrymidine kinase gene of <u>Herpes</u> <u>simplex</u> virus. It is noteworthy that the G-C rich sequences of the latter genes are known to be the binding sites of a <u>trans</u>-acting protein factor called SP1. The -202 (C to G) and -196 mutations are associated with high levels of HbF (15-20%), expressed in a pancellular fashion, whereas the -202 (C to T)and -198 mutations are associated with lower levels of HbF (3.0-6%) expressed in a heterocellular fashion.

The second region containing a mutation associated with nondeletion HPFH is located at position -175 (Surrey et al, 1988; Ottolenghi et al, 1988; Stoming et al, 1989). A single point mutation at this position has the same phenotype as the C to G mutation at position -202. This region of DNA is noteworthy because it contains an octanucleotide sequence which is present in the promoter region of a number of genes, in particular the immunoglobulin genes and is the binding site of another <u>trans</u>-acting factor. The point mutation at position -175 changes the last base of the conserved octanucleotide.

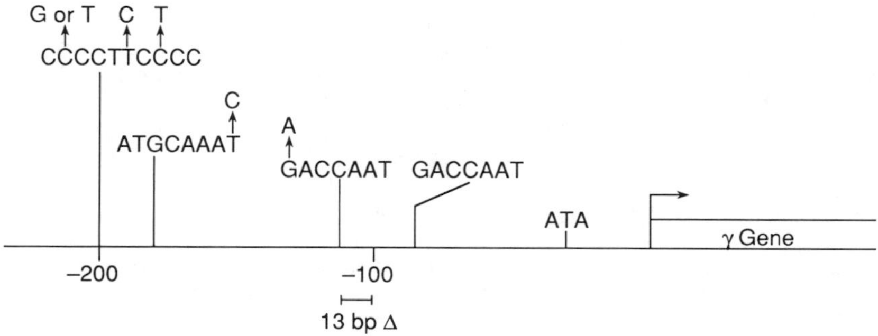

Figure 1. Relative locations and types of mutations associated with nondeletion forms of HPFH.

The third region affected by a point mutation in ndHPFH is in the area of a well known regulatory element of globin and other genes: the CCAAT box sequence. In the γ genes, the CCAAT sequence is duplicated and the mutation associated with ndHPFH is located at position -117, 2 bases upstream of the distal CCAAT box (Gelinas et al, 1985; Collins et al, 1985). The base change disrupts a pentanucleotide sequence that is highly conserved immediately upstream of the CCAAT sequence in all animal fetal and embryonic genes. Another mutation with a similar phenotype involves the deletion of 13 base pairs of DNA encompassing the distal CCAAT box and adjacent 3' DNA (Gilman et al, 1988b). The CCAAT box region is known to be the binding site of a number of trans-acting factors.

The unifying model by which these various mutations affect hemoglobin switching proposes that these base changes alter the binding of a number of different trans-acting factors to critical regions of the γ gene promoters and thereby prevent the normal postnatal suppression of γ gene expression. The mutations could prevent the binding of negative regulatory factors or enhance the binding of positive regulatory factors. Either mechanism could be operative in different mutations. Further insights into this fascinating problem is being obtained with the characterization of the various trans-acting factors that are involved in the regulation of globin gene expression and by functional studies of the mutant genes in various gene transfer systems.

Studies of DNA/Protein Interactions

Studies of DNA/protein interactions have revealed the presence of a number of different proteins, in nuclear extracts of erythroid and non-erythroid cells, that are capable of binding to the γ globin gene promoter (Mantovani et al, 1987, 1988, 1989; Gumucio et al, 1988; Superti-Furga et al, 1988; Metherall et al, 1988; Martin et al, 1989; Tsai et al, 1989). At least two proteins (or activities) normally bind to the -175 region of the γ promoter. One is present in nonerythroid as well as erythroid cells and binds to the octamer consensus sequence; the -175 mutation markedly decreases the binding of this protein (Mantovani et al, 1988; Gumucio et al, 1988; Martin et al, 1989). The second protein is erythroid-specific and binds to either side of the octamer sequence; its binding affinity is either unaffected (Gumucio et al, 1988; Martin et al, 1989) or somewhat enhanced (Mantovani et al, 1989) by the -175 mutation. The mutation also alters the DNase I "footprint" pattern of the protein/DNA complex (Martin et al, 1989). In the case of the -117 region, there are a number of different proteins that bind at or near the CCAAT boxes of the γ gene promoter (Montovani et al, 1988; Superti-Furgna et al, 1988). The binding of one of these proteins, which is erythroid specific, is reduced by the base substitution at -117 (Superti-Furga et al, 1988), whereas the binding affinity of a second ubiquitous CCAAT binding protein is somewhat enhanced (Gumucio et al, 1988; Superti-Furga et al, 1988).

These various studies have not yet elucidated the precise mechanism by which the mutations cause deregulated γ gene expression, but they clearly demonstrate an effect of the mutations on the binding of trans-acting factors to the γ gene promoter.

Functional Studies of Mutant Genes Following Gene Transfer

Functional studies of mutant nondeletion HPFH γ genes or their promoters following gene transfer into tissue culture cells have provided evidence for moderately increased gene expression associated with the mutant genes or promoters, but the increases were only 2 to 5 fold compared to the normal genes or promoters (Martin et al, 1989; Charney and Henry, 1986; Collins et al, 1986; Stoeckert et al, 1987; Rixon and Gelinas, 1988,; Nicolis et al, 1989), whereas the *in vivo* effect of the mutations is a 40 fold increase over normal. The cell culture systems therefore do not appear to constitute a faithful model of hemoglobin switching.

Transgenic mice may provide a more faithful model for hemoglobin switching, although mice do not have a truly fetal hemoglobin: they switch from production of embryonic hemoglobins in yolk-sac derived erythroid cells during early embryogenesis to the production of definitive adult hemoglobins during later intrauterine fetal development (reviewed by Chada et al, 1986). When individual normal human globin genes are transferred into transgenic mice, the γ globin genes are expressed predominantly or exclusively in yolk-sac derived erythroid cells, whereas the β globin gene is highly expressed in fetal liver as well as adult erythroid tissues (Chada et al, 1985, 1986; Magram et al, 1985; Townes et al, 1985; Kollias et al, 1987). However, more recent studies (Tanaka et al, 1989) utilizing as the transgene a large (40kb) DNA fragment of the β cluster containing the linked γ, δ and β genes, indicate that these genes are expressed in transgenic mice in a manner more closely resembling their pattern of expression in man. It is conceivable therefore that the normal switching process involves competition between fetal and adult promoters and/or enhancer sequences for various *trans*-acting factors that are required for optimal globin gene expression (Figure 2). Such a model has been previously proposed for the regulation of the embryonic to adult hemoglobin switch in the chicken (Choi and Engel, 1988; Gallarda et al, 1989).

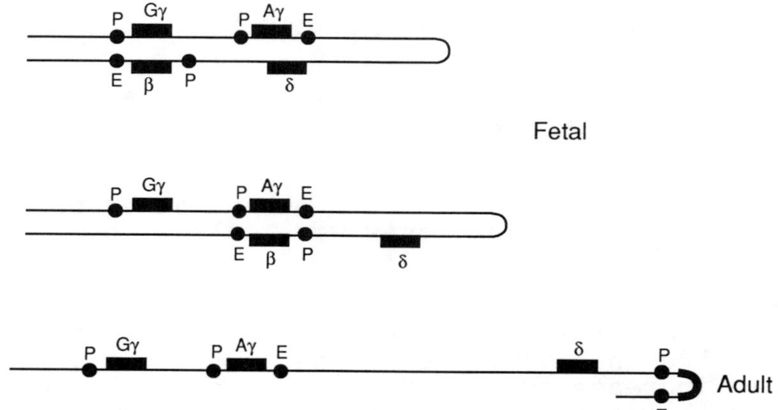

Figure 2. Model of globin gene regulation by promoter (P)/enhancer (E) competition.

Functional studies of mutated nondeletion HPFH genes in transgenic mice have yielded varied results. The -196 Aγ HPFH globin gene, as an isolated transgene, was not expressed in fetal or adult tissues but only in yolk sac derived erythroid cells (Trudel et al, 1987). On the other hand, the -202 Gγ HPFH globin gene as part of a 40 kb transgene containing the linked γ, δ and β globin genes, was highly overexpressed in relation to the normal, linked Aγ globin gene of the transgene, in both fetal and adult tissues (Tanaka et al, 1989).

In summary, the study of the downstream repeats in transgenic mice of nondeletion HPFH mutations and of large DNA fragments containing both fetal and adult globin genes holds the promise of providing an animal model system for the study of the molecular mechanisms that regulate hemoglobin switching in man.

ACKNOWLEDGMENTS

The author's research was supported in part by grants from the National Institutes of Health.

REFERENCES

Bunn HF, Forget BG (1986). Hemoglobin: Molecular, genetic and clinical aspects. WB Saunders, Inc., Philadelphia.

Chada K, Magram J, Raphael K, Radice G, Lacy E, Costantini F (1985). Specific expression of a foreign β-globin gene in erythroid cells of transgenic mice. Nature 314:377-380.

Chada K, Magram J, Costantini F (1986). An embryonic pattern of expression of a human fetal globin gene in transgenic mice. Nature, 319:685-689.

Charnay P, Henry L (1986). Regulated expression of cloned human fetal Aγ-globin genes introduced into murine erythroleukemia cells. Eur J Biochem 159:475-478.

Choi, OB,Engel, JD (1988). Developmental regulation of β-globin gene switching. Cell 55:17-26.

Collins, FS, Stoeckert CJ Jr, Serjeant GR, Forget BG, Weissman SM (1984). $G\gamma\beta^{+}$ hereditary persistence of fetal hemoglobin: Cosmid cloning and identification of a specific mutation 5' to the Gγ gene. Proc Natl Acad Sci USA 81:4894-4898.

Collins FS, Metherall JE, Yamakawa M, Pan J, Weissman SM, Forget BG (1985). A point mutation in the Aγ-globin gene promoter in Greek hereditary persistence of fetal hemoglobin. Nature 313:325-326.

Collins F, Bodine D, Lockwood W, Cole J, Mickley L, Ley T (1986). Expression analysis of the human fetal globin gene promoter in hereditary persistence of fetal hemogloblin. Clin Res 34:454a.

Gallarda JL, Foley, KP, Yang Z, Engle, DE (1989). The β-globin stage selector element factor is erythroid-specific promoter/enhancer binding protein NF-E4. Genes Dev 3:1845-1859.

Gelinas R, Endlich B, Pfeiffer C, Yagi M, Stamatoyannopoulos G (1985). G to A substitution in the distal CCAAT box of the Aγ globin gene in Greek hereditary persistence of fetal hemoglobin. Nature 313:323-325.

Gelinas R, Bender M, Lotshaw C, Waber P, Kazazian H Jr, Stamatoyannopoulos G (1986). Chinese $^{A}\gamma$ fetal hemoglobin: C to T substitution at position -196 of the $^{A}\gamma$ gene promoter. Blood 67:1777-1779.

Giglioni B, Casini C, Mantovani R, Merli S, Comi P, Ottolenghi S, Saglio G, Camaschella C, Mazza U (1984). A molecular study of a family with Greek hereditary persistence of fetal hemoglobin and β-thalassemia. EMBO J 3:2641-2645.

Gilman, JG, Mishima, N, Wen, XJ, Kutlar, F, Huisman, THJ (1988). Upstream promoter mutation associated with a modest elevation of fetal hemoglobin expression in human adults. Blood 72:78-81.

Gilman, JG, Mishima, N, Wen, XJ, Stoming, TA, Lobel, J, Huisman, THJ (1988). Distal CCAAT box deletion in the $^{A}\gamma$ globin gene of two black adolescents with elevated fetal $^{A}\gamma$ globin. Nucl Acids Res 16:10635-10642.

Gumucio D, Rood K, Gray T, Riordan M, Sartor C, Collins F (1988). Nuclear proteins that bind the human γ-globin gene promoter: alterations in binding produced by point mutations associated with hereditary persistence of fetal hemoglobin. Mol Cell Biol 8:5310-5322.

Kollias G, Wrighton N, Hurst J, Grosveld F (1986). Regulated expression of human $^{A}\gamma$-, β-, and hybrid $\gamma\beta$-globin genes in transgenic mice: manipulation of the developmental expression patterns. Cell 46:89-94.

Magram J, Chada K, Costantini F (1985). Developmental regulation of a cloned adult β-globin gene in transgenic mice. Nature 315:338-340.

Mantovani R, Malgaretti N, Giglioni B, Comi P, Cappellini N, Nicolis S, Ottolenghi S (1987). A protein factor binding to an octamer motif in the γ-globin promoter disappears upon induction of differentiation and hemoglobin synthesis in K562 cells. Nucl Acids Res 15:9349-9364.

Mantovani R, Malgaretti N, Nicolis S, Ronchi A, Giglioni B, Ottolenghi S (1988). The effects of HPFH mutations in the human γ-globin promoter on binding of ubiquitous and erythroid specific nuclear factors. Nucl Acids Res, 16:7783-7797.

Mantovani, R, Superti-Furga, G, Gilman, J, Ottolenghi, S (1989). The detection of the distal CCAAT box region of the $^{A}\gamma$-globin gene in black HPFH abolishes the binding of the erythroid specific protein NFE3 and of the CCAAT displacement protein. Nucl Acids Res 17:6681-6691.

Martin D, Tsai S, Orkin S (1989). Increased γ-globin expression in a nondeletion HPFH mediated by an erythroid-specific DNA-binding factor. Nature 338:435-438.

Metherall J, Gillespie F, Forget B (1989). Nuclear proteins of a human erythroleukemic cell line that bind to the promoter region of normal and nondeletion HPFH γ-globin genes. Stamatoyannopoulos, G, Nienhuis, AW (eds): "Hemoglobin Switching, Part A: Transcriptional Regulation," New York: Alan R. Liss, pp 247-260.

Nicolis, S, Ronchi, A, Malgaretti, N, Mantovani, R, Giglioni, B, Ottolenghi, S (1989). Increased erythroid-specific expression of a mutated HPFH γ-globin promoter requires the erythroid factor NFE-1. Nucl Acids Res 17:5509-5516.

Ottolenghi, S, Giglioni, B, Pulazzini, Comi, P, Camaschella, C, Serra, A, Guerrasio, A, Saglio, G (1987). Sardinian $\delta\beta^{O}$-thalassemia: A further example of a C to T substitution at position -196 of the $^{A}\gamma$ globin gene promoter. Blood 69:1058-1061.

Ottolenghi S, Nicolis R, Taramelli N, Malgaretti R, Mantovani P, Comi P, Giglioni B, Longinotti M, Dore F, Oggiano L, Pistidda P, Serra A, Camaschella C, Saglio G (1988). Sardinian $^{G}\gamma$-HPFH: A T -> C substitution in a conserved "octamer" sequence in $^{G}\gamma$-globin promoter. Blood 71:815-817.

Rixon M, Gelinas, R (1988). A fetal globin gene mutation in $^{A}\gamma$ nondeletion hereditary persistence of fetal hemoglobin increases promoter strength in a nonerythroid cell. Mol Cell Biol 8:713-721.

Stamatoyannopoulos G, Nienhuis AW. (1987) Hemoglobin switching. In Stamatoyannopoulos G, Nienhuis AW, Leder P, Majerus PW (eds): "The Molecular Basis of Blood Diseases," Philadelphia: Saunders, pp 66-105.

Stoeckert CJ Jr, Metherall JE, Yamakawa M, Eisenstadt JM, Weissman SM, Forget BG (1987). Expression of the affected Aγ globin gene associated with Greek nondeletion hereditary persistence of fetal hemoglobin. Mol Cell Biol 7:2999-3003.

Stoming, TA, Stoming GS, Lanclos, KD, Fei, YJ, Altay, C, Kutlar, F, Huisman, THJ (1989). An $^{A}\gamma$ type of nondeletional hereditary persistence of fetal hemoglobin with a T->C mutation at position -175 to the cap site of the $^{A}\gamma$ globin gene. Blood 73:329-333.

Superti-Furga G, Barberis A, Schaffner G, Busslinger M (1988). The -117 mutation in Greek HPFH affects the binding of three nuclear factors to the CCAAT region of the γ-globin gene. EMBO J 7:3099-3107.

Surrey S, Delgrosso K, Malladi P, Schwartz E (1988). A single-base change at position -175 in the 5'-flanking region of the $^{G}\gamma$-globin gene from a black with $^{G}\gamma$-β^{+} HPFH. Blood 71:807-810.

Tanaka M, Chamberlain J, Bhargava A, Nolan J, Collins F, Forget B, Weissman S (1989). Expression of human globin genes in transgenic mice carrying $G\gamma$-, $A\gamma$-, δ- and β-globin gene cluster of $G\gamma\beta^{+}$ and $A\gamma\beta^{+}$ hereditary persistence of fetal hemoglobin (submitted).

Tate VE, Wood WG, Weatherall DJ (1986). The British form of hereditary persistence of fetal hemoglobin results from a single base mutation adjacent to an S1 hypersensitive site 5' to the $^{A}\gamma$ globin gene. Blood 68:1389-1393.

Townes T, Lingrel J, Chen H, Brinster R, Palmiter R (1985). Erythroid-specific expression of human β-globin gene in transgenic mice. EMBO J 4:1715-1723.

Trudel M, Magram J, Chada K, Wilson R, Costantini F (1987). Expression of normal, mutant and hybrid human globin genes in transgenic mice. In Stamatoyannopoulos G, Nienhuis AW (eds): "Developmental Control of Globin Gene Expression," New York: Alan R. Liss, pp 305-321.

Tsai S, Martin D, Zon L, D'Andrea A Wong G, Orkin S (1989). Cloning of cDNA for the major DNA-binding protein of the erythroid lineage through expression in mammalian cells. Nature 339:446-451.

Weatherall DJ, Clegg JB (1981). The Thalassemia Syndromes, 3rd edition. Blackwell Scientific Publications, Oxford.

The Biology of Hematopoiesis, pages 323–328

GLOBIN GENE SWITCHING: INSIGHTS FROM STUDIES IN SOMATIC HETEROSPECIFIC HYBRIDS AND IN TRANSGENIC MICE.

Thalia Papayannopoulou, Martha Brice, Tariq Enver and George Stamatoyannopoulos
Departments of Hematology and Medical Genetics, University of Washington, Seattle, Washington 98195

BRIEF OVERVIEW

The precise mechanism by which the sequential globin gene activation (from embryonic → fetal → adult) is achieved during development remains elusive. Previous in vitro studies (using clonal erythroid cultures) as well as experiments in vivo with fetal to adult transplants have suggested a control that is intrinsic to cells at each developmental stage, rather than a dependence on external environmental stimuli. More recent studies in transgenic mice and in transient heterokaryons (fusion of cells with different cytoplasmic factors) have expanded this concept and suggested the presence of stage-specific transcriptional factors. Whether positive or negative regulators are involved in each stage, however, is unclear. Moreover, the contribution of chromatin structure or position effects; (i.e. deletions, substitutions) within the β locus, deemed important from naturally existing mutations, have been difficult to study in all previous models.

To expand previous observations and address several unsettled issues regarding globin switching we have used somatic cell hybrids as models for the cellular and molecular analysis of globin switching. This approach provides a unique opportunity to study the behavior of globin genes within their native chromosomal environment, as they interact with a changing regime of transcriptional factors.

Through fusion mediated chromosomal transferring we have established continuously proliferating synkaryons containing a human erythroid chromosome 11 from discrete developmental stages (first or second trimester fetal liver or adult bone marrow) introduced into a MEL (adult murine) cell environment. The properties of these hybrids (1), summarized below, have validated their use as surrogate erythroid cells in the molecular analysis of switching; their human globin phenotype reflects the phenotype of the parental human erythroid cell used for fusion. Hybrids from first trimester fetal liver produce predominantly fetal globin, whereas those from adult erythroblasts produce adult globin; with time in culture, hybrids with a "fetal" phenotype switch to an "adult" phenotype, providing an in vitro reconstruction of the fetal to adult switch. This switch entails the progressive generation of adult (β) globin only containing cells from fetal (γ) only containing cells. Thus at a cellular level, much like in vivo, only one of the two globins is dominant at any given time; the rate of γ to β switching is roughly proportional to the gestational age of the parent human erythroid chromosome. Hybrids from second trimester fetal liver erythroid cells switch faster than the ones from the first trimester.

Using these hybrids as surrogate erythroid cells for the developmental fetal to adult switch we were able to test several questions pertaining to the mechanism of switching, which are difficult to study with primary erythroid cells. For example, what is the relationship between DNA methylation and globin gene switching? Is methylation the cause or the consequence of globin gene switching? To answer this question we have obtained, in hybrids, the chronological order in which transcriptional silencing and DNA methylation occur. We have found (2) that γ-globin gene inactivation precedes DNA methylation, implying that the transcriptional activity of the gene dictates the methylation pattern rather than vice versa. Thus methylation does not appear to be a primary event in γ-gene inactivation during human development.

If the switching is controlled by stage specific transcriptional factors, what chromosome is responsible for this? We have carried out extensive chromosomal studies (using both DNA probes and cytogenetics) in our hybrids to test the chromosomal composition of preswitched and switched hybrids. These studies (3) have shown that chromosome 11 (harboring the β-locus) is not only necessary, but sufficient for the switching process; no other human chromosome, besides 11, needs to be present. These data suggested either a control *cis* to the β-locus or a *trans* mechanism dependent on chromosome 11.

Since adult erythroid chromosomes express within the MEL cell environment only adult (β) globin, whereas fetal erythroid chromosomes, within the same environment (i.e. the same MEL cell line), express mainly fetal globin, the β-globin in these fetal chromosomes must be actively repressed. To test whether the *trans* environment of MEL cells has changed as a result of the incoming fetal chromosome, as well as the nature of the globin gene sequences that are required for interaction with positive or negative *trans* factors, we have introduced cloned γ or β-gene constructs into parental MEL cells used as fusion partners, or in established fetal liver x MEL hybrids, before and after their switching. Using a marked 3.3 kb Hind III Aγ fragment or a 5.2 kb Bgl II fragment, either individually or linked together, we have found that these constructs were expressed at all stages of hybrid development, in a manner discordant to the endogenous (chromosomal) gene, regardless of whether the chromosome was introduced into the MEL cells before or after the construct was introduced. These data suggested an independent control of the endogenous compared to exogenous β or γ-genes and, if the *trans* control hypothesis is correct, they implied a *trans* mechanism that is working outside the sequences used. These ideas are being tested with further ongoing experiments.

In addition to adult erythroid x MEL hybrids we have made a series of observations using hybrids made from human non-erythroid cells. Hybrids between MEL cells and non-erythroid cells express only adult globin regardless of whether the non-erythroid cells are derived from adults or fetuses (4). These data suggested that the MEL cell environment can reactivate only the β-globin from non-erythroid cells. Using DNAse 1 sensitivity assays we asked whether the expression of the previously silent β-globin gene in MEL x human lymphoid hybrids is accomplished through a limited activation of the chromatin surrounding the β-gene, or whether activation of the whole β-locus domain is required. We found that in addition to the 5′ (promoter) hypersensitive sites (HSs) of the β-gene, HSs 5′ to ϵ locus have now appeared in these lymphoid chromosomes. These results suggested that the region 5′ to ϵ gene contains sequences which interact with the MEL erythroid environment and lead to activation of the whole β-domain (5). This region has been named Locus Activation Region (LAR) and is deleted in $(\gamma\delta\beta)^{\circ}$ thalassemia mutations, in which all remaining, structurally intact, globin genes downstream from deletion are now silenced. Hybrids containing chromosome 11 from three of these mutations (Hispanic, Dutch or English $(\gamma\delta\beta)^{\circ}$ thalassemia) also fail to activate, within the MEL cell environment any intact globin genes downstream from LAR deletion (Th. Papayannopoulou unpublished).

In contrast to normal lymphoid x MEL hybrids, which express β-globin, lymphocytes from heterozygotes with HPFH mutations (i.e. deletion HPFH-I, deletion HPFH-II, -117Aγ HPFH, -196Aγ) give rise to hybrids which reflect the phenotype of the HPFH mutation; that is, in contrast to the wild type γ-genes, HPFH γ-globin is now activated within these hybrids (6). Since the hybrids are erythroid and hemizygous they provide an opportunity for further functional studies which require erythroid nuclei.

In addition to experiments with hybrid cells, several experiments were carried out in transgenic mice to explore the role of intergenic globin sequences, as well as the role of LAR in the developmental regulation of embryonic (ϵ), fetal (γ) or adult (β) genes. In these experiments, ϵ, γ or β are attached directly to a construct containing all five HSs′ present in LAR, but in a truncated form (μLAR). These experiments showed that γ or β genes attached to LAR are not developmentally regulated (i.e. they are present in both primitive and definitive murine erythroid cells), in contrast to previous experiments done without the use of LAR. These data suggested that either additional sequences in the globin locus are necessary for developmental control of γ or β-globin genes, or that the function of LAR is different in its native position several kb away from the fetal γ or β genes than in the construct. Whereas μLAR can override the developmental control of the attached γ or β gene, it fails to do so when it is linked to ϵ gene. The expression of the latter, even in the μLAR presence, is under developmental control, since it is expressed only in primitive (embryonic) erythroid cells. Candidate sequences within the ϵ gene responsible for this control are currently being tested. In concurrent experiments, the role of intergenic (between γ and $\delta\beta$) sequences in the developmental globin switch is also being explored. Preliminary evidence from these experiments indicates that when both γ and β promoters are present, developmental regulation (i.e. globin switching) occurs. These results imply a stage-specific differential promoter utilization which is mutually exclusive.

Taken together the data with either the transgenic mice or the hybrids suggest that the switch is likely accomplished through complex interactions between several areas within the β locus and stage specific transcriptional factors.

REFERENCES

Papayannopoulou Th, Brice M, Stamatoyannopoulos G (1986). Analysis of human hemoglobin switching in MEL x human fetal erythroid cell hybrids. Cell 46:469-476.

Enver T, Zhang J, Papayannopoulou Th, Stamatoyannopoulos G (1988). DNA methylation: a secondary event in globin gene switching? Genes & Dev 2:698-706.

Melis M, Demopulos G, Najfeld V, Zhang J, Brice M, Papayannopoulou Th, Stamatoyannopoulos G (1987). A chromosome 11-linked determinant controls fetal globin expression and the fetal to adult globin switch. Proc Nat Acad Sci 84:8105-8109.

Takegawa S, Brice M, Stamatoyannopoulos G, Papayannopoulou Th (1986). Only adult hemoglobin is produced in fetal nonerythroid x MEL cell hybrids. Blood 68:1384-1388.

Forrester WC, Takegawa S, Papayannopoulou Th, Stamatoyannopoulos G, Groudine M (1987). Evidence for a locus activation region: The formation of developmentally stable hypersensitive sites in globin-expressing hybrids. Nucleic Acids Res 24:10159-10177.

Papayannopoulou Th, Enver T, Takegawa S, Anagnou NP, Stamatoyannopoulos G (1988). Activation of developmentally mutated human globin genes by cell fusion. Science 242:1056-1058.

The Biology of Hematopoiesis, pages 329–337

INSERTIONAL MUTAGENESIS AND TRANSFORMATION OF HEMATOPOIETIC STEM CELLS

James N. Ihle, Kazuhiro Morishita, Takayasu Matsugi and Christopher Bartholomew

Department of Biochemistry, St. Jude Children's Research Hospital, 332 N. Lauderdale, Memphis, TN 38105

INTRODUCTION

Mature myeloid cells are derived from the proliferation and differentiation of pluripotential stem cells. During the last several years, research has focused on the identification and isolation of a variety of hematopoietic growth factors that support the proliferation and allow the differentiation of stem cells and committed myeloid progenitors. Among these factors interleukin-3 (IL-3) uniquely supports the proliferation of early stem cells as well as the committed progenitors of a number of the myeloid lineages (Ihle, 1989a). This has been most amply demonstrated by the ability of IL-3 to support the differentiation of early stem cells to a variety of mature myeloid cells in vitro in the absence of other hematopoietic growth factors.

While considerable information is available on the growth factors that support committed myeloid progenitors, relatively little is known about the genes that regulate lineage commitments and differentiation. Knowledge of these genes is important because, in acute myelogenous leukemia, transformation has altered the capacity of the cells to terminally differentiate. This kind of transformation often occurs without any detectable alterations in the growth factor requirements of the cells and is best demonstrated by a series of IL-3-dependent myeloid leukemia cell lines that were isolated from retroviral induced leukemias (Holmes et al.1985; Ihle and Askew, 1989b). These cell lines require IL-3 for maintenance of viability and have phenotypes comparable to normal intermediates in IL-3 supported myeloid differentiation. Unlike their normal counterparts however, the cells cannot be induced to terminally differentiate. Using these cell lines, we have begun to identify the genes that are associated with this type of transformation. Knowledge of the structure and function of these genes can be expected to provide important insights into the normal regulation of hematopoietic stem cell differentiation.

RETROVIRAL INSERTIONAL ACTIVATION OF THE C-MYB GENE IN AN IL-3-DEPENDENT MYELOID LEUKEMIA CELL LINE

The IL-3-dependent cell lines were initially isolated from retrovirus induced myeloid leukemias (Holmes et al.1985; Ihle et al.1984). Since replication competent retroviruses cause transformation by insertional mutagenesis (Clurman and Hayward, 1988), it is possible to identify genes whose expression may have been by retroviral integration. Initially we examined the cell lines for the rearrangement of a number of potential transforming genes. Using a number of cell lines and examining for the rearrangement of a variety of known oncogenes, two cell lines were found to have a retroviral insertions in the c-myb locus (Weinstein et al.1986; Weinstein et al.1987). The rearrangements of the gene involved the integration of proviruses in the middle of the gene near the sixth viral related exon. As a consequence of the insertions, the NFS-60 cells produce a carboxyl-truncated c-myb protein of 45 kDa. This truncated gene product is produced at levels approximately 10 times that of the gene product from the normal allele due to either an enhancer effect of the provirus on transcription or due to stabilization of the transcripts from the rearranged locus. No detectable alterations were found in the amino terminal domain of the protein.

The significance of the carboxy-truncated c-myb gene product is not known. However, it is significant the carboxyl deletion is comparable to that which occurred during the transduction of the avian gene into the myeloid transforming retroviruses AML and E26. Unlike the transduced avian genes however, there were no additional alterations in the amino terminal domain of the gene. Based on the biological properties of the cells and the biochemical properties of the altered c-myb gene product, we have hypothesized that the myb gene plays a role in normal myeloid differentiation and carboxyl-truncations of the protein can block this function. In particular, it can be hypothesized that c-myb is a transcriptional factor that is specifically required for the expression of myeloid genes that control differentiation. The amino terminal region of the gene product is required for DNA binding while the carboxyl domain is required to interact with other factors for appropriate transcriptional regulation. In NFS-60 cells, the carboxyl deletion, while not interfering with DNA binding, does alter its ability to form a competent transcriptional complex. This model is currently being explored through the use of retroviral vectors.

RETROVIRAL INSERTIONS IN THE CB-1/FIM3 AND EVI-1 COMMON SITES OF INTEGRATION

Rearrangements of known oncogenes were not detectable in the majority of the IL-3-dependent myeloid leukemia cell lines suggesting the possibility that new, novel transforming genes were involved in their transformation. One approach to identify these genes involves the cloning and characterization of proviral integration sites from individual cell lines. Using flanking cellular sequences, it can be determined whether a particular site is a "common" site of integration and thus suggesting the possible presence of a transforming gene which provided a selective advantage for the growth of the cells (Clurman and Hayward, 1988). Alternatively, individual loci can be genetically mapped to determine whether they map to regions that have been implicated in myeloid leukemias by chromosomal rearrangements. Lastly, expression from the locus can be examined to determine whether transcription has been altered in a manner that would be consistent with a transforming event.

The Evi-1 common site of integration was identified in a series of retrovirus induced myeloid leukemias in mice and was shown to be rearranged in a number of the IL-3-dependent cell lines (Mucenski et al.1988). The CB-1 locus was identified as a common integration site in two of the IL-3-dependent cell lines (Bartholomew et al.1989) but was subsequently found to have a restriction enzyme map that was nearly identical to that of another common integration site termed FIM3. The FIM3 locus has been identified as a common site of viral integrations in a series of retrovirus induced myeloid leukemias (Bordereaux et al.1987). To determine the possible relationship between these loci and to other transforming genes, they were genetically mapped. Remarkably, the Evi-1 and CB-1/FIM3 loci were genetically tightly linked on chromosome 3 (Bartholomew et al.1989). Indeed no recombinants were found between the loci in over 150 backcrossed mice.

In order to determine the possible physical relationship of the Evi-1 and CB-1/FIM3 loci, chromosomal walking in phage vectors was undertaken. These studies demonstrated that the two loci were approximately 90 kb apart and that the proviruses were predominantly integrated in opposite orientations in the two loci (Bartholomew et al., in preparation).

INSERTIONAL ACTIVATION OF THE EVI-1, ZINC FINGER TRANSCRIPTIONAL FACTOR

To study the potential significance of the proviral insertions in the Evi-1 locus, flanking cellular probes were used to identify a transcriptional unit whose expression was altered. This approach identified a region of the locus that was transcribed in cells with viral insertions in either the Evi-1 locus (Morishita et al.1988) or the CB-1/FIM3 locus (Bartholomew et al.1989) but which was not expressed in other, comparable, myeloid leukemia cell lines. Sequencing of cDNAs demonstrated that the Evi-1 gene that was activated encoded a member of the zinc finger family of transcriptional factors (Miller et al.1985; Evans Hollenberg, 1988). In particular, the open reading frame of the cDNA encoded a 120 kDa protein containing two domains with the characteristic 28-30 amino acid repeats of the zinc finger motif. Seven domains, six of which were contiguous, were found in the amino terminal domain while three contiguous repeats were found in the carboxyl domain. In addition, a highly acidic domain was present in the carboxyl region which had similarity to comparable domains in other transcriptional factors. Taken together, the structure of the cDNAs strongly suggested that the Evi-1 gene would encode a nuclear, DNA binding protein which might function in transcriptional regulation.

The biochemical characterization of the gene product has been perused by the preparation of polyvalent antisera to various regions of the gene product by using bacterial expression vectors (Matsugi et al.1989). Using these antisera it has been shown that the protein is a 145 kDa phosphoprotein that is predominantly found in the nucleus of myeloid cells in which the gene is activated. The difference between the predicted size of 120 kDa and the observed size of 145 kDa is likely due to anomalous migration in SDS-PAGE sizing gels due to the acidic domain and secondary modifications such as phosphorylation. Using immunological approaches it was also demonstrated that the 145 kDa Evi-1 gene product binds DNA and the DNA-binding requires metal ions such as zinc. Studies are currently in progress to try to determine the whether DNA binding is sequence specific and to determine the specific sequences that are recognized.

THE EVI-1 GENE IS NORMALLY EXPRESSED IN KIDNEY AND OVARY

Retroviral integrations in the CB-1/FIM3 or Evi-1 locus activate the expression of the Evi-1 gene. The Evi-1 gene is not found expressed in comparable myeloid cell lines or in hematopoietic tissues such as bone marrow, spleen or fetal liver. These results suggest therefore that the gene does not normally function in hematopoiesis but rather that its expression in myeloid cells interferes with their ability to differentiate normally. In order to determine the normal function of the gene, various tissues were screened for the expression of the gene (Morishita et al.1989c). Among a variety of tissues, transcripts were only detected in the kidney and in the ovary. Among a variety of cell lines that were examined, most were negative with the exception of fibroblasts which contained low levels of transcripts. In contrast, one endometrial carcinoma cell line, HEC-1-B, contained levels of transcripts that were comparable to those found in myeloid cells in which the gene is activated. The basis for the high levels of expression in this one cell line are currently being examined.

To determine the sites of expression of the Evi-1 gene in kidney and ovary, where it is normally expressed, immunological approaches were pursued. Using immunoperoxidase staining, the expression of the Evi-1 gene product was found to be limited to the tubules between the cortical and medullary boundaries in the kidney (Morishita et al.1989a). In the ovary, the expression was predominantly found in the developing oocytes and the cytoplasm was found to contain extremely high levels of the protein. These results suggest the possibility that the

Evi-1 gene product may play a role in early oocyte or embryo development. This is particularly striking since a number of the zinc finger transcriptional factors have been implicated in gene regulation during early development.

THE EVI-1 GENE MAPS TO HUMAN CHROMOSOME 3q25 AND IS INVOLVED IN SOME CASES OF AML INVOLVING THIS REGION

The activation of the Evi-1 gene is one of the most common events associated with myeloid transformation in retrovirus induced leukemia in mice. It was therefore of importance to determine the potential involvement of the Evi-1 gene in human myeloid leukemias. To address this, we have cloned the human gene from HEC-1-B cells and genetically mapped the human Evi-1 locus. A comparison of the human and murine Evi-1 cDNA sequences demonstrate that the gene is highly conserved. Within the coding region there is 91% homology in nucleotide sequence and 94% homology in the amino acid sequence. Remarkably, within the zinc finger repeats there are only three amino acid differences between the human and murine gene.

The human Evi-1 gene was mapped to chromosome 3q25 by using somatic cell hybrids and in situ hybridization (Morishita et al.1989b). This region was of particular importance because inversions and translocations of this region of chromosome 3 have been implicated in human myeloid leukemia (Raimondi et al.1989; Bitter et al.1985). To determine whether the Evi-1 gene was involved in these leukemias we have looked for expression of the gene in several cases. The Evi-1 gene was not found to be expressed in the first case of AML examined which involved in a t(3;5)(q25;q34). However, expression of the Evi-1 gene has been detected in another case of involving a complex t(3;5), an AML with an inv(3)(q21q27) and an AML with a t(2;3) (p21;q27). The pattern of transcripts in these cells is consistent with activation of transcription by a translocation. Experiments are currently in progress to identify the chromosomal breakpoints and to determine the mechanisms involved in the activation of the expression of the gene.

SUMMARY

The mechanisms that are involved in the control of the normal differentiation of hematopoietic progenitor cells are largely unknown. Moreover, little is known concerning the types of genes that can alter the ability of hematopoietic progenitors to differentiate and cause transformation. One approach to the latter has been to use retroviral induced IL-3-dependent myeloid leukemia cell lines to identify transforming genes by their activation through insertional mutagenesis. This approach has implicated alterations in c-myb in transformation and has identified a novel transcriptional factor of the zinc finger family that is frequently activated in murine myeloid leukemias and in some cases of human AML. Using this approach it should be possible to identify additional myeloid transforming genes. The identification and characterization of the genes will provide important information and approaches to the study the of regulation of differentiation in normal hematopoiesis.

REFERENCES

Bartholomew C, Morishita K, Askew D, Buchberg A, Jenkins NA, Copeland NG, Ihle JN (1989). Retroviral insertions in the CB-1/Fim-3 common site of integration activate expression of the Evi-1 gene. Oncogene 4: 529-534.

Bitter MA, Neilly ME, LeBeau MM, Pearson MG, Rowley JD (1985). Rearrangements of chromosome 3 involving bands 3q21 and 3q26 are associated with normal or elevated platelet counts in acute nonlymphocytic leukemia. Blood 66: 1362-1370.

Bordereaux D, Fichelson S, Sola B, Tambourin PE, Gisselbrecht S (1987). Frequent involvement of the fim-3 region in Friend murine leukemia virus-induced mouse myeloblastic leukemias. J.Virol. 61: 4043-4045.

Clurman B.E., Hayward W.S. (1988). Insertional activation of proto-oncogenes previously identified as viral oncogenes. In: Cellular Oncogene Activation, edited by Klein, G. New York: Marcell Dekker, Inc., pp 55-94.

Evans RM, Hollenberg SM (1988). Zinc fingers: gilt by association minireview. Cell 52: 1-3.

Holmes KL, Palaszynski E, Fredrickson TN, Morse HC 3d, Ihle JN (1985). Correlation of cell-surface phenotype with the establishment of interleukin 3-dependent cell lines from wild-mouse murine leukemia virus-induced neoplasms. Proc.Natl.Acad.Sci.USA 82: 6687-6691.

Ihle JN, Rein A., Mural R. (1984). Immunological and virological mechanisms in retrovirus induced murine leukemogenesis. In: Advances in Viral Oncology Vol. 4, edited by Klein, G. New York: Raven Press, pp 95-137.

Ihle J.N. (1989a). The molecular and cellular biology of interleukin-3. In: The Year in Immunology 1988, edited by Cruse, J.M. and Lewis Jr., R.E. New York: Karger, pp 59-102.

Ihle JN, Askew D (1989b). Origins and properties of hematopoietic growth factor-dependent cell lines. Int J Cell.Cloning. 1: 1-30.

Matsugi T, Morishita K, Ihle JN (1989). Identification, nuclear localization and DNA binding activity of the zinc finger protein encoded by the Evi-1 murine myeloid transforming gene. Mol.Cell.Biol.: in press

Miller J, McLachlan AD, Klug A (1985). Repetitive zinc-binding domains in the protein transcription factor IIIA from Xenopus oocytes. EMBO.J. 4: 1609-1614.

Morishita K, Parker DS, Mucenski ML, Copeland NG, Ihle JN (1988). Retroviral activation of a novel gene encoding a zinc finger protein in IL-3-dependent myeloid leukemia cell lines. Cell 54: 831-840.

Morishita K, Parganas E, Parham D, Matsugi T, Ihle JN (1989a). The Evi-1 zinc finger myeloid transforming gene is normally expressed in the kidney and in developing ooctyes. submitted

Morishita K, Parganas E, Bartholomew C, Sacchi N, Valentine MB, Raimondi SC, LeBeau MM, Ihle JN (1989b). The human evi-1 gene is located on chromosome 3q24-q28 but is not rearranged in three cases of acute nonlymphocytic leukemias containing t(3;5)(q25;q34) translocations. Oncogene Res.: in press

Morishita K, Parganas E, Douglass EC, Ihle JN (1989c). Unique expression of the human Evi-1 gene in an endometrial carcinoma cell line: Sequence of cDNAs and structure of alternatively spliced transcripts. submitted

Mucenski ML, Taylor BA, Ihle JN, Hartley JW, Morse HC 3d, Jenkins NA, Copeland NG (1988). Identification of a common ecotropic viral integration site, Evi-1, in the DNA of AKXD murine myeloid tumors. Mol.Cell Biol. 8: 301-308.

Raimondi SC, Dube ID, Valentine MB, Mirro J, Watt HJ, Larson RA, Le Beau MM, Rowley JD (1989). Cliniopathologic manifestations and breakpoints of the t(3;5) in patients with acute nonlymphocytic leukemia. Leukemia 3: 42-47.

Weinstein Y, Ihle JN, Lavu S, Reddy EP (1986). Truncation of the c-myb gene by a retroviral integration in an interleukin-3 dependent myeloid leukemia cell line. Proc.Natl.Acad.Sci.USA 83: 5010-5014.

Weinstein Y, Cleveland JL, Askew DS, Rapp UR, Ihle JN (1987). Insertion and truncation of c-myb by MuLV in a myeloid cell line derived from cultures of normal hematopoietic cells. J.Virol. 61: 2339-2343.

The Biology of Hematopoiesis, pages 339–346

HUMAN GENE THERAPY--PLAYING GOD?

Frank D. Seydel

Department of Obstetrics and Gynecology, Georgetown University School of Medicine, Washington, DC 20007

INTRODUCTION

The concept of playing God is a major recurrent theme in the long-standing and continuing controversy regarding biomedical technology in general and genetic manipulation in particular. The extent of this theme can be quickly grasped just by looking at publications which incorporate this theme into their titles. Thus, during the last two decades five such books have appeared, and a search of BIOETHICSLINE, an on-line data base which is part of MEDLARS at the National Library of Medicine, revealed an additional 16 articles containing some variation of the phrase "play God" in their titles. In addition, an untold number of newpaper articles and popular magazine articles use this phrase within the text, and I often hear the phrase used in discussions of genetic technology by various religious groups.

Perhaps because of my training in both biochemistry and ministry, the issue of playing God with science has always interested me. To my mind the charge of playing God is the most serious charge that can be made about current recombinant DNA research and human gene therapy. Implicit in our Judaeo-Christian heritage is the understanding of the sovereignty of God, and its corollary that human beings should not play God. Thus, the effect, if not the intent, of such an assertion is often to preclude serious debate on the subject.

Unfortunately, despite the number of books and articles alluding to the subject of playing God, the concept is not well delineated. Indeed, usually the concept is barely mentioned or not even discussed. Rather, it appears to function symbolically as an expression of anxiety about current and future technology. Thus before we can begin to discuss the wide range of prudential ethical issues before us in contemporary human gene therapy, we must first address the fundamental theological question of what it means to play God and we must address the anxiety of the ordinary citizen regarding the status and intent of current biomedical technology.

APPLICATION OF THE THEME "PLAYING GOD" TO BIOMEDICAL TECHNOLOGY

Come let Us Play God by Leroy Augenstein (1969) was the first work to ascribe the role of "playing God" to modern biomedical activity, and it framed the terms of the subsequent debate. Augenstein, himself a biochemist, in fact wrote sympathetically about prospective biomedical possibilities. His concern was to acquaint people to the unprecedented range of decision-making power on the horizon. The neologism *bioethics*, which encapsulates many of these same concerns, was not created until the subsequent year (Potter).

After suggesting that every significant action, from applying pesticide in one's own garden to procreating life is "playing God," Augenstein states (p. 12) "The big change is that the ante in this poker game has gone sky-high." Continuing, he writes:

> Must we play God deliberately and extensively by making such awesome decisions? The answer is a definite yes. In fact we no longer have any option as to whether we will or will not "play God." Once these new tools become available, no matter what we do, we *shall* be playing God.

Approximately a fourth of the subsequent books and articles in the bioethics literature echo the Augenstein theme of the awesome power of modern biomedical technology and the choices it engenders, e.g., *Should Doctors Play God?* (Frazier), *When Doctors Play God* (Scully and Scully), and *"Playing God": the Ethics of Biotechnical Intervention* (Varga). An additional one half of the works narrow this theme specifically to those actions relating to seriously ill or dying patients, e.g., *On Playing God: the Theological Center of Daniel Maguire's Death by Choice* (Allsopp), *I Had to Play God* (Anon.), *Who Shall Live? Who Shall Die? Who Shall Play God? Some Reflections on Euthanasia* (Derr), and *Playing God in the Nursery* (Lyon).

Playing God was first linked to genetics in 1977 in two separate works: *Playing God: Genetic Engineering and the Manipulation of Life* (Goodfield) and *Who Should Play God? The Artificial Creation of Human Life and What It Means for the Future of the Human Race* (Howard and Rifkin). Only a handful of works have continued this theme.

Four observations are apparent regarding usage of the phrase "to play God." First, despite an abundance of articles on the topic in the bioethics literature, including those judging this concept serious enough to feature the phrase in their titles, there is very little substantive discussion of the concept. The vast majority of works either do not mention the concept in the body of the text, or they mention the phrase only in passing. Thus, for example, both books concerning genetic manipulation (Goodfield; Howard and Rifkin) mention this phrase only once. Second, most of the texts are either dispassionate or sympathetic to the dilemmas they are raising. Again, for example, physician and bioethicist Pellegrino (1987), in discussing cessation of treatment to dying patients, states "I don't think we were playing God." Yet, I would suggest, his article is provocatively titled: *Life and Death Decisions: Do you Trust Yourself to Play God?* Third, as Van Eys (1982) noted, the question of "Should one play God?" is always asked in such a way as to evoke a negative answer. Fourth, the major intellectual effort on this theme was done in the first decade after its introduction (1968-1977); as time progressed the phrase has been employed in a perfunctory manner.

The overwhelming conclusion from these observations is that the phrase has degenerated into mainly a symbolic way of expression of concern over the extensive power of contemporary biomedical technology. In support of this conclusion is the paucity of discussion of this issue in church policy statements. In a 1975 document by the World Council of Churches (Birch and Abrecht), after nearly a decade of books and articles on "playing God," this theme is mentioned only once in passing (p. 208). As recently as

1986, in the face of the enormous increase in biomedical power, a National Council of Churches policy statement on the religious issues related to genetics does not include "playing God" (National Counil of the Churches of Christ in the U.S.A.).

The notable exception to the dispassionate treatment of this theme is the polemic activity of Jeremy Rifkin and colleagues (e.g., Howard and Rifkin). Even here it should be noted that explicit reference to "playing God" occurs only once in the text (p. 33). Thus the prominence of the phrase in the title serves primarily as a catch-phrase to crystallize concern. Nevertheless, neither the potency of the argument or the arguers should be underestimated. Rifkin, through his deceptively named Foundation on Economic Trends, has been extremely successful in impeding the application of recombinant DNA technology (Van Biema).

THEOLOGICAL ISSUES IN "PLAYING GOD"

Although Rifkin may be fighting a rear-guard action against the implementation of new genetic technology, the remarkable success of his efforts suggests a considerable amount of shared objection to the new technology. Thus, in order to successfully implement the new technology, it becomes necessary for proponents of human gene therapy to direct attention to the theological and ethical arguments involved in playing God and to the underlying anxiety of typical citizens. I will first outline a response to the two specific theological implications of playing God, usurpation of God's role and the creation of new species. Then, I will briefly address the slippery slope argument and alteration of the natural order.

Usurpation of God's Role

A legitimate concern of the majority of authors raising the issue of "playing God" is the need for accountability of persons and society employing the powerful technology of genetic manipulation. Unfortunately, Augenstein, like numerous others throughout the history of technology, incorrectly framed the debate with his equation of this new power with playing God. If this were so, then any new genetic technology, no matter how carefully regulated, would be inherently usurpatious and evil.

The verb "play" in the phrase "play God" is a word rich in meaning; over 39 meanings have been identified (Oxford Eng. Dict., and Birchfield, Suppl. to the Oxford Eng.Dict.). However, in the current debate the usage is restricted to the meaning of "act the part of" and carries the negative connotation of "to impersonate." Moreover, since "play" is typically contrasted with "work," to "play God" implies a frivolous attitude. Regrettably a number of scientists and other proponents have contributed to a sense of arrogance and frivolity regarding genetic technology with overly optimistic, incautious, or irresponsible statements, such as admiration of the new *homo autofabricus* (Fletcher).

In his book *Fabricated Man*, Paul Ramsey is by no means an enthusiast for biomedical technology. Nevertheless, he "regrets" the equating "of any vital decision that is risk-filled for ourselves and others with playing a divine role," and he implores that "this loose use of language must be given up if we are to search out the meaning of being men who know not to play God as a regulative norm in the 'awesome business' that is before us" (Ramsey, p. 172).

Both the Old Testament and the New Testament have stories which are instructive here. In Genesis (Ch. 11) God destroyed the Tower of Babel and scattered the people over all the earth. Genesis tells us that it wasn't the new-found technology that displeased God, but rather the people's effort, by building a tower unto heaven, which is God's domain, to make a name for themselves. In Matthew (Ch. 4) Jesus is tempted by the devil to use his great power for his own glorification, but Jesus refuses: "Get away, Satan! For it is written, 'you shall worship the Lord your God, and him only shall you serve'" (RSV trans.).

Creation of New Species

The biological issue of exactly what constitutes a new species is too complex to pursue here. Let me concede for the moment that that transgenic organisms are new species. Underlying the charge that the creating of new species is playing God is the assumption that this activity is reserved to God. However, there is no explicit Biblical injunction against the creation of new species (cf. Varga).

The issue hinges on the interpretation of the Creation narrative in Genesis. What does it mean to be made in the image of God and what does it mean to subdue the earth and have dominion over all living things? Are we but stewards of our power (Hammes), or are we co-creators with God, as the theologians who advised the 1982 President's Ethics Commission asserted (President's Commission, p. 53)? Co-creation can, of course, be a dangerous cocept, and we are back to the issue of accountability.

The Slippery Slope Argument

Perhaps the most difficult accusation to refute is that initial efforts at recombinant DNA place us on a slippery slope towards the loss of our natural humanity and undetertmined ecological damage. Any appearance of good is only seductive, leading towards the edge of disaster. "Is guaranteeing our health worth trading away our humanity? asks Rifkin (1983). The appeal of the Slippery Slope argument is that it conforms to our every-day experience, but the great danger of the argument is its over-simplification. By ignoring the risks and problems of conventional medical therapy, antagonists to human gene therapy prejudice the discussion against gene therapy. In reality we are beset with multiple slopes at once. Withdrawing too far in one direction only increases our risk of tumbling down the opposite slope. Thus one might well ask if guaranteeing our humanity necessitates trading away our health.

Alteration of the Natural Order

I believe that an anxiety even deeper than the fear of irresponsible action lurks, perhaps unconsciously, behind the phrase "playing God." Genetic technology is not the only technology with enormous potential to alter the structure of society or create life or death decisions. But genetic technology appears unique in its capability to alter both human nature and the biological world. The fear is that at last the power of technology will get out of hand and allow us to destroy the preestablished harmony of the universe (Ledley). Faith in this static harmony has been a major tenet of the world view that has dominated Western civilization since the revolutionary discoveries of

Copernicus. In this world view, science is seen as passive; it discloses natural laws but does not alter the nature of things. According to Ledley, "Human activity, however compatible with natural precepts, when taken to its logical and logistical extremes often obscures the distinction between what we perceive as man's natural interaction with his environment and his meddling with natural events."

The critical problem that occurs with deriving ethics from a concept of naturalism is that it is impossible to determine what should be from what is. Howard and Rifkin (1977) ask: How can we be sure that in our tinkering and fixing with three billion years of evolutionary wisdom, we do not inadvertently join the 98 million species that have passed from the earth?" In fact, all reproductive actions, whether intentional or not, have genetic and evolutionary consequences. Moreover, extensive conventional medical treatment, by enabling persons with genetic disorders to survive to reproductive age, poses a risk to the human gene pool that seems as equally unknown as gene therapy. Note also the assumption in the above quote that evolution has reached an end-point; such an assumption betrays an ignorance of the very concept of evolution that the authors invoke.

CONCLUSION

In conclusion, there is no fundamental theological objection to genetic manipulation in general or human gene therapy in particular. The accusation of playing God in this controversy functions symbolically as an expression of anxiety 1) over potential human irresponsibility and 2) over the extent to which such manipulation might irreversibly and unforseeably change the world. Proponents of human gene therapy must address these anxieties with persistence, openness, patience, and careful language if this therapy is to proceed.

REFERENCES

Allsopp, ME (1985). On playing God: the theological center of Daniel Maguire's Death by Choice. Linacre Quarterly 52: 343-348.

Anon. (1978). I had to play God. Med Econom 55: 53-57.

Augenstein, L (1969). Come, let us play God. Evanston, IL: Harper and Row.
Birch, C, Abrecht, P, eds. (1975). Genetics and the quality of life. Potts Point, NSW, Austral.: Pergamon Press.
Derr, P (1982). Who shall live? Who shall die? Who shall play God? Some reflections on euthanasia. Thought 57: 422-437.
Fletcher, J (1974). The ethics of genetic control--ending reproductive roulette. Garden City, NY: Anchor Books.
Frazier, CA, ed. (1971). Should doctors play God? Nashville, TN: Broadman Press.
Goodfield, J (1977). Playing God: Genetic engineering and the manipulation of life. New York: Random House.
Howard, T, Rifkin, J (1977). Who should play God? The artificial creation of life and what it means for the future of the human race. New York: Delacorte Press.
Ledley, FD (1983). Recombinant DNA and the Copernican world view. Perspect in Biol and Med 26: 245-260
Lyon, J (1985). Playing God in the nursery. New York: W. W. Norton.
National Council of the Churches of Christ in the U.S.A. (1986). Genetic science for human benefit: a policy statement. New York.
The Oxford English Dictionary (1933). Oxford: Oxford Univ. Press. Vol. 7: 974-978.
Pellegrino, ED (1987). Life and death decisions: do you trust yourself to play God? U.S. Catholic 52: 6-13.
Potter, VR (1971). Bioethics: Bridge to the Future. Englewood Cliffs, NJ: Prentice Hall.
President's Commission for the Study of Ethical Problems in Medicine and Biomedical and Behavioral Research (1982). Splicing life. Washington: GPO.
Ramsey, P (1970). Fabricated man. The ethics of genetic control. New Haven: Yale Univ. Press.
Rifkin, J (1983). Whom do we designate to play God? Engage/Social Action 11(10): 22-28.
Scully, T, Scully, C (1987). Playing God: The new world of medical choices. New York: Simon and Schuster.
Supplement to the Oxford English Dict. (1982). Birchfield, RW, ed. Oxford: Oxford Univ. Press. Vol. 3: 567-570.
Van Biema, D (1988). Biotech gadfly buzzes Italy. The Washington Post Magazine (Jan. 17): 13-38.
Van Eys (1982). Should doctors play God? Perspect in Biol and Med 25: 481-485.
Varga, AC (1985). "Playing God": the ethics of biotechnical intervention. Thought 60: 181-195.

The Biology of Hematopoiesis, pages 347–353

AN ETHICAL ANALYSIS OF GENE THERAPY AS MOLECULAR SURGERY

Matthew J. Temple, O.Carm., Ph.D.
Department of Biology
Nazareth College of Rochester
4245 East Avenue
Rochester, NY 14610

"Genetic engineering" still conjures up Orwellian notions of a brave new world. But a brave new world approach to human genetic engineering exaggerates what is new - the technology - and is blind to what is familiar - the ethical assessment of clinical acts that are both risky and beneficial. We have just taken a guided tour of the present and future landscape of human gene therapy under the direction of Dr. Anderson, and have seen the promise and limits of both somatic and germ line therapy. Building on Dr. Anderson's tour, I would like to explore two areas with you:

1) the manipulation of DNA in human cells as molecular surgery, from both empirical and ethical viewpoints; and

2) the particularly praiseworthy and problematic aspects of this surgery identified in recent Roman Catholic moral writings.

GENE THERAPY AS MOLECULAR SURGERY

Human gene therapy is the deliberate introduction of selected DNA sequences into human cells to ameliorate or cure a disease, or to improve health. Gene therapy of human cells resembles surgery: the physical, invasive manipulation of body components to remove, repair, replace or enhance bodily structures. Despite the pain, physical risks, and unclear prognoses that may attend surgery, society justifies surgery when its benefits to the patient are proportionate to its risks. Society condemns surgery on humans for purely experimental intentions - despite the good that might accrue to others - because risks and benefits of such procedures are no longer proportionate for the patient.

Consider the three kinds of genetic therapy identified by Friedmann: replacement, correction, and augmentation (Friedmann, 1989). Accept for the time being that each could be performed for either somatic or germ line therapy. Replacement gene therapy intends removal of a dysfunctional gene and its replacement by a donated gene. Correction therapy would incorporate external DNA to replace existing mutant sequences within the cell, as in site-directed mutagenesis. Gene augmentation, which is most immediately practical, would add a correct gene(s) to mutant target cells to compensate for the inborn mutation.

All three approaches - whether practicable or not - are analagous to surgery. Gene replacement parallels the logic of tissue and organ transplants: removal of diseased components and replacement by functioning tissue. Gene correction resembles reconstructive surgery in which externally supplied tissue, such as skin or vessel grafts, is used to replace a portion of otherwise healthy, functional tissue. And finally, gene augmentation resembles that surgery which compensates for diseased tissues or organs by the addition of external structures, such as implantable bone splints, cardiac pacemakers, or limb prostheses.

There are obvious differences in the size of what is manipulated: grams of tissue or picograms of DNA. There are obvious differences in the importance of location in these techniques: good surgery demands clear visualization of the actual site for removal, replacement or correction, whereas precise localization of defective and correcting DNA sequences within microscopic cell nuclei is still an unsolved problem. And whereas the results of surgery are often known within hours and almost always within weeks, the results of gene therapy might take years to become apparent in somatic cases, and decades in germ line cases. Nonetheless, the same basic ethical paradigms we apply to surgical cases are also applicable to gene therapy cases.

Patterns set by the weighing of surgical risks and benefits could help the ethical assessment of human gene therapy protocols. For example, prosthetic surgery poses short- and long-term risks for disruption of normal tissue function and toleration of the grafted material. Augmentation gene therapy with retroviral vectors raises parallel questions about disruption of normal cellular genes and control of the transferred genes. The benefits of removing diseased multifunctional tissues such as endocrine glands are offset by the loss of other vital unimpaired functions. Replacement gene therapy for a mutant pleiotropically acting gene would similarly need to account for maintenance of essential gene functions in all tissues which normally express this gene. Finally, corrective surgery generally minimizes the loss or destruction of normal tissue. Site-directed mutagenesis in corrective gene therapy would need similar safeguards against unplanned "correction" of non-targeted genes.

SPECIFIC ROMAN CATHOLIC CONCERNS.

I find nothing in Roman Catholic official teaching or mainstream moral theology which regards human gene therapy - somatic or germinal - as instrinsically objectionable. Rather, there appears to be a consensus that such therapy is justifiable and indeed desirable when that therapy is attempted with the explicit intention of reducing disease or promoting health of the patient, respects the patient´s rights and human freedom, and has taken risks and benefits into account (John Paul II, 1983; Ashley, 1989).

The 1987 Vatican instruction on human reproduction states that science has a positive imperative to do what it reasonably and morally can to relieve the burden of genetic disease (Congregation, 1987). I suggest that there is a tone of cautious optimism in Catholic thought about the principle and promise of gene therapy.

Church officials and theologians also stress that care of the poor - including those physically, mentally, socially and economically impoverished by genetic defects - remains a positive moral obligation of society and its health care providers. Diverse Catholic writers emphasize that technological treatment of some genetically affected patients must not lead to the neglect or elimination of those whose genetic diseases remain untreatable (Haring, 1978; Ashley, 1989).

Two major ethical problems dominate current Roman

Catholic moral appraisals of human gene therapy. The first is the appropriate care of the human embryo in germ line therapy. The second in the safeguarding of human freedom as human gene therapy becomes practical.

Although human germ line therapy is only speculative at this point, it would most likely involve gene transfer into early embryos. Many commentators are dubious about practical prospects for human germ line therapy because of its technical and ethical complexities (Muller, 1987; Anderson, 1984; Friedmann, 1989). However, Walters notes that demand for germ line therapy may increase with the success of somatic therapy for two reasons: first, successful somatic cell therapy will enable more treated individuals to pass on their mutant germ line genes to their children, increasing the chances of genetically affected offspring; and second, genetically-diseased brain and liver tissues will probably remain refractile to somatic cell gene therapy by methods currently envisioned (Walters, 1986). The only genetic cure for these diseases will be ones in which early embryonic cells are cured prior to organ differentiation and development. Therefore, gene therapy of gametes or, more likely, early embryos will be indicated.

The moral end, or intention, of such germ line therapy is the elimination of genetic disease in the embryo and its potential offspring. The object of such therapy would be the embryo itself, and any exogenous DNA introduced into its cells. The means would include the mode of fertilization leading to formation of the embryo, its diagnosis as genetically affected and successfully treated, its implantation back into the uterus, and its disposition if not re-implanted. It is the latter point of the analysis - means - that has evoked official Church concern.

There are several moral issues relating to the embryo: some directly concern gene therapy and others are prior to it. Vatican statements addressing gene therapy explicitly condemn any manipulation of human embryos except for their own direct benefit (John Paul II, 1983; Congregation, 1987). Hence, gene therapy experiments cannot be performed on a human embryo from an official Catholic viewpoint because it would be exposing a human individual to physical risk without proportionate direct benefit to that individual and without regard for that individual's rights to develop unimpeded and in freedom. Nor could the risks of gene therapy on a human embryo be justified by the probable benefit to its offspring or society, according to this teaching.

Underlying concerns about the embryo as the object of gene therapy are deeper concerns about the states of the embryo itself in the hands of medicine. The 1987 Vatican instruction condemns _in vitro_ fertilization, on the grounds that conception of a human individual - to be truly human - must necessarily arise from the physical sexual union of spouses united in marriage (Congregation, 1987). _In vitro_ fertilization disrupts this fundamental union by the technical intervention of a third party: this intervention threatens to make such embryos appear as mere objects - the product of human ingenuity - rather than as individuals ultimately deriving their origin and dignity from God through marriage.

Obviously, Vatican opposition to _in vitro_ fertilization has generated debate within Catholic theological circles. A major point of dissent asserts that human technical intervention in the biological origin of an individual through _in vitro_ fertilization does not necessarily deprive that individual of his or her personal dignity as the Vatican contends (McCormick, 1987). The point of concern here, however, is that germ line therapy of human embryos would demand ready physical access to a very early embryo, in order to diagnose a potentially treatable genetic defect, perform gene transfer into some or all of the embryonic cells, presumably verify the success of the gene transfer, and then implant the treated embryo into a receptive uterine lining. Such timely access is virtually impossible by _in vivo_ fertilization but is guaranteed by _in vitro_ fertilization.

Thus, even if proportionately beneficial gene therapies could be developed without human embryo experimentation, _in vitro_ fertilization could not be justified by official Church teaching in order to treat embryos which could benefit from those therapies. A reasonable theological speculation is that germ line therapy of "naturally" conceived embryos recovered before implantation, or of post-implantation embryos _in utero_, might be justifiable.

Finally, Catholic theologians and official Church statements stress that human gene therapy - whether somatic or germinal - must be ordered towards the good of the individual, either by reducing or preventing disease or by achieving genuine improvement for the patient. Any procedure which promotes domination or subjugation, or contributes to discrimination must be avoided. What is true of medical procedures in general is to be true of gene therapy in particular: it is to be used to pursue health in human freedom, and never to constrain humans into positions of inhuman subservience, docility or profitability for others.

CONCLUSIONS.

Human gene therapy, by its logic and physical manipulation of matter, is ethically analagous to surgery. I suggest that somatic and germ line gene therapy proposals be submitted to the same kind of risk/benefit analyses used to accept or reject surgical proposals. Indeed, inclusion of surgeons on institutional review boards for gene therapy protocols could be effective. The major ethical difference in gene therapy cases will be in weighing potential benefits to as yet unconceived offspring against risks to as yet unborn embryos subjected to germ line therapy.

Roman Catholic moral appraisal of human gene therapy has been favorable in principle, and suggests a positive imperative to pursue and apply new techniques because of their power to cure and prevent genetic disease. However, Catholic moral reasoning upholds the right of the human embryo to be treated as a human person: as such, it is not to be subjected to experimentation, disproportionate risks, or treated in any way which denies its personal dignity. These strictures certainly narrow - if not close - practical possibilities in official Catholic teaching for making the human embryo the legitimate object of germ line gene therapy. At the same time, Catholic moral thought agrees with many other ethical viewpoints in asserting that human gene therapy must never be used to restrict the physical development or personal freedom of some in order to serve the political or economic objectives of others.

REFERENCES.

Anderson WF (1984). Prospects for Human Gene Therapy.

Science 226:401-09.
Ashley B, O'Rourke K (1989). "Health Care Ethics. A Theological Analysis." 3rd ed St. Louis: Catholic Hospital Association, pp 316-19.
Congregation for the Doctrine of the Faith (1987). Instruction on Respect for Human Life in Its Origin and on the Dignity of Procreation. Origins 16:698-711.
Friedmann T (1989). Progress Towards Human Gene Therapy. Science 244:1275-81.
Haring BF (1978). "Free and Faithful in Christ." Vol 3 New York: Seabury, pp 25-26.
John Paul II (1983). The Ethics of Human Genetic Manipulation. Address to the 35th Assembly of the World Health Association. Origins 13:386-89.
McCormick RA (1987). The Vatican Document on Bioethics. America 156:247.
Muller HJ (1989). Human Gene Therapy: Possibilities and Limitations. Experientia 43:375-78.
Walters L (1986). The Ethics of Human Gene Therapy. Nature 320:225-27.

The Biology of Hematopoiesis, pages 355–364

ETHICAL CONSIDERATIONS REGARDING POTENTIALS OF HUMAN GENE THERAPY:

Ethical Dilemmas in Serendipity

Terry R. Bard,

Director, Pastoral Care and Coordinator the Ethics Program, Beth Israel Hospital, Boston, MA. Clinical Instructor in Pastoral Counseling, Department of Psychiatry, Harvard Medical School, Boston, MA

Joseph Fletcher, one of the earlier contemporary ponderers of **Morals and Medicine** [1954] noted that "...we can say with good reason that Gresham's law -- that bad money tends to drive out good -- can operate in genetics too!" (p. 170) Fletcher's primary focus in this comment was on emerging possibilities afforded by artificial insemination. Watson and Crick's findings had not yet received scientific review. Likewise, they had not gained public attention. Nonetheless, the issues which have framed discussions about genetic research were formulated by this early thinker. He distinguished between the therapeutic, the eugenic, and the punitive possibilities of artificial insemination and sterilization. These categories, especially the eugenic and therapeutic, have bracketed much of the philosophical reflection on genetic research and its clinical applications. This meeting takes place in Cambridge where, just a few years ago, frightened citizens protested recombinant DNA investigations. One prime contributor to these protests was fear fed by ignorance. Were these protestors at potential risk by such research? What about their progeny? As with many modern scientific advancements, new findings errupted in advance of any clear thinking about the potentials these findings bore. These findings had not been open to public debate and scrutiny because, in many instances, their practical impact had not been reviewed by researchers themselves. The challenges they found in these serendipitous occurrences focused on understanding genetic mechanics, the structure, the form, and the potential. Few reflected on the meaning such serendipitous discoveries had either for science or for society.

As genetic research continues, more and more is understood about the basic building blocks of life, where problems emerge, how good and bad mutations effect the total organism. The potentials have became more obvious, and the public occasionally expresses its concern and fear that life could be generated artifically, by chemicals. Cloning heightens these potentials and has accelerated public fears. The production of recombinant DNA generated a frenzy. Advocates of orthodox religions have condemned researchers, claiming that scientists are taking over the perogatives of God. For them, the dangers outstrip the benefits.

This climate has forced genetic researchers to ask additional questions about their scientific queries. Although most scientists resist asking teleological questions about their investigations, pure research should not be undertaken for outcome alone, those involved in genetic research today cannot avoid addressing teleological issues. In fact, I take it that, in part, questions about meaning and purpose are why I was invited to address this assembly. It would be considered unconscionable and irresponsible to exclude ethical considerations from a symposium on genetic research in 1989.

This afternoon, I will not present a detailed philosophical treatise on the ethics of gene research and gene therapy. Exhaustive discussions of these issues abound, and I think that I have little to add to the considerations which other ethicists have adumbrated. Some thinkers reflect on the ethics of the eugenic possibilities inherent in genetic research;

others on the therapeutic merits. Most discuss the epistemological groundings for their arguments and the distinctions between deontological and utilitarian modes of thinking. On the basis of these discussions, some argue for limitations in funding research which may lead to deleterious outcomes. Others discuss whether government should support such research, asking whether it is in the benefit of the commonweal. These discussions and arguments are important, and they must continue to provide a backdrop of dispassionate reflection. Nonetheless, I suggest that such philosophical discussions are essentially heuristic and do not provide workable guidelines for the researcher in genetics.

I base this conclusion on an observation of the research climate today and the nature of genetic research itself. Despite the recent announcements about projected government restrictions on research funds to universities, the fact remains that, beginning with the President Reagan's administration, government funding of scientific research has seriously eroded. But Reagan's goal became realized; scientific advancement did not stop. Funding for scientific research began to be absorbed by the private sector. Researchers, themselves, began to incorporate, and many have now added "businessman" to their academic profiles. This new dimension is also receiving current governmental scrutiny as steps are underway to undo what government overseers call inappropriate and unacceptalbe conflicts of interest. The values and motives, the teleological issues, of research became compounded by issues of entrapreneurship and its necessary drive to survive by claiming its share of the market. No matter how one frames the philosophical questions about whether the government should fund genetic research, such research **will** continue. Moreover, genetic research has made too much of a contribution to agriculture and to human health to justify additional restrictions. Consequently, the theoretical questions about whether such research should continue or be restricted are moot. They become paper windmills for ivy-towered jousting.

Furthermore, most scientists acknowlege that often the most useful finds have been serendipitous. Researchers attempt to demonstrate X; Y occurs and has far more applicability than X ever would have. Curiosity, creativity, and serendipity are primary elements of scientific discovery. These are also elements comprising the very core of our humanity. Curbs on these capacities will not occur no matter how many philosophical treatises are written about whether or not researchers should pursue certain avenues of inquiry.

Consequently, I suggest diverting the ethical debate regarding genetic research and genetic therapies to a different track. Given this reality that genetic research **will** continue and grow in ensuing years, and given the likelihood that serendipitious occurrences will arise, the more pressing theoretical and practical issues facing genetic research in the '90s and beyond concern the ethical issues inherent in the **management** of serendipity.

Ethical management is not pure ethics; it is applied ethics. Research is pure until it is applied; so too is ethics. Applied sciences are far more complex than their purer points of origin. **Pure thinking** and **applied thinking** face this same dilemma. For some, pure socialism is an ideal system. Its many applications have fallen far short of the ideal. This dichotomy applies to genetic research as well.

Ethical management considers context and outcome as significant and equally important to the scientific discovery which is to be managed. A scientific discovery and any practical application it may have cannot be considered separately from the context out of which it emerged or the potential(s) for its use. Although this conclusion may be reasonable, it threatens to alter a primary scientific premise, the purity of scientific investigation unimpeded by external pressures, concerns or implications. Most scientific discoveries and their applications in the last half of this century demonstrate that a goal of pure genetic research, while desirable, is potentially immoral. The advent of nuclear fission beneath the football stadium at the University of Chicago fifty years ago was serendipitous; the management of this discovery has been focal ever since. Recent scientific discoveries arise out of a context and could potentially be used in a context. The identification of the polypeptide chains of genetic construction in E-coli does not stand in isolation from the possible applications of this knowledge. The natural envirnoment and the human enterprise are inextricably intertwined.

Genetic research raises these questions at every turn. When one investigates genetic constitution, the natural context is the living organism. Understanding the nature of genetic structure, its beauty, logic, its "simple complexity" may fulfill a cognitive quest and perhaps even an aesthetic desire. The yields of such research, however, have rarely stopped at understanding. Part of human curiosity is not only to know but also to manipulate and to control. Much of the understanding in genetic research has also unleashed the desire to test this understanding out, to replicate what is in nature, and perhaps to attempt some "unnatural" experiments as well. The question "should we do these investigations or clinical trials?" is, in effect, irrelevant. Sanctions are unrealsitic; someone is going to do such studies, and some industry will fund them. Enacting laws which impose limits on this process simply do not work.

Two different conclusions emerge from this scenerio. The more libertarian conclusion is that genetic research and therapies are the private purview of the researchers, clinicians, and potential recipients. Anything goes; those who can benefit by them will receive them on the basis of whatever criteria the marketplace affords. A second conclusion is that a system of management should be employed which helps to direct the nature and the application of genetic research and therapy. This system would not be imposed but itwould be so pursuasive that few if any would wish to move beyond the pale of this framework for ethical management.

The debate continues about whether genetic research should proceed unbounded or constrained. A model can be constructed, however, which can provide for unbounded research within a managed context. To create such a model would mean that society and scientists together begin to discuss the directions for research. Since serendipity will occur regardless of the research, it may as well emerge out of investigations which have a teleogical focus. A current example is research undertaken to cure AIDS. The AIDS epidemic began to channel research and funding. The teleological goal is to irradicate this disease.

In the early 1960's Science, Scientific American, The New York Times, and The Wall Street Journal all reported the new developments in cell and molecular biology in sensational fashion. The headlines read, "Scientists learn the keys to life." These reports led to concern about the goals of genetic research and whether limits on such studies should be imposed. Since that time, little formal attention has been given to these concerns by the scientific community.

The ethical management of scientific research, and specifically, of genetic research, can be viewed against this backdrop. Considering growing potentials, more scientists are troubled by outcome questions. Consequently, the time has come for clarification of the goals of research. Those involved in genetic research need to frame some general and fundamental questions about genetics. Too often, such questions are raised only after significant breakthroughs rather than when the research is initiated. Although genetic research is quite advanced and treatment modalites are underway, there is still time to reflect on generic ethical issues. I suggest that the following questions could help to shape the environment for addressing the ethical potentials of human gene therapy:

1. What are the **scientific goals** of

genetic research on humans?
2. What are the **social goals** of this research?
3. What consitutes the cost/loss ratios in such research?
4. What constitutes the risk/benefit ratios in such research?
5. How are these goals evaluated?
6. How are these goals viewed within the scientific community?
7. How are these goals viewed within the general community?
8. How are these goals to be implemented?

These questions apply both generally and specifically, to the entire discipline of genetic research as well as to any specific study. Similarly, they can apply to most areas of medical research.

1. **What are the scientific goals of genetic research on humans?**
This question frames the enterprise. Is human genetic research undertaken simply to better understand the human genome? Is this research focused on obtaining information which can be applied for human welfare? Is the focus to correct diseases or malfunctions? Is the focus to create more resilliant human phenotypes? Is the creation of stronger genotypes one of the foci of such research?

No clarity currently exists regarding primary therapeutic or eugenic goals of genetic research and application. Discussions need be undertaken. A consensus on goals will help to shape the ethical issues which emerge. Many of the concerns which have been expressed by society and by some scientists center on the potential eugenic use of genetic therapies. Deep-seated fears arise as comparisons are drawn between eugenics and some of the Nazi "experiments". If most or all researchers conclude that the eugenic use of genetic information is unacceptable, this limitation will help to shape the direction of genetic research. These and other potential goals should be similarly scrutinized. Until the scientific community is able to wrestle with its broadly articulated goals, it will be unable to share them with society at large.

2. **What are the social goals of this research?** Many scientific endeavors are justified by their purity, their detachment from external forces. Such claims can no longer be attributed to human genetic research. For all of the reasons mentioned above, the funding for genetic research and the implications of its findings make genetic research a social endeavor? Have geneticists articulated any clear social goals such as the irradication of a disease or the development of a safer environment. Geneticists and their fellow citizens, alike, remain unaware of any clearly articulated social goals which impel current genetic research. As mentioned before, one goal, alone, the irradication of AIDS, has been endorsed as common.

3. **What are the cost/loss ratios of such research?** In the context of clearly defined goals, at what point is the cost of research outstripped by the losses it creates in unfocused research, financial expenditures, and inability to contribute toward the fulfillment of the goals? The scientific merit of the research should also be evaluated.

4. **What are the risk/benefit ratios of such research?** Risk and benefit are concepts used to evaluate the effects of clinical research on subjects, but they can also be applied to the research module itself. The question of risks and benefits also relates to the scientific merit of the research. The protestors in Cambridge a few years ago concluded that the perceived risk to the community was greater than the potential benefit the researchers tauted. The concern here is not whether the protestors were right, but had the risk/benefit ratios been assessed? If so, how had they been communicated with the community?

5. How are these goals evaluated? **Who evaluates these goals and the method by which they are evaluated are both important. Should research**

peers evaluate these goals, should outsiders to this process evaluate them, should there some mixture of the two? Ad hoc methods for such evaluation exist in the governmental grant application process. Such does not routinely take place in private industry. Moreover, no process exists to develop overarching goals for genetic research as suggested by question #1. Any assessment of these goals and the ethical issues which they may engender are thwarted by a lack of general evaluative principles.

6. How are these goals shared within the scientific community? Is there a forum within the genetic research community which has been charged with communicating general information about the field of genetic research? Symposia like this one are replicated throughout the country and world; papers are offered on topics of specific scientific interest, but little attention is given to general philosophical and ethical concerns as they relate to genetic research. In order to manage the ethical issues around genetic research, a method of sharing information needs to be created. I think that many people in this room harbor some of the concerns which I have articulated, but some of my friends involved in different areas of research have lamented that they have no formal place to channel such questions and concerns.

7. How are these goals viewed in the general community? Because issues of genetic research have proven so potentially volatile, what is the researchers responsibility to consider community concerns? Because the geneticist can no longer be deluded into thinking that the research is pure and beyond the interest or investment of the community, social concerns must be addressed.

8. How are these goals to be implemented? One of the ethical management goals is how to implement these goals in such a way as to benefit the enterprise, society, and its citizens. Just as it is unethical to impose any specific medical treatment on a person without obtaining consent, so, too, it is unethical to unleash scientific discoveries without appropriate preparation and

information. Too often, the scientific community has been sanguine about how society greets its discoveries. Because of the profound implications of genetic research and its potential applications, a process for providing information to society should be developed.

The above questions can be applied to specific scientific protocols and serendipitous occurrances in a manner similar to their application to the entire field of genetic research. Each of these questions is designed to look not only at the scientific goals but at the philosophical/ethical implications of these goals, to place them into a broader spectrum. As geneticists and society begin to struggle with these issues together in a more open fashion, the ethical issues inherent in genetic research and application will emerge, be addressed, and managed.

The Biology of Hematopoiesis, pages 365–374

BIOLOGICAL EFFECTS OF RECOMBINANT HUMAN GM-CSF

Richard K. Shadduck, Sandra S. Kaplan, Theresa L. Whiteside and Edward J. Wing

Pittsburgh Cancer Institute, Montefiore Hospital, Department of Medicine, University of Pittsburgh School of Medicine and the Department of Pathology, University of Pittsburgh School of Medicine

INTRODUCTION

The colony stimulating factors are a group of glycoproteins that are responsible for the proliferation and maturation of hemopoietic progenitor cells. The effects of these growth factors were discovered by their ability to induce colonies of granulocytes and macrophages by bone marrow cells in vitro (Wing and Shadduck, 1985).

The purification, sequencing and cloning of these factors has provided sufficient materials for clinical trials. The most widely used factor, GM-CSF, has been evaluated in patients with the acquired immune deficiency syndrome (Groopman et al., 1987), myelodysplasia (Vadhan-Raj et al., 1987), aplastic anemia (Vadhan-Raj et al., 1988) and in patients with a variety of malignancies (Herrman, et al., 1989; Phillips et al., 1989). These clinical trials have indicated marked stimulation of granulopoiesis in response to GM-CSF.

Recently the CSF's have been shown to bind to and stimulate mature granulocytes or macrophages (Gasson et al., 1984; Wing et al., 1982). Thus, in addition to their role in stimulating the growth of hemopoietic progenitor cells, they appear capable of activating mature cells. Studies suggest that such activated cells may be useful in augmenting host defense against certain infections or stimulating endogenous antitumor activity (Wing et al., 1982; Grabstein et al., 1986). Although these effects are seen after in vitro exposure to GM or M-CSF, little data is available concerning in vivo activation of the phagocytic system. The present studies explored the kinetics of hemopoiesis and the activation of mature granulocytes and monocyte-macrophages after a single bolus and during daily continuous infusions of GM-CSF.

PATIENTS AND METHODS

Ten patients with metastatic carcinoma received GM-CSF as a potential biological response modifier (Phillips et al., 1989). They were given continuous intravenous infusions of recombinant human GM-CSF (Immunex Corporation) - at 100 $\mu g/M^2$ or 500 $\mu g/M^2$ per 24 hours. Each patient received 5% of the total dose by IV bolus injection on day 0. Six days later a 24 hour intravenous infusion was initiated and was reinstituted each day for 14 days.

Blood samples (100 ml) were obtained on two occasions prior to the bolus injection, two days after the bolus, prior to starting the continuous infusion and then on days 3 and 10 of the continuous infusion for evaluation of neutrophil and monocyte activity.

Blood monocytes were obtained by Ficoll-Hypaque density gradient centrifugation. Adherent monolayers were prepared that consisted of 80 to 90% monocytes (Wing et al., 1989). ADCC activity was measured using antibody coated chicken erythrocytes with a chromium release assay. Monocyte production of TNF alpha and interferon was measured after incubation of 2 x 10^6 cells with 10 μg/ml of E. coli LPS (Wing et al., 1989).

Neutrophils were separated following Ficoll-Hypaque centrifugation. Superoxide release was measured from resting cells and after stimulation with 10^{-7} or 10^{-8} M fMLP or 1 μg/ml of phorbol myristate acetate (PMA) (Kaplan et al., 1989). Chemotaxis was evaluated in response to Zymosan activated plasma (ZAP) or fMLP.

RESULTS

There was a marked decrease in leukocyte count within 5 minutes after injection of 25 $\mu g/M^2$ of GM-CSF. The total leukocyte count declined from 8250 to 1150/µl (Figure 1).

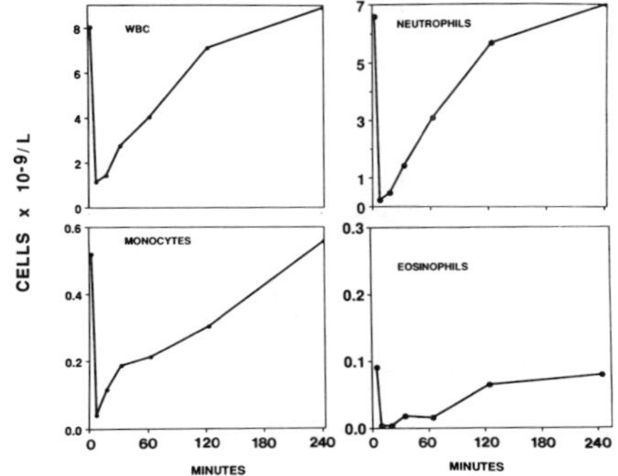

Figure 1. Acute leukocyte responses to 25 µg/M^2 of GM-CSF. Reprinted by permission from Blood 74:26,1989.

There was a virtual disappearance of circulating neutrophils, monocytes and eosinophils. Leukocytes returned to baseline values within 2 hours after injection. It is of interest that the band/segmented neutrophil ratio was increased from 30 to 240 minutes after administration of GM-CSF. In two patients marrow aspirates were obtained 30 minutes after the injection. The total number of band and segmented cells in the marrow declined from 22% to 9% in the first patient and from 36% to 17% in the second patient.

This acute leukopenia appeared to result from activation of the MO1 receptor on neutrophils and monocytes. As judged by flow cytometry the number of neutrophils reactive with the MO1 monoclonal antibody (Freyer et al., 1988) increased from 75% to 95% within two hours after injection. Moreover, there was a two-fold increase in fluorescence units indicating up regulation of this receptor.

With a continuous intravenous infusion of GM-CSF, the leukocyte count rose within 24 hours with a second increase in leukocytes approximately 5 days into the infusion

(Figure 2). This was due to an increase in the number of

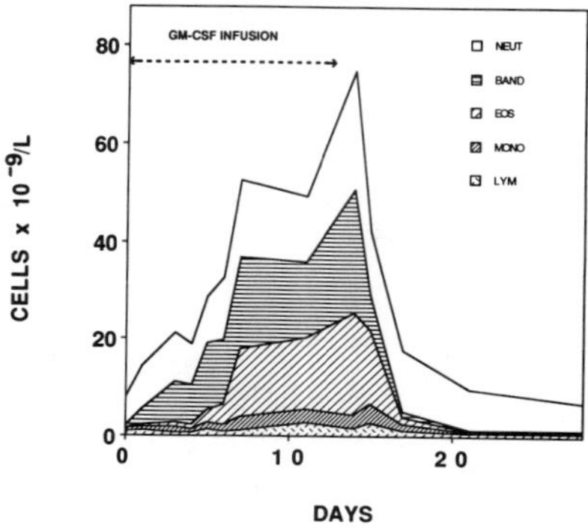

Figure 2. Leukocyte responses to infusion of 500 µg/M^2/day of GM-CSF. Reprinted by permission from Blood 74:26,1989.

neutrophils, bands, eosinophils and a modest increase in the number of monocytes. There was also a modest increase in myelocytes and metamyelocytes with approximately 1,000 cells/µl at 100 µg/M^2 and approximately 2700 cells/µl at 500 µg/M^2 on day 8 of the infusion. There was also a dramatic increase in eosinophils to as high as 21,000 cells/µl on the last day of treatment.

Monocyte ADCC activity was increased in 8 out of 10 patients two days after the bolus injection of GM-CSF, however, these changes were not significant. There was essentially no difference in the results obtained with patients receiving 100/µg or 500/µg/M^2 of GM-CSF; results of all patients were pooled. ADCC activity was increased on days 3 and 10 of the constant GM-CSF infusion.

Table 1

Monocyte ADCC Activity

Baseline	Continuous Infusion Day 3	Continuous Infusion Day 10
45 ± 5	66 ± 7	68 ± 8

Values are % cytotoxicity. Day 3 and 10 values are significantly increased at the 1% level. (Wilcoxon signed rank test).

TNF alpha release by LPS appeared greater after 3 days of continuous infusion, however, the values did not reach statistical significance. TNF activity was, however, increased after 10 days of continuous GM-CSF therapy. Similar findings were noted with interferon (IFN) secretion in response to LPS. Values were unchanged on day 3 but were increased significantly 10 days after continuous GM-CSF therapy.

Table 2

Monocyte TNF and INF Secretion

	Baseline	Continuous Infusion Day 3	Continuous Infusion Day 10
TNF	2.2 ± 1.0	7.3 ± 3.0	16.1 ± 4.6
IFN	<5.0	20.1 ± 11.6	94.6 ± 77.6

Values are units/ml. Both TNF and IFN were increased on day 10 at the 1% level. (Wilcoxon signed rank test).

Serum levels of TNF were measured in 3 patients on days 5, 10 and 11 of the GM-CSF infusion. The ELISA assay indicated no increase in TNF activity over baseline levels, however, all patients had increased activity as judged by the bioassay. Baseline levels ranged from 1.2 to 3.3 ng/ml whereas levels of 4.0 to 9.2 ng/ml were detected during continuous GM-CSF treatment.

There was no consistent effect of GM-CSF on baseline neutrophil superoxide release (Figure 3). Those cells

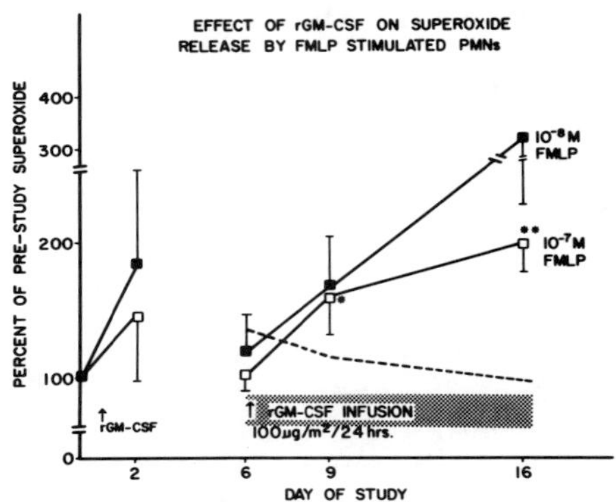

Figure 3. Neutrophil superoxide release during treatment with GM-CSF.

stimulated with 10^{-7} M fMLP showed significant enhancement of superoxide release on day 3 (146%) and on day 10 (204%) of continuous IV infusion. Owing to a wider variation on day 10 the results with 10^{-8} M fMLP did not reach significance. When PMA was used to induce superoxide release, no increase was seen after the bolus injection or after 3 days of GM-CSF therapy. All 4 patients had enhanced production of superoxide on day 10 of continuous therapy.

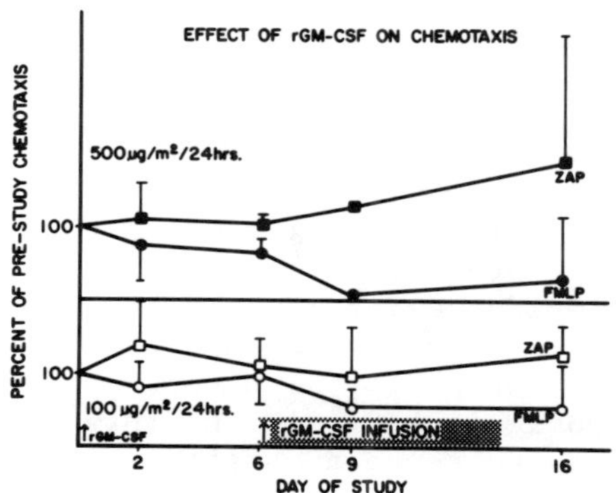

Figure 4. Neutrophil chemotaxis during treatment with GM-CSF

In contrast to the stimulation of superoxide release, there was no enhancement of chemotaxis following the bolus injection of GM-CSF. Chemotaxis in response to fMLP was depressed throughout the 3 and 10 day continuous infusion of GM-CSF (Figure 4).

DISCUSSION

These studies show that GM-CSF has striking effects on leukopoiesis. There is an early dramatic leukopenia that appears to be secondary to activation or up regulation of the MO1 receptor on neutrophils and monocytes. This receptor is a plasma membrane glycoprotein, also known as CD11b - a member of the CD18 family of leukocyte adhesion glycoproteins (Freyer et al., 1988). It would appear that such activation serves to localize neutrophils and monocytes at the site of inflammation and to effect neutrophil aggregation, chemotaxis, phagocytosis and respiratory burst activity. The dramatic early neutropenia resulted in a secondary release of band and segmented neutrophils from the marrow. This effect could serve to stimulate myelopoiesis by removal of a negative feedback system. It appears, however, that GM-CSF also stimulates hemopoietic progenitor cells directly as this agent is effective in accelerating myelopoiesis after high dose chemotherapy (Antman et al., 1988) or autologous bone marrow transplant (Nemunaitis et al., 1988). In these circumstances there are ordinarily no mature cells in the bone marrow that would be responsive to this factor.

A second major effect of GM-CSF is to stimulate the function of mature monocytes and neutrophils. Although the CSFs are quite active in vitro, there has been little information to support their activity in vivo. The present studies show that there are modest direct effects on these cells as well as evidence for marked sensitization. Monocyte ADCC activity is increased during continuous IV infusion and secretion of TNF alpha and interferon is augmented in response to LPS. In the three patients studied there appeared to be a modest increase in circulating levels of TNF as well.

There was a mild increase in neutrophil superoxide release during the continuous infusion of GM-CSF. With addition of fMLP there was evidence for augmented superoxide release. It is of interest that there was either no change or a modest decrease in neutrophil chemotaxis in response to fMLP. This finding may result from activation of the M01 receptor and a tendency for cells to adhere or localize rather than to respond to migration signals. In this regard, reduced migration of neutrophils to skin windows has been found in patients receiving GM-CSF after autologous bone marrow transplantation (Peters et al., 1988). Further studies will be necessary to determine whether this can be overcome by other chemotactic stimuli.

These studies suggest that GM-CSF may be useful in a variety of clinical situations. This growth factor is useful in accelerating recovering of myelopoiesis following high dose chemotherapy or autologous bone marrow transplantation. By stimulating mature neutrophils, monocytes and macrophages, GM-CSF may also augment the function of the few circulating or fixed tissue cells during severe bone marrow aplasia. As such it may boost the phagocytic system during the hypoplastic interval after chemotherapy. Stimulation of neutrophils and monocytes may also be expected to have a potential antitumor effect. Further studies in patients with minimal residual disease or in the adjuvant setting may be warranted.

ACKNOWLEDGMENT

The authors gratefully acknowledge the supply of recombinant human GM-CSF by the Immunex Corporation. These studies were supported in part by NIH grants A124121, CA15237 and American Cancer Society grant PDT337 and grants from the Immunex Corporation and the Pathology Education and Research Foundation.

REFERENCES

Antman KS, Griffin JD, Elias A, Socinski MA, Ryan L, Cannistra SA, Oette D, Whitley M, Frei E III, Schnipper LE (1988). Effect of recombinant human granulocyte-macrophage colony-stimulating factor on chemotherapy-induced myelosuppression. N Engl J Med 319:593-598.

Freyer DR, Morganroth ML, Rogers CE, Arnaout MA, Todd RF III (1988). Modulation of surface CD11/CD18 glycoproteins (Mo1, LFA, p150,95) by human mononuclear phagocytes. Clin Immunol Immunopath 46:272-283.

Gasson JC, Weisbart RH, Kaufman ST, Clark SC, Hemick RM, Wang GG, Golde DW (1984). Purified human granulocyte-macrophage colony-stimulating factor: direct action on neutrophils. Science 226:1339.

Grabstein KH, Urdal DL, Tushinski RJ, Mochizuki DY, Price VL, Cantrell MA, Gillis S, Conlon PJ (1986). Induction of macrophage tumoricidal activity by granulocyte-macrophage colony-stimulating factor. Science 232:506.

Groopman JE, Mitsuyasu RT, Deleo MJ, Oette DH, Golde, DW (1987). Effect of recombinant human granulocyte-macrophage colony-stimulating factor on myelopoiesis in the acquired immunodeficiency syndrome. N Engl J Med 317:593-598.

Herrman F, Schulz G, Lindemann A, Meyenburg W, Oster W, Krumwiek D, Mertelsmann R (1989). Hematopoietic responses in patients with advanced malignancy treated with recombinant human granulocyte-macrophage colony-stimulating factor. J Clin Oncol 7:159-167.

Kaplan SS, Basford RE, Wing EJ, Shadduck RK (1989). The effect of recombinant human granulocyte macrophage colony-stimulating factor on neutrophil activation in patients with refractory carcinoma. Blood 73:636-638.

Nemunaitis J, Singer JW, Buckner CD, Hill R, Storb R, Thomas ED, Applebaum FR (1988). Use of recombinant human granulocyte-macrophage colony-stimulating factor in autologous marrow transplantation for lymphoid malignancies. Blood 72:834-836.

Peters WP, Stuart A, Affronti ML, Kim CS, Coleman RE (1988). Neutrophil migration is defective during recombinant human granulocyte-macrophage colony-stimulating factor infusion after autologous bone marrow transplantation in humans. Blood 72:1310-1315.

Phillips N, Jacobs S, Stoller R, Earle M, Przepiorka D, Shadduck RK (1989). Effect of recombinant human granulocyte-macrophage colony stimulating factor on myelopoiesis in patients with refractory metastatic carcinoma. Blood 74, 26-34.

Vadhan-Raj S, Keating M, LeMaistre A, Hittelman WN, McCredie K, Trujillo JM, Broxmeyer HE, Henney C, Gutterman JU (1987). Effects of recombinant human granulocyte-macrophage colony-stimulating factor in patients with myelodysplastic syndromes. N Engl J Med 317:1545-1552.

Vadhan-Raj S, Buescher S, Broxmeyer HE, LeMaistre A, Lepe-Zuniga JL, Ventura G, Jeha S, Horwitz LJ, Trujillo JM, Gillis S, Hittelman WN, Gutterman JO (1988). Stimulation of myelopoiesis in patients with aplastic anemia by recombinant human granulocyte-macrophage colony-stimulating factor. N Engl J Med 319:1628-1634.

Wing EJ, Waheed A, Shadduck RK, Nagle LS, Stephenson BA (1982). Effect of colony stimulating factor on murine macrophages: Induction of anti-tumor activity. J Clin Invest 69:270-276.

Wing EJ, Magee DM, Whiteside TL, Kaplan SS, Shadduck RK (1989). Recombinant human granulocyte/macrophage colony-stimulating factor enhances monocyte cytotoxicity and secretion of tumor necrosis factor α and interferon in cancer patients. Blood 73:643-646.

Wing EJ, Shadduck RK (1985). Colony stimulating factor. In "Biological Response Modifiers" Torrence PF (ed.). New York: Academic Press, pp 219-243.

The Biology of Hematopoiesis, pages 375–384

THE BIOLOGY OF HUMAN GRANULOCYTE-MACROPHAGE COLONY-STIMULATING FACTOR (GM-CSF)

Judith C. Gasson, Gayle C. Baldwin, Kathleen M. Sakamoto and John F. DiPersio

Division of Hematology-Oncology, Department of Medicine, UCLA School of Medicine, Los Angeles CA 90024 and Department of Pediatrics, Children's Hospital of Los Angeles (KMS), Los Angeles CA 90054

INTRODUCTION

Human granulocyte-macrophage colony-stimulating factor (GM-CSF) was originally identified and characterized by its ability to support proliferation and maturation of bone marrow-derived myeloid progenitor cells in semi-solid media. The colonies formed in response to this factor primarily consist of neutrophilic granulocytes and monocytes; hence, the name GM-CSF. Work by a number of groups over the past six years has resulted in the purification and molecular cloning of both murine and human GM-CSF (rev. 1,2). Considerable information is now available about the production and biological activities of GM-CSF. Due to the rapid progress made in this field, GM-CSF is currently employed in numerous clinical trials to enhance host defense of patients in a variety of disorders. Research today focuses upon the role of GM-CSF in three critical areas: physiologic regulation of white blood cell production, pathophysiologic involvement in autoimmune and inflammatory disorders, and therapeutic use in cancer treatment and immunodeficient patients.

BIOLOGICAL ACTIVITIES OF GM-CSF

All blood cell elements are derived from pluripotent progenitor cells in the bone marrow (Figure 1). Regulation of this process appears to be controlled by production of a family of stimulatory cytokines known as the colony-stimulating factors and interleukins, as well as expression of specific cell surface receptors on the maturing blood cells.

Figure 1: GM-CSF Stimulates Proliferation of Myeloid Progenitors

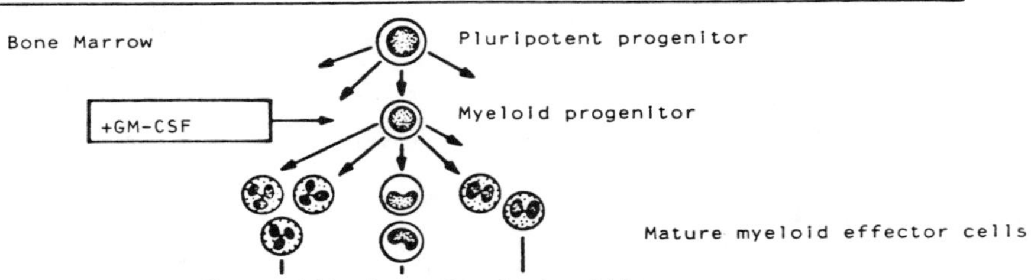

Stimulation of bone marrow progenitors with GM-CSF *in vitro* leads primarily to production of colonies consisting of neutrophils, monocytes, and eosinophils (3). In addition, GM-CSF has been implicated in the stimulation of both erythroid progenitors and megakaryocytes. *In vivo* affects of GM-CSF closely mirror those observed in the laboratory (4-8). A dose-dependent increase in white blood cells is observed in patients treated with GM-CSF. The increase is primarily in neutrophils, monocytes, and eosinophils. GM-CSF also stimulates proliferation of fresh myeloid leukemia cells, as well as a variety of human myeloid cell lines. Since GM-CSF clearly stimulates proliferation of myeloid progenitors both *in vivo* and *in vitro*, it is critical to evaluate its role both in the homeostatic regulation of white cell production, as well as in response to infection.

In addition to its role as a hematopoietic growth factor, GM-CSF also enhances the function of terminally differentiated cells such as neutrophils, monocytes, macrophages, and eosinophils (Figure 2). The direct effects of GM-CSF on human neutrophils include membrane ruffling, degranulation, and increased expression of cell surface adhesion proteins (9). In addition, GM-CSF increases the number and/or affinity of neutrophil receptors for f-Met-Leu-Phe and IgA (10). GM-CSF has also been shown to enhance the function of eosinophils and monocytes.

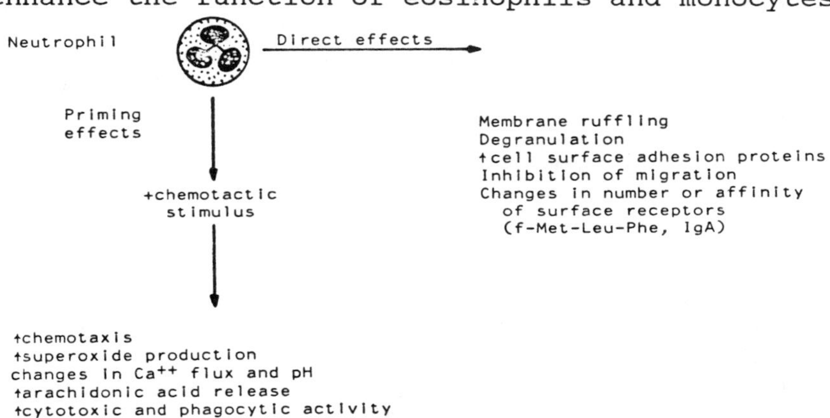

Figure 2: GM-CSF Enhances Host Defense Cell Function

GM-CSF has priming effects on neutrophils which are not observed unless the cells are subsequently stimulated with a chemotactic agent. Neutrophils primed with GM-CSF show enhanced chemotaxis, increased production of superoxide, enhanced release of arachidonic acid, and subsequent production of 5-lipoxygenase products, as well as increased cytotoxic and phagocytic activities (11,12).

Neutrophil function has been evaluated in AIDS patients treated with GM-CSF, and the results confirmed that cells produced in response to GM-CSF were, in every case, fully functional. In a few cases, enhanced function in specific *in vitro* assays was suggested (13). Taken together, the effects of GM-CSF on differentiated myeloid effector cells would result in retention of cells at local areas of inflammation, as well as enhanced ability of the cells to combat invading micro-organisms.

GM-CSF RECEPTORS

The mechanism by which GM-CSF induces such diverse biological responses is of considerable interest. We initially identified the presence of GM-CSF receptors on myeloid leukemia cell lines, as well as primary human neutrophils (14). The GM-CSF receptor is present in a low number on all responsive cells, including bone marrow neutrophils, eosinophils, monocytes, and myeloid leukemia cells (Table 1). The affinity of the GM-CSF receptor on all hematopoietic cells is in the range of 20-50 pM, which is in excellent agreement with the range of concentrations which elicit biological response. Covalent cross-linking of ^{125}I-labeled GM-CSF to cells yields a complex which suggests an apparent molecular weight of 84 kilodaltons (kD) for the GM-CSF receptor. Thus, GM-CSF seems to exert its effects on both proliferation and function through an 84 kD high-affinity receptor.

Table 1. Human GM-CSF Receptors

Primary	Cell Lines
Hematopoietic Origin	
Bone marrow	HL-60
Neutrophils	KG-1
Eosinophils	U937
Monocytes	
Chronic myelogenous leukemia	
Acute myelogenous leukemia	
Non-hematopoietic Origin	
Melanoma	M14 (melanoma)
Paraganglioma	M101
	H-128 (SCCL)
	H-69

We have subsequently observed the presence of GM-CSF receptors on cells of non-hematopoietic origin, and particularly, those derived from the neural crest (15). Small cell carcinoma of the lung cell lines express a low number of high-affinity GM-CSF receptors. We have also observed specific binding of GM-CSF to primary melanoma cells and melanoma cell lines, as well as primary paraganglioma tumor cells. Cross-linking of GM-CSF to receptors on cells of neural crest origin yields a complex which co-migrates with the receptor on hematopoietic cells. However, GM-CSF receptors expressed on melanoma cells appears to be of a lower affinity (Kd approximately 500 pM) than that observed on hematopoietic cells. It is important to determine the molecular differences between the high- and low-affinity GM-CSF receptors, as well as to substantiate the activity of the low-affinity receptor. It is, at this point, critical to determine whether GM-CSF receptors are present on normal cells of neural crest origin, and if so, what role GM-CSF might play in the development or function of these cells.

A considerable amount of effort has gone into trying to understand the biochemical events elicited by binding of GM-CSF to its receptor (Figure 3). GM-CSF does not directly stimulate a calcium flux, nor is any change in pH observed in neutrophils. Several investigators have suggested that GM-CSF may exert its effects through a pertussis toxin-sensitive G-protein. However, we and others have demonstrated that treatment of neutrophils with GM-CSF results in release of arachidonic acid and synthesis of potent inflammatory products of the 5-lipoxygenase pathway, including leukotriene B_4. For this reason, it is difficult to determine from inhibitor studies whether the effects observed are directly blocking GM-CSF action or interfering with subsequent metabolic events which serve to amplify the biological response (12).

Figure 3: GM-CSF Mechanism of Action

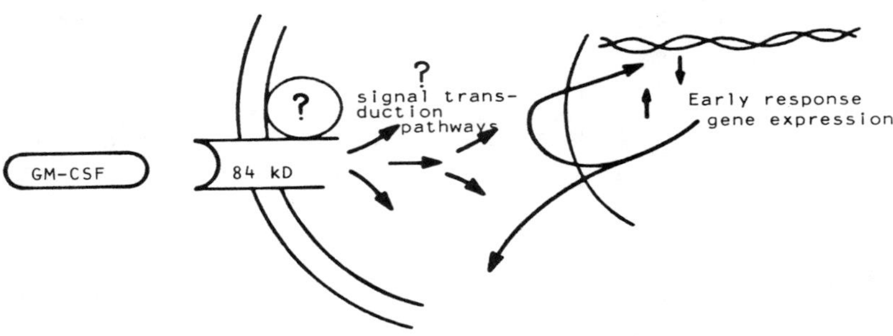

GM-CSF INDUCES EXPRESSION OF PRIMARY RESPONSE GENES

In order to understand the biochemical events which mediate the activities of hematopoietic growth factors in inducing proliferation, it is useful to examine the induction of primary response genes as an indicator of cellular stimulation. Primary response genes are those whose expression is induced independently of protein synthesis.

We have explored induction of primary response genes using a family of genes induced in Swiss 3T3 cells by the tumor promotor, TPA (16). The pattern of early response response genes induced by GM-CSF both in proliferating and terminally differentiated cells was compared by studying the effects of GM-CSF on a factor-dependent murine cell line, 32D clone 3, and terminally differentiated human neutrophils (17). In these studies, we examined induction of three primary response genes, TIS1, which is a member of the nuclear receptor gene superfamily; TIS8, also known as EGR-1, a putative transcription factor; and TIS11, which has no sequence motifs indicating function. We showed that while TIS1 can be induced in either 3T3 fibroblasts or PC12 cells by a variety of factors including TPA, EGF, or NGF, neither TPA nor GM-CSF could induce TIS1 in the proliferating or terminally differentiated myeloid cells. However, both TIS8 and TIS11 were induced by TPA or GM-CSF in the 32D clone 3 cells as well as neutrophils (Table 2).

Table 2. GM-CSF Induces Expression of Early Response Genes

	32D clone 3 (murine)		Neutrophils (human)	
	+TPA	+GM-CSF	+TPA	+GM-CSF
TIS1 (member of nuclear receptor gene superfamily)	-	-	-	-
TIS8 (zinc finger-containing protein)	+	+	+	+
TIS11 (no sequence motif indicating function)	+	+	+	+

The restricted pattern of TIS gene expression in different cell types may confer some degree of specificity of hormone action on different cells. Similarly, the pattern of genes induced by GM-CSF in proliferating versus post-mitotic cells is the same, suggesting that GM-CSF may exert its diverse biological actions through similar mechanisms.

FUTURE DIRECTIONS

Clinical trials currently underway employing GM-CSF revolve around three basic therapeutic uses. The first is to enhance the effectiveness of currently existing therapies for treatment of solid tumor patients by alternating the use of GM-CSF with radiation or chemotherapy. The second therapeutic use is to enhance recovery following bone marrow transplantation or in marrow failure states such as aplastic anemia. Third, the use of GM-CSF is currently being explored to augment host defense in immunocompromised patients. The best clinical settings in which GM-CSF can be utilized remain to be defined. A likely outcome of current clinical trials will be that specific combinations of hematopoietic growth factors will be administered in different situations in order to manipulate the types of cells that are produced. Because of the dual roles of colony-stimulating factors on proliferating and terminally differentiated cells, proper therapeutic administration should greatly enhance the patient's ability to resist infections, and may be beneficial in destruction of tumor cells as well.

In addition to exploring potential therapeutic uses of the colony-stimulating factors, much remains to be determined about their role in the physiologic regulation of hematopoiesis. It is important to understand which CSFs and interleukins play a role in day-to-day maintenance of hematopoiesis in the bone marrow, and what series of events lead to increased white blood cell counts in response to infection. These are the most basic regulatory events in hematopoiesis and host defense. Finally, from a broader perspective, many current questions centering around hormone and receptor interactions and stimulation of cellular proliferation can readily be addressed using the hematopoietic system as a model. The availability of primary target cells, both normal and neoplastic, makes studies on the mechanism of action of the hemopoietins especially suitable for experimental manipulation. Results of such work may yield insights into the unregulated growth of myeloid leukemia cells as well as physiologic regulation of myelopoiesis.

ACKNOWLEDGEMENTS

We are pleased to acknowledge the contributions of our collaborators at UCLA on the biological activities of GM-CSF, David Golde and Richard Weisbart. We are grateful to Wendy Aft for preparation of this manuscript.

REFERENCES

1. Clark SC, Kamen R (1987). Science 236:1229-1236.
2. Golde DW, Gasson JC (1988). Scient Am 259:62-70.
3. Tomonaga M, Golde DW, Gasson JC (1986). Blood 67:31-36.
4. Groopman JE, Mitsuyasu RT, DeLeo MJ, Oette DH, Golde DW (1987). New Engl J Med 317:593-598.
5. Antman KS, Griffin JD, Elias A, Socinski MA, Ryan L, Cannistra SA, Oette D, Whitley M, Frei E III, Schnipper LE (1988). New Engl J Med 319:593-598.
6. Brandt SJ, Peters WP, Atwater SK, Kurtzberg J, Borowitz MJ, Jones RB, Shpall EJ, Bast RC, Gilbert CJ, Oette DH (1988). New Engl J Med 318:869-876.
7. Champlin RE, Nimer SD, Ireland P, Oette D, Golde DW (1989). Blood 73:694-699.
8. Vadhan-Raj S, Keating M, LeMaistre A, Hittelman WN, McCredie K, Trujillo JM, Broxmeyer HE, Henney C, Gutterman JU (1987). New Engl J Med 317:1545-1552.
9. Weisbart RH, Golde DW, Clark SC, Wong GG, Gasson JC (1985). Nature 314:361-363.
10. Weisbart RH, Kwan L, Golde DW, Gasson JC (1987). Blood 69:18-21.
11. Weisbart RH, Golde DW, Gasson JC (1986). J Immunol 137:3584-3587.
12. DiPersio JF, Billing P, Williams R, Gasson JC (1988). J Immunol 140:4315-4322.
13. Baldwin GC, Gasson JC, Quan SG, Fleischmann J, Weisbart R, Oette D, Mitsuyasu RT, Golde DW (1988). Proc Natl Acad Sci USA 85:2763-2766.
14. DiPersio J, Billing P, Kaufman S, Egtesady P, Williams RE, Gasson JC (1988). J Biol Chem 263:1834-1841.
15. Baldwin GC, Gasson JC, Kaufman SE, Quan SG, Williams RE, Avalos BR, Gazdar AF, Golde DW, DiPersio JF (1989). Blood 73:1033-1037.
16. Lim RW, Varnum BC, Herschman HR (1987). Oncogene 1:263-270.

17. Varnum BC, Lim RW, Kujubu D, Luner S, Kaufman SE, Greenberger JS, Gasson JC, Herschman H (1989). Mol Cell Biol 9:3580-3583.

The Biology of Hematopoiesis, pages 385–390

GROWTH FACTORS CONTROLLING THE DEVELOPMENT OF HEMOPOIETIC CELLS

Frank Lee

Department of Molecular Biology, DNAX Research Institute of Molecular and Cellular Biology, 901 California Avenue, Palo Alto, California 94304-1104

INTRODUCTION

Recent studies have documented the function of a variety of colony stimulating factors and interleukins which control the growth and differentiation of hemopoietic cells. Many of these factors were first characterized as biological activities produced by cultured cell lines including fibroblasts, T lymphocytes and various tumor cell lines. In many cases, particularly T cell lines, the production of hemopoietic growth factors is strictly regulated and produced only when the cells are activated.

Several years ago we began to investigate the role of growth factors in controlling the steady state production of hemopoietic cells. In these studies we focused on the contribution of cells in the bone marrow, the major site of hemopoiesis in the adult. As first developed by Dexter and co-workers, long-term bone marrow cultures can mimic many of the events of bone marrow including the prolonged maintenance of hemopoietic progenitor cells coupled with their continuous maturation and differentiation(1). As shown by a number of investigators, the adherent cells in these cultures, also called stromal cells, are crucial for the long-term maintenance of hemopoietic *in vitro*. In our studies we have characterized the growth factors produced by stromal cells.

Summarized in Table 1 are the hemopoietic growth factors which are produced by a panel of mouse bone marrow stromal cells isolated from long term bone marrow cultures. From analysis of several cell lines M-CSF, the growth factor specific for the monocyte/macrophage cell lineage is produced constitutively by all stromal cell lines examined. This growth factor is also produced by many tissues of the mouse in a constitutive fashion. Several other growth factors are produced in an inducible fashion. GM-CSF, G-CSF and interleukin-6 are all produced at low basal levels in untreated stromal cells, but their synthesis is significantly up-regulated when the cells are exposed to the cytokine IL-1, a product of activated macrophages(2).

Table 1. Hemopoietic Growth Factors Made by Stromal Cells

M-CSF	IL-6
G-CSF	IL-7
GM-CSF	LIF

Interleukin-6

IL-6 was independently characterized in several laboratories on the basis of various biological activities. The cDNA was cloned on the basis of protein sequence derived from a B cell stimulatory factor (BSF-2) characterized by Kishimoto and co-workers(3). cDNA clones encoding the same molecule had been isolated earlier based on the finding that the mRNA was coordinately induced in human fibroblasts with the mRNA encoding fibroblast or beta interferon(4). It was therefore designated beta-2-interferon, and some studies indicated that the protein possessed weak anti-viral properties in interferon assays. Independent studies showed that IL-6 also is involved in the inflammatory response by mediating the induction of acute phase proteins by liver cells(5). These multiple activities establish IL-6 as a major biological mediator in various inducible responses.

In our studies, we wished to determine whether IL-6 was involved in the regulation of steady state hemopoiesis. cDNA libraries from stromal cells treated with IL-1 were screened with a probe from the human IL-6 cDNA. Cross hybridizing clones were isolated and sequenced and shown to encode a polypeptide homologous to the human polypeptide(6). Analysis of the mRNA from several stromal cells indicated that IL-6 mRNA is also inducible by IL-1; thus the IL-6 gene responds similarly to the genes for G-CSF and GM-CSF. This data suggests a similar role for IL-6 in regulating hemopoiesis.

The cDNA clone was then expressed in COS monkey cells and the recombinant protein purified for biological studies. Initial studies confirmed that the murine protein shared the same biological activities with the human molecule. It is active in supporting the growth of transformed B cell lines and in inducing the production of acute phase proteins from hepatoma cell lines <u>in vitro</u>. We also found that IL-6 can be a growth factor supporting the growth of factor dependent myeloid cell lines, first isolated as IL-3 dependent cell lines(6).

In assays with normal bone marrow progenitor cells, IL-6 can induce the growth of colonies in semisolid medium(6). These colonies are composed of cells with granulocyte or macrophage morphology. When combined with other growth factors such IL-3 or GM-CSF, IL-6 can enhance the response of primitive hemopoietic cells to these factors(7). In all of these <u>in vitro</u> assays, IL-6 stimulates the growth and differentiation of myeloid populations of progenitor cells. IL-6 also has the somewhat unique activity of inducing terminal differentiation of certain myeloid leukemia cells[8]. The M1 leukemic tumor cell line grows in a factor independent fashion in vitro, but when exposed to IL-6, these cells undergo rapid terminal differentiation and exhibit the morphological and functional properties of mature macrophages. Although the differentiation inducing activity of IL-6 on these leukemic cells is quite potent, the role of IL-6 in the differentiation of normal myeloid progenitor cells and its role as a growth factor for these cells is still unclear. It is likely, however, that IL-6 acts coordinately with other factors such as GM-CSF and G-CSF in the generation of myeloid cells in the bone marrow.

Leukemia Inhibitory Factor

The studies of Gearing, et al.[9], initially identified another cytokine with the ability to induce differentiation of myeloid leukemic cells. This factor, termed leukemia inhibitory factor or LIF, was purified from the medium of Krebs cells and cloned from a cDNA library made from a helper T cell clone. Using the polymerase chain reaction technique we were able to detect LIF cDNA clones in libraries made from several stromal cell clones, results also confirmed by the detection of LIF mRNA by S-1 nuclease analysis.

LIF does not appear to have activity on normal progenitor cells, however, despite the presence of cellular receptors on macrophage lineage cells[9]. LIF appears to be as potent as IL-6 in its ability to induce differentiation of the M1 leukemic cell line, but as for IL-6, its role in the differentiation of normal cells is unclear. LIF is also reported to be involved in bone metabolism[10]. In addition, LIF, like IL-6, can induce the expression of acute phase proteins by liver cells[11]. Thus, LIF shares several properties with IL-6, although it may not have the complete hemopoietic growth and modulating activity of IL-6. The other described activity of LIF which is significant is its ability to act on embryonic stem (ES) cells. LIF is apparently identical to the differentiation inhibitory factor made by fibroblast feeder cells normally used to maintain the undifferentiated phenotype of ES cells. The role of both IL-6 and LIF in embryonic development will be discussed further.

Interleukin-7

Whitlock and Witte modified long term bone marrow cultures to permit the growth of early lymphoid cells, predominantly pre-B cells[12]. Using a cloned bone marrow stromal cell line, Namen, et al described the purification and cloning of a cDNA encoding a pre-B cell growth factor[13]. We have isolated IL-7 cDNA clones from stromal cell cDNA libraries using PCR amplification of cDNAs. The IL-7 cDNA was expressed in COS monkey cells and used for biological studies.

IL-7 can support the long-term growth of pre-B cell clones derived as stromal cell-dependent clones. It can support the growth of both IL-3 responsive and IL-3 non-responsive pre-B cells. The studies of Namen originally showed that thymus is an abundant source of IL-7 mRNA[13].

Our own mRNA analysis demonstrated that IL-7 mRNA is expressed in stromal cells isolated from bone marrow and also stromal cells isolated from thymus(14). IL-7 biological activity could also be detected in medium from thymic stromal cells. We thus examined the growth factor activity of IL-7 on various populations of thymocytes.

IL-7 appears to be a potent growth factor for the most immature population of thymocytes(14). These cells can be identified in adult thymus as those lacking expression of both the CD4 and CD8 cell surface antigens. Cells which are either CD4+ or CD8+ exhibit a somewhat weaker proliferative response to IL-7 while the double positive population does not respond at all. The proliferative response of the double negative thymocytes is not accompanied by any obvious differentiation. Unlike the response of thymocytes to several other cytokines, the response to IL-7 does not require co- stimulation by other cytokines or mitogens. IL-7 is likely to play a role in the growth and development of normal thymocytes as well as B lymphocytes.

Hemopoietic Growth Factors in Development

The studies described above address the function of growth factors in the maintenance of hemopoiesis during steady state hemopoiesis in the adult. Growth factors made by stromal cells in bone marrow and thymus can account for the production of most of the hemopoietic cell lineages arising from each of these sites. We wish to understand the process by which hemopoietic stem cells first arise in the embryo at the onset of hemopoiesis.

During mouse embryonic development hemopoiesis can first be detected in the blood islands of the extra-embryonic yolk sac at about day seven of gestation. At this time there are easily visualized erythroid cells expressing distinct embryonic forms of globin. Following this stage hemopoiesis shifts to the fetal liver which is an active site for both erythropoiesis and lymphopoiesis, and finally the fetal bone marrow which continues as the predominant site of hemopoiesis in the adult. We are particularly interested in the events in the embryo immediately preceding the appearance of hemopoiesis in the yolk sac, because differentiation events ocurring at this time may contribute directly to the development of hemopoietic stem cells.

Our initial approach to this problem has been to examine the expression of known hemopoietic growth factors in the preimplantation mouse embryo. Blastocysts can be isolated at about three and a half days of development. At this point these embryos consist of about 50-60 cells; an outer layer of trophoblasts and the inner cell mass of stem cells. This stage precedes by about four days the beginning of hemopoiesis. Thus, growth factor expression at this stage could provide us with clues concerning factors which are involved in the development of the first hemopoietic stem cells.

Our analysis uses PCR to amplify mRNA sequences into DNA because of the limited amount of cellular RNA available from embryos. Using oligonucleotide primers specific for the detection of several cytokines known to have biological effects on primitive hemopoietic cells or embryonic cells, we find evidence for the expression of two hemopoietic factors, IL-6 and LIF. We were unable to detect mRNA for IL-3 and GM-CSF. We have evidence for the presence of both IL-6 and LIF in the medium of blastocysts cultured for one day _in vitro_. We could dectect an activity which could stimulate an IL-6 responsive cell line and which could be neutralized by a specific antibody against IL-6, while an activity which could stimulate the proliferation of a LIF responsive myeloid cell line, DA-1a, was also detectable.

These results suggest that these two molecules, which share a number of biological activities are expressed in the pre-implantation embryo several days before the beginning of hemopoiesis. Further studies will be required to determine if they are involved in the differentiation events leading to hemopoietic cells or if they control the growth or differentiation of other primitive embryonic cell types.

REFERENCES

Dexter, TM et al., (1977). Stromal cell associated haemopoiesis. J Cell Physiol 91:335-344.

Rennick, D et al., (1987). Control of hemopoiesis by a bone marrow stromal cell clone: Lipopolysaccharide - and Interleukin-1-inducible production of colony-stimulating factors. Blood, 69:682-691.

Hirano, T et al. (1986). Complementary DNA for a novel human interleukin (BSF-2) that induces B lymphocytes to produce immunoglobulin. Nature 324:73-76.

Sehgal, PB et al., (1987). Human β_2 interferon and B-cell differentiation factor BSF-2 are identical. J Science 235:731-732.

Gauldie, J et al., (1987). Interferon β_2/B-cell stimulatory factor type 2 shares identity with monocyte-derived hepatocyte-stimulating factor and regulates the major acute phase protein response in liver cells. Proc Nat Acad Sci USA 84:7251-7255.

Chiu, C-P et al., (1988). Multiple biological activities are expressed by a mouse Interleukin-6 cDNA clone isolated from bone marrow stromal cells. Proc Nat Acad Sci USA 85:7099-7103.

Rennick D et al., (1989). Interleukin-6 interacts with Interleukin-4 and other hematopoietic growth factors to selectively enhance the growth of megakaryocytic, erythroid, myeloid, and multipotential progenitor cells. Blood 73:1828-1835.

Chiu, C-P, Lee, F (1989). IL-6 is a differentiation factor for M1 and WEHI-3B myeloid leukemic cells. J Immunol 142:1909-1915.

Gearing, DP et al. (1987). Molecular cloning and expression of cDNA encoding a murine myeloid leukaemia inhibitory factor (LIF). EMBO J 6:3995-4002.

Metcalf, D, Gearing, DP (1989). Fatal syndrome in mice engrafted with cells producing high levels of the leukemia inhibitory factor. Proc Nat Acad Sci USA 86:5948-5942.

Baumann H, Wong, GG (1989). Hepatocyte-stimulating factor III shares structural and functional identity with leukemia-inhibitory factor. J Immunol 143:1163-1167.

Whitlock, CA, Witte, ON (1982). Long-term culture of B-lymphocytes and their precursors from murine bone marrow. Proc Nat Acad Sci USA 79:3608-3612.

Namen, AE et al., (1988). B cell precursor growth-promoting activity. Purification and characterization of a growth factor active on lymphocyte precursors. J Exp Med 167:988-1002.

Murray, R et al., (1989). IL-7 is a growth and maintenance factor for mature and immature thymocyte subsets. Int Immunol 1:526-531.

The Biology of Hematopoiesis, pages 391–407

KINETIC RESPONSE OF HAEMOPOIETIC CELL LINEAGES TO GROWTH FACTORS IN VIVO: THEIR RELATIONSHIP TO THE MICROARCHITECTURE OF THE TISSUE AND ITS MICROENVIRONMENT

Brian I. Lord

Departments of Experimental Haematology, Paterson Institute for Cancer Research, Christie Hospital and Holt Radium Institute, Manchester M20 9BX, United Kingdom

The Structure of Haemopoietic Bone Marrow

The microarchitecture/cellular organization of haemopoietic tissue, disregarded as an anatomical feature by some experimental and many clinical haematologists, has periodically been invoked as an important feature (a) historically from the anatomical point of view and (b) more recently from the point of view of tissue regulation. In 1938, Weinbeck reported a non-uniform distribution of the maturer granulocytic cells which he found were more concentrated in the vicinity of the central venous sinuses of the marrow spaces, the point from which they are released into the circulation. In 1968, van Dyke observed the ordered reconstruction of the marrow populations outwards from the bone surfaces after clearing the marrow space in experimental myelofibrosis. Lambertsen and Weiss (1984) later made similar but more sophisticated stereoscan observations on endogenous recovery following sublethal irradiation. Meanwhile, Schackney *et al* (1975, 1976) had observed greater kinetic activity in cells closer to the bone surfaces implying a greater proportion of the less mature cells in those regions. Prior to that time, Lord and Hendry (1972) described first the distribution of pluripotent CFU-S across the radial diameter of a mouse femur in which the CFU-S were most highly concentrated close to the bone surfaces and then Lord *et al* (1975) described a discontinous distribution of *in vitro* colony-forming cells which showed a peak concen-tration at a fixed distance from the bone surface. Confirmation of this high concentration of CFU-S in the endosteal regions of the bone surface was provided by Gong (1978) further corroborated this principle.

Furthermore, we now know that the structural distributions of both CFU-S and the in vitro CFC are established by the age of the weaning (Mason et al, 1989). In addition, we have also demonstrated a non-uniform distribution for erythroid progenitor cells (Frassoni et al, 1982) which was also corroborated by Lambertsen and Weiss (1984).

These characteristic distributions for the individual cell types can thus be used to build up a three-dimensional image of the microarchitectural relationship between the haemopoietic cell populations. The fact that the "remote-from-bone" axial CFU-S have a very low proliferative activity and high self-renewal probability compared with marginal CFU-S in close proximity to the bone (Lord, 1978; Lord and Schofield, 1980) suggests that the primitive stem cells are likely to be found more centrally placed while the more mature ones are situated close to the bone surface. Together with the shapes of the differentiated and maturing cell distributions, this, in turn, suggests movement of the stem cell population towards the bone where the cells encounter the greatest differentiation pressures before progressing back towards the central venous sinus for release as mature functional cells.

The observations of van Dyke (1968) and of Lambertsen and Weiss (1984) support this principle for the morphologically recognizable cells. For the progenitor cells, there is of course no direct evidence for this image of cellular migration other than what may be termed a logical description of the cell distributions and their relationships with each other. However, the fact that such distributions can be defined indicates that bone marrow does conform to a precise anatomical structure and is not merely a conglomeration of loosely associated, mutually independent cells. In order to maintain this structure therefore, the system must be fully regulated.

Limited investigations indicate that comparable distributions exist also in human marrow (Testa et al, 1985). Marrow flushed from human ribs contained fewer in vitro colony-forming cells than brushings of the remaining trabecular surface and these in turn contained more colony formers than cells from the ground trabeculae.

Microenvironmental Regulation of Haemopoiesis

There now seems little question that the haemopoietic microenvironment plays a major role in the proper functioning of haemopoietic tissue. Early work on the role of the microenvironment in determining the performance and direction of development (Wolf and Trentin, 1966, 1968; Trentin, 1970) met with mixed support and opposition, but the development of the long-term marrow culture (Dexter *et al*, 1973, 1977) with its dependence on the formation of a stromal adherent layer (Dexter, *et al*, 1977; Allen and Dexter, 1983) expelled most of those early doubts. Whilst intrinsic "housekeeping" functions undoubtedly play a role in maintaining the integrity of the cells it then became clear that external influences, in the form of environmental factors, are instrumental in regulating the performance of the culture.

The establishment, for example, of a long-term bone marrow culture requires an initial 3 week period during which the stromal adherent layer develops and before significant new haemopoiesis can be detected. However, an established culture, irradiated sufficiently to kill haemopoiesis will promote new haemopoiesis immediately on reseeding with fresh marrow (Schofield and Dexter, 1985).

In 1978, Schofield proposed the existence of a stem cell niche in which a self-renewing stem cell is protected from the pressures of commitment and differentiation. It seems no coincidence, therefore, that the best quality stem cells (CFU-S with the highest self-renewal probability) are found within the matrix of the adherent stromal layer (Dexter, 1979) and it appears likely that this adherent layer is equivalent to comparable structures *in situ* in the bones as described by Weiss (1976). It is probably no coincidence either, that the cells making up this microenvironment, which includes macrophages, fibroblastoid and endothelial cells are also the cell types which produce the variety of colony stimulating factors (CSFs) or growth factors (GFs) required for the recognition *in vitro* of haemopoietic progenitor cells. From a study on the effects of these growth factors, singly and in combination, on purified populations of CFU-S (Heyworth *et al*, 1988) it became clear that the nature of the response is more dependent on the external signals rather than on stochastic processes operating independently within the cells themselves (Dexter, 1989). Furthermore, in an excellent review on the microenvironment, Zippori (1988) came to the conclusion that "the spatial positioning of stem cells and progenitors relative to stromal tissues determines their response to growth and differentiation signals".

Spatial Distribution of the Microenvironmental Stroma

Assays for factor producing cells which, in the main, are produced by more than one cell type, are more problematic, making assessment of the distribution less definitive. Only the fibroblastoid cells can be assayed as a colony forming unit (CFU-f) and thus, Xu and Hendry (1981) using the same technique as for haemopoietic cells were able to define a specific distribution. This distribution, confirmed later by Yang et al (1984) has its highest concentration in the center of the bone spaces, coincident with the more primitive stem cells and lending support for the idea that the CFU-f may be an integral part of the stem cell niche.

The only other distribution we have been able to investigate are those for a CFU-S proliferation inhibitor (Lord et al, 1976) and stimulator (Lord et al, 1977) both of which are products of macrophage subpopulations (Wright et al, 1980), 1982; Simmons and Lord, 1985). In these cases, the reverse approach was made, assaying the distribution of factor producing capacity. Inhibitor production, like the CFU-f, was most concentrated in the axial zone associating it also, as a possible niche component, with the low proliferative activity of the primitive CFU-S while stimulator production was largely restricted to the subendosteal zones, associating it with the less primitive and more rapidly proliferating, maturer CFU-S (Lord and Wright, 1984). The microenvironment is, therefore, also continously distributed across the marrow space, rather than existing as a collection of microenvironmental units spread randomly about that space.

By defining the distributions of in vitro colony-forming cells which respond to the specific purified growth factors (our preliminary results suggest that different populations can be resolved - Testa and Lord, unpublished observations) and also by measuring the responses of haemopoietic tissue to those specified growth factors it should be possible, therefore, to define variations in the microenvironment.

The first step in this direction came when Chan and Metcalf (1972) found that flushed bone conditioned medium is a richer source of CSA than is whole bone marrow conditioned medium. It was then too early to say which or what combination of the growth factors this bone conditioned medium contained, but it did serve to illustrate the non-uniform distribution of CSF production by non-haemopoietic cells.

We have now embarked on a study of the effects of the pure growth factors on the kinetics of haemopoiesis in humans and mice. From these studies, it may be possible to use a responsive population to get further insight into the microarchitecture of the stromal microenvironment.

Effect of rh-CSF on Human Myelopoiesis

These studies were carried out as part of a clinical trial program using rhG-CSF to ameliorate the granulocytopenia caused by chemotherapy. Earlier studies had shown that continuous infusion of G-CSF elicits a rapid influx of mature neutrophils into the peripheral blood within 2-8 hrs, rising 10 fold over the normal level (Bronchud et al, 1988). Furthermore, this elevated level is maintained as long as the G-CSF infusion is continued. The proportion of cycling haemopoietic progenitors is only slightly raised and although the overall myeloid/erythroid ratio is significantly increased, the ratio of GM-CFC to BFU-E is unchanged. They concluded therefore that most of the expansion in cell numbers probably occurs after the GM-CFC stage.

We (Lord et al, 1989) have extended these observations to an auto-radiographic study of the maturing granulocytic cells in two patients with metastatic breast cancer (the patients informed consent and approval by the South Manchester Ethical Committee were obtained). The protocol of treatment is shown in Figure 1.

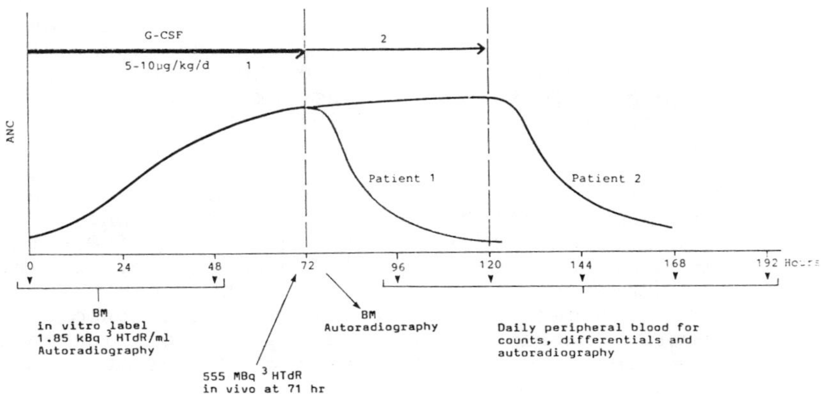

Figure 1: Diagrammatic change in peripheral neutrophil counts (ANC) with continous infusion of G-CSF to patients 1 and 2. Bone marrow samples were taken at 0 and 48 hrs for _in vitro_ ^{3}HTdR labelling and at 72 hrs - 1 hr after _in vivo_ labelling with ^{3}HTdR. Daily peripheral blood was collected from d.4. Cytospin preparations of bone marrow and blood were prepared for autoradiographic analysis.

(a). Peripheral Blood

Figure 2 confirms the original observations on the appearance and loss of mature neutrophils relative to G-CSF treatment. Following ^{3}HTdR _in vivo_, labelled cells were maximal by 24 hrs and have all disappeared by 2 to 3 d after stopping G-CSF with half clearance times of 11.1 and 5.7 hrs for the two patients respectively. These compare well with a normal value of about 8 hours (Vincent, 1977). The kinetics of neutrophil influx were independent of the continued G-CSF treatment since the wave of labelled cells (Figure 3) was the same for both patients.

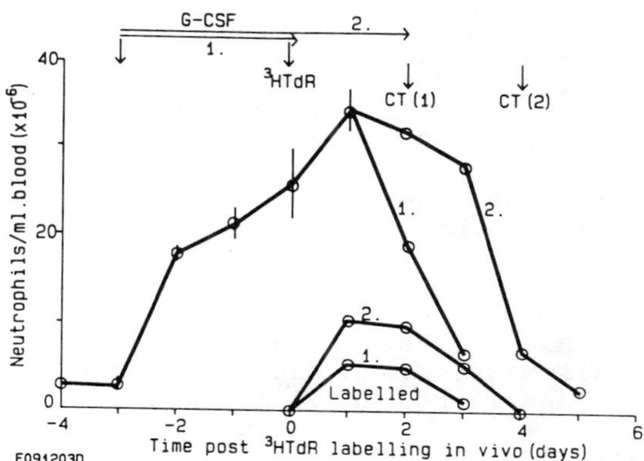

Figure 2: G-CSF induced neutrophilia and emergence of labelled cells after injection of ^{3}HTdR in patients 1 and 2. Arrows indicate times of injection of ^{3}HdR and start of subsequent chemotherapy (CT) cycles.

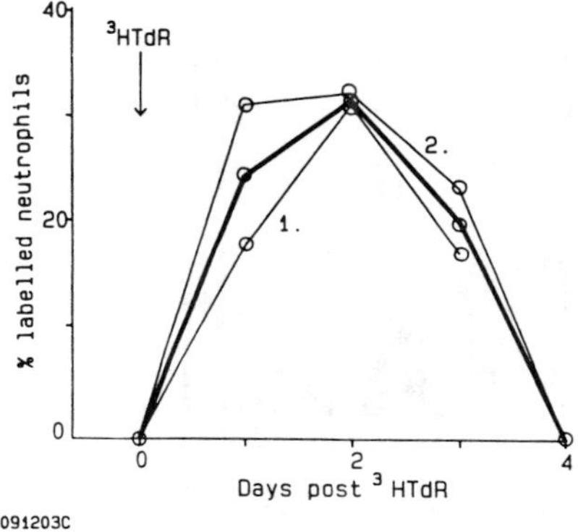

Figure 3: Emergence of labelled neutrophils in pheripheral blood of G-CSF treated patients 1 and 2 following injection of ^{3}HTdR. The heavy line is the mean of the individual patients.

From the calculated half lives, assays of neutrophil function (Bronchud et al, 1988) and sequestration studies using 99Tc^m labelling (Lord et al, 1989), the peripheral neutrophils appear normal in all respects. It is possible, then, using the calculated half-life to correct for the apparent rate of production and to compare this with the normal rate. Thus, from Figure 2, taking the 24 hr increase from the time of labelling and correcting it for loss, a production rate of 31 x 10^6 cells/ml/d is obtained. In the normal steady state, the comparable figure is 3.25 x 10^6 cells/ml/d so that the net production amplification is 9.54 times normal which is equivalent to 3.25 extra cell cycles in the bone marrow.

It is worthwhile pointing out that this is a very modest demand on the proliferative capacity of bone marrow and the thought that G-CSF-stimulated granulopoiesis might drain the stem and progenitor populations is probably unfounded.

(b) Bone Marrow

Differential bone marrow labelling is shown in Figure 4, averaged for both patients. Overall, there was an increase in granulocytic cells at the expense of erythroid cells as with earlier patients (Bronchud _et al_, 1988). The myeloblast and promyelocyte labelling indices for

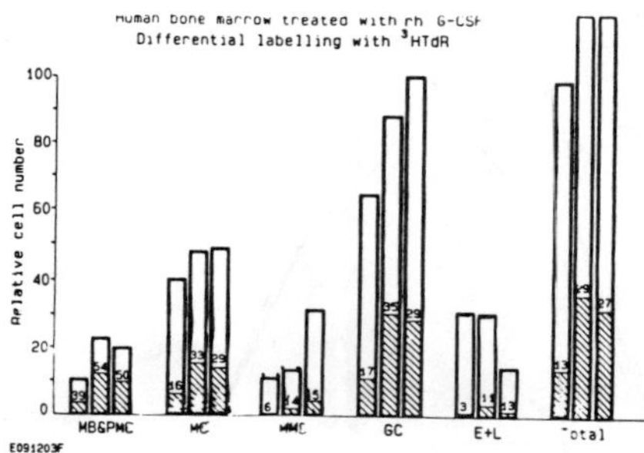

Figure 4: The first and second columns are for 0 and 48 hrs _in vitro_ ^{3}HTdR labelling and the third column for _in vivo_ labelling. Shaded areas represent total labelled cells and the numbers are the precent labelled. MB + PMC = myeloblasts + promyelocytes; MC = myelocytes; MMC = metamyelocytes; GC = total granulocytic; E + L = erythroid + lymphoid cells.

all stages of granulocytic cells were increased 50 to 100% and grain counts were approximately doubled (Figure 4 and Table 1). Elevated autoradiographic indices indicate increased proliferative activity but the increased myeloblast compartment size without subsequent increase in myelocyte numbers suggests that, in addition to increased rate of proliferation, the net maturation time is also proportionately reduced, thus accounting for the early appearance of mature neutrophils in the peripheral blood. Table 1 shows the relative overall cycle times of the proliferating granulocytic cells assuming a normal DNA synthesis time of 13 hrs (Stryckmans et al, 1966). The reduction in average cycle time to about one third of its normal duration represents a very significantly elevated production rate which, coupled with a shortened transit time, rapidly generates large numbers of neutrophils.

The doubling of the myeloblast + promyelocyte compartment, together with the small increase in proliferative activity of GM-CFC (Bronchud et al, 1988 probably indicates that one of the extra 3 divisions occurs before the myeloblast stage while the increased labelling in the metamyelocyte compartment suggests that another occurs late in the maturation program. Thus, G-CSF appears to extend the range of proliferative activity. Taken with the poor direct colony stimulating activity of G-CSF, however, the range of action of G-CSF would appear to be limited mainly to the maturation stages.

The location of this range of cells can clearly be defined in the distributions as residing between the peak of in vitro colony-forming cells and the central venous sinus. Since in long-term cultures it is difficult to detect any G-CSF, it is considered that it exerts its effect at a local level as a product of the local environment (Dexter, 1989). It is tempting, therefore, to speculate that in situ the appropriate G-CSF producing cells will be similarly located. The increasing concentration of in vitro colony-forming cells in the subendosteal marrow would similarly mitigate against G-CSF production in those regions.

Mouse Studies

A comparable series of studies was carried out using rhG-CSF, rmGM-CSF and rmIL-3, injected repeatedly over 4 d into mice. In vivo ^{3}HTdR labelling studies on the marrow and subsequently on the blood were carried out in each case. The data for these experiments will be published elsewhere (with G. Molineux) but in essence, G-CSF produces the same reaction as in humans. The maximum neutrophil count was 14 times the control level substantiating previous work in mice and primates (Moore and Warren, 1987; Welte et al, 1987a, 1987b; Fujisawa et al, 1986; Podja et al, 1989) and their peripheral half-life was about 10 hrs. As in humans, the blood labelling data showed that cells were emerging in the circulation more quickly than normal, peaking by 24 hrs instead of emerging slowly over about 5 days. From the production and loss rates, an amplification factor of 13.3 compared to normal was calculated for G-CSF treated mice; equivalent to 3.7 extra cell cycles (cf. 3.25 in humans) during neutrophil development.

In the marrow, assuming a DNA synthesis phase of 5 hrs (Maloney et al, 1962) the increased labelling indices and grain counts suggested cell cycle time reductions from 10.4 to 7.2 hrs for myeloblasts and promyelocytes and from 27.8 to 13.2 hrs for myelocytes (19.1 to 10.9 hrs average for proliferative granulocytic cells). Erythropoiesis was almost completely suppressed, the G : E ration increasing from 3 to 46.

By contrast, GM-CSF and IL-3 had relatively little effect in mice (for IL-3 see also Lord et al, 1986). Maximum neutrophil counts were less than twice normal and their release was advanced by less than one day. There was little effect on bone marrow labelling or transit though IL-3 stimulated erythroid cell proliferation slightly. G : E ratios were 3.5 and 4.3 respectively, increased only a small amount over the control level of 3.0. The results for GM-CSF appear somewhat at odds with human experience. Anglietta et al (1989) reported a three-fold increase in neutrophils, that both granulocytic and erythroid progenitors are stimulated but that of the maturation lineages, only granulocytic cells are the target, these cells exhibiting shortened DNA-S phases and cell cycle times.

The human/mouse discrepancy is so far unexplained but taking the human comparisons, the production of GM-CSF, with its effect on the progenitor compartments, might be expected primarily to coincide spatially with the growing population of GM-CFC in the regions close to the bone. A minor structural difference between human and mouse may limit its production to this region in the latter thus accounting for its lack of effect on the maturing granulocytic cells in mice.

IL-3 is more problematical. Although it clearly stimulates a wide variety of cells, over a wide range of maturity *in vitro*, it has not been detected as a circulating molecule (Dexter, 1989) nor is there any evidence for a role in bone marrow stromal cell-mediated blood cell production (Whetton and Dexter, 1989). Its physiological role is therefore still in some doubt.

Conclusion

Haemopoietic tissue, like all other tissues in the body is well structured and regulated. Cell lineages conform to specific spatial distributions and there is evidence from direct measurement and from the requirements of a long-term culture system that an equally well structured microenvironment is required for proper functioning of the tissue, probably by the direct action of locally produced growth regulatory factors. A knowledge of the specific cell types affected by defined growth factors may tentatively be used to define better the function and localization of the microenvironment. For example, the proliferation stimulating effects of G-CSF, limited primarily to the maturing granulocytic cells which are located distant from the bone, may well indicate a lack of G-CSF producing cells in the close vicinity of bone surfaces.

Acknowledgements

rhG-CSF was kindly supplied by AMGEM. rmIL-3 and rmGM-CSF was kindly supplied by BIOGEN. This work was supported by grants from the Cancer Research Campaign.

TABLE 1: CELL CYCLE PARAMETERS OF PROLIFERATING GRANULOCYTIC CELLS

[1]Time of Labelling (hrs)	Percent Labelled Cells	Mean Grains Per Labelled Cell	DNA Synthesis Time, ts (hrs)	Cell cycle Time tc (hrs)
0	21	49	13	61.9
48	39	92	[2]7.2	18.5
71	35	[3]92	7.2	20.6

1. Relative to start of rhG-CSF infusion.

2. Calculated in proportion to increase in grain count.

3. Normalized for difference in labelling intensities: in vitro (48 hr) vs in vivo (71 hr) labelling.

References

Weinbeck, J. (1938). Die Granulopese des Kindlichen Knockenmarkes und ihre Reaktion auf Infectione. Beit. z. Path. Anat. Alg. Path. 101, 268-283.

van Dyke, D.C. (1968). Distribution of spleen colony forming units in bone marrow. In: Biology & Medicine, Donner Laboratory, UCRC-18793. Berkeley, U.C., p. 38.

Lambertsen, R.H. and Weiss, L. (1984). A model of intramedullary hematopoietic microenvironments based on stereologic study of the distribution of endocloned marrow colonies. Blood 63, 287-297.

Shackney, S.E., Ford S.S. and Whitting, A.B. (1975). Kinetic microarchitectural correlations in bone marrow of the mouse. Cell Tissue Kinet. 8, 505-516.

Shackney, S.E., Bunn P.A. and Ford S.S. (1976). The effects of colcemid on the mouse bone marrow. Cell Tissue Kinet. 9, 363-369.

Lord, B.I. and Hendry J.H. (1972). The distribution of haemopoeitic colony-forming units in the mouse femur and its modification by X-rays. Brit. J. Radiol. 45, 110-115.

Lord, B.I., Testa, N.G. and Hendry, J.H. (1975). The relative spatial distributions of CFU-S and CFU-C in the normal mouse femur. Blood 46, 65-72.

Gong, J.F. (1978). Endosteal marrow: a rich source of hematopoietic stem cells. Science 199, 1443-1445.

Mason, T.M., Lord, B.I. and Hendry, J.H. (1989). The development of spatial distributions of CFU-S and *in vitro* CFC in femora of mice of different ages. Brit. J. Hematol. 73, In press.

Frassoni, F., Testa, N.G. and Lord, B.I. (1982). The relative spatial distributions of erythroid progenitor cells (BFU-E and CFU-E) in the normal mouse femur. Cell Tissue Kinet. 15, 447-455.

Lord, B.I. (1978). Cellular and architectural factors influencing the proliferation of hematopoietic stem cells. In: Differentiation of Normal and Neoplastic Hematopoietic Cells. Eds. Clarkson, B., Marks, P.A. and Till, J.E. Cold Spring Harbor Laboratory 5, 775-788.

Lord, B.I. and Schofield, R. (1980). Some observations on the kinetics of haemopoietic stem cells and their relationship to the spatial cellular organization of the tissue. In: Biological Growth and Spread. Eds. Jager, W., Rost, H. and Tautu, P. Lecture Notes in Biomaths. 38, 9-22.

Testa, N.G., Hendry, J.H. and Molineux, G. (1985). Long-term marrow damage in experimental systems and in patients after radiation or chemotherapy. Anticancer Res. 5, 101-110.

Wolf, N.S. and Trentin, J.J. (1966). Fate of hemopoietic colony forming units present in intravenously injected suspensions of bone marrow. Fed. Proc. 26, 746.

Wolf, N.S. and Trentin, J.J. (1968). Hemopoietic colony studies vs. effects of hemopoietic organ stroma on differentiation of pluripotent stem cells. J. Exp. Med. 127, 205-214.

Trentin, J.J. (1970). Influence of hematopoietic organ stroma (hematopoietic inductive microenvironments) on stem cell differentiation. In: Regulation of Hematopoiesis. Vol. 1. Ed. Gordon, A.S., pp. 161-186, New York, Meredith.

Dexter, T.M., Allen T.D., Lajtha, L.G., Schofield, R. and Lord, B.I. (1973). Stimulation of differentiation and proliferation of haemopoietic cells *in vitro.* J. Cell Physiol. 82, 461-474.

Dexter, T.M., Allen T.D. and Lajtha, L.G. (1977). Conditions controlling the proliferation of haemopoeitic stem cells *in vitro*. J. Cell Physiol. 91, 355-344.

Allen, T.D. and Dexter, T.M. (1983). Long-term bone marrow cultures: an ultrastructural review. Scanning Elect. Microsc. 4, 1851-1866.

Schofield, R. and Dexter, T.M. (1985). Studies on the self-renewal ability of CFU-S which have been serially transfered in long-term culture or in vivo. Leuk. Res. 9, 305-313.

Schofield, R. (1978). The relationship between the spleen colony forming cell and the haemopoietic stem cell. Blood Cells 4, 7-25.

Dexter, T.M. (1979). Cell interactions in vitro. In: Cellular Dynamics of Haemopoiesis. Ed. Lajtha, L.G., 8, 453-468. W.B. Saunders Co. Ltd., London, Philadelphia, Toronto.

Weiss, L. (1976). The hemopoietic microenvironment of the bone marrow: an ultrastructural study of the stroma in rats. Anat. Rec. 186, 161-184.

Heyworth, C.M., Pointing, I.L.O. and Dexter, T.M. (1988). the response of haemopoietic cells to growth factors: developmental implication of synergistic interactions. J Cell Sci. 91, 239-247.

Dexter, T.M. (1989). Regulation of hemopoietic cell growth and development: Experimental and clinical studies. Leukemia 3, 469-474.

Zippori, D. (1988). Hemopoietic microenvironments. In: Hematopoiesis: Long-term Effects of Chemotherapy and Radiation. Eds. Testa, N.G. and Gale, R.P., pp 27-62, Marcel Dekker Inc., New York.

Xu, C.X. and Hendry, J.H. (1981). The radial distribution of fibroblastic colony-forming cells in the mouse femoral marrow. Biomed. Exp. 353, 119-122.

Yang, E.D., Rooney, P. and Wright, E.G. (1984). The radial distribution of fibroblastic colony-forming cells in mouse femoral marrow. IRCS Med. Sci. 12, 1141-1142.

Lord, B.I., Mori, K.J., Wright, E.G. and Lajtha, L.G. (1976). An inhibitor of stem cell proliferation in regenerating bone marrow. Biomed. Exp. 27, 223-226.

Lord, B.I., Mori, K.J. and Wright, E.G. (1977). A stimulator of stem cell proliferation in regenerating bone marrow. Biomed. Exp. 27, 223-226.

Wright, E.G., Garland, J.M. and Lord, B.I. (1980). Specific inhibition of haemopoetic stem cell proliferation: Characteristics of the stimulator producing cells. Leuk. Res. 6, 531-539.

Simmons, P.J. and Lord, B.I. (1985). Enrichment of CFU-S proliferation inhibitor-producing cells based on their identification by the monoclonal antibody F4/80. J Cell Sci. 78, 117-131.

Lord, B.I. and Wright, E.G. (1984). Spatial organization of CFU-S proliferation regulators in the mouse femur. Leuk Res. 8, 1073-1083.

Chan, S.H. and Metcalf, D. (1972). Local production of colony stimulating factor within the bone marrow: Role of non-hematopoietic cells. Blood 40, 646-653.

Bronchud, M.H., Potter, M.R., Morgenstern, G., Blasco, M.J., Scarffe, J.H., Thatcher, N., Crowther, D., Souza, L.M. Alton, N.K., Testa, effects of recombinant human granulocyte colony-stimulating factor in patients. Brit. J. Cancer 58, 64-69.

Lord, B.I., Bronchud, M.H., Owens ,S., Chang, J., Howell, A., Souza, L. and Dexter, T.M. (1989). The kinetics of human granulopoiesis following treatment with G-CSF *in vivo*. Proc. Acad. Sci. USA. In press.

Vincent, P.C. (1977). Granulocyte kinetics in health and disease. Clinical Haemat. 6, 695-717. W.B. Saunders Co. Ltd., London.

Stryckmans, P., Cronkite, E.P., Fache, F., Fliedner, T.M. and Ramos, J. (1966). Deoxyribonucleic acid synthesis time of erythropoietic and granulopoietic cells in human beings. Nature (Lond.) 211, 717-720.

Moore, M.A.S. and Warren, D.J. (1987). Synergy of interleukin 1 and granulocyte colony-stimulating factor: *In vivo* stimulation of stem cell recovery and hemopoietic regeneration following 5-fluorouracil treatment of mice. Proc. Natl. Acad. Sci. USA 84, 7134-7138.

Welte, K., Bonilla, M.A., Gabrilove, J.L., Gillio, A.P., Potter, G.K., Moore, M.A.S., O'Reilly, R.S., Boone, T.C. and Souza, L.M. (1987a). Recombinant human granulocyte colony stimulating factor: In vitro and in vivo effects on myelopoiesis. Blood Cells 13, 17.

Welte, K., Bonilla, M.A., Gillio, A., O'Reilly, R.J., Gabrilove, J.L., Potter, G., Boone, T. and Souza, L.M. (1987b). In vivo effects of recombinant human G-CSF in therapy induced neutropenias in primates. Exp. Hematol. 15, p. 460.

Fujisawa, M., Kobayashi, Y., Okabe, T., Takaku, F., Komatsu, Y. and Itoh, S. (1986). Recombinant human granulocyte colony stimulating factor induces granulocytosis in vivo. Jpn J. Canc. Res. 77, 866.

Pojda, Z., Molineux, G. and Dexter, T.M. (1989). Hemopoietic effects of short-term in vivo treatment of mice with various doses of rhG-CSF. Exp. Hematol. 17, In press.

Maloney, M.A., Patt, H.M. and Weber, C.L. (1962). Estimation of DNA synthetic period for myelocytes in dog bone marrow. Nature 193, 134.

Lord, B.I., Molineux, G., Testa, N.G., Kelly, M., Spooncer, E. and Dexter, T.M. (1986). The kinetic response of haemopoietic precursor cells, in vivo, to highly purified, recombinant interleukin 3. Lymphokine Res. 5, 97-104.

Aglietta, M., Piacibello, W., Sanavio F., Stacchini, A., Apra, F., Schena, M., Moscetti, C., Carnino, F., Caligaris-Cappio, F. and Gavosto, F. (1989). Kinetics of human granulocyte macrophage colony-stimulating factor. J. Clin. Invest. 83 551-557.

Whetton, A.D., and Dexter, T.M. (1989). Myeloid haemopoietic growth factors. Biochim. Biophys. Acta. In press.

The Biology of Hematopoiesis, pages 409–416

TERMINAL TRANSFERASE AS A THERAPEUTIC TARGET IN LEUKEMIA CELLS

Ronald McCaffrey, Robert Duff, Kyran Bulger, Zachary Spigelman, Karl Flora, Raymond Schinazi, and C.K. Chu

Boston University Medical Center (R.M., R.D., K.B., Z.S.), National Cancer Institute (K.F.), Emory University(R.S.), and University of Georgia(C.K.C.)

INTRODUCTION

Terminal deoxynucleotidyl transferase (TdT, EC2.7.7.31) is an unusual enzyme which catalyzes the polymerization of deoxyribonucleotides on the 3'-hydroxyl ends of preformed oligo- or polydeoxynucleotide initiators, in a template-independent manner (McCaffrey et al., 1973). Its expression is restricted, in normal animals, to pre-B and pre-T cells in bone marrow and thymus. In disease states TdT expression is found in a variety of hematopoietic neoplasms. It is found in the blast cells of almost all adults and children with acute lymphoblastic leukemia; in essentially all cases of diffuse lymphoblastic lymphoma; in lymphoblastic blast-crisis of chronic myelogenous leukemia; and, in a subset of patients with multiple myeloma, TdT is found in the neoplastic cells from which the immunoglobulin producing cells arise (McCaffrey et al., 1981; Grogan et al., 1987).

The precise function which this enzyme plays in the cells in which it is expressed is unknown. Whatever that function (or functions) may be, we now have a considerable body of preliminary data which suggests that its role is in some way critical to the viability of the cells in which it is found, in that perturbation of the function of TdT appears to constitute a lethal event for such cells. Our data, which we summarize here, show that the anti-viral dideoxynucleosides are recognized as substrate analogues by TdT and are, as a consequence, cytotoxic for TdT-positive cells. These observations have prompted us to consider TdT as a novel therapeutic target in neoplastic lymphoid cells, and to suggest that the compounds which we have so far studied may be prototypes for potentially new, specific therapeutic agents for the management of those lymphoblastic malignancies which express this unique DNA synthetic enzyme.

DIDEOXYNUCLEOSIDES

Our interest in the dideoxynucleosides (ddNs) as agents capable of perturbing the function of TdT had its intellectual origin in their use as anti-retroviral agents in HIV-infected states. DdNs lack the 3'-OH group present on normal 2'-deoxyribonucleosides. Retroviral DNA polymerase (reverse transcriptase) utilizes the ddN triphosphates (ddNTPs) as substrates. Following incorporation of ddNMP residues, further chain elongation is impossible due to the absence of the 3'-OH group required to form the next 5'->3' phosphodiester bond. Through this process of chain termination, proviral DNA synthesis is prevented, thus inhibiting retroviral proliferation(Mitsuya and Broder, 1987).

TdT also recognizes the ddNTPs as substrate analogs. As with reverse transcriptase, the addition of ddNMP residues to nascent DNA by TdT results in chain termination. In contrast, DNA polymerase alpha, the major replicative polymerase of mammalian cells, does not recognize ddNTPs as substrates. Because of this lack of recognition of ddNTPs by DNA polymerase alpha, we exposed a series of TdT-positive and TdT-negative cell lines to a representative ddN, dideoxyadenosine (ddA), to determine the effects of additions of ddAMP to genomic DNA by TdT. In these cellular studies non-phosphorylated ddA was used to allow transport across cytoplasmic cell membranes. Anabolic intracellular conversion from ddA to ddATP provides a chain-terminating substrate recognized by TdT. Our data showed that ddA was specifically cytotoxic for multiple TdT-positive cell lines, and was especially so in the co-presence of corformycin, which protected the ddA from deamination by adenosine deaminase. (Corformycin alone, at the concentrations we used, had no cytotoxic effects). At 48 hours, continuous exposure to 250uM ddA, preceded by a 30 minute exposure to 30uM Corformycin, resulted in cell death (as defined by trypan blue dye exclusion) which ranged from 85%-95% for 7 human TdT-positive cell lines. Likewise, when we exposed fresh, TdT-positive leukemic blast cells from patients with acute lymphoblastic leukemia to ddA _ex vivo_, significant cytotoxicity was noted at 72 hours. In contrast, blast cells from patients with TdT-negative acute leukemia were not affected by ddA exposure under identical _ex vivo_ conditions. For six TdT-positive ALL samples cell death ranged from 80%-88% (by trypan blue). For six TdT-negative ANLL samples viability ranged from 91%-100% at 72 hours (Spigelman et al.,1988).

To establish that TdT was the central determinant of the ddN cytotoxicity we were seeing, we added ddA to a normally TdT-negative murine cell line, PD-31, after it had been rendered TdT-positive by a DOL retroviral expression vector containing TdT cDNA. The parental, TdT-negative PD-31 cells were insensitive to the ddA. However, the PD-31 cells rendered TdT-positive by the DOL vector showed 90% cell death at 48 hrs. in the presence of ddA. To establish that _enzymatic_ TdT activity was critically related to the toxicity we observed with ddA, we also studied a PD-31 cell line infected with a DOL vector containing a TdT cDNA with several point mutations so that an enzymatically inactive TdT was expressed. In this PD-31 line there was no increased sensitivity to ddA (Spigelman et al.,1988).

These experiments suggest that TdT *per se* plays a central role in the ddA cytotoxicity we observe and is not simply a marker for cells that are sensitive on some other basis. For example, lymphoid cells in general, and T cells in particular, are known to be sensitive to killing by adenosine and deoxyadenosine. The mechanisms responsible for this "purine cytotoxicity" are poorly understood. Although ddA cytotoxicity theoretically may be a variant of the purine cytotoxicity produced by adenosine and deoxyadenosine, it should be emphasized that adenosine and deoxyadenosine can produce purine cytotoxicity in TdT-negative, mature lymphoid cells (Kefford and Fox, 1982). As we show, ddA cytotoxicity is confined to TdT-positive lymphoid cells, making it unlikely that it is mechanistically related to conventional purine cytotoxicity.

DIDEOXYADENOSINE DERIVATIVES

The concentrations of ddA required for cytotoxic damage to TdT-positive leukemia cells *ex vivo* (250 uM for 48 hours) would likely exceed the range of what would be clinically tolerable. Based on our current experience with ddNs in HIV-infected individuals, clinically relevant ddN dosage in neoplastic disease will need to be in the 1-10 uM range. Hence we continue to seek a ddN derivative with cytotoxic activity in this range.

To date we have studied modifications of ddA in the 2-position and the 6-position. Substitutions at either position have major effects on both the substrate recognition and biologic properties of ddA. A halogen in the 2-position (2-chloro-ddA) results in continued recognitions by TdT (Ki < 2uM, Figure 1), whereas a substitution in the 6-position (6-n-methyl-ddA) results in loss of substrate analogue properties (Ki > 500uM, Figure 1).

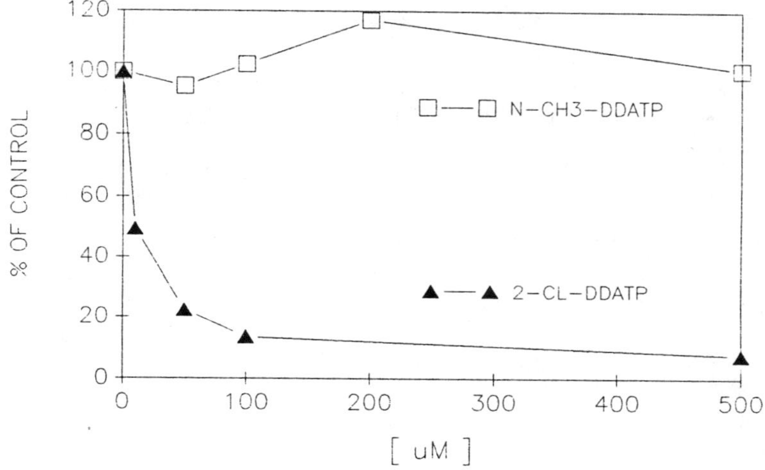

FIGURE 1. Comparison of 2-chloro-ddA and 6-N-Methyl-ddA as substrate analogues for TdT, assayed as previously described (McCaffrey, et al 1981).

These substrate recognition properties are mirrored by the results of cellular experiments. The 6-N-methyl-ddA, which is not recognized by TdT, is not cytotoxic, at concentrations up to 500uM, for TdT-positive cells. In contrast, the 2-chloro-ddA derivative, which is recognized as a substrate by TdT, has enhanced cytotoxicity for TdT-positive cells. As summarized in Table 1 below, at 72 hours, 2 chloro-ddA is cytotoxic for almost all TdT-positive cell lines tested, at concentrations between 5uM-10uM. TdT-negative cell lines are largely unaffected. Adenosine deaminase does not recognize 2-chloro-ddA (Ki>500uM), thus there is no requirement for coformycin in these experiments. Further structural modifications of ddA, particularly at the 2-position, should enhance its cytotoxicity for TdT-positive cells beyond what we show here.

TABLE 1

EFFECT OF 2-CHLORO-ddA ON
TDT(+) AND TdT(-) CELL LINES

CELL LINES	TdT STATUS	% INHIBITION 5uM	10uM
SUP-B#2	+	70	89
SUP-T#3	+	34	67
SUP-T#1	+	63	92
NALM-6	+	16	13
MOLT-4	+	20	45
298-26	+	17	64
B-244	+	11	44
L-1210	-	0	6
U-937	-	10	54
K-562	-	5	14
EL-4	-	0	5
702	-	0	10

Effect of a 72 hour exposure to 2-chloro-ddA on various TdT-positive and TdT-negative cell lines in culture. Growth inhibition was defined as the ratio of viable cells in the durg-exposed cultures to control cultures. Each determination reflects the mean of triplicate or quadruplicate flasks from a single experiment representative of at least three independent experiments.

CONCLUSIONS

Although the precise cellular function(s) of TdT remain to be established, our data suggest a critical role for it in maintaining the viability of the cells in which it is transiently expressed. The perturbation of its activity by dideoxyadenosine results in specific cytotoxic damage in TdT-positive cells. The basis for this cytotoxic damage remains to be established, but very likely involves DNA fragmentation following chain-terminating additions of ddAMP residues to genomic DNA by TdT. Substituted ddA derivatives, which are cytotoxic at the 5-10uM Range may represent a departure point for the development of novel therapeutic agents in TdT-positive neoplasia. Murine disease model studies are now in progress.

The significance of TdT as a novel therapeutic target deserves comment. Based on the data we have presented, it is very likely that the agents we identify as cytotoxic for TdT-positive cells will not distinguish between TdT-positive neoplastic cells and TdT-positive normal cells. Thus, the clinical application of TdT-specific cytotoxic agents will very likely eliminate TdT-positive normal pre-B and pre-T cell populations while eliminating neoplastic TdT-positive cells. We would envision, however, such a depletion of normal pre-B and pre-T cell compartments to be transient in nature, since the "feeder population" for bone marrow pre-B and pre-T cells is TdT-negative. Thus, repopulation of those normal TdT-positive marrow compartments, from the TdT-negative precursor compartment, would be the expected outcome. We therefore expect the clinical use of agents specifically cytotoxic for TdT-positive cells will produce a only self-limited, transient depletion of normal TdT-positive cell populations. These normal TdT-positive populations will be renewed from their TdT-negative precursor compartments which will have suffered no cytotoxic damage from these agents. We look forward to experiments aimed at verifying this hypothesis over the next several months.

REFERENCES

Grogan TM, Durie BG, Lomen C, Spier C, Wirt DP, Nagle R, Wilson GS, Richter L, Vela E, Maxev V,et al(1987). Delineation of a novel pre-B cell component in plasma cell myeloma:immunochemical,immunophenotypic, genotypic, cytologic, cell culture, and kinetic features, Blood 70:932-42.

Kefford RF, Fox RM (1982). Purine deoxynucleside toxicity in nondividing human lymphoid cells. Cancer Res 42:324.

McCaffrey, RP, Smoler DF, and Baltimore D (1973). Terminal deoxynucleotidyl transferase in case of childhood acute lymphoblastic leukemia. Proc Natl Acad Sci USA 70:521-525.

McCaffrey RP, Lillquist A, Sallan S, Cohen E, and Osband M (1981). The clinical utility of leukemia cell terminal transferase measurements. Cancer Research 41:481-482.

Mitsuya H, Broder S (1987). Strategies for antiviral therapies in AIDS. Nature 325:773.

Spigelman Z, Duff, R Beardsley GP, Broder S, Cooney D, Landau NR, Mitsuya H, Ullman B, McCaffrey RP (1988). 2',3'-Dideoxyadenosine is selecitvely toxic for TdT-positive cells. Blood 71:1601-1608

The Biology of Hematopoiesis, pages 417–422

DEVELOPMENTAL REGULATION OF NORMAL AND LEUKEMIC HUMAN B CELL PRECURSORS

Tucker W. LeBien

Department of Laboratory Medicine and Pathology, University of Minnesota Medical School, Minneapolis, MN 55455

Acute lymphoblastic leukemia (ALL) strikes 2-3/100,000 children/year in western countries (Linet, 1985). Fortunately, treatment of pediatric ALL is one of the more dramatic success stories in oncology. Not withstanding this success, it is still painfully clear that we have few clues regarding the etiology of this disease. Greaves has recently developed a hypothesis that implicates the enzymatic machinery (i.e., recombinase(s), terminal deoxynucleotidyl transferase) involved in immunoglobulin (Ig) and T cell receptor (TCR) gene rearrangement in the sequential generation of mutations that could culminate in malignant transformation of normal B and T cell precursors into ALL (Greaves, 1988). A simple extension of this hypothesis implicates the accumulated mutations in uncontrolled growth of leukemic cells. Uncontrolled growth in ALL could manifest as autocrine growth factor production, mutation in a growth factor receptor, constitutive growth factor receptor expression, etc. I am currently unaware of published data that definitively implicates any of these potential perturbations in growth regulation in the pathogenesis of ALL.

Monoclonal antibody phenotyping and Southern blotting with Ig and TCR probes clearly indicate that the vast majority (~80%) of pediatric ALL, (historically designated non-T, non-B), are malignant B cell precursors. A large data base supporting this conclusion has been generated in many laboratories (reviewed in Foon and Todd, 1986; Griesser et al., 1989). Although there are phenotypic/genotypic variations that result in considerable heterogeneity, the overwhelming majority (if not all) of B cell precursor ALL express the B cell restricted cell surface molecule CD19, have rearranged Ig heavy chain genes, but do not express surface Ig. This can be viewed as a minimal immunologic definition of B cell precursor ALL. The precise placement of the various B cell precursor ALL phenotypes in a scheme of normal B cell ontogeny is compromised by the difficulty in growing normal B cell precursors in vitro (see below). In order to delineate the perturbations in proliferation or differentiation that contribute to or characterize B cell precursor ALL, it is essential to characterize the patterns of gene expression and growth factor requirements that epitomize normal B cell precursors. The intent of this contribution is to overview some of the recent data on normal, human B cell precursors, with a particular emphasis on recent work from my laboratory.

If B cell precursor ALL manifests a perturbation in growth control, then a thorough analysis of growth control in normal bone marrow B cell precursors is an obvious necessity. Although progress has been made in characterizing B cell precursor surface antigen expression by multiparameter flow cytometry (Ryan et al, 1986; Loken et al, 1987; Kansas and Dailey, 1989; Law et al, 1989; LeBien et al, 1989c), we know very little about the growth factor requirements and differentiative potential of normal human B cell precursors. The major reason for this dearth of information is the absence of short-term or long-term assays for maintaining these cells in vitro (LeBien, 1989a). This is in contrast to the highly successful Whitlock-Witte long-term bone marrow culture that supports the selective growth of murine B cell precursors (Whitlock and Witte, 1982). Whitlock-Witte cultures have been used by numerous investigators, and have been instrumental in unraveling the cells and molecules that regulate B cell development in the mouse. Many laboratories have attempted to establish a human equivalent of the murine Whitlock-Witte culture system, without success. As I have discussed elsewhere (LeBien, 1989a), human bone marrow plated under Whitlock-Witte conditions is characterized by a complete loss of $CD19^+$ B cells by 2-3 weeks, concomitant with a rather florid overgrowth of fibroblasts. We have preliminary data indicating that suppression of fibroblast overgrowth substantially facilitates the survival of CD10$^+$/surface Ig$^-$ and CD10$^+$/surface Ig$^+$ bone marrow-derived B cells for up to 3 weeks in culture (M. Wolf and T LeBien, unpublished observations). We are currently assessing the self-renewal and differentiative capacity of the CD10$^+$/ surface Ig$^-$ cells. A recent report has shown that bone marrow-derived cells with a mature B cell phenotype (CD19$^+$/CD20$^+$/surface Ig$^+$) can be maintained for up to 8 weeks using human long-term bone marrow cultures (Berneman et al., 1989). Interestingly, this long-term culture system was "Dexter-like" containing horse serum, hydrocortisone, and 33° C culture conditions. The inclusion of hydrocortisone is notoriously toxic to most lymphoid cells (Whitlock and Witte, 1982), so that this result is somewhat of a surprise. Continuing development of bone marrow culture systems that support early human B cell development is vital.

We have recently undertaken a series of studies to examine Ig/TCR gene rearrangements and differentiation of normal human B cell precursors, an area in which there is very little published data. Since many B cell precursor ALL express a CD10$^+$/surface Ig$^-$ immunologic phenotype, we purified fetal bone marrow lymphoid cells with this phenotype by cell sorting, and examined their differentiative capacity in vitro. We initially sought to confirm a report which suggested that IL-4 could induce pre-B -> B cell differentiation in fetal bone marrow lymphoid cells (Hofman et al, 1988). Although we failed to observe IL-4-mediated differentiation, a consistent and dramatic increase in surface Ig was observed in CD10$^+$/surface Ig$^-$ cells cultured in tissue culture medium alone (Villablanca et al, 1989). A detailed analysis of this developmental transition revealed that active rearrangement of kappa light chain genes, and expression of surface kappa or lambda light chain proteins was occurring in these cells. Differentiation occurred within 2 days in the absence of exogenous cytokines and growth factors. Growth factor/cytokine-independent normal human pre-B cell differentiation suggests that a stimulus-independent differentiative inertia might characterize these cells in vivo. Our culture system should hasten cellular and molecular studies of this critical transition point in B cell ontogeny, and may facilitate comparative studies of pre-B ALL. The growth factor/cytokine-independent differentiation of normal pre-B cells bears a resemblance to that observed in a leukemic cell line, BLIN-1, recently established in this laboratory (Wörmann et al., 1989). The hallmark characteristic of BLIN-1 is its propensity to undergo spontaneous pre-B -> B cell differentiation, characterized by functional rearrangement and expression of kappa light chain genes. Differentiation cannot be enhanced by several cytokines tested to date, but is enhanced by culturing BLIN-1 cells in low serum, or serum-free medium. The recombinase enzyme(s) and transcriptional factors that mediate rearrangement and expression of kappa light chain genes may be under similar control in normal pre-B cells and the BLIN-1 pre-B ALL cell line. It is also notworthy that murine $B220^+$/surface mu^- cells have recently been reported to spontaneously differentiate in vitro (Simons and Zharhary, 1989).

In a related study we have begun to examine Ig/TCR gene rearrangement in subsets of normal B lineage cells. Little information is available on normal B lineage cells, whereas a vast body of data exists on B lineage ALL (Griesser et al., 1989). $CD10^+$/surface Ig^- fetal bone marrow lymphoid cells purified by cell sorting had a high frequency of Ig heavy chain rearrangements, as one would predict if these cells are at various stages of early B cell development. Surprisingly, analysis of these same cells failed to reveal rearrangement of TCR-γ and TCR-δ genes (LeBien et al., 1989b). This is in sharp contrast to the high frequency of TCR-γ,δ rearrangements present in B lineage ALL (Greenberg et al, 1986; Griesinger et al, 1989), and suggests a potentially significant difference in patterns of gene rearrangement that may distinguish normal and leukemic B cell precursors. This observation needs to be extended using the more sensitive polymerase chain reaction. We ultimately hope to delineate TCR gene rearrangement at the single cell level in normal B cell precursors. This will provide us with a thorough data base on TCR gene rearrangements during normal ontogeny, and facilitate interpretation of TCR gene rearrangement in B cell precursor ALL.

REFERENCES

Berneman ZN, Chen ZZ, van Bockstaele D, Ramael M, Korthout M, Peetermans ME (1989). The nature of the adherent hemopoietic cells in human long-term bone marrow cultures (HLTBMCs): Presence of lymphocytes and plasma cells next to the myelomonocytic population. Leukemia 3:648-661.

Foon KA, Todd RF (1986). Immunologic classification of leukemia and lymphoma. Blood 68:1-32.

Greaves MF (1988). Speculations on the cause of childhood acute lymphoblastic leukemia. Leukemia 2:120-125.

Greenberg JM, Quertermous T, Seidman JG, Kersey JH (1986). Human T cell γ chain gene rearrangements in acute lymphoid and nonlymphoid leukemia. Comparison with the T cell receptor β chain gene. J Immunol 137:2043-2049.

Griesinger F, Greenberg JM, Kersey JH (1989). T cell receptor gamma and delta rearrangements in hematologic malignancies. J Clin Invest 84:506-516.

Griesser H, Tkachuk D, Reis MD, Mak TW (1989). Gene rearrangements and translocations in lymphoproliferative diseases. Blood 73:1402-1415.

Hofman FM, Brock M, Taylor CR, Lyons B (1988). IL-4 regulates differentiation and proliferation of human precursor B cells. J Immunol 141:1185-1190.

Kansas GD, Dailey MO (1989). Expression of adhesion structures during B cell development in man. J Immunol 142:3058-3062.

Law C-L, Wörmann B, LeBien TW (1989). Analysis of expression and function of CD40 on normal and leukemic human B cell precursors. Submitted for publication.

LeBien TW (1989a). Growing human B cell precursors in vitro: the continuing challenge. Immunol Today 10: 296-298.

LeBien TW, Elstrom RL, Kersey JH, Griesinger F (1989b). Analysis of Ig and TCR gene rearrangements in normal human fetal bone marrow (FBM) B lineage cells. Blood 74:abstract (in press).

LeBien TW, Wörmann B, Villablanca JG, Law C-L, Shah VO, Loken MR (1989c). Multiparameter flow cytometric analysis of human fetal bone marrow B cells. Submitted for publication.

Linet MS (1985). "The leukemias: epidemiologic aspects." New York: Oxford University Press.

Loken MR, Shah VO, Dattilio KL, Civin CI (1987). Flow cytometric analysis of human bone marrow: II. Normal B lymphocyte development. Blood 70:1316-1324.

Ryan D, Kossover S, Mitchell S, Frantz C, Hennessy L, Cohen H (1986). Subpopulations of common acute lymphoblastic leukemia antigen-positive lymphoid cells in normal bone marrow identified by hematopoietic differentiation antigens. Blood 68:417-425.

Simons A, Zharhary D (1989). The role of IL-4 in the generation of B lymphocytes in the bone marrow. J Immunol 143:2540-2545.

Villablanca JG, Elstrom RL, Anderson JM, LeBien TW (1989). Differentiation of normal human pre-B cells in vitro. Submitted for publication.

Whitlock CA, Witte ON (1982). Long-term culture of B lymphocytes and their precursors from murine bone marrow. Proc Natl Acad Sci USA 79:3608-3612.

Wörmann B, Anderson JM, Liberty JA, Gajl-Peczalska K, Brunning RD, Silberman TL, Arthur DC, LeBien TW (1989) Establishment of a leukemic cell model for studying human pre-B to B cell differentiation. J Immunol 142:110-117.

The Biology of Hematopoiesis, pages 423–437

SURVIVING HEMATOLOGICAL MALIGNANCIES: STRESS RESPONSES AND PREDICTING PSYCHOLOGICAL ADJUSTMENT

LYNNA M. LESKO, M.D., PH.D.

Psychiatry Service, Department of Neurology

Memorial Sloan-Kettering Cancer Center

INTRODUCTION

Given the advancement of innovative procedures such as bone marrow transplantation and the progress in combination chemotherapy, some patients with hematologic malignancies can expect a lengthened or near normal life span. This improvement in long-term survival has altered the perception of cancer from a uniformly fatal illness in all to a chronic illness for several age groups. This alteration in perception of hematological malignancies has, in turn, changed the role that mental health professionals serve in an oncology setting. Rather than helping family members deal with the inevitable death of the patient, a greater focus is being placed on the long-term psychosocial and mental health needs of this new and growing population of survivors.

However, increased survival may be associated with an increased risk for delayed medical complications, including organ failure, central nervous system dysfunction, sterility, secondary malignancies, and decreased physical stamina. (Meadows, 1985; Meadows, 1986; Byrd 1988). In addition, as a result of the stressors inherent in illness and treatment, survivors can experience prolonged psychological, interpersonal and vocation dysfunction.

Clinical reports and empirical studies have emphasized the following psychosocial sequelae: fears of disease recurrence, diminished self-esteem, preoccupation with death, heightened psychological distress, job-related difficulties, social isolation, and difficulties re-entering school, family and friendship networks (Cella, 1986; Koocher, 1981; Teta, 1986; Wasserman, 1987). In short, cancer and its treatment has been associated with psychosocial disruptions in school, peer, vocational, familial and mental health domains. Paradoxically, having been successfully treated for cancer may also represent a stressful period in the course of the cancer experience.

These psychological findings, though, are primarily from studies that have looked at middle aged adult survivors or adult survivors of childhood cancers. Special attention to adolescent and young adult survivors is needed for a number of crucial reasons. First, healthy adolescents and young adults are normally at increased risk for psychosocial difficulties by virtue of the rapid changes associated with their developmental state. Though most negotiate developmental milestones quite adequately (Offer, 1981), research suggests that if too many stressors occur simultaneously, psychosocial adjustment may be threatened (Peterson, 1982). Thus, when a cancer diagnosis precedes or occurs during this time, the potential for psychosocial dysfunction is increased. Adolescents who have been treated for cancer not only have the substantial physical, cognitive, emotional, and interpersonal tasks faced by all adolescents, but have the added burden of integrating a life-threatening disease into their experiences. Persistent body image concerns, somatic preoccupation, disruptions in heterosexual relationships, and deficits in social competence have all been documented in this age group (Fritz, 1988; Mulhern, 1989). Second, assessment during adolescence young adulthood rather than later adulthood, allows for attention to potential problems that may surface closer to the original stressor of the diagnosis and treatment.

Considering the variability in previous research findings, there is increasing importance in studying the psychosocial functioning of survivors by specific disease site and treatment regimen and developmental/life cycle stage (Cella, 1986; Freidenbergs, 1982; Wellisch, 1984). However, with few exceptions (Fobair, 1986; Cella, 1986; Lesko, 1989) existing studies of the post-treatment psychosocial status including hematologic malignancy patients have generally been conducted with heterogeneous small patient samples (Wolcott, 1986; Andrykowski, 1987; Daiter, 1988). There are suggestions that illness or treatment-related variables, such as time since treatment or stage of disease, may predict the level of psychological distress in survivors and the breadth of functional areas effected (Cella, 1986; Fobair, 1986). In addition, studies thus far, have ignored the specific impact of leukemia on various areas of functioning among survivors as well as the possible differential impact of treatment modality, bone marrow transplantation vs. conventional chemotherapy. Likewise, using measures of psychosocial functioning with established reliability and validity is paramount.

The specific aims of this research are 1) to ascertain the prevalence of psychosocial difficulties among adolescent and young adult cancer survivors; 2) to explore specific vulnerability and resiliency factors that may be associated with off-treatment adjustment and 3) to highlight the pivotal role oncologists can play in promoting the mental health of off-treatment cancer patients.

METHOD

Several studies assessed the quality of life of adolescents and young adults successfully treated for hematological malignancies. Patients were treated with conventional multidrug regimens and 30% of the young adults received an additional allogeneic bone marrow transplantation.

All patients received their cancer treatment at MSKCC and were at least 1 year from termination of treatment. Soicodemographic and disease/treatment characteristics are reported in Figure 1.

Subjects completed several well-validated psychosocial inventories chosen to reflect both positive and negative markers of psychosocial adjustment. Function was assessed (depending on the study) in five general areas: global psychological distress (The Brief Symptom Inventory (Derogatis, 1982), Mental Health Inventory (Veit,1983)), illness-related distress (The Impact of Events Scale (Horowtiz, 1979)), work/social/leisure activities (Social Adjustment Scale (Weissman, 1976) Achenbach Behavior Check List, (Achenbach, 1986)), psychosexual functioning (The Derogatis Sexual

Functioning Inventory (Derogatis, 1975)) and <u>family functioning</u> (Family Adaptability and Cohesion Scale (Olson, Wilson, 1985)).

Variables investigated as possible predictors of adjustment outcome were divided into two major categories: Sociodemographic/patient characteristics and disease and treatment related variables.

RESULTS

a. Global Psychological Distress and Illness-Related Distress

Due to the extensive hospitalization of the transplantation procedure, it was hypothesized that young adult BMT patients would report higher levels of psychosocial distress than those patients who had received conventional chemotherapy only. Multivariate analysis of variance (MANOVA) revealed no significant mean differences between the BMT and CO groups on either the global or illness-specific measures of psychological distress. Data from both treatment groups was then combined to form a combined sample of acute leukemia survivors. It was expected that leukemia survivors would report less psychological distress than psychiatric outpatients and more psychological distress than nonpatients. Tests for mean differences in the Global Severity Index (GSI) revealed significant differences between the combined leukemia survivors and nonpatients $t(787) = 8.8$, $p < .001$ as well as between the leukemia survivors and the psychiatric outpatients, $t(1070) = 2.0$, $p < .05$. In general, leukemia survivors were more psychologically distressed than nonpatients; however, they reported distress levels well below that of psychiatric outpatients.

Degree of illness-related distress in this group was represented by the Avoidant and Intrusive cognition subscales of the Impact of Events Scale (IES). Female leukemia survivors reported significantly less intrusive ($t(84)$ - 3.26, $p < .001$) and avoidant ($t(84) = 2.36$, $p < .01$) cognitions than a comparison sample of female psychiatric outpatients referred for the treatment of stress-related disorders. Male leukemia survivors also reported significantly less intrusive cognitions ($t(48) = 3.41$, $p < .001$) than the male stress-related disorder outpatients; however, there were no differences in the level of avoidant cognitions.

To evaluate global psychological distress in adolescents survivors, tests for mean differences between adolescent cancer survivors and normative samples of healthy adolescents on the MHI were performed. Though not of psychopathological proportions, adolescent survivors did report significantly more global psychological distress ($t(56) = 3.18$, $p < .001$) and less overall mental health ($t(56) = 2.44$, $p < .01$) than their healthy counterparts. Likewise, a majority of patients reported persistent, intrusive thoughts about their illness and treatment.

b. Psychosocial Adjustment

The Social Adjustment Scale (SAS) was used to assess the family, vocational and social/leisure functioning of the young adult leukemia survivors. The marital, parental, family unit and extended family subscales of the SAS were used to assess various facets of family adjustment. Due to sex differences in family disruption, SAS values are separated by gender for comparisons with normative samples. In general, young adult acute leukemia survivors reported family adjustment levels that were comparable to nonpatient standard norms. Female leukemia survivors reported significantly more disruption in the SAS Extended Family, $t(317) = 3.37$ $p < .001$, and the Family Unit subscales, $t(292) = 3.11$ $p< .01$, then the female nonpatient sample. In contrast, male survivors reported family adjustment levels that were similar to levels reported by the male nonpatient sample. The SAS Work subscales was used to assess vocation adjustment. Considering that sex differences in vocational adjustment have been found in previous studies, analyses were conducted separately for males and females. Female leukemia survivors and female nonpatients were comparable in vocational functioning ($p >.10$). However, male leukemia survivors reported more vocational destruction than male nonpatients ($t(155) = 3.70$ $p < .01$. No significant differences in leisure functioning, were found between the leukemia survivors and the nonpatient sample.

The adolescent cancer survivors did not perceive themselves differently than a healthy comparison group on functional indicators of adjustment. More specifically, as measured by the Achenbach Youth Self-Report, there were no significant differences in social competence, number of behavior problems, or school achievement. Our data suggest that while adolescent cancer survivors experience psychosocial difficulties, the difficulty is within the particular domain of emotional distress, both global and illness-specific, and not seen in behavorial markers of adjustment.

c. Psychosexual Adjustment

Assessment of psychosexual function in the young adult subjects included frequency of sexual activity, satisfaction, body image, gender role identity, and adjustment in sexual relations. Despite the greater additional strain, longer hospitalization and high probability of gonadal impairment associated with bone marrow transplantation and compared to conventional chemotherapy, there was no difference in present psychosexual function among these individuals. Women survivors as a whole generally reported decreased sexual frequency and satisfaction compared to community norms, while both men and women reported poorer body image. Greater time since treatment significantly predicted poorer body image ($p < .03$). Decreased drive, lower satisfaction and poor body image were associated with increased psychological distress and and decreased energy level. These data suggest that bone marrow transplantation does not place the patient at higher risk for psychosexual dysfunction but that both treatments carry a psychological burden that should be recognized in the total care of the patient and requires further intensive investigation.

d. Family Milieu

Current trends in adolescent mental health research emphasize the importance of social-ecological factors in negotiating normative development milestones and coping with non-normative stressful life events. Among these contextual variables, much attention has been given to the importance of family milieu in shaping adolescents' psychosocial adjustment and attainment of age-appropriate developmental milestones. These tasks typically require a familial context of tolerance of increased autonomy, continued support and connectedness, and reorganization of family roles and resources. However, the family context for developing peer relationships, self-concept and further orientation has receive limited attention among adolescent cancer survivors. (Michael, 1987; Kazak, 1989).

Several studies have emphasized openness of communication, living in the present, cohesion, flexibility, extrafamilial social support and other family members emotional well-being as related to adolescent's global adjustment. (Barbarian, 1985; Greenberg, 1989; Kupst 1988; Spinetta, 1981; Spinetta, 1987; Rait, 1989) These aspects of family milieu are hypothesized as facilitative of adolescents' post-treatment re-entry. However, no empirical work has been conducted looking at the role of family context in promoting this important transition.

In terms of family context, we found that adolescent survivors who perceived their families as balanced in adaptability and cohesion report less psychological distress (t (68) = 2.04, $p < .05$) and greater positive well-being (t (68) = 2.56, $p < .05$) than adolescents who described their families as nonbalanced. In these domains there was also a trend towards adolescents who perceived their families as balanced in adaptability and cohesion to report higher levels of self-esteem (t (68) = 1.96, $p < .10$). In addition, adolescents' report of the quality of parent-child communication was strongly associated ($p < .001$) with the psychological adjustment of adolescent cancer survivors. According to interview data, 71% reported that their families were crucial in dealing with stressors of cancer; though, 70% stated that unfortunately open discussions of cancer-related concerns ended with the termination of active treatment. These findings strongly support the notion that family context is an integral component of adolescents' transition to non-illness, developmentally appropriate activities.

e. Predictors of Adjustment

For adults, sociodemographic, disease/treatment and psychological distress variables were treated as three sets of predictor variables used to explain variance in social, family and vocational adjustment. Neither the sociodemographic nor the disease/treatment variables were strongly associated with vocational and household responsibility adjustment. Psychological distress was the best predictor of social ($p < .001$), family ($p <. 05$) and vocational ($p <. 001$) adjustment. More analyses are underway to determine other predictors for psychological, distress, social and sexual adjustment in adults.

We attempted to identify cofactors that would aid in the identification of adolescent cancer survivors most at-risk for experiencing psychosocial sequelae. Preliminary correlational analyses showed that there were no differences in adjustment found on the basis of gender, family constellation, religion, or family socioeconomic level. Likewise, neither diagnosis nor type of treatment were associated with psychosocial difficulties. However, patients who were older at the time of assessment and at the time of diagnosis, and who were more recently off-treatment reported heightened psychological distress ($p < .01$).

Hierarchical setwise multiple regression was used in order to further understand the relative contribution of medical, sociodemographic, and family parameters as predictors of adolescent psychosocial adjustment. In the first equation, positive well-being was treated as the criterion variable and disease/treatment and family variables were used as predictor variable sets. At Step 1, with age at diagnosis, months in active treatment and months post-treatment entered into the equation, 12% of the variance in positive well-being was accounted for (F (3,49) = 2.21, $p < .09$). At Step 2, with adolescent-mother communication, adolescent-father communication and family structure entered into the equation, an additional 21% of variance was explained (F 3,49)= 4.70, $p < .006$). Overall, these variables accounted for 33% of the variance in positive well-being (F (6,46) = 3.70, $p < .004$. In the second equation, psychological distress was treated as the criterion variable and disease/treatment and family variables were used as predictor variables. At Step 1, with age at diagnosis, months in active treatment, and months post-treatment entered, only 6% of the variance in psychological distress was accounted for (F (3,46) = 1.04, n.s.). At Step 2, with the family parameters entered, 19% of the variance in psychological distress was explained (F (3,46) = 2.43, $p < .08$). Overall, these variables account for 20% of the variance in psychological distress (F (6,46) = 1.78, $p = .12$). Thus, much of the variability in outcome remains unexplained.

SUMMARY

Within the adolescent survivor sample, the psychosocial response of having been diagnosed and successfully treated for cancer is not universal as evidenced by the variability in psychosocial adjustment. Data from the MHI suggests that adolescent cancer survivors do experience more global psychological distress than a comparison group of healthy adolescents. In addition, the majority of these patients reported persistent, intrusive thoughts about their illness and its treatment. Conversely, the adolescent cancer survivors did not differ from a normative sample on social competence, manifestation of problems behaviors, or school achievement. Thus, our data suggest that adjustment in this population is multi-dimensional with variability. While they are functioning quite adequately at school and in social situation, they continue to experience heightened and persistent distress of both a global and illness-specific quality. A number of factors that are conducive to psychosocial intervention appear to be related to adjustment. Family communication and family cohesion were significantly related to the mental health of the adolescent survivors, suggesting a need to further explore the family context of adolescent adjustment.

The present work also represents the first attempt to directly examine the psychosocial functioning of young adult, acute leukemia survivors. When compared with normative samples of nonpatients, these survivors (taken as a whole group), reported heightened levels on several indicators of psychological distress. While not entirely consistent across different psychological measures, these young people were generally one standard deviation above the mean for psychological distress. But when compared to normative samples of psychiatric outpatients, our survivors reported significantly less psychological distress. For instance, leukemia survivors reported less intrusive and avoidant cognitions associated with the stressor of being diagnosed and treated for cancer than those associated with patients experiencing traumatic stress disorders. In aggregate, these findings again suggest that the psychosocial adjustment of leukemia survivors is quite variable.

Finally, while group comparisons shed light on the psychosocial functioning of leukemia survivors, in general, wide variability in psychosocial adjustment may mask identification of a cohort of cancer survivors most at-risk for psychosocial dysfunction. Sociodemographic, disease/treatment and psychological distress variables only partially explain this variability.

The findings from our data suggest several clinical recommendations. First, the prevalence of persistent, psychiatric comorbidity is quite low among long-term survivors of hematologic malignancies survivors. Second, if survivors do experience some psychological distress, usually, it is of non-psychopathological proportions. Furthermore, the severity of the stress associated with undergoing rigorous research regimens such as BMT appears to be no greater than that associated with convention chemotherapy treatment. Many patients will be reassured to be told that it is normal to have concerns about 1) fear of relapse, 2) feeling different, 3) or feeling behind their peers in obtaining developmental tasks, 4) sharing their experiences with non-cancer friends, 5) dating and 6) having satisfying sexual experiences. Finally, it appears that a subset of leukemia survivors experience relatively poor psychosocial adjustment. Our findings suggest that young women, who have had extensive hospitalization and are recently off-treatment may be most at-risk for aversive psychosocial sequelae. Most notably, these patients experienced greater mood disturbance and difficulties in family adjustment and intimate relationships. This subset of patients may particularly benefit form psychosocial interventions aimed at the prevention and amelioration of such psychological dysfunction.

FIGURE 1

SUBJECT CHARACTERISTICS

	Adolescents	Adults
Total Patients (N)	58	70
Sex		
Male (%)	74	54
Female (%)	26	51
Age at Dx (Years)	9±4	23±7
Current Age (Years)	16±2	31±8
Ethnicity (% White)	71	90
Marital Status (% Married)	---	43
Family Income % < $30,000	59	70
Disease/Tx (%)		
Hodgkin's Disease	31	---
Non Hodgkin's Lymphoma	31	---
Acute Leukemia	38	100
BMT	---	30
Karnofsky > 90%	100	100
Time off Treatment (Months)	49±34	61±37

REFERENCES

Achenbach, T. (1986). Youth Self-Report. Burlington: University Associates in Psychiatry.

Andrykowski M, Henselee P, Farrall M: (1987). Physical and psychosocial functioning of adult survivors of allogeneic bone marrow transplantation. Bone Marrow Transplantation 4:

Barbarin, O., Hughes, D., and Chesler, M. (1985). Stress, coping, and marital functioning among parents of children with cancer. Journal of Marriage and the Family, 46: 473-480.

Byrd, R. (1985). Late effects of treatment of cancer in children. Pediatric Clinics of North America, 32 (3): 835-857.

Cella, D., and Tross, S. (1986). Psychological adjustment to survival from Hodgkin's disease. Journal of Consulting and Clinical Psychology, 54, 616-622.

Daiter, s., Larson, R. Weddington, W., and Ultmann, J. (1988). Psychosocial symptomatology, personal growth, and development among young adult patients following the diagnosis of leukemia or lymphoma. Journal of Clinical Oncology, 6 (4), 613-617.

Derogatis L. (1975). Derogatis sexual functioning inventory. Baltimore MD: Clinical Psychometric Research.

Derogatis L, Spencer P. (1982). The brief symptom inventory (BSI): Administration, scoring and procedures Manual I. Baltimore, Clinical Psychometric Research.

Fobair P, Hoppe R, Bloom F, et al (1986). Psychosocial problems among survivors of Hodgkin's Disease. Journal of Clinical Oncology 4:805-814.

Freidenbergs I, Gordon W, Hibbard M, et al (1982). Psychosocial aspects of living with cancer: A review of the literature. Int'l Journal Psychiatry in Medicine 11:303-329.

Fritz, B., and Williams, J. (1988). Issues of adolescent development for survivors of childhood cancer. Journal of the American Academy of Child and Adolescent Psychiatry, 27(6): 712-715.

Greenberg, J., Kazak, A., and Meadows, A. (1989). Psychologic functioning in 8-to 16-year old cancer survivors and their parents. Journal of Pediatrics. 114: 488-493.

Horowitz, M., Wilner, N., and Alvarez, W. (1979). Impact of Events Scale: A measure of subjective distress. Psychosomatic Medicine, 41(3): 209-218

Kazak, A. (1989). families of chronically ill children: A systems and social-ecological model of adaptation and challenge. Journal of Consulting and Clinical Psychology, 57: 25-30.

Koocher, G., and O'Malley, J. (Eds.) (1981). The Damocles Syndrome: Psychological consequences of surviving childhood cancer. NY: McGraw-Hill.

Kupst, M., and Schulman, J. (1988) Long-term coping with pediatric leukemia: A six-year follow-up study. Journal of Pediatric Psychology, 13(1): 7-22.

Lesko, L.M., Ostroff, J.S., Mumma, G.H., Mashberg, D.E., Holland, J.C. (1989). Long-term psychological adjustment acute leukemia survivors: Impact of bone marrow transplantation vs chemotherapy (manuscript submitted for publication).

Meadows, A., and Silber, J. (1985). Delayed consequences of therapy for childhood cancer. CA-A Cancer Journal for Clinicians 35 (5): 271-285

Meadows, A., and Hobbie, W. (1986). The medical consequences of cure. Cancer 58: 524-528.

Michael, B. and Copeland, D. (1987). Psychosocial issues in childhood cancer. American Journal of Pediatric Hematology/Oncology 9 (1): 73-83

Mulhern, R., Wasserman, A., Friedman, A., and Fairclough, D. (1989). Social competence and behavioral adjustment of children who are long-term survivors of cancer. Pediatrics, 83(1): 18-25.

Offer, D., Ostrov, E., and Howard, K. (1981). The Adolescent: A Psychological Self-Portrait. NY: Basic Books.

Olson, D., and Wilson, M. (1985). Family Inventories. St. Paul, MN: Family Social service, University of Minnesota.

Peterson, A., and Spiga, R. (1982) Adolescence and stress. In L. Goldberger and S. Breznitz (Eds.), Handbook of Stress, NY: Free Press.

Rait, D., Ostroff, J., Smith K., Cella, D., & Lesko, L. (1989). Perceptions of family functioning and psychosocial adjustment among adolescent cancer survivors. Society of Behavioral Medicine Meeting.

Spinetta, J.E., and Deasy-Spineta, P. (Eds.) (1981). Living with Childhood Cancer. St. Louis: Hosby.

Spinetta, J., Murphy, J., Vik, P. Day, J., and Mott, M. (1987). Long-term adjustment in families of children with cancer. Paper presented at the American Cancer Society conference. Los Angels, CA. January 31st

Teta, M., Del Po, M., Kasl, S., Meigs, J., Myers, M., and Mulvihill, J. (1986). Psychosocial consequences of childhood and adolescent cancer survival. Journal of Chronic Disease, 3 (9): 751-759.

Veit, C., and Ware, J. (1983). The structure of psychological distress and well-being in general populations. Journal of Consulting and Clinical Psychology, 51: 730-742.

Wasserman, A., Thompson, E., Willimas, J., and Fairclough, D. (1987). The psychological status of survivors of childhood/adolescent Hodgkin's disease. Archives of Diseases of Children, 141: 626-631.

Weissman M, Bothwell S: Assessment of social adjustment by patient self-report. Arch Gen Psychiatry 33:1111-1115, 1976.

Wellisch D, (1984). Work, social, recreation, family, and physical status. Cancer 53:2290-2302.

Wolcott D, Wellish D, Fawzy F, et al (1986). Adaptation of adult bone marrow transplant recipient long-term survivors. Transplantation 41: 478-483.

The Biology of Hematopoiesis, pages 439–448

IS NATURAL BACKGROUND OR RADIATION FROM NUCLEAR POWER PLANTS LEUKEMOGENIC?*

Eugene P. Cronkite

Medical Department, Brookhaven National Laboratory
Upton, New York 11973

Life originated on this planet and evolved in a radiation field that was more intense than today. Despite pollution, man-made radiation sources in medicine and industry, human beings in developed countries are living longer (up 4 years since 1970) are healthier and have more productive lives in general than ever before. The quest of many activists, well-doers, and environmentalists for a risk-free environment is an illusion. Radiation-free is an impossibility. The major exposure of human beings is natural radiation. Radiation exposure from generation of electricity by fossil and nuclear fuels will inevitably increase radiation exposure as the world's population expands and underdeveloped countries deserve and demand a higher standard of living through the use of more electricity. Solar and geothermal energy are attractive, must be expanded, but produce their own environmental problems.

The question of whether very low-level exposure to radiation is leukemogenic or carcinogenic is foremost in the minds of many because of the morbid fear of radiation that has permeated society. On the other hand, no one seems concerned about 3 millirem received from a transatlantic flight (voluntary) but 3 millirem caused by the fallout from Chernobyl caused great anxiety in Western Europe (Gonzalez and Anderer, 1989). The objective in this review is to provide some facts about normal hemopoietic cell proliferation relevant to leukemogenesis, physical, chemical, and biological facts about radiation effects with the hope that each person will be able to decide for themselves whether background radiation or emissions from nuclear power plants and facilities significantly add to the spontaneous leukemia incidence. A very simplistic approach will be used.

Berenblum and Shubik (1949) demonstrated that cutaneous carcinogenesis consists of two phases. First is initiation, in which a genetic change is induced in the target cells and then there is a long period during which the initiated cells are promoted to a diagnosable cancer. In modern parlance, a protooncogene is activated by mutation, translocation, adduct formation or by the inactivation of a suppressor gene. Promotion takes place over a prolonged period of time as a result of internal physiological processes that are not clearly defined.

Leukemia is a monoclonal disease. This was first demonstrated for chronic granulocytic leukemia when the pH 1 chromosome was found to be present in erythrocytic megakaryocytic and granulocytic precursors (Nowell and Hungerford, 1960). Since this initial observation many studies with G6DP, immuno- globulins, immunoglobulins, restriction fragment polymorphism of x-linked genes, and IgG rearrangement have demonstrated the monoclonality for almost all human leukemia. In other words, a specific lesion is induced somewhere in the human genome of 3.0×10^9 base pair which initiates the leukemic process.

Through the studies of Cronkite et al. (1960), and Fliedner et al. (1960, 1964) on the kinetics of granulocytopoiesis and determination of the time for DNA synthesis in granulocytic precursors by Stryckmans et al. (1967), and an analytical review on granulopoiesis by Cronkite and Vincent (1969), one can calculate the number of base pairs that must be replicated per minute in the course of granulocyte production.

Vincent (1989) has calculated base pair replication during granulopoiesis and suggested that acute myeloblastic leukemia may be the result of an error in base substitution or deletion in the appropriate exon. Analogous calculations follow.

Neutrophil production rate in average human being is 7.92×10^7 per minute
Average number of base pairs per genome, 3.0×10^9
DNA synthesis time in granulocytic precursors, 12 hours

Therefore, the production of 7.92×10^7 neutrophils per minute requires a replication of 3.0×10^{14} base pairs per minute. The fidelity with which polymerases accomplish this enormous task is remarkable, but it is likely that some errors in substitution may occur spontaneously.

The amplification of the stem cell input is equal to or greater than 16. Thus, the base pair replication in unidentifiable precursor cells, the putative target cell for leukemogenesis, is equal to or less than 1.9×10^{13} per minute. If one assumes that 10^{-5} of the DNA codes for regulatory genes, then 1.9×10^8 base pairs are replicated per minute in these genes and annually 9.9×10^{13} base pairs are replicated in these genes. One can make an argument that most leukemia is the result of deletion or substitution in a regulatory gene during normal cell proliferation thus initiating the leukemic process. An interesting question is whether acute myeloblastic and chronic granulocytic leukemia are due to spontaneous mutation resulting from an error in base insertion during hemopoiesis. The incidence of acute myeloblastic leukemia in the United States is three cases per 10^5 persons per year (Ellis and McCredie, 1989). It can be calculated assuming amplification of stem cell input into neutrophil-dividing compartment of 16 that there are a maximum of 2.6×10^{17} stem cell mitoses per year in 10^5 persons. This is an upper limit. The number of base pair replications in progenitor cells are 7.8×10^{26}, an enormous number indeed. It has been shown that in about 25% of persons with acute myeloblastic leukemia that there is a single base substitution in a codon of the N-ras oncogene (Bos et al., 1985; Shen et al., 1987). In view of the enormous number of base pair replications per annum, it is conceivable, perhaps likely that an error will on occasion be made in a vulnerable spot in DNA by chance alone, suggesting that most acute myeloblastic leukemia may be spontaneous. Of course, many factors may increase the incidence of leukemia, of which ionizing radiation is one.

The best documented example of radiation-induced leukemia is the exposure of the Japanese to the atomic bomb. In this case the exposure was very short, only a few seconds. There was a long latent period of 18 months to 20 or more years before the initiated cell was promoted to proliferate and be expressed as a diagnosable leukemia (Ishimaru et al., 1979). The maximum incidence occurred at about 7 1/2 years after exposure to the bomb radiation.

Radiation induction of leukemia is an extremely infrequent cellular event. This was first demonstrated by Mole (1975). The incidence of leukemia in the Japanese reached a maximum at exposure of 200 rad. Of 283,498 survivors with an average dose of 16.1 rad, the total leukemia through 1978 was 387 with an estimated excess of 190.6. All estimates of dose-effect relationships are basically based on these 190 excess cases. Since leukemia is monoclonal and 200 rad produces 1% of excess leukemia, one can estimate the frequency of initiation in the bone marrow cells. The average adult has about 10^{12} bone marrow cells. Only one cell in 100 persons is initiated and promoted to leukemia, that is one cell in 10^{14} bone marrow cells by induction of gene rearrangement, translocation, deletion, mutation, adduct formation to activate a protooncogene or inactivate a suppressor gene. This is truly a very rare event at the cellular level.

Simplistically, ionizing radiation produces its deleterious effects by a photon hitting an orbital electron and knocking it out of its orbit. This Compton electron does the damage directly and indirectly. First by the production of chemical bond breaks and second by the production of free radicals, activated oxygen species and peroxides. Direct and indirect effects may produce a loss of base or base exchange at the rate of about 5 per rad exposure, single-strand breaks at about 5 per rad, double-strand at about 0.2. Thus these lesions occur at random in DNA. It is of interest to calculate the number of Compton electrons per cell volume as function of dose of 100 KeV X ray as has been done by Feinendegen et al. (1985). The one rad exposure results in an average of 10 Compton electrons per average cell volume. With higher energies, for example, ^{60}Co (1.2 MeV γ) there would be about 20 electrons per cell. Leukemia incidence is known to be statistically increased by single doses in excess of 25 rad, which gives a shower of 250 electrons per cell about 125 base changes, 125 single strand breaks, and 5 double strand breaks. The maximum incidence of leukemia is after a single dose of 200 rad which produces a shower of 2000 electrons per cell producing 8 times as many aberrations in DNA. It is evident from the studies of Feinendegen et al. (1985) that 10 mrad results in results in an average of 1 electron per 10 cells. In other words, 9 of 10 cells are not affected at all. With the low doses of environmental interest, many cells are not hit. The probability of a single electron hitting the leukemogenic spot in 3.0 x 10^9 base pairs appears vanishingly small.

In considering the possible effects of background radiation, it is first important to recognize that the unavoidable radiation to which human beings are exposed vary substantially throughout the world from approximately 50 to 1000 mrem per annum (NCRP Report 94, 1987), it is interesting to estimate the number of cells that are hit per year in the 70 kg person from an average background radiation of 100 mrad/year or 0.27 mrad per day. The fraction of cells hit per day is rounded out to 10^{-3} and since the number of cells in a 70 kg person is about 10^{14}, around 10^{11} cells will be hit per day, the nuclei will be hit less frequently. The time to hit all cells is therefore about 1000 days. Considering Poisson statistics, a few cells will have been hit more than once and a few spared.

The time between hits varies with the dose rate. For example, at 100 mrad/day, the interval between hits is about three days. With 1 rad per day about 8 hours, 10 rad per day about 50 minutes, and 100 rad per day 5 minutes, thus as the dose rate goes up the time for repair decreases rapidly. At doses of environmental interest, however, there is one more day between hits to allow repair.

In addition to the above purely physical factors concerned with radiation and its effect as a function of dose rate, there are biochemical protective mechanisms (Hall, 1988). The indirect effects of radiation can be modified by scavengers for free radicals such as glutathione and other glycols, superoxide dismutase that inactivates superoxide, and the DNA repair enzymes which excise and replace defective DNA with a generally high fidelity.

The sparsity of hits by electrons in cellular DNA at low-dose rates and the biochemical protective mechanisms along with the DNA repair enzymes makes one wonder whether there may be a dose rate at which inactivation of radiation products and/or repair is totally complete. This is in the realm of possibility but has not as yet been shown to be the case.

Many analyses on the relationship between dose of radiation and incidence of leukemia have been performed by diverse groups (United Nations Scientific Committee, 1972) analyzes these data exhaustively without experimental proof it has been assumed that the relationship is linear with dose, there is no threshold and that a single dose of one rad will induce 1-2 extra cases of leukemia for 10^6 persons exposed per year. This assumption errs on the conservative side. There is no epidemiological confirmation of this assumption. One can, then, using this assumption, estimate how many cases of leukemia are being induced in the United States by an average background of 100 mrem per year. The probability of inducing excess leukemia is 2×10^{-6} per rad per year. Thus, background-induced leukemia will be: $0.1 \times 2 \text{x} 10^{-6} \times 10^6$ or 0.2 cases of leukemia per year per 10^6 at risk. Since in the United States about 60 cases of all types of leukemia are observed per year per 10^6 population at risk, 59 cases are therefore due to genetics, diet, drugs,chemicals, other radiation, other diseases, smoking or most probably just due to errors in replication of an enormous number of base pairs during normal cell division.

In the United States about 15,000 cases of acute myeloblastic, chronic granulocytic and acute lymphocytic leukemia are observed. An additional 10 mrem to the entire population of the United States would produce 5 additional cases which for statistical reasons simply could not be detected in a background of 15,000 cases.

The population exposure in the United States comes from several sources. Background radiation accounts for 82%. Man-made radiation accounts for 18% of which 11% is from medical uses of radiation. Consumer products contribute 3% and the residual by a combination of occupational, fallout, and nuclear power (Gonzalez and Anderer, 1989).

There are many epidemiological studies. Some show no effect of high-level background. For example, in the Han peasants in China 200 mG compared to 70 mGy, there is a lesser incidence of cancer in the high exposure (Luxin et al., 1987). On the Colorado plateau with high natural radiation, the cancer incidence is less than the low-level natural radiation on the West Coast or East Coast. There is also no detectable effect in the people living in high-level Kerala India or monazite sands in Brazil (United Nations, 1972).

There are many studies in smaller groups showing effects or no effects such as American soldiers exposed at the Nevada test site to 0.5 rad and followed for 22 years. Four cases of leukemia were expected and 10 were observed, giving a relative risk of 2.5 (Caldwell et al., 1980). Relative risks may be misleading because of the statistics of small numbers. Webster (1981) has used counting rates of radioisotopes at low levels as an example to illustrate the effect of Poisson statistics. The counting rates of radioisotopes like cancer events follow Poisson statistics. In his example, illustrated in Table 1, in 20 successive periods the counting rates varied from zero to 8 per minute. The observed frequency is shown in the 2nd column. The theoretical expected frequency is shown in the 3rd column and the ratio of the observed to the expected is shown in the 4th column. This ratio is analogous to relative risk and varied from 0.6 to 2.8. Numbers greater than unity imply an effect, and the numbers less than unity no effect or perhaps a reduction in incidence.

Table 1. Poisson Statistics:* The Problem of Small Number Observations

	No. Observed	Actual %	Prob. %	Occur. Prob.
Actual counts Observed 20 Consecutive Accounting Periods	6,3,5,4 2,2,4,4 7,3,8,6 6,2,0,5, 2,3,6,1			
Theoretical Expections with Poisson Distribution	0	5.0	1.8	2.8
	1	5.0	7.3	0.63
	2	20.0	14.6	1.37
	3	15.0	19.5	0.77
	4	15.0	19.5	0.77
	5	10.0	15.6	0.64
	6	20.0	10.4	1.90
	7	5.0	5.9	0.85
	8	5.0	3.0	1.60

*Modified from Webster (1981)

It is possible that the sum of all relative risks of all epidemiological studies on exposure of human populations to less than 1 rad might well be unity. Lewis Thomas

(1983) has emphasized that epidemiologic studies of non-infectious disease have produced their own adverse side effects in an "epidemic of apprehension" based on questionable alarm in daily life. The non-scientific and in part the scientific public is unable to distinguish between alarms and the true hazards.

An incomprehensible paradox is the fact that the public is relatively unconcerned about the major source of population exposure, that is, natural unavoidable radiation (82%) and medical uses of radiation are prudently accepted (11%) and radiation from consumer products (3%) is desired, whereas nuclear energy (<1%) causes the most apprehension.

Since the world's population is expanding, there will be an ever-increasing need for greater amounts of electricity to meet the requirements of the developed and developing countries. It is of some interest to compare population radiation exposures from burning fossil and nuclear fuels. It may be a surprise that the population exposure from burning fossil fuels with its inherent radioactivity is 8.5 man Sv per year per gigawatt year compared to 3.973 man Sv from nuclear fuels (Gonzalez and Anderer, 1989).

The culprits in order of decreasing exposure of the population to radiation are:

Natural radioactivity - unavoidable
Medical uses - beneficial
Consumer products - beneficial and desired
Fossil fuel generation of electricity - unavoidable
Nuclear generation of electricity - ultimately unavoidable

It is postulated that at doses of radiation below 1 rad exposure radiation-induced leukemia or cancer in general cannot be detected for statistical reasons or excess cancer is not induced.

SUMMARY AND CONCLUSIONS

In view of the enormous number of base pair replications per annum in hemopoietic stem cells with the likelihood of coding errors, the rarity of the leukemogenic event at the cellular level after high doses of radiation, the infrequent occurrence of radiation events in cells at low-level exposure (large fraction of cells uninvolved), biological protective mechanisms and the realization that exposure of human populations to radiation from nuclear power plants is a very small fraction of natural radioactivity and will for the foreseeable future remain small and that populations exposed to high natural background radiation show no detectable harmful effects, it is concluded that either there is no effect, or for statistical reasons one cannot detect an effect.

REFERENCES

Berenblum I, Schubik P (1949). The persistence of latent tumor cells induced in the mouse's skin by a single application of 9,10-di-methyl-1,2-benzanthracene. Brit J Cancer 3:384-386.

Bos JL, Toksoz D, Marshall CJ et al. (1985). Amino acid substitutions at codon-13 of the N-ras oncogene in human acute myeloid leukemia. Nature 315: 726-730.

Caldwell GG, Kelley DB, Heath CW, Jr. (1980). Leukemia among participants in military maneuvers at a nuclear bomb test. JAMA 244:1575-1578.

Cronkite EP, Vincent PC (1969). Granulocytopoiesis Series. Hematologica 2:3-43.

Cronkite EP, Bond VP, Fliedner TM, Killman SA. The use of tritiated thymidine in the study of hemopoietic cell proliferation. CIBA Foundation Symposium on Hemopoiesis, Churchill, London, 1960.

Ellis LD, McCredie KB (1989). Acute myelogenous leukemia. Public Education Dept., Leukemia Society of American, Inc.

Feinendegen LE, Booz J, Bond VP, Sondhaus CA (1985). Microdosimetric approach to the analysis of cell responses at low dose and low-dose rate. Radiat Prot Dosimetry 13:299-306.

Fliedner TM, Cronkite EP, Robertson, JS (1960) Granulocytopoiesis I. Senescence and random loss of neutrophilic granulocytes in human beings. Blood 24:402-414.

Fliedner, TM, Cronkite EP, Killman SA, Bond VP (1964). Granuylocytopoiesis II. Emergence and pattern of labeling of neutrophilic granulocytes in human beings. Blood 24:683-700.

Gonzalez AJ, Anderer J (1989). Radiation versus radiation: Nuclear Energy in Perspective. IAEA Bulletin 31:21-31.
Hall EJ, Radiobiology for the Radiologist. Chapters 7 and 10, J.P., Lipincott Company, Philadelphia, 1988.
Ishimaru T, Otake M, Ichimaru M (1979). Dose-response relationship of neutrons and gamma rays to leukemia incidence among atomic bomb survivors at Hiroshima and Nagasaki by type of leukemia, 1950-71. Radiat Res 77:377-394.
Luxin W, Yongru Z, Zufan T, Weihui H, Deqing C, Rongling Y (1987). Cancer mortality study in high background radiation areas of Yangjiang, China. In "Epidemiological Investigations on Health Effects of Ionizing Radiation", Proc. International Colloquium, Institute fur Strahlenschutz der Berufsgenossenschaft der Feinmechanik und Elektrotechnik Gustav-Heinemann-Ufer, 130, 5000 Koln 51, West Germany.
Mole RH (1975). Ionizing radiation as a carcinogen. Practical questions in academic pursuits. Brit J Radiol 48:157-169.
NCRP Report No. 94, "Exposure of a Population in the United States and Canada from Natural Background Radiation". National Council on Radiation Protection and Measurements, 7910 Woodmont Avenue, Bethesda, MD 20814, 1987.
Nowell PC, Hungerford DA (1960). A minute chromosome in human chronic granulocytic leukemia. Science 132:1497.
Shen WPV, Aldrich TH, Venta-Perez G, Franza DR Jr., Firth ME (1987). Expression of normal and mutant ras proteins in human acute myeloid leukemia. Oncogene 1:157-165.
Stryckmans P, Cronkite EP, Fache J, Fliedner TM, Ramos J (1967). Deoxyribonucleic acid synthesis time of erythropoietic granulopoietic cells in human beings. Nature (London) 211:717-720.
Thomas L (1983). Discover 4:78.
United Nations Scientific Committee on the Effects of Atomic Radiation. Ionizing Radiation: Levels and Effects. Vol. 2, Effects, New York, United Nations, pp. 427-428, 1972.
Vincent PC (December 1989). Acute myeloblastic leukemia: Epidemiology, etiology and pathogenesis. Bull Postgrad Comm Med, University of Sydney, 45.
Webster AW (1981). On the question of cancer induction by small x-ray doses. AJR 137:647-666.

The Biology of Hematopoiesis, pages 449–458

BONE MARROW PROLIFERATION AFTER PASSAGE THROUGH AN IRRADIATED HOST

G. Brecher, S. Neben and M. Yee

University of California, Lawrence Berkeley Laboratory, Cell and Molecular Biology Division, Berkeley, CA 94720

Serial bone marrow transfusions through irradiated hosts have long been known to be impractical, because after 5 or 6 transfers, the bone marrow, though never irradiated itself, loses its normal capacity of rescuing irradiated mice by replacing their marrow. A number of attempts had been made to circumvent the exhaustion of the marrow on serial transfusion (Wolf et al., 1983). I found the idea attractive that exposure to the microenvironment of the irradiated host could affect the non-irradiated marrow. In 1957 Fred Stohlman (Stohlman et al. 1957) infused normal red cells intramuscularly into irratiated dogs. The red cells that reached the general circulation had a markedly shortened life span, while irradiated red cells so transfused into normal dogs, survived normally, clear evidence of an adverse effect of the irradiated microenvironment. More recently, Micklem showed (Ross et al., 1982, Micklem, 1983) that a single passage of marrow through an irradiated host will indeed reduce its subsequent proliferation. In pursuing and somewhat extending these studies, we found some perplexing results. The size of the initial inoculum into the irradiated host appeared of overriding importance for its subsequent performance. This appears surprising since we are generally counting on the bone marrow being capable to expand extensively without loss of functional capacity.

MATERIAL AND METHODS

All experiments employed CBA/Ca mice which are homozygous for Pgk-1^{b} and Gpi-1s^{b} and the congenic strains CBA/Ca-Pgk-1^{a} and CBA/Gpi-1s^{a}, bred at the University of California. The congenic strains had been originally backcrossed on the standard CBA/Ca strain (Ansell and Micklem, 1986) in the laboratory of H. S. Micklem who generously supplied breeder pairs to us. Three enzyme markers were thus available to us, phosphoglycerate kinase A and B (PGK-A and B)and glucose phosphate isomerase A (GPI-A). (GPI-B could not be used simultaneously since both CBA/Ca-Pgk-1^a and 1^b are GPI-B positive.) The markers will be referred to as A, B, and G.

First or primary transfusions used mice homozygous for PGK-A as donors and PGK-B as recipients or vice versa. Marrows from such primary hosts were re-transfused into secondary hosts which were generally GPI-A, so that cells originating from primary donors and primary hosts could still be identified in the secondary hosts. The ratios of donor to host cell enzymes were determined electrophoretically on red blood cells of the peripheral blood, obtained at 4 week intervals by bleeding from the orbital sinus. The methodology of enzyme determination followed the recommendation of Ansell and Micklem (Ansell and Micklem, 1986). Donors and hosts were of the same sex to avoid incompatibilities that occurred in syngeneic hosts that were not sex matched (Raveche et al., 1985).

Mice were irradiated with a ^{60}Co source at 1 m and a dose rate of between 80 and 90 cGy per minute computed from the ^{60}Co decay course and checked with a Victoreen dosimeter. Animals were irradiated either to explore the effect of passage through an irradiated host, or to test proliferation of bone marrow so passaged in a secondary host. In all cases mice received a uniformly lethal dose of 1050cGy from the ^{60}Co source and were given bone marrow transfusions within 2 hours of irradiation. The marrows to be tested for the effect of passage through the irradiated host were harvested 1 to 3 months later and were designated as "exposed." Exposed and control marrows were transfused into irradiated and non-irradiated hosts as indicated in the individual experiments. Before re-transfusion into irradiated secondary hosts, exposed marrows were sometimes mixed with equal numbers of normal marrow cells. That approach duplicated Micklem's (Micklem et al., 1972) competitive repopulation assay. In it, cells with proliferative capacity inferior to normal cells would gradually be lost from the secondary host, because the normal cells replaced others thanks to their superior self renewal.

Suspensions of bone marrow were prepared in phosphate-buffered saline and counted in a Coulter Counter. The desired number of cells was injected intravenously in 0.5 ml phosphate buffered saline. When 200×10^6 cells were to be injected, 50×10^6 cells were given in the morning and repeated that afternoon and the following morning and afternoon. CFU-S determinations were performed following the standard method of Till and McCullouch (Till and McCullouch, 1961).

RESULTS

Experiment 1. Thirty A mice were irradiated with a uniformly lethal dose and given $10x10^6$ B bone marrow cells. One month later, the marrows of these animals, now 100% B, and marrows of normal B controls were harvested and tested for their content of CFU-S. The exposed marrows contained only 2/3 the concentration of CFU-S of the normal mice. To equalize the number of CFU-S in the exposed and control marrows, $300x10^6$ exposed B cells were transfused into each of 4 non-irradiated A mice and $200x10^6$ normal B cells into another 4 non-irradiated A hosts. (It should be noted that $200x10^6$ cells approach the total content of marrow cells of the average normal adult mouse, estimated at $260x10^6$ by Boggs (Boggs, 1984). The results are shown in Fig. 1. The normal donor cells reached 30% in the control group, well within the range of similar prior experiments (Brecher et al., 1982). The exposed marrow cells failed to proliferate permanently. They averaged 15% at 4 weeks, gradually dropped to 0 by 20 weeks, and remained at the 0 level until the experiment was terminated at 24 weeks. In contrast, 1.5 million cells from the same suspension of exposed marrows repopulated 3 of 4 irradiated secondary hosts entirely and donor cells reached 60% in a fourth. Normal donor cells repopulated 100% of the marrow of all lethally irradiated hosts. Thus exposed marrow cells lagged only slightly, if at all, behind the normal cells in repopulating an irradiated host. The marked defect in the repopulating ability of the exposed marrows was evident, however, when such marrows were re-transfused into normal hosts. The defect was present, even though the exposed and control normal cells were matched for CFU-S.

Experiment 2. Wolf et al. (Wolf et al., 1983) suggested that the serially transferred marrow is severely stressed as it must repopulate a series of marrows depleted by irradiation. We wished to test whether progressively larger inocula would indeed reduce any unfavorable effect of passage through an irradiated host. We did so by using the competitive repopulation assay. Six A mice were irradiated with 1050cGy and 2 each were given 10^6, $10x10^6$, and $200x10^6$ B cells. After 1 month all animals were 100% B. Their marrows were harvested and mixed with equal numbers of normal A cells. On electrophoresis the mixtures were confirmed to contain $50 \pm 5\%$ B cells and were given to groups of 5 irradiated G hosts, each animal receiving $10x10^6$ cells. After 14 weeks the secondary hosts that had contained 50% exposed cells from the initial inocula of 200, 10, and 1 million cells now had been replaced by normal cells to the extent of 10%, 50% and 100%. In terms of a repopulation assay, the initial inoculum of 200 million cells was only minimally inferior to the normal cells and only 10% was replaced. In contrast the lowest, 1 million inoculum could not compete with normal cells at all and was entirely replaced by them.

Experiment 3: Fifteen G animals were used as primary hosts, given 1050cGy and 100 million A cells each. After 1 month, 200 million of the exposed cells were transfused into each of 3 normal, non-irradiated B hosts. Another 10 million of the exposed cells were mixed with 10 million normal G cells and transfused into lethally irradiated B mice. The exposed cells derived from an initial inoculum of 100 million cells did circulate in normal hosts for less than 8 weeks, although these cells did well in the competitive repopulation assay. The 50% of normal cells increased to only 65% after 30 weeks, thus replacing only 15% of the exposed marrow cells

Experiment 4: The experiment was aimed at maximizing the effect of transfusion of exposed cells into normal, non-irradiated hosts. Lethally irradiated G mice were given a mixture of 300 million B and G cells. From these mice, 4 non-irradiated A mice received 200 exposed B+G cells each. For comparison, a typical experiment in which 200 million normal cells were transfused into non-irradiated hosts is depicted. It may be seen that the proliferation of exposed cells was indeed maximized when an initial inoculum of 300 million marrow cells was passed through an irradiated host and 200 million of the exposed cells transfused into a non-irradiated host. The results were comparable to the effect of 200 normal cells in normal hosts as standardized in this laboratory.

DISCUSSION

Experiment 4 demonstrated that very large initial inocula of bone marrow cells passaged through a lethally irradiated hosts could perform about as well as non-exposed cells transfused into normal hosts. Thus exposure to an irradiated environment did not necessarily impair the subsequent proliferation of the exposed cells. Yet it must be realized that 200 and 300 million marrow cells are equal to, or exceed the total complement of hemopoietic cells of a mouse (Boggs, 1984). Thus they represent amounts of marrow not ordinarily employed experimentally or clinically.

At lower, though at times still considerable volumes of exposed cells, a definite impairment of proliferation of exposed marrow cells was always noted. That was true when the competitive repopulation assay was employed as in experiments 2 and part of 3, or when exposed cells were re-transfused into a non-irradiated host as in part of experiment 3. The improved proliferation in secondary hosts when the initial inoculum was increased was particularly clear in experiment 2. In summary, proliferation of exposed cells was impaired whether the exposed cells were re-transfused into irradiated or non-irradiated secondary hosts and at different levels of initial inocula. However, the impairment was lessened with increased initial inocula with normalization of proliferation when the number of exposed cells approached or exceeded the total hemopoietic complement of the mouse.

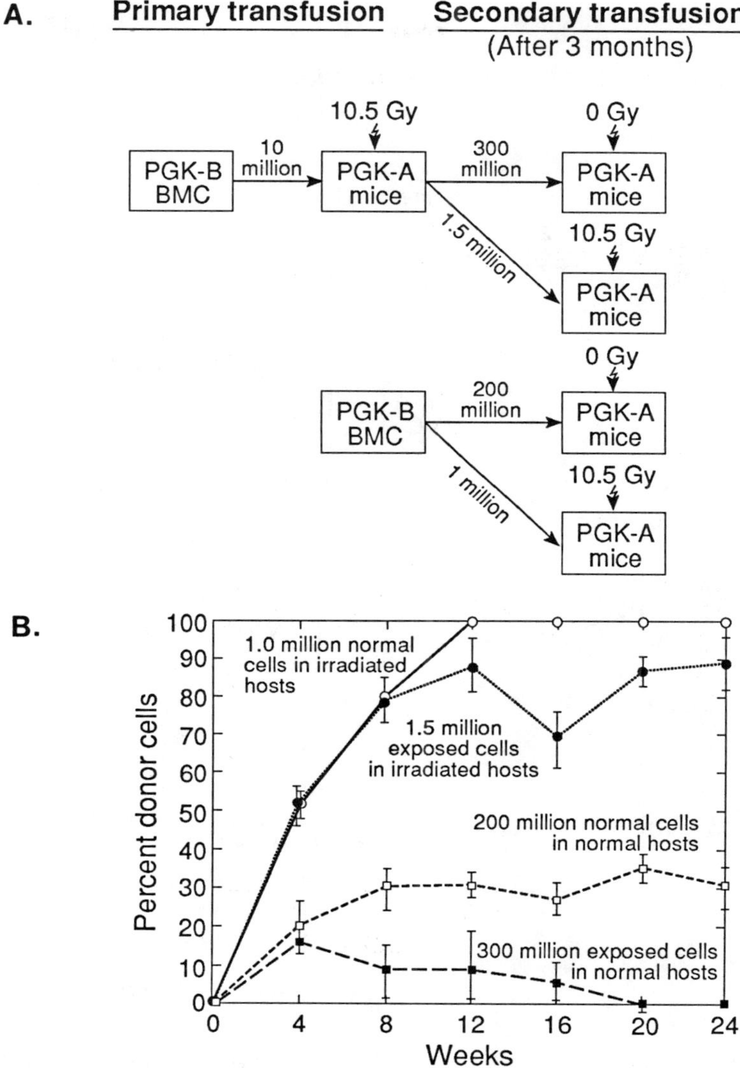

Figure 1. A: Lower curves. 300 million exposed cells (initial inoculum10 million marrow cells) and 200 million normal cells, matched for CFU-S transfused into normal, non-irradiated hosts. B: Upper curves. 1.5 million exposed cells and 1 million normal cells, matched for CFU-S, transfused into irradiated hosts.

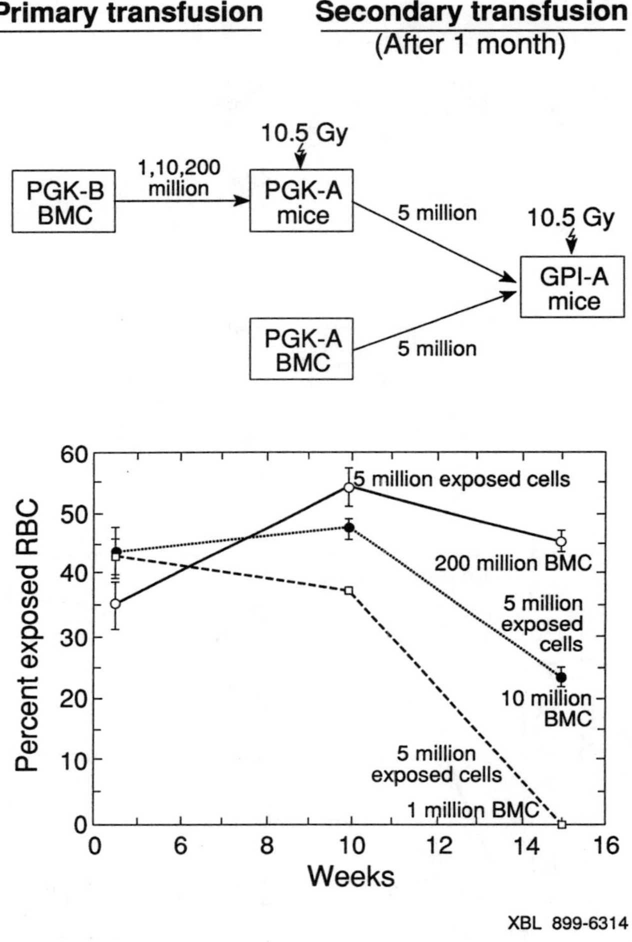

Figure 2. Five million exposed cells (initial inocula 1,10, and 200 million cells) mixed with 5 million normal cells and transfused into irradiated hosts. (Competitive repopulation assay.) Normal cells replace all, 50% and 10 % of exposed cells.

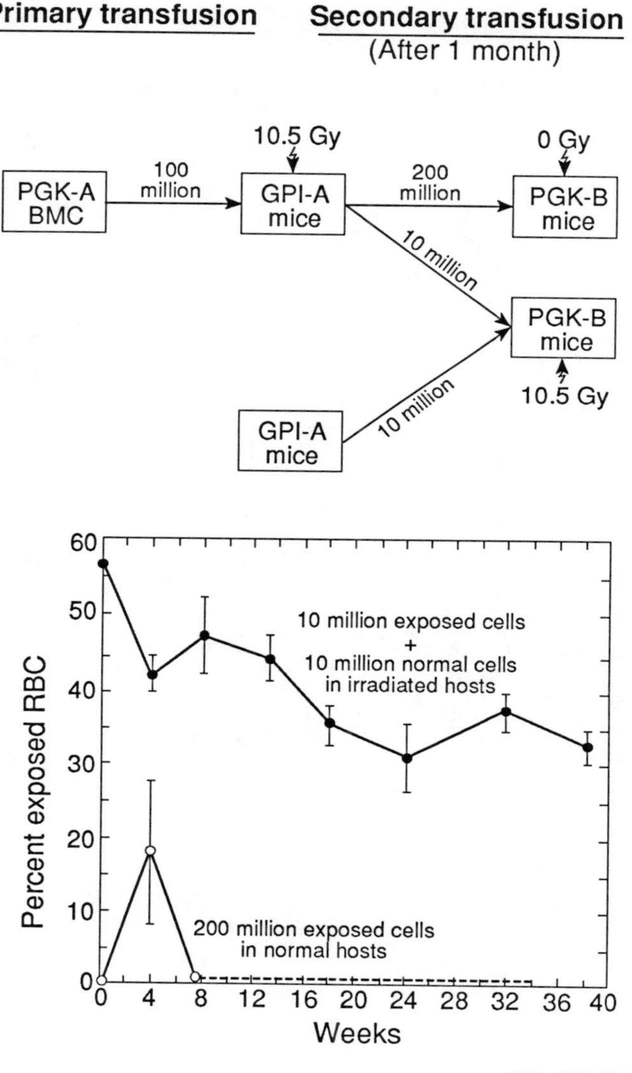

Figure 3. Two hundred million exposed cells (initial inoculum 100 million cells) into normal hosts. 10 million exposed cells of the same suspension mixed with 10 million normal cells. (Competitive repopulation assay). Normal cells replace 60% of exposed cells.

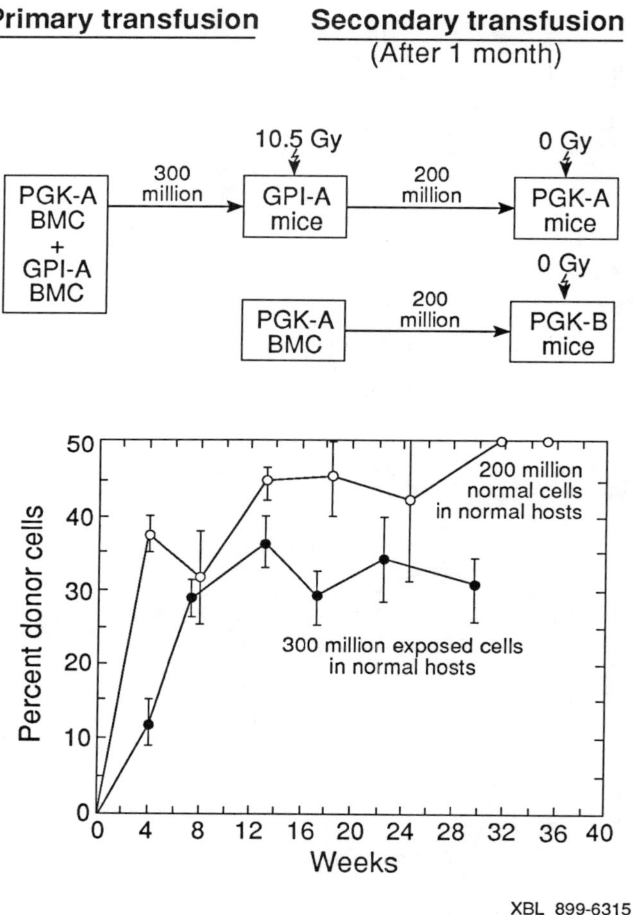

Figure 4. Two hundred million exposed cells (initial inoculum 300 million cells) into normal hosts.200 million normal cells into non-irradiated hosts for comparison.

The results of exposure of marrow cells to an irradiated host may be misleading. For example, Mauch and Hellman (Mauch and Hellman, 1989) observed "Loss of hemopoietic stem cell self-renewal after bone marrow transplantation." As lethally irradiated mice were given 10^5, 10^6, or 10^7 marrow cells, their CFU-S contents improved From these data and their concept of the bone marrow structure, the authors deduced the need for optimizing stem cell number in clinical bone marrow transfusions. From our experiment 1 it does not appear that CFU-S are reliable guides to gauge self renewal of murine stem cells. Based on experiment 4, the optimal number of murine donor cells may be 2 or $3x10^8$ rather than 10^7. Most importantly, the reduced cell self renewal of stem cells is a function of exposure to an irradiated host. Transfusion itself does not alter bone marrow survival and proliferation. This was shown in our lab when normal animals were transfused with normal, non-irradiated marrow and their marrow re-transfused into a second set of normal mice. The percentage take of donor cells remained unchanged. (To be published.)

Conclusions: Passage through a irradiated host reduces bone marrow proliferation in secondary irradiated or unirradiated hosts. Proliferation is normalized when the initial inoculum into the irradiated primary host is increased to match the total complement of marrow cells. At lower levels poor proliferation of transfused bone marrow has been erroneously ascribed to the transfusion itself rather than the passage through an irradiated host.

ACKNOWLEDGMENTS

Sponsored by NIH grant DK27454. Research conducted at Lawrence Berkeley Laboratory, which is supported by the U. S. Department of Energy under contract DE-AC 03-76SF00098.

REFERENCES

Ansell JD, Micklem HS (1986). Genetic markers for following cell populations. In: Weir DM, Herzenberg LA, Blackwell CC (eds) Handbook of experimental immunology, 4th ed vol 2 ch 56. Edinburgh, Blackwell Publishers.

Brecher G, Ansell JD, Micklem HS, Tjio JH, Cronkite EP (1982). Special proliferative sites are not needed for seeding and proliferation of transfused marrow cells in normal syngeneic mice. Proc Natl Acad Sci USA 79:5085-5087.

Boggs DR (1984). Total marrow mass of the mouse. AJ Hematol 16:277-286.

Mauch P. and Hellman S (1989). Loss of hematopoetic stem cell self-renewal after bone marrow transplantation. Blood 74:872-875.

Micklem HS, Ford CE, Evans EP, Ogden DA, Papworth DS (1972). Competitive *in vivo* proliferation of faetal and adult haematopoitic cells in lethally irradiated mice. J Cell Physiol 79:293-298.

Micklem HS (1983). Factors influencing serially transplanted marrows. Blood Cells 9:527-531.

Raveche ES, Santoro T, Brecher G, Tjio JH (1985). Role of T cells in sex differences in syngeneic bone marrow transfusions. Exp Hematol 13:975-980.

Ross EAM, Anderson N, Micklem HS (1982). Serial depletion and regeneration of the murine hematopoietic system. J Exp Med 155:432-444.

Stohlman FJr, Brecher G, Schneiderman M, Cronkite EP (1957). The hemolytic effect of ionizing radiations and its relationship to the hemorrhagic phase of radiation injury. Blood 12:1061-1085.

Till JE, McCullouch EA (1961). Direct measurement of radiation sensitivity of normal bone marrow cells. Radiation Research 14:213.

Wolf NS, Macmillan JR, Priestley GV (1983). Decline of colony forming units with serial bone marrow passage: intrinsic or extrinsic causation? Blood Cells 9:515-525.

The Biology of Hematopoiesis, pages 459–470

PREDICTION OF CLINICAL OUTCOME OF RADIATION ACCIDENT VICTIMS*

Fliedner, T.M., Maiwald, M.**, Weinsheimer, W., Szepesi, T.***

Institute of Occupational and Social Medicine
University of Ulm
D - 7900 Ulm (Donau)

INTRODUCTION

It is the purpose of this presentation to draw first conclusions from the synoptic review of more than 370 persons who received homogeneous as well as inhomogeneous but in all cases total body exposure to ionizing radiation in the course of radiation accidents. We were able to record in our data bank a total of 25 accidents that involved more than 600 persons with clinical signs and symptoms of "radiation sickness" during 1945 and 1987. Of these, so far 55 were analysed in detail with respect to their clinical symptomatology, especially their blood cell changes

* The scientific work was supported by the European Community and the Federal Ministry for the Environment

** Present address: Staatliches Medizinal-, Lebensmittel- und Veterinäruntersuchungsamt Südhessen, Abt.I: Allgemeine Seuchen- und Umwelthygiene, Wilhelminenstr. 2, D - 6100 Darmstadt

*** Present address: Allgemeines Krankenhaus der Stadt Wien Abt. für Strahlentherapie und Strahlenbiologie, Alser Str. 4, A - 1090 Wien

(Fliedner et al. 1988; Szepesi et al. 1988 and Fliedner et al. 1989). The granulocyte patterns were analysed using a computer simulation model in order to calculate the number of "stem cell units" that must have remained in the organism to allow hemopoietic regeneration or not (Fliedner et al. 1988). On this basis it appears possible to describe the early hematological changes (first 5-10 days after accidental exposure) that will predict a spontaneous hemopoietic recovery (with or without "replacement therapy") or that most likely will require a "stem cell substitution therapy" to accomplish hematopoietic reconstitution. Due to the advances made in hematology during the past 2-3 decades, it is possible to utilize appropriate therapeutic measures for these two situations. The transient hematopoietic failure (in case of a situation in which the stem cell pool is damaged but not eradicated) with granulocytopenia as well as thrombocytopenia can be treated by antibiotics, granulocyte as well as platelet tranfusions. The irreversible hematopoietic failure due to destruction of the stem cell pool can - in principle - be overcome by autologous or allogeneic stem cell transplantation. Thus, the key hematological question for the physician in charge seeing a patient that has received an unknown quantity and quality of ionizing radiation exposure is: Does this patient suffer from a reversible or an irreversible hematopoietic stem cell damage?

TYPICAL BLOOD CELL PATTERNS AFTER ACCIDENTAL RADIATION EXPOSURE

It is of great interest to note that there are only a very few principle patterns of blood cell changes seen after accidental whole body radiation exposure. This is not very surprising considering the physiology and pathophysiology of hematopoiesis (Bond et al. 1965). The hematopoietic bone marrow is spread throughout the more than 200 skeletal bones of the human organism. It is very rare to observe in radiation accidents a truely homogeneous whole body irradiation. In most cases, there was a total body exposure but a marked inhomogeneity as far as the effects on the bone marrow in the different skeletal bones is concerned. The blood cell changes observed are the result of the ratio of the influx of newly formed cells from all skeletal sub-units of the bone marrow and the cell efflux from the blood determined by cell emigration or cell death. Thus, if there is any degree of inhomogenous radiation exposure, it is quite likely to assume that cells in the blood have come from unirradiated or less irradiated bone marrow sites and their presence indicates continued cell production in some parts of the marrow. There are two basic hematological response patterns in radiation accidents resulting in whole body exposure.

There is little or no chance for a spontaneous hemopoietic recovery of hemopoiesis if the granulocytes disappear nearly completely by day 6-8 after irradiation, if the platelets show a marked depletion by day 10-12 and if the lympohocytes decrease to very low levels within 1-3 days after exposure. (Fig. 1) ("Irreversible Damage to the Stem Cell Pool").

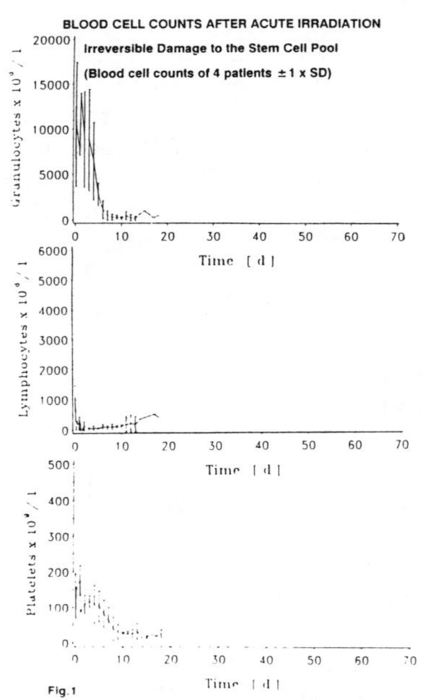

Fig.1

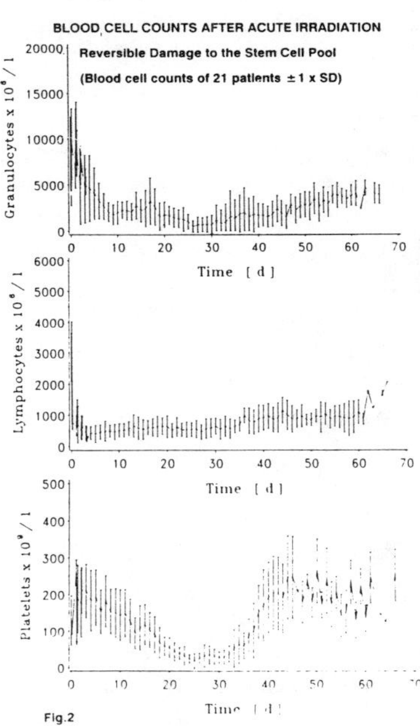

Fig.2

On the other hand, if the granulocyte concentration decreases during the first 10 days after exposure but does not go down to very low levels on day 6-8 (less than 200 per mm^3 blood), then a spontaneous recovery can eventually be expected (using replacement therapy)(Fig. 2). In this case, there is usually seen an "abortive rise"-phase between days 10 and 20 after exposure, and a nadir around day 30 followed by a granulocyte recovery. In these patients, the platelet count does not go down to thrombopenic values during the first 10-12 days but reaches a nadir only after 25-35 days, followed by a spontaneous recovery. In these patients, the lymphocytes demonstrated an early decline to values between 200-700 per mm^3 followed by a slow recovery. ("Reversible Damage to the Stem Cell Pool")

It goes without saying, that one may encounter other radiation accident response patterns. There were a very few patients that had received an extreme radiation exposure involving most likely doses in excess of 3000-4000 cGy (Fliedner et al. 1988, Szepesi et al. 1988). Such a dose causes severe CNS damage and any medical treatment can only aim at the relief of symptoms before the death occurs within 3-5 days (Bond et al. 1965). In such a case, severe skin reactions can be observed and an initial extensive granulocytosis with counts up to 30.000 to 50.000 per mm^3. On the other hand, many "mild" cases have been observed. ["Survival probable category" (Bond et al. 1965)]. In these patients, a total body exposure occurred, but there was hardly any typical pattern of blood cell changes. Blood cell counts performed at around day 30 may reveal in some but not in all cases a certain degree of granulocyte as well as platelet depression but without the no necessity of a symptomatic or prelacement therapy.

COMPUTER SIMULATION MODEL TO CALCULATE THE REMAINING STEM CELLS AVAILABLE FOR HEMOPOIETIC RECONSTITUTION

The pattern of typical granulocyte changes after significant radiation exposure can be simulated by a biomathematical computer model of human granulocytopoiesis that has been described in extenso elsewhere (Fliedner et al. 1987, Fliedner et al. 1988) and that was found to be suitable to describe in the dog several completely different perturbances of the granulocytic cell renewal system (Steinbach et al. 1980). This model consists of several cellular and two regulatory compartments (Fig.3).

Fig. 3

MODEL OF GRANULOCYTOPOIESIS

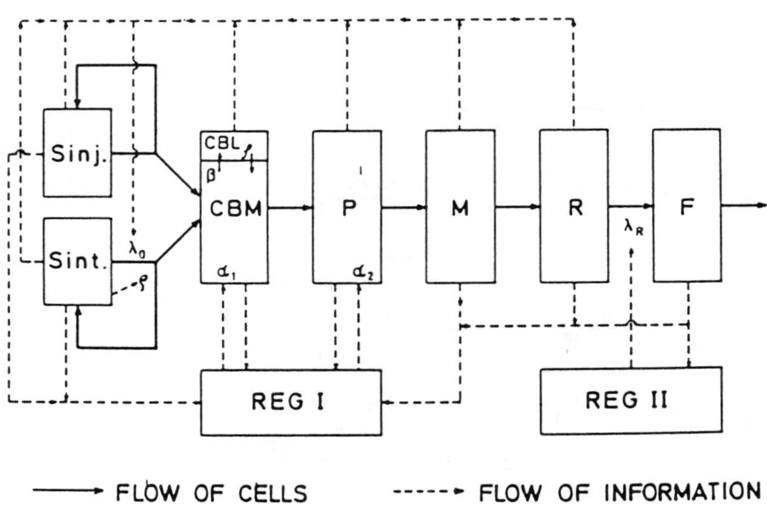

It is based on the assumption that a certain number of granulocytes are at any one time in the blood pool "F" characterized by a transit time of 10 hours. Any cell entering the blood compartment will be replaced by a cell from the reserve compartment "R" which in turn is replaced by a cell from the maturation compartment "M". There is a corresponding production of new cells in the proliferative compartment "P". The compartment transit times for man and the renewal characteristics have been measured previously by radioactive labeling methods (Bond et al. 1965). There is a compartment of committed stem cells in the bone marrow ("CBM") which is in equilibrium with a compartment of circulating stem cells ("CBL"). This stem cell compartment is balanced by a compartment of pluripotent stem cells "S". After total body exposure, it is assumed that some stem cells remain intact or an repaired ("int"), and some are qualitatively injured (inj) so that their replicative potential is limited. The relationship of injured to intact or repaired stem cells will depend on the degree of homogeneity or inhomogeneity of radiation exposure and on other factors, such as radiation quality. It is also assumed that there are - in principle - 2 regulator compartments (Reg. I and II).

Tab. 1 Computer Derived Calculations of Stem Cell Pool Sizes

Radiation Response Category	Remaining Intact Stem Cells % (Cell number)	Remaining Injured Stem Cells % (Cell number)	Destroyed Stem Cells %	Ranges of Physical Dose Estimates in cGy
Category II Pat. 4,5,38	0.008 (1.0×10^5)	24.0 (3.0×10^8)	76	127 - 236
Category III Pat. 1, 3	0.0024 (3.0×10^4)	4.8 (6.0×10^7)	95	339 - 365
Category IV Pat. 11,12,13	0.0008 (1.0×10^4)	2.4 (3.0×10^7)	97.6	323 - 426
Category V Pat. 17, 37	0 (0)	0.0006 (7.7×10^3)	99.9994	1.114 - 1.200

In table 1 it is shown, that the pattern of granulocyte changes seen in 3 patients of "Category IV" ("reversible stem cell pool injuriy") can be simulated if one assumes, that the number of stem cells that remained intact or were repaired to allow a spontaneous hematopoietic recovery was 1.0 x 10 or 0.008% of normal. In the case of 2 patients classified in "Category V" ("irreversible stem cell pool injury"), there was no evidence of intact or repaired stem cells but a very few injured cells.

The details of the analyses made were described elsewhere (Fliedner et al. 1988). It appears sufficient in this paper to indicate that the observed granulocyte values as a function of time after exposure in the Categories V and IV (irreversible or reversible stem cell pool damage, respectively) can be simulated by computer desived curves (solid line) fitting the points using the biomathematical model described (Figs. 4 and 5). The patients assigned to category V were exposed in Los Alamos 1946 and in Brescia 1975, those in category IV in Vinca 1958.

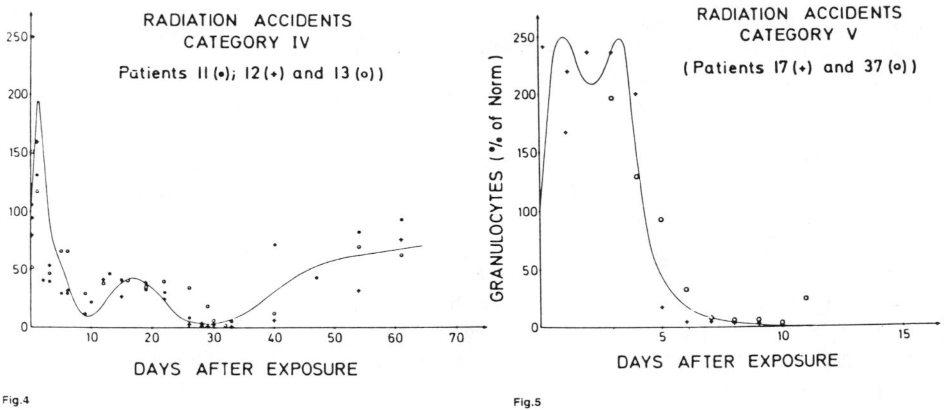

Fig.4

Fig.5

HEMATOLOGICAL PREDICTORS OF THE ACUTE RADIATION SYNDROME

The decisive question for the clinical management of accidentally radiation exposed persons is whether or not one might expect a spontaneous recovery of the hematopoietic cell renewal systems or not. There are of course a variety of other variables to be considered, such as the question of the extend of the involvement of the central nervous system or of the skin (as was the case in a number of persons involved in the Chernobyl accident) (Gustokova et al. 1986). In these cases, it is of course necessary to find answers to the question, whether there is a chance of successful treatment of the resulting symptomatology or not (CNS-syndrome, skin burns). The mortality in Chernobyl, for instance, was due largely to the severe skin burns while it was evident that the hematopoietic systems received a reversible radiation injury, not requiring stem cell substitution therapy (Gustokova et al. 1986).

In all instances, however, in which patients presented themselves as "uncomplicated" radiation accident victims (i.e. not complicated by additional chemical or physical injury such as burns or cuts) it is important to obtain as soon as possible an answer to the question, whether a reversible or an irreversible damage to the stem cell pool must be assumed.

The analysis of the 373 radiation accident victims registered in our data bank is in accordance with the following conclusions:

An irreversible damage to the stem cell pool is likely, if the following constellation of blood cell changes is observed during the first 6-8 days after exposure: (Fig. 1)the granulocyte changes are characterized by an initial granulocytosis during days 1-3, followed by a rather abrupt granulocyte decline during days 4-6 to low values of less than 200-400 per mm^3 on days 6-8. This pattern is in accordance with a complete interruption of cell replication, and proliferation in the precursor and progenitor cell pools in the marrow but a "maturing out" of cells residing in the maturing and the reserve pool of cells. The platelet pattern with a progressive decline of platelet numbers reaching a nadir already at day 10-12 is compatible also with a cessation of new platelet formation in the megakaryocyte pools. The life span of platelets is known to be about 10 days so that a platelet nadir at this time indicates the disappearance of platelets according to their age without replenishment from precursor pools. The lymphocytes show very low values of less than 10-20% of normal within 24 hours. This decline can be attributed to the high radiation sensibility of lymphocytes but also to the perturbation of the physiological mechanisms of recirculation. The pathophysiological mechanisms resulting in this pattern were described in extenso previously (Bond et al. 1965).

It is this pattern of blood cell changes clearly recognizable within 6-8 days after exposure but to be suspected on this basis of the severe lymphopenia accompanied by a pronounced granulocytosis within 24-48 hours that is compatible with the diagnosis of an <u>irreversible stem cell pool change.</u> The computer calculations used indicate that the fraction of stem cells that remained intact in less than 0.0008% of normal and that more than 98% of the stem cell pool was destroyed (Table 1).

In such a situation, the only therapy that may result in a survival of the patient would be stem cell substitution. Usually, the stem cells might come from the bone marrow or peripheral blood of histocompatible donors (allogeneic transplantation). It is important to consider adequate conditioning regimens in analogy to the treatment of patients with severe aplastic anemia (Storb et al. 1974). In some cases, autologous stem cells might be available collected from bone marrow or blood from persons "at risk" for accidental radiation exposure (Körbling et al. 1986). In the future, there may be opportunities for the use of fetal liver derived stem cells, the use of which at the present time must be considered as highly experimental (Prümmer and Fliedner 1986).

Such a pattern compatible with an irreversible damage to the stem cell pool is clearly distinguishable from blood cell changes compatible with a <u>reversible damage to the stem cell pool</u> (Fig. 2). In all patients that showed a spontaneous hematopoietic recovery starting 30 - 40 days after accidental radiation exposure, the following initial changes are characteristic: the granulocytes may show a moderate initial granulocytosis (1-3 days) and a subsequent decline with a first nadir around 8-10 days. However, it is evident that on days 5-8, there are always a few granulocytes present in the blood (at least 300-600 per mm^3). The examination of leukocyte cell concentrates may indicate the presence of granulocytes with "mitotically connected abnormalities" (giant cells) (Bond et al. 1965). Such a pattern is compatible with the assumption of some granulocyte production and maturation somewhere in the skeletal bone marrow and any degree of inhomogeneity of exposure will favour such a pattern. The granulocyte course in all these cases of "reversible stem cell pool damage"is characterized by an "abortive" granulocyte recovery (days 10-20) followed by a secondary decline with a nadir around day 25-35. This abortive rise was explained on the basis of the "injured cell"-hypothesis advanced previously (Bond et al. 1965) and discussed recently (Fliedner et al. 1988). It appears likely, that the time of the occurrence of the secondary nadir is related to the degree of stem cell pool injury. The platelet pattern corresponding to a "reversible" stem cell pool damage is characterized by a platelet nadir around 25-35 days. The initial pattern during the first 10 days does not show a progressive decline. The number of platelets at day 6-10 is usually above 100.000 per mm^3. The lymphocyte count that corresponds to this pattern shows an initial decline to about 50% of normal within one day, and values of about30% of normal at day 2 but not the extreme decline seen in the "irreversible damage" category. The calculation presented in table 1 indicate that the fractions of stem cells remaining intact or that are repaired must be more than 0.0008% of normal.

The assignment of a patient to the "reversible stem cell pool damage"-category does not mean, of course, that no specific therapy is needed. It means that it is likely that a "replacement therapy" in a sterile environment using antibiotics, granulocyte and platelet transfusions is sufficient to bridge the phase of a transient hematopoietic failure.

THE NEED FOR BIOLOGICAL INDICATORS IN RADIATION ACCIDENT MANAGEMENT

The data presented indicate a renewed approach to define "hematological indicators" to characterize the "strain" to the hematopoietic tissue distributed throughout the skeleton inflicted by the "stress" to the organisms due to whole body exposure. Since hemopoiesis is such a complex organ system, it will be impossible or improbable in radiation accident situations to describe any "radiation dose" in any term meaningful to the clinical management. Rather, it should be the goal to describe the biological consequences in terms that are used in "biological monitoring" in occupational medicine after exposure to toxic chemicals. The data presented indicate that "hematological indictors" are of central importance and are available early after exposure to predict the later biological consequences and to develop plans for appropriate clinical management. Furthermore, the data and concepts presented will allow one to develop an "expert system" to support the clinical decision making in radiation accident handling.

SUMMARY

On the basis of the analysis of more than 350 individuals that were exposed to ionizing radiation in the course of more than 25 radiation accidents reported world wide since 1945, a biomathematical computer model was developed that simulates the pattern of granulocyte changes seen. It allows one to calculate the number of stem cells remaining intact to initiate recovery. It is shown that the major question to be asked is whether a spontaneous stem cell recovery can be expected or not. This question can be readily answered within 3-5 days after radiation exposure on the basis of the constellation of hematopoietic findings and desived stem cell pool size calculations.

REFERENCES

Bond VP, Fliedner TM, Archambean JO (1965). Mammalian Radiation Lethality, A Disturbance in Cellular Kinetics. Academic Press, New York and London.

Fliedner TM, Steinbach KH (1987). Simulationsmodelle von Perturbationen des granulozytären Zellerneuerungssystems. In: Doerr W, Schipperges H (Hrsg.): Modelle der Pathologischen Physiologie, Springer Verlag, Heidelberg.

Fliedner TM (1989). Steinbach KH, Szepesi T (1988). Hematological Indicators in the Determination of Clinical Management Strategies in Radiation Accidents. Proceedings of the International Conference on Biological Effects of Large Dose Ionizing and Non-ionizing Radiation, pp 60-91.

Fliedner TM. Hematological Indicators to Predict Patient Recovery after Whole Body Irradiation as a Basis for Clinical Management. In Ricks RC, Fry SA (eds): The Medical Basis for Radiation Accident Preparedness, Second Edition, Elsevier Science Publishing Company, Inc., New York, in press.

Gustkova B, Baranov V (1986). Chernobyl Radiation Accident 1986. Medical-Biological Problems. Size of the dose received and consequences for health. Experience of Treatment. Expert Meeting, IAEA, Vienna.

Körbling M, Dörken B et al. (1986). Autologous Transplantation of Blood-Derived Hemopoietic Stem Cells After Myeloablative Therapy in a Patient With Burkitt's Lymphoma. Blood 67:529-532.

Prümmer O, Fliedner TM (1986). The fetal liver as an alternative stem cell source for hemolymphopoietic reconstitution. Int J Cell Cloning 4:237-249.

Steinbach KH, Ruffler H, Pabst G, Fliedner TM (1980). A mathematical model of canine granulocytopoiesis. J Math Biol 10, 1.

Storb R, Thomas ED, Buckner CD et al. (1974). Allogeneic Marrow Grafting for Treatment of Aplastic Anemia. Blood 43: 157-180.

Szepesi T, Fliedner TM, Steinbach KH (1988). Hematological Responses after Accidential Exposure to Ionizing Radiation: A Review of 22 reported Accidents. In: Proceedings of the International Conference on Biological Effects of Large Dose Ionizing and Non-ionizing radiation, pp 30-60, 1988. Eds. Zhang Qing-XI and Wu De-Chang, Society of Radiation Medicine and Protection Beijing, 1988.

The Biology of Hematopoiesis, pages 471–478

RADIOPROTECTION AND THERAPY OF RADIATION INJURY WITH CYTOKINES

Ruth Neta

Department of Experimental Hematology
Armed Forces Radiobiology Research Institute
Bethesda, Maryland 20814

INTRODUCTION

Inflammatory agents, such as bacterial lipopolysacharides (LPS), were shown 30 years ago to enhance host defenses against the damaging effects of ionizing radiation (Ainsworth and Chase, 1959). Because LPS (and similar agents) induces a multitude of inflammatory pathways, it is difficult to determine the mechanisms leading to radioprotection. The finding that interleukin 1 (IL 1), a cytokine induced by LPS, is radioprotective (Neta et al., 1986a) allows more direct studies of the radioprotective pathways, based on the defined functions of IL 1 and its action on specific cellular receptors.

RADIOPROTECTION WITH INTERLEUKIN 1

Our previous work has shown that administration of IL 1 protects mice from radiation death in the dose range that results in hematopoietic failure. This protection depends on the dose and time of administration of IL 1 (Neta et al., 1986b; 1986d). With doses ranging from 0.1 μg to 1.0 μg, optimal protection was obtained when IL 1 was administered 20 hrs before irradiation. The necessity for a lag period between IL 1 treatment and irradiation suggests that radioprotection is mediated by other agents induced with IL 1.

Pharmacological doses of prostaglandin confer radioprotection. However, radioprotection with IL 1 does not depend on prostaglandin induction, because indomethacin and aspirin do not reduce the radioprotective effect of IL 1 (Neta et al., 1986c). IL 1 induces production of metallothionein and ceruloplasmin, two acute phase proteins with scavenging properties, that may contribute to radioprotection. IL 1 also induces manganese superoxide dismutase (Mn/SOD), an antioxidant enzyme that converts superoxide into hydrogen peroxide (Wong and Goeddel, 1988). The importance of this enzyme in resistance to radiation has been demonstrated in several systems (Marklund et al., 1984). However, much higher doses of IL 1 were required to enhance production of Mn/SOD in the liver than to induce radioprotection within 20 hrs (10 μg vs. 0.1 μg) (Vaishnav et al., 1989). Whereas a 0.1 μg dose of IL 1 was most effective when given 20 hrs before irradiation, a 10 μg dose of IL 1 was equally effective when given 20 hrs or 3 hrs before irradiation. Thus, SOD may be one of several factors that contribute to radioprotection with IL 1.

Because the survival of irradiated mice parallels the recovery of the hematopoietic system, the effect of IL 1 on bone marrow cells was assessed in irradiated and normal mice. In irradiated mice, bone marrow cellularity in control and IL 1 treated mice declines similarly during the first 3 days after irradiation, to reach only 0.2% to 0.3% of the original cell numbers (Neta et al., 1986b). Whereas the irradiated control group showed only small increases in cell numbers, viable cell counts increased gradually from day 5 to day 12 in the IL 1 treated group. A comparison of colony forming cells in the two groups at day 12 showed an 8-fold increase in CFU-E, 20-fold increase in GM-CFU, and 3-4-fold increase in day 8 CFU-s in the IL 1 treated group over irradiated control mice (Schwartz et al., 1987).

Treatment of normal, non-irradiated mice with radioprotective doses of IL 1 did not induce an increase in the numbers of CFU-s, CFU-E, BFU-E, or GM-CFU within 20 hrs. However, within hours of injection with IL 1, enhanced cycling of GM-CFU and BFU-E have been observed (Schwartz et al., 1989). These results indicate that although IL 1 does not increase the number of progenitor cells in the marrow, the cycling of these cells was greatly increased. The late S-phase of the cell cycle was reported by several researchers to be the most radioresistant phase of the cell cycle. Therefore, it is possible that more cycling cells in IL 1 treated mice survive radiation. However, these cells cannot be accounted for in colony assays carried out immediately after irradiation. Further studies are required to explain the accelerated recovery of the hematopoietic system in irradiated IL 1 treated mice.

INTERACTION OF INTERLEUKIN 1 WITH OTHER CYTOKINES

IL 1 acts as a pleiotropic cytokine, probably because of the divergent activities of the numerous responding cell types. Hematopoietic stem cells and progenitor cells, endothelial cells, hepatocytes, fibroblasts, macrophages, and neutrophils are some of the cells that exhibit characteristic responses to IL 1 (Dinarello, 1989). IL 1 induces many of these cells to produce other cytokines, including CSFs, IL 6, and TNF. IL 1 also interacts with these newly induced cytokines to augment and further diversify its biological effects. Therefore, we have conducted experiments to establish the interaction of IL 1 with TNF, CSFs, and IL 6 in radioprotection of mice.

Our initial experiments established that from a battery of recombinant cytokines, including IL 1, GM-CSF, G-CSF, IL 6, and TNF, only IL 1 and TNF are radioprotective when used alone prior to lethal irradiation of mice (Neta et al., 1986c; 1988a; 1988b). Of the two, IL 1 was more efficacious, as it was required in lower doses and achieved a greater degree of protection (dose reduction factor (DRF) for IL 1 was 1.25 and for TNF 1.15 in B6D2F1 mice). Despite a similar range of biological effects, the two cytokines in combination had a synergistic effect on survival, suggesting that the two may employ different pathways.

GM-CSF or G-CSF given alone in doses ranging from 1 to 10 μg/mouse had no significant protective effect against lethal doses of radiation (Neta et al., 1986c). However, administration of these growth factors in combination with suboptimal doses of IL 1 resulted in synergistic radioprotection (Neta et al., 1988a). Thus, in the presence of IL 1, both G-CSF and GM-CSF are radioprotective. A similar situation occurred using IL 6. This cytokine shares with IL 1 a number of biological effects, such as induction of fever, neutrophilia and the acute phase response (Wong and Clark, 1988). In the absence of IL 1, IL 6 administration resulted in a higher death rate for irradiated mice but with suboptimal doses of IL 1, IL 6 was radioprotective (Neta et al. 1988b). Thus, as with G-CSF and GM-CSF, IL 6 interacts synergistically with IL 1 to confer radioprotection.

Administration of IL 1 results in the presence of high titers of CSF in circulation (Vogel et al., 1986). Similarly, IL 1 induces high titers of IL 6 in circulation (Neta et al., 1988b). Thus, the presence of the hematopoietic growth factors, which interact with IL 1, may expand the proliferative capacity of hematopoietic stem cells. This interaction may be the basis for the increased number of cycling cells in the bone marrow of IL 1 treated mice (Neta et al., 1987).

In conclusion, the radioprotective effect of IL 1 may depend on the induction of and interaction with TNF, CSF's, and IL 6, all induced with IL 1.

RESTORATION OF RADIATION INDUCED MYELOTOXICITY WITH IL 1

Our initial work has shown that IL 1 given before, but not after, lethal irradiation ($LD_{100/30}$) protects mice from death. However, sublethally irradiated mice that received IL 1 after irradiation showed accelerated bone marrow recovery (Neta et al., 1986c). Because IL 1 induces CSF and has hematopoietin 1 activity (Moore and Warren, 1987), i.e. it promotes proliferation of early progenitor cells, we reasoned that IL 1 may be useful in promoting bone marrow recovery and survival of irradiated animals. To test this hypothesis we examined two systems for the effect of IL 1 given after irradiation. First, IL 1 was tested in irradiated ($LD_{95/30}$) mice and second, IL 1 was given with syngeneic or allogeneic bone marrow transplants to lethally irradiated mice.

Reversal of radiation induced myelotoxicity

IL 1 promoted survival of mice in a dose-dependent manner when given within 24 hrs after an $LD_{95/30}$ dose of radiation (Neta and Oppenheim, 1988). Doses of 0.15 μg of IL 1 resulted in 30% survival while 10 μg of IL 1 were required to achieve 100% survival. Thus, much higher doses of IL 1 were necessary to restore hematopoiesis after irradiation than to protect the hematopoietic system. Because IL 1 was not effective in treating mice receiving radiation doses higher than the $LD_{95/30}$, IL 1 probably acts on a few surviving stem cells or progenitor cells to expand them. IL 1 production was reported to be induced by irradiation (Ansel et al., 1983), suggesting that endogenously produced IL 1 may aid in prevention or repair of damage. The greater effectiveness of high (rather than low) doses of IL 1 suggests that induction of intracellular Mn/SOD may contribute to a higher rate of recovery of bone marrow progenitor cells.

Interleukin 1 in bone marrow transplantation

The apparent ability of IL 1 to promote proliferation

of bone marrow cells suggested that IL 1 may be beneficial when used with bone marrow transplantation. We conducted experiments to evaluate (1) whether IL 1 treatment combined with syngeneic or allogeneic bone marrow cell transplantation results in enhanced mice survival, (2) whether fewer allogeneic bone marrow cells will be sufficient for survival under these conditions, and (3) whether bone marrow engraftment can be enhanced with IL 1.

IL 1 treatment before and after 15 Gy irradiation of C3H/HeN mice ($LD_{100/30}$ = 8.5 Gy) did not affect survival. Transplantation of syngeneic bone marrow cells to these mice resulted in 50% survival. Combined use of 10 μg IL 1, given either before or after irradiation, with bone marrow cells resulted in 90% survival of mice (Neta et al., 1989). Thus, at doses of radiation that approach death due to gastro-intestinal failure, treatment with IL 1 enhances survival. It remains to be determined whether IL 1 treatment may be beneficial at the doses of radiation that result in the gastrointestinal syndrome.

IL 1 was also tested in combination with allogeneic bone marrow transplantion. C57Bl/6 mice ($H\text{-}2^b$) were given suboptimal numbers (<15×10^6) of T depleted Balb/c ($H\text{-}2^d$) bone marrow cells (Oppenheim et al., 1989). Following a 12 Gy dose of irradiation, all untreated $C57Bl/_6$ mice or mice given 10 μg IL 1 following irradiation, died with a median survival time of 11 days. Similarly, mice receiving 2.5×10^6 bone marrow cells, with and without IL 1, died with mean survival time of 12 days. Mice that received 5×10^6 bone marrow cells without IL 1 died with a mean survival time of 15 days. In contrast, 75% of mice given IL 1 in addition to 5×10^6 bone marrow cells survived >20 weeks. Similarly, addition of IL 1 to 10×10^6 transplanted bone marrow cells promoted survival from 40% of those given bone marrow alone to 92% of those given bone marrow plus IL 1.

Phenotypic analysis of spleen cells obtained from mice 1.5 to 5 months after treatment with 10×10^6 bone marrow cells and IL 1 revealed that all mice (8 out 8) were reconstituted predominantly (74% to 92%) with donor ($H\text{-}2^d$) cells. However, 4% to 23% of recipient phenotype cells were still present. These mixed chimeric mice were also examined for their capacity to generate in vitro cytotoxic T-lymphocyte reactivity against host ($H\text{-}2^b$), donor ($H\text{-}2^d$), and third-party ($H\text{-}2^k$) target cells. Pooled spleen cells from $C57Bl/_6$ recipient mice reconstituted with more than 86% Balb/c phenotype did not generate a lytic effect for donor or recipient, H-2^b or H-2^d cells, but lysed allogeneic H-2^k target cells. This suggests that the T-cells in the chimeric mice that survive for more than 6 weeks were not only tolerant to both donor and recipient MHC antigens, but were also immunologically competent.

Similarly, enhanced survival of mice could be reproduced at even higher doses of recipient irradiation. For example, whereas only 8% of mice given 13.5 Gy irradiation and 10×10^6 bone marrow cells alone survived, 75% of mice treated with 10×10^6 bone marrow cells and IL 1 survived more than 45 days. However, the degree of chimerism of these mice was similar to that observed after 12 Gy irradiation, indicating that some recipient stem cells survived after a dose of 13.5 Gy.

SUMMARY AND CONCLUSIONS

Our results demonstrate that IL 1 promotes hematopoiesis in normal and radiation-compromised animals. IL 1 protected mice from lethal hematopoietic syndrome when given before irradiation. Given therapeutically after irradiation, IL 1 promoted recovery from radiation injury.

Several activities of IL 1 may explain its bone marrow restorative properties. The induction with IL 1 of several hematopoietic growth factors (GM-CSF, G-CSF, M-CSF, IL 3, and IL 6) clearly contributes to the accelerated growth and differentiation of hematopoietic progenitor cells. The induction of scavenger proteins may reduce oxidative damage after irradiation.

Our work raises a number of additional questions concerning the potential therapeutic utility of IL 1. The ability of IL 1 to promote engraftment of allogeneic bone marrow cells will require further study. The optimal dosage, schedule, and route for IL 1 induction of hematopoiesis will need to be established. The observed synergy of IL 1 with TNF, IL 6, or CSF's may be useful in reducing the requisite doses of cytokines from pharmacological to physiological levels, thus reducing toxic effects. The observation that the cyclooxygenase inhibitor, indomethacin, does not inhibit IL 1 radioprotection may allow us to combat some of the toxic manifestations of IL 1 and to preserve its beneficial actions.

Clinical trials with IL 1 in patients, now in progress, should establish whether this cytokine may be useful in reversing the myelotoxic effects of radiotherapy and chemotherapy in humans.

ACKNOWLEDGEMENTS

I thank Dr. G. D. Ledney for review of this manuscript. This work was supported by the Armed Forces Radiobiology Research Institute, Defense Nuclear Agency, under Research Work Unit 4440-00129. The opinions contained herein are the private views of the author; no endorsement by the Defense Nuclear Agency has been given or should be inferred. The research was conducted according to the principles enunciated in the "Guide for the Care and Use of Laboratory Animals" prepared by the Institute of Laboratory Animal Resources, National Research Council.

REFERENCES

Ainsworth EJ, Chase HB (1959). Effect of microbial antigens on irradiation mortality in mice. Proc Soc Exp Biol Med 102:483-485.

Ansel JC, Luger TA, Green I (1983). The effect of in vitro and in vivo UV irradiation on the production of ETAF by human and murine keratenocytes. J Invest Dermatol 81:519.

Dinarello CA (1989). Interleukin-1 and its biologically related cytokines. Adv Immunol 44:153-205.

Marklund SL, Westman NG, Roos G, Carlsson J (1984). Radiation resistance and the CuZn superoxide dismutase, Mn superoxide dismutase, catalase, and glutathione peroxidase activities of seven human cell lines. Radiat Res 100:115-123.

Moore MAS, Warren DJ (1987). Synergy of interleukin-1 and granulocyte colony stimulating factor; In vivo stimulation of stem cell recovery and hematopoietic regeneration following 5-fluorouracil treatment of mice. Proc Natl Acad Sci USA 84:7134-7138.

Neta R, Douches SD, Oppenheim JJ (1986a). Interleukin-1 is a radioprotector. J Immunol 136:2483-2485.

Neta R, Douches SD, Oppenheim JJ (1986b). Radioprotection by interleukin-1. In: Immunoregulation by Characterized Polypeptides. UCLA Symposia on Molecular Biology, eds. G Goldstein, JF Bach, H Wigzal, 41:429-441.

Neta R, Oppenheim JJ, Douches SD, Giclas PC, Imbra RJ, Karin M (1986c). Radioprotection with IL-1. Comparison with other cytokines. In: Progress in Immunology, eds B Cinader and RG Miller, Academic Press, New York, VI:900-909.

Neta R, Vogel SN, Oppenheim JJ, Douches SD (1986d). Cytokines in radioprotection. Comparison of the radioprotective effects of IL-1 to IL-2, GM-CSF, and IFN. Lymphokine Res 5:S105-S110.

Neta R, Sztein MB, Oppenheim JJ, Gillis S, Douches SD (1987). In vivo effects of IL-1. I. Bone marrow cells are induced to cycle following administration of IL-1. J Immunol 139:1861-1866.

Neta R, Oppenheim JJ (1988). Cytokines in therapy of radiation injury. Blood 72:1093-1095.

Neta R, Oppenheim JJ, Douches SD (1988a). Interdependence of the radioprotective effects of human recombinant IL-1, TNF, G-CSF, and murine recombinant G-CSF. J Immunol 140:108-111.

Neta R, Vogel SN, Sipe JD, Wong GG, Nordan RP (1988b). Comparison of in vivo effects of human recombinant IL 1 and human recombinant IL 6 in mice. Lymphokine Res 7:403-412.

Neta R, Tiebergen P, Gress R, Kenny J, Longo DL, Oppenheim JJ (1989). Tumor necrosis factor, interleukin 1, and interferon γ enhance survival of lethally irradiated mice. Exp Hematol 17:712.

Oppenheim JJ, Neta R, Tibergen P, Gress R, Kenny J, Longo DL (1989). Interleukin 1 enhances survival of lethally irradiated mice treated with allogeneic bone marrow cells. Blood, in press.

Schwartz GN, MacVittie TJ, Vigneulle RM, Patchen ML, Douches SD, Oppenheim JJ, Neta R (1987). Enhanced hematopoietic recovery in irradiated mice pretreated with interleukin-1 (IL-1). Immunopharmacol Immunotoxicol 9:371-389.

Schwartz GN, Patchen ML, Neta R, MacVittie TJ (1989). An increase in the number of spleen colony-forming units (CFU-s) at the time of irradiation is not necessary for the radioprotection of mice pretreated with interleukin-1. Radiat Res 119:101-112.

Vaishnav YN, Kumar KS, Weiss JF, Neta R (1989). Induction of superoxide dismutase: A mechanism for radioprotection by interleukin-1 (IL-1)? 37th Annual Meeting of the Radiation Research Society, Seattle, Washington, p. 185.

Vogel SN, Douches SD, Kaufman EN, Neta R (1987). Induction of colony stimulating factor in vivo by recombinant interleukin-1 α and recombinant tumor necrosis factor α. J Immunol 138:2143-2148.

Wong GG, Clark SC (1988). Multiple actions of interleukin 6 within a cytokine network. Immunology Today 9:137-139.

Wong GHW, Goeddel DV (1988). Induction of manganous superoxide dismutase by tumor necrosis factor. Possible protective mechanism. Science 242:941-944.

The Biology of Hematopoiesis, pages 479–491

FACTORS INFLUENCING RECONSTITUTION BY BONE MARROW TRANSPLANTATION.

Radiobiological Institute, P.O. Box 5815, 2280 HV Rijswijk, The Netherlands [1],
and
Dept. Radiobiology of the Erasmus University Rotterdam [2].

D.W. van Bekkum[1) 2)], J.J. Wielenga[1)], F. van Gils[2)] and G. Wagemaker[2)].

Introduction.

Bone Marrow Transplantation (BMT) is most commonly practiced to treat patients suffering from irreversible bone marrow aplasia. The aplasia may be spontaneous, drug induced, or caused by exposure to a lethal dose of Total Body Irradiation (TBI). In the treatment of leukemia patients, a combination of chemotherapeutic agents and high-dose TBI is employed to eradicate malignant cells and BMT is subsequently required to rescue the patient by way of reconstitution of hemopoiesis. The latter can be achieved with an allogeneic BM graft or with autologous bone marrow collected during remission and cryopreserved until needed.

Reconstitution of hemopoiesis is dependent on a take of the grafted stem cells, which in the case of allogeneic grafts requires a sufficiently strong immunosuppression of the recipient to prevent rejection.

Timely reconstitution is dependent on the number of BM (stem) cells grafted in the case of both allogeneic and autologous grafts; more cells being needed of allogeneic than of autologous bone marrow. At a symposium on _In vitro Culture of Hemopoietic Cells_ in 1971 in the Radiobiological Institute TNO at Rijswijk, The Netherlands, the crucial role of pluripotent stem cells in providing reconstitution was stressed by Fred Stohlman as follows: "You measured takes of bone marrow grafts in terms of thrombocyte and reticulocyte recovery. So I would infer that you have contamination there with a more pluripotent stem cell than that which gives rise to the colonies in agar, although you think they are both the same" (1). It is interesting that < 25 years (1971-1990) later we employ the rate of recovery of peripheral blood cells as one of the most reliable measures of the number of pluripotent stem cells grafted, as will be described later in this paper.

The take of allografts is negatively influenced by increasing immunogenetic difference between donor and recipient, by decreasing the number of T-lymphocytes in the grafted marrow and by gastro-intestinal decontamination of the recipient (Table 1).

As compared to single-dose TBI, fractionation of TBI necessitates a substantial adjustment (increase) of total dose of radiation (Table 2). Graft rejection is generally ascribed to surviving T-lymphocytes of the recipient. Given the small shoulder of the published survival curves for lymphocytes, another factor than recovery from sublethal radiation damage has to account for this effect of fractionation.

Recent attempts to fit the experimental data in the mouse to lymphocyte survival curves with varying Do and shoulders have led us to the conclusion that repopulation of surviving lymphoid cells at a rate of 2 cells divisions per 24 hours could explain the larger total dose required upon fractionation (3).

When optimal conditions for a take of allogeneic grafts are established, the major set-back has been the development of Graft-versus-Host-Disease (GvHD) during or after hemopoietic reconstitution. GvHD is accompanied by severe immune deficiency, and immune reconstitution only occurs after the acute GvHD has subsided. Chronic GvHD is characterised by a dysfunction of the immune system (4).

Even in the case of MHC identical sibling donor marrow, the incidence of acute GvHD has been high (up to 50%) with a significant mortality (25% of all recipients) mostly due to severe infections. These figures apply to patients given post-transplantation immunosuppressive therapy, such as methotrexate or cyclosporin A. In Rhesus monkeys, not given such prophylactic immunosuppressive agents, mortality from GvHD following transplantation of Rhesus LA matched sibling marrow was 85% (5).

It was demonstrated as early as 1964 that lymphocytes in the grafted bone marrow are inducing acute GvHD. In irradiated recipient mice, the severity of GvHD was shown to increase linearly with the number of lymphocytes added to the graft (6). In later years T cells have been identified as the effector cells of acute GvHD. The high incidence of acute GvHD in primates as compared to rodents is explained by the higher proportion of T-lymphocytes (20-30%) in primate punctate bone marrow as compared to rodent bone marrow (2-3%).

As a logical consequence of these observations, attempts were made to remove or inactivate the T-lymphocytes from the graft before transplantation. Initially this was done with discontinuous density gradient centrifugation which depleted about 1 log of T cells, sufficient to nearly completely prevent acute GvHD in MHC-matched combinations, but only partly effective in mismatched combinations (7).

Methods of T cell depletion have improved over the years by the introduction of a variety of other physical methods such as rosetting and elutriation, and of monoclonal antibodies directed at T-lymphocytes.

T cell depletion has virtually eliminated GvHD as a complication of matched BM grafting (8) and greatly reduced its severity in partially matched combinations. This is best illustrated by the fact that a recent inventory of results with BM grafted SCID patients shows that long term survival of patients grafted with T cell depleted mismatched marrow equals that of patients who received HLA identical sibling marrow (9). Grafting of T cell depleted marrow does not delay the recovery of immune competence as compared to patients treated with unmodified marrow.

However, when applied to treatment of leukemic and aplastic patients, several transplant teams have experienced delayed hematological recovery and an increased incidence of take failures with T cell depleted grafts. This problem will be the subject of the first part of this paper. In the second part we shall discuss the role of recombinant hemopoietic growth factors in the promotion of the hemopoietic reconstitution of bone marrow graft recipients and of monkeys exposed to high dose TBI.

Causes and prevention of take failure with T cell depleted bone marrow grafts.

Soon after the introduction of T cell depletion to prevent acute GvHD we observed an increase of take failures in mismatched unrelated Rhesus monkey combinations (10) and later also in matched dog combinations (11). This problem was not encountered in matched monkey transplants, probably because the routinely employed dose of TBI was higher in monkeys than in dogs.

Acting on the assumption that the acute GvHD reaction eliminates residual T cells of the host, we increased the TBI dose in the monkey from 8.8 Gy (X-rays) single dose to 2 x 6 Gy (interval 24 hrs) or 2 x 7 Gy (72 hrs) and in dogs from 7.5 Gy (single dose) to 2 x 4.5 Gy, and these increases eliminated the take failures (5, 12). The introduction of split irradiation was necessary because higher single doses were not tolerated. These observations demonstrated that consistent takes of T cell depleted marrow requires increased immunosuppression of the recipient prior to grafting. Since the minimal TBI dose required for 100% takes of unmodified MHC identical marrow has not been determined accurately in these species (as a matter of fact also not in humans) we have to rely on best guesses as to the extra TBI dose actually needed. Some useful information is obtained from experiments with mismatched marrow combinations in mice. In early experiments with supralethally irradiated mice we showed that the addition of 4×10^5 host type lymph node cells completely prevented the protective effect of a graft of rat bone marrow (13). Such experiments have recently been repeated with a H2 mismatched mouse combination in which we used graded numbers of host type (CBA) spleen cells and C57BL bone marrow grafts. The range between 100% and 0% graft failures was between 10^4 and 10^6 spleen cells (14). The incidence of take failures observed in patients treated with T cell depleted marrow was at most 50% but usually 20-30% as compared to less than 5% with full bone marrow. This implies that T cells in the graft are roughly capable of eliminating one log of residual host T cells. With a Do of T-lymphocytes estimated at 0.7 Gy, this would be equivalent to an additional dose of 2 Gy TBI. Clinical experience appears to be in accordance with this estimate. Löwenberg et al. (8) reported no graft failures in 18 leukemia patients grafted with T cell depleted matched marrow following conditioning with Ara-C, cyclophosphamide and 2 x 5 Gy TBI (interval 72 hrs., maximal total lung dose 8.5 Gy). Their regimen with T cell replete marrow was 8.5 Gy single dose TBI and cyclophosphamide. Even more elucidating are the data published by Burnett et al. (15). When they switched to T cell depleted marrow, using the conditioning employed for normal marrow grafts (cyclophosphamide and 6 x 2 Gy

TBI over 3 days), 5 out of 8 patients had graft failure. Following the addition of one extra TBI fraction of 2 Gy, 26 out of 27 patients engrafted with T cell depleted marrow.

Employing experimental data obtained with the BNML leukemia model in the rat, Hagenbeek et al. (16) calculated that the increased relapse rate of leukemia patients reported for T cell depleted bone marrow grafts can also be prevented by increasing the conditioning dose of TBI with 2 Gy.

In view of the well-documented production of hemopoietic growth factors by activated T-lymphocytes it has been suggested (17) that the take failures observed with T cell depleted grafts are to be ascribed to the absence of such a trophic influence.

This issue was approached in Rhesus monkeys using normal and T cell depleted autologous bone grafts (18). Autologous bone marrow grafts were used to avoid the influence of immunological factors. The monkeys were subjected to lethal TBI (2 x 6 Gy) and the rate of reconstitution was measured by recording the time when the reticulocytes reached 1% or when the leukocyte count reached 10^9 cells/l. Grafting of graded numbers of autologous bone marrow between 10^6 and 10^8 cells/kg yielded a linear relationship between log numbers of cells/kg body weight grafted and time in days until peripheral blood cell recovery. The data recorded for reticulocytes were more useful than those for leukocytes or thrombocytes due to smaller variation and a steeper slope of the regression. T cell depletion (2-3 log) with Campath I or other anti-human T-lymphocyte MCA crossreacting with Rhesus monkey lymphocytes did not affect the predicted rate of recovery (Table 3).

In the complimentary experiment, purified autologous stem cells were administered. It was found that peripheral blood cell reconstitution was similar to that observed following an equivalent number of whole bone marrow cells. Consequenty, these results do not lend support to a trophic function of grafted T-lymphocytes on hemopoietic reconstitution.

The influence of treatment with hemopoietic growth factors on reconstitution.

Recombinant human (rh) G-CSF and GM-CSF have been shown in clinical trials to enhance peripheral blood recovery in patients following treatment with high-dose chemotherapeutic agents and in patients treated with TBI followed by bone marrow transplantation. The administration of rh GM-CSF was reported to result in a faster recovery of peripheral blood cells in lethally irradiated Rhesus monkeys grafted with supra-optimal amounts of low density fraction, autologous bone marrow cells (17, 19) and G-CSF was found to have a similar effect in cynomolgus monkeys made cytopenic by a nonlethal dose of cyclophosphamide (20).

In sublethally irradiated mice the administration of rh G-CSF or rm GM-CSF accelarated the recovery of WBC and platelets in the peripheral blood and the repopulation of a variety of committed precursor cells and CFU-S in the bone marrow (21).

The experiments performed in our laboratory employed irradiated Rhesus monkeys and rh GM-CSF (Glaxo).

The objective of these experiments was to determine the lower limit of residual hemopoietic stem cells which permit stimulation of blood cell formation by this hemopoietic growth factor (22). In the first series of experiments, monkeys were subjected to sublethal TBI doses between 4 and 8 Gy and treated with 30 micro-g/kg/day subcutaneously for a period of 14 days after irradiation; control monkeys received placebo injections.

Peripheral leukocyte, reticulocyte and platelet counts and differentiated leukocyte counts were measured daily. At 4 and 5 Gy TBI, neutropenia was completely prevented by GM-CSF, but at 8 Gy TBI the effect of GM-CSF was no longer demonstrable in a significant shortening of neutropenia.

In this experiment, the sum of all values for each blood cell type obtained during the observation period was plotted against the TBI dose for both groups of animals. The results showed a rapid decline of the response of GM-CSF with increasing doses of irradiation. Most prominent was the effect on leukocytes (in fact: neutrophilic and eosinophilic granulocytes). For these cells, the GM-CSF effect was insignificant at a dose of 8 Gy. It was concluded that GM-CSF is most effective at a TBI dose that results in a 2-log stem cell kill and ineffective at doses which result in > 3 log stem cell kill.

The second series of experiments involved TBI with a lethal dose of irradiation (2 x 6 Gy/day) followed by transplantation of 10^7 autologous bone marrow cells which were pretreated with Campath I to deplete T cells. This amount of bone marrow is relatively small: the time to reach $10^9/l$ for leukocytes being 16-21 days and for reticulocytes to reach 1% being 19-23 days. rh GM-CSF was administered for a period of 30 days once daily s.c., at doses of 3, 10, 30 or 100 micro-g/kg body weight. Two or more monkeys were employed per dose point. In nearly all monkeys treated with GM-CSF an enhancement of leukocyte recovery occurred only at the time when a rise of counts had begun in the controls. The leukopenic period defined as $<10^9$ leukocytes/l was nonetheless shortened somewhat by 4-6 days on the average for all GM-CSF dose levels. A GM-CSF dose dependent peak value of leukocyte counts was observed up to 30 micro-g/kg/day.

In these situations the stimulatory effect of GM-CSF was considerably less pronounced than in experimental set-ups reported in the literature so far. Similar results as we describe here for GM-CSF have been recorded in preliminary experiments with recombinant Rhesus monkey IL-3. We set out to produce Rhesus monkey IL-3 for studies in monkeys (23) after we noted that human IL-3 was much less effective for Rhesus monkey bone marrow cells than for human bone marrow cells.

The two series of experiments discussed above suggest that a benificial effect of GM-CSF and IL-3 is restricted to counteracting chemotherapy and/or irradiation doses which result in not more than 3-log stem cell kill. Since a 2-log stem cell kill or less hardly result in pancytopenia, these experiments set the therapeutic window of the hemopoietic growth factors.

In other words, HGF are not effective when the stem cell population is below a certain critical number. Further investigations are required to establish whether the response obtained from short-term administration of HGF may reflect the actual number of surviving stem cells in lethally irradiated subjects and if the occurrence or absence of such responses are of practical value in predicting the capacity for autochtonous regeneration of hemopoiesis.

Summary.

Reconstitution of levels of pheripheral blood cells following bone marrow tranplantation is dependent on the engraftment of the pluripotent hemopoietic stem cells of the transplant. In the case of allogeneic tranplants, a successful engraftment carries a high risk of the development of GvHD, which is a serious and often life-threatening complication. T cell depletion of the allogeneic bone marrow graft can completely prevent GvHD provided a sufficient degree of depletion is achieved. Experiments with laboratory animals and clinical experience have shown that the higher rate of graft failure that occurs with T cell depleted marrow grafts can be avoided by increasing the conditioning dose of TBI with approximately 2 Gy. Experiments with T cell depleted autologous bone marrow grafts and with grafts of autologous purified stem cells in monkeys demonstrate that the decreased engraftment of T cell depleted bone marrow cannot be ascribed to a trophic function of T lymphocytes, e.g. via production of hemopoietic growth fractors.

Using sublethally irradiated Rhesus monkeys, the effect of post-irradiation treatment with GM-CSF or with Rhesus monkey r IL-3 was studied. Enhancement of blood cell regeneration was only recorded within a relatively small TBI dose range. When the dose of TBI induces more than approximately a 3-log stem cell kill, treatment with growth factors becomes ineffective. Comparable results are obtained when supralethally irradiated monkeys given relatively small grafts of T cell depleted autologous bone marrow were treated with the hemopoietic growth factors.

References

1. "In Vitro culture of hemopoietic cells". Proceedings of a workshop held at Rijswijk, The Netherlands, October 1971. Eds.: DW van Bekkum and KA Dicke (1972). Published by the Radiobiological Institute TNO, 224.
2. Van Bekkum DW (1963). Foreign bone marrow transplantation following fractinated whole-body irradiation in mice. In Radiation Effect in Physics, Chemistry and Biology (M Ebert and A Howard, eds.), North Holland, Amsterdam, 362.
3. Symposium at Schloss Reisenburg Sept. 28 - Oct. 1, 1989.
4. Van Bekkum DW (1985). Graft versus Host Disease, 147-213, "Bone Marrow Transplantation: biological mechanisms and clinical practice", eds.: DW van Bekkum and B Löwenberg. Marcel Dekker, Inc. New York.
5. Wagemaker G, Heidt PJ, Merchav S and Van Bekkum DW (1982). Abrogation of histocompatibility barriers to bone marrow transplantation in Rhesus monkeys. In:

Baum SJ, Ledney GD and Thierfelder S (eds.): Experimental Hematology Today. Basel, Karger, p. 111-118.

6. Van Bekkum DW (1964). The selective elimination of immunological competent cells from bone marrow and lymphatic cell mixtures. Transplantation 2:393-404.
7. Van Bekkum DW, Dicke KA (1972). Treatment of immune deficiency disease with bone marrow stem cell concentrates. In: Ontogeny of Acquired Immunity. Amsterdam Elsevier, 223-247.
8. Löwenberg B, Wagemaker G, Van Bekkum DW, Sizoo W, et al. (1986). Graft-versus-Host-Disease following transplantation of 'one lo' versus 'two log' T-lymphocyte-depleted bone marrow from HLA-identical donors. Bone Marrow Transplantation 1:133-140.
9. Fischer A, Friedrich W, Levinsky R, et al. (1986). Bone Marrow Transplantation for immunodeficiencies and osteopetrosis: European Survey, 1968-1985. Lancet: 1080-1086.
10. Van Bekkum D.W., Wagemaker G. and Vriesendorp H.M. (1979) Mechanism and avoidance of graft-versus-host-disease. Tranplant. Proc. 11:189-195.
11. Vriesendorp HM, Klapwijk WM, Heidt PJ, Hogeweg B, Zurcher C and Van Bekkum DW (1982). Factors controlling the engraftment of transplanted dog bone marrow cells. Tissue Antigens 20:63-80.
12. Walma EP, Vriesendorp HM, Zurcher C and Van Bekkum DW (1987). Engraftment of stem-cell-enriched bone marrow fractions in MHC-identical dogs after fractionated total-body irradiation. Transplantation 43:818-823.
13. Van Bekkum DW and Vos O (1957). Immunological aspects of homo- and heterologous bone marrow transplantation in irradiated animals. J. Cell Comp. Physiol. 50, Suppl. 1:139.
14. Van Bekkum DW and Hagenbeek A (1988). Immunohematological aspects of Total Body Irradiation and bone marrow transplantation for the treatment of leukemia. Radiotherapy and Oncology, in press.
15. Burnett AK, Han IM, Roberson AG, et al. (1988). Prevention of graft-versus-host-disease by ex vivo T cell depletion and graft failure with augmented total body irradiation. Leukemia 2:300-303.
16. Hagenbeek A, Martens A and Schultz FW (1988). How to prevent a leukemia relapse after bone marrow transplantation in acute leukemia: preclinical and

clinical model studies. Experimental Hematology Today, Springer-Verlag, New York, 147-151.

17. Nienhuis AW, Donahue RE, Karlsson S, Clark SC, Agricola B, et al. (1987). Recombinant human granulocyte-macrophage colony-stimulating factor (GM-CSF) shortens the period of neutropenia after autologous bone marrow transplantationin a primate model, The Journal of Clinical Investigation, Inc. 80:5723-577.
18. Gerritsen WR, Wagemaker G, Jonker M, Kenter MJH, Wielenga JJ, Hale G, Waldmann H and Van Bekkum DW (1988). The repopulation capacity of bone marrow trafts following pretreatment with monoclonal antibodies against T lymphocytes in Rhesus monkeys. Transplantation No 2, 45:301-307.
19. Monroy RL, Skelly RR, MacVittie TJ, Davis TA, Sauber JJ, Clark SC and Donahue RE (1987). The effect of recombinant GM-CSF on the revovery of monkeys transplanted with autologous bone marrow. Blood, No 5, 70:1696-1699.
20. Welte K, Bonilla MA, Gillio AP, et al. (1987). Recombinant human granulocyte colony-stimulating factor. Effects on hematopoiesis in normal and cyclophosphamide-treated primates. J. Exp. Med. 165:941-948.
21. Tanikawa S, Nakao I, Tsuneoka K and Nara N (1989). Effects of recombinant granulocyte colony-stimulating factor (rG-CSF) and recombinant granulocyte-macrophage colony-stimulating factor (rGM-CSF) on acute radiation hematopoietic injury in mice. Exp. Hematol. 17:883-888.
22. Wielenga JJ et al. Manuscript in preparation.
23. Burger H et al. Manuscript in preparation.

Table 1

MAJOR FACTORS INFLUENCING TAKE AND GRAFT VERSUS HOST DISEASE FOLLOWING ALLOGENEIC BM GRAFTING

	TAKE	GvHD
matching for MHC	facilitated	less
conditioning of recipient	facilitated	more
more cells	facilitated	more
lymphocyte depletion	less	less
g.i. decontamination	less	less
ALG	facilitated	less
Cyclosporin A	facilitated	less

Table 2

EFFECT OF FRACTIONATION OF TOTAL BODY X-IRRADIATION ON LD 50/30d AND TOTAL DOSE REQUIRED FOR FULL ENGRAFTMENT OF RAT BONE MARROW IN MICE. *)

Nr of daily fractions	LD 50 (cGy)	Total dose that permitted engraftment (cGy)
1	650	800
2	825	1000
3	1000	1200
4	1100	1300
5	1200	1500

*) Data from reference 2.

Table 3

REGENERATION TIME OF RETICULOCYTES AND LEUKOCYTES OF LETHALLY IRRADIATED RHESUS MONKEYS FOLLOWING INCUBATION OF AUTOLOGOUS MARROW GRAFTS WITH MONOCLONAL ANTIBODIES DIRECTED AGAINST T LYMPHOCYTES AND COMPLEMENT.[1)]

MCA	Nr of bm cells grafted per kg bwt [2)]	Reticulocyte > 1% (day)		Leukocytes > 10^9/l (day)	
		observed	expected	observed	expected
Campath I	10^7	19	18-21	19	16-21
	10^8	10	8-13	8	10-18
B9-pool	10^7	20	18-21	21	16-21
	10^8	10	8-13	9	10-18
OKT_4 + 4a	10^7	19	18-21	18	16-21
WT_1	10^7	22	18-21	21	16-21
Anti.DR cocktail[3)]	10^8	21; >22	8-13	21; >22	10-18

1) Data from reference 23.

2) Pre-incubation counts.

3) To inactivate multipotent stem cells, as a control test.

The Biology of Hematopoiesis, pages 493–504

SERUM IMMUNOREACTIVE ERYTHROPOIETIN IN PATIENTS WITH END STAGE RENAL DISEASE

L.F. Gimenez, A.J. Watson and J.L. Spivak

Divisions of Nephrology and Hematology, The Johns Hopkins University School of Medicine, Baltimore, Maryland.

INTRODUCTION

Erythropoietin, a glycoprotein produced primarily in the kidneys in adults, is an obligatory growth factor for erythroid cells. Erythropoietin recruits erythroid progenitor cells into cycle, maintains their survival and facilitates their differentiation (Spivak, 1986). Presumably, because of its vital role in erythropoiesis, erythropoietin production in the kidneys is both constitutive and inducible (Koury et al., 1989). There are no preformed stores of erythropoietin in the kidneys (Schooley et al., 1972) and tissue hypoxia, due either to anemia or a decrease in available oxygen, enhances erythropoietin production while erythrocytosis suppresses it but never completely (Moccia et al., 1980). Thus, a feedback relationship exists between tissue oxygenation and erythropoietin production, and as a corollary, there is normally an inverse linear correlation between the concentration of erythropoietin in the circulation and the hemoglobin level (Garcia et al., 1982).

Since erythropoietin is produced in the kidneys, renal disease can have a profound impact on erythropoietin production and patients with end-stage renal disease are usually severely anemic. In this paper, we describe serum immunoreactive erythropoietin levels, using a sensitive and specific radioimmunoassay employing recombinant reagents (Egrie et al., 1987), in patients with end-stage renal disease being treated by hemodialysis or continuous ambulatory peritoneal dialysis (CAPD). Our data indicate that while immunoreactive erythropoietin is always present in the circulation of patients with end-stage renal disease, even when anephric, the normal inverse relationship between the circulating erythropoietin level and the hemoglobin level is absent.

MATERIALS AND METHODS

Patients

The patient population studied consisted of 143 patients with end stage renal disease. Seventy-eight patients were maintained on chronic hemodialysis and eight of these were anephric. The other fifty-seven patients were treated by CAPD. The demographic characteristics of the patients with respect to gender and age are depicted in Table 1.

Table 1
Patient Demographics

	Sex		Age (years)*
	Male	Female	
Hemodialysis	48	30	55.7 ± 1.7 (21-80)
C.A.P.D.	29	28	51.7 ± 1.8 (26-85)
Anephric	6	2	40.1 ± 4.2 (21-57)

* Mean ± S.E.M.
( ) Range

Erythropoietin Assay

Serum erythropoietin was measured by a sensitive and specific commercially available radioimmunoassay (Smith-Kline Bio-Science, Van Nuys, CA) in which immunologically detectable erythropoietin is equivalent to biologically active erythropoietin (Egrie et al., 1987). With this assay, the range of normal values in nonanemic men and women is 4-26 mU/ml with an interassay coefficient of variation of 14.5% at a level of 9.6 mU/ml to 8.6% at a level of 99.3 mU/ml.

Statistical analysis was performed using the t test for unpaired, normally distributed data and Wilcoxon's nonparametric rank sum test for nonnormally distributed data.

RESULTS

Table 2 lists the serum immunoreactive erythropoietin, hemoglobin and serum creatinine levels of the three patient groups.

Table 2
Serum Immunoreactive Erythropoietin (S.I.E.) In Patients With End-Stage Renal Disease

	S.I.E.* (mU/ml)	Hemoglobin (gm%)	Serum Creatinine (mg%)
Hemodialysis (n = 78)	18.8 ± 2.3 (2-119)	7.9 ± 0.2 (4.4-148)	13.2 ± 0.5 (5.2-23.8)
C.A.P.D. (n = 57)	17.1 ± 2.0** (5-97)	9.2 ± 0.3+ (5.4-14.3)	11.8 ± 0.6 (5.5-23.5)
Anephric (n = 8)	11.0 ± 3.5 (5-35)	7.2 ± 0.8 (44-11.3)	13.8 ± 1.5 (6.6-19.7)

*Mean ± S.E.M.
( ) Range
** $p < 0.02$ for CAPD versus anephric patients; for hemodialysis versus anephric patients, the differences were just at the level of significance ($p = 0.058$)
+ $p < 0.001$ for CAPD versus the other groups

There was no statistical difference amongst the three groups with respect to serum creatinine. However, there was a significant difference in the mean hemoglobin level between the CAPD group and the other two groups. The mean serum erythropoietin levels were higher also for the hemodialysis and CAPD groups than the anephric group; the differences were statistically significant for the CAPD group but just reached the level of significance for the hemodialysis patients due to the broad range of values in that group. For all groups, however, the mean serum erythropoietin level was not outside the range of normal and was thus inappropriately low for the degree of anemia. The wide range of erythropoietin levels observed was not related to dialysis per se since measurements of serum immunoreactive erythropoietin before and after dialysis were not different (data not shown) nor, in contrast to the observations of others (Walle, 1987, Chandra et al., 1988b) was there any clinical evidence of hypoxia or hemorrhage to account for the high levels of serum immunoreactive erythropoietin observed in some of the hemodialysis patients which were not persistent.

Figures 1 and 2 illustrate the relationship between serum immunoreactive erythropoietin, hemoglobin and serum creatinine in all 143 dialysis patients. Although there is normally an inverse correlation between the circulating erythropoietin level and the hemoglobin or hematocrit, this relationship was absent in patients with end-stage renal disease regardless of the type of dialysis with which they were treated or whether or not they were anephric. Furthermore, there was no correlation between serum erythropoietin and serum creatinine (Figure 2), indicating that renal excretory and endocrine functions were not directly related, at least in patients whose renal function was as severely compromised as those described in this study. There was also no correlation between hemoglobin and serum creatinine (data not shown) but the fact that many of the patients required red cell transfusions reduces the relevance of this observation.

DISCUSSION

Anemia is a common feature of end-stage renal disease and can have many causes including folic acid deficiency, iron deficiency, blood loss, hemolysis, hypersplenism, renal osteodystrophy, infection, inflammation, and aluminum toxicity. The most important cause, however, is a deficiency of erythropoietin. Studies utilizing a bioassay for the detection and quantitation of plasma erythropoietin suggested that uremic patients generally had low circulat-

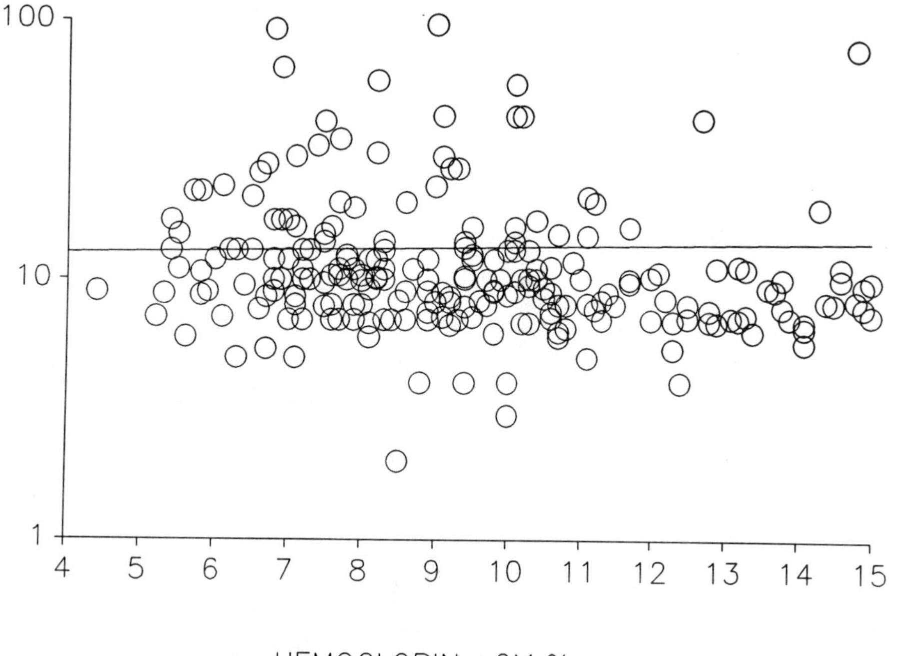

Figure 1. The relationship between hemoglobin and the log serum erythropoietin levels in all 143 patients with end-stage renal disease. ($r = 0.02$; $p = 0.83$)

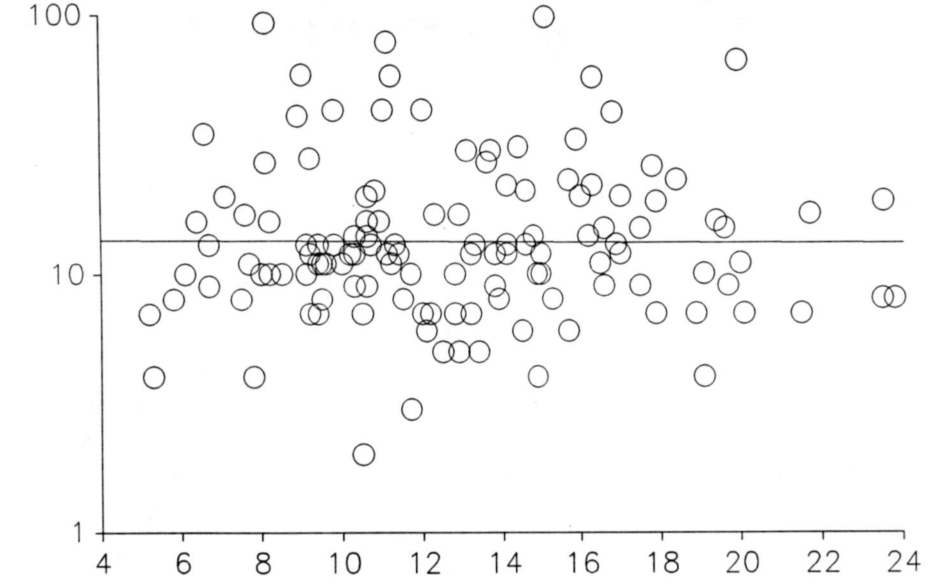

Figure 2. The relationship between serum creatinine and the log serum erythropoietin levels in all 143 patients with end-stage renal disease. ($r = 0.04$; $p = 0.61$)

ing levels of the hormone (Eschbach et al., 1967, Zucker et al., 1976, Caro et al., 1979). More recently, when sensitive radioimmunoassay techniques have been used, normal or even elevated levels of erythropoietin were found in patients with end-stage renal disease (McGonigle et al., 1984a, McGonigle et al., 1984b, Chandra et al., 1988b). Indeed, several studies have demonstrated that this residual (and presumably renal) endocrine function was important in the maintenance of even the limited extent of erythropoiesis in these patients (Eschbach et al., 1970, Walle et al., 1987). This is exemplified by the lower hematocrit levels that anephric patients demonstrate and the higher hematocrit levels of some patients with polycystic kidney disease (Chandra et al., 1985, Pavlovi'c-Kentera et al., 1987) as well as the suppression of erythropoiesis and erythropoietin levels in some patients by transfusion (Eschbach et al., 1970, Walle et al., 1987).

In normal individuals, an inverse correlation exists between the hematocrit or hemoglobin level and serum erythropoietin. Thus, with progressive anemia, erythropoietin levels, as measured by radioimmunoassay can increase over 1,000 times above the baseline value. In the present study, using a sensitive radioimmunoassay technique, serum erythropoietin levels in anemic patients with end-stage renal disease were generally in the "normal range," but must be considered low when the concomitant degree of hemoglobin reduction is considered. In addition, the normal inverse relationship between hemoglobin and serum erythropoietin level was absent, nor was there any correlation between hemoglobin, erythropoietin and serum creatinine.

Our findings are similar to those of other investigators using either a bioassay (Eschbach et al., 1967, Zucker et al., 1976, Caro et al., 1979) or a radioimmumoassay (McGonigle et al., 1984a and 1984b, Walle et al., 1987, Chandra et al., 1988a, Chandra et al., 1988b) to measure circulating erythropoietin.

Because elevations in serum erythropoietin have been observed in patients with end-stage renal disease who were hypoxic or bleeding, it was postulated that the feedback relationship between renal erythropoietin production and tissue oxygenation persists in these patients but with an altered threshold and a blunted response due to loss of functional tissue (Chandra et al., 1988a). However, Sherwood et al. (1988) have identified multiple forms of immunoreactive erythropoietin in the circulation of patients with end-stage renal disease as well as normal individuals, suggesting that elevated levels of erythropoietin as measured by radioimmunoassay in some patients may not reflect biologically active erythropoietin. This observation has not yet been confirmed.

The possibility that an elevated serum erythropoietin level in a patient with end stage renal disease may reflect the presence of congenital or acquired cystic disease must also be considered. Renal cysts may be associated with higher erythropoietin levels and higher hemoglobin levels (Shalhoub et al., 1982, Chandra et al., 1985, McGonigle et al., 1984b, Pavlovi'c-Kentera et al., 1987, Eckardt et al., 1989). Six of our patients had polycystic kidney disease, only one of whom was receiving CAPD. None had elevated serum erythropoietin levels but four of the six had hemoglobin levels greater than 10 gm%.

Higher erythropoietin and hematocrit or hemoglobin levels have been noted in some patients treated with CAPD (Zappacosta et al., 1982, Chandra et al., 1988b) but not others (Salahudeen et al., 1983, McGonigle et al., 1984b). In some cases, the hematocrit elevation was actually due to a reduction in plasma volume (De Paepe et al., 1983) while in one study, the serum erythropoietin levels were inappropriately high for the degree of anemia (Chandra et al., 1988b) suggesting either autonomous erythropoietin production or production of immunoreactive but non-biologically active erythropoietin. Although our CAPD patients had higher hemoglobin levels than the hemodialysis or anephric patients, their erythropoietin levels were not different from the hemodialysis patients, once again emphasizing the lack of correlation between these measurements which is so characteristic of end-stage renal disease.

Erythropoietin released from the liver could provide another explanation for variations in circulating erythropoietin which are not explainable on clinical grounds by tissue hypoxia or hemorrhage. Indeed, during the course of toxic or infectious hepatitis some patients with end-stage renal disease develop an increase in serum erythropoietin and have an amelioration of their anemia (Brown et al., 1980, Meyrier et al., 1981). Although acquisition of infectious hepatitis is common in dialysis patients, none of our patients had clinically overt hepatitis.

Other factors which could be responsible for the lack of correlation between hemoglobin and circulating erythropoietin in patients with end-stage renal disease include alterations in red cell 2,3 DPG which can be elevated in renal failure and thereby enhance oxygen delivery by hemoglobin (Blumberg et al., 1973), the presence of inflammation or infection which could suppress erythropoietin production (Hochberg et al., 1988, Spivak et al., 1989), renal osteodystrophy or hypersplenism. Although there is no evidence that the uremic state alters erythropoietin catabolism (Steinberg et al., 1986), it is possible that carbamylation of erythropoietin might occur which could inactivate it. Carbamylation of hemoglobin is known to occur in end-stage renal disease (Smith et al., 1988). Finally, it is also worth emphasizing the inhomogeneity of the population under scrutiny as well as the limited extent of the observation period in each patient. Renal damage and, therefore, renal function varies from patient to patient over time as does nutritional status and transfusion status, all of which will affect serum erythropoietin and hemoglobin levels.

Whatever the basis for variations in circulating erythropoietin and their lack of correlation with the hemoglobin level, it is clear that in most patients with end-stage renal disease, erythropoietin production is insufficient for the degree of anemia, and it is this failure to increase erythropoietin production in a commensurate and sustained fashion as the red cell mass declines which is primarily responsible for the anemia of end-stage renal disease.

REFERENCES

Blumberg A, Keller H, Marti HR (1973). Effect of altitude on erythropoiesis and oxygen affinity in anaemic patients on maintenance dialysis. Europ J Clin Invest 3:93-97.

Brown S, Caro J, Erslev AJ, Murray TG (1980). Spontaneous increase in erythropoietin and hematocrit value associated with transient liver enzyme abnormalities in an anephric patient undergoing hemodialysis. Am J Med 68:280-284.

Caro J, Brown S, Miller O, Murray T, Erslev AJ (1979). Erythropoietin levels in uremic nephric and anephric patients. J Lab Clin Med 93:449-458.

Chandra M, Miller ME, Garcia JF, Mossey RT, McVicar M (1985). Serum immunoreactive erythropoietin levels in patients with polycystic kidney disease as compared with other hemodialysis patients. Nephron 39:26-29.

Chandra M, Clemons GK, McVicar MI (1988a). Relation of serum erythropoietin levels to renal excretory function: evidence for lowered set point for erythropoietin production in chronic renal failure. J Pediatr 113:1015-1021.

Chandra M, Clemons GK, McVicar M, Wilkes B, Bluestone PA, Maillous LU, Mossey RT (1988b). Serum erythropoietin levels and hematocrit in end-stage renal disease: influence of the mode of dialysis. Am J Kid Dis 12:208-213.

De Paepe MBJ, Schelstraete KHG, Ringoir SMG, Lameire NH (1983). Influence of continuous ambulatory peritoneal dialysis on the anemia of endstage renal disease. Kid Intl 23:744-748.

Eckardt K-U, Mollmann M, Neumann R, Brunkhorst R, Burger H-U, Lonnemann G, Scholz H, Keusch G, Buchholz B, Frei U, Bauer C, Kurtz A (1989). Erythropoietin in polycystic kidneys. J Clin Invest 84:1160-1166.

Egrie JC, Cotes PM, Lane J, Gaines Das RE, Tam RC (1987). Development of radioimmunoassays for human erythropoietin using recombinant erythropoietin as a tracer and immunogen. J Immunol Meth 99:235-241.

Eschbach JW, Funk D, Adamson J, Kuhn I, Scribner BH, Finch CA (1967). Erythropoiesis in patients with renal failure undergoing chronic dialysis. N Engl J Med 276:653-658.

Eschbach JW, Adamson JW, Cook JD (1970). Disorders of red blood cell production in uremia. Arch Intern Med 126:812-815.

Garcia JF, Ebbe SN, Hollander L, Cutting HO, Miller ME, Cronkite (1982). Radioimmunoassay of erythropoietin: circulating levels in normal and polycythemic human beings. J Lab Clin Med 99:624-635.

Hochberg MC, Arnold CM, Hogans BB, Spivak JL (1988). Serum immunoreactive erythropoietin in rheumatoid arthritis: impaired response to anemia. Arth Rheuma 31:1318-1321.

Koury ST, Koury MJ, Bondurant MC, Caro J, Graber SE (1989) Quantitation of erythropoietin-producing cells in kidneys of mice by in situ hybridization: correlation with hematocrit, renal erythropoietin mRNA, and serum erythropoietin concentration. Blood 74:645-651.

McGonigle RJS, Wallin JD, Shadduck RK, Fisher JW (1984a). Erythropoietin deficiency and inhibition of erythropoiesis in renal insufficiency. Kid Intl 25:437-444.

McGonigle RJS, Husserl F, Wallin JD, Fisher JW (1984b). Hemodialysis and continuous ambulatory peritoneal dialysis effects on erythropoiesis in renal failure. Kid Intl 25:430-436.

Meyrier A, Simon P, Boffa G, Brissot P (1981). Uremia and the liver. Nephron 29:3-6.

Pavlovi'c-Kentera V, Clemons GK, Djukanovi'c L, Biljanovi'c-Paunovic L (1987). Erythropoietin and anemia in chronic renal failure. Exp Hematol 15:785-789.

Moccia G, Miller ME, Garcia JF, Cronkite EP (1980). The effect of plethora on erythropoietin levels. Proc Soc Exp Biol Med 163:36-38.

Salahudeen AK, Hawkins T, Keavey PM, Wilkinson R (1983). Is anaemia during continuous ambulatory peritoneal dialysis really better than during haemodialysis? Lancet 2:1046-1048.

Schooley JC, Mahlmann LF (1972). Evidence for the de novo synthesis of erythropoietin in hypoxic rats. Blood 40:662-670.

Shalhoub RJ, Rajan U, Kim VV, Goldwasser E, Kark JA, Antoniou LD (1982). Erythrocytosis in patients on long-term hemodialysis. Ann Intern Med 97:686-690.

Sherwood JB, Carmichael D, Goldwasser E (1988). The heterogeneity of circulating human serum erythropoietin. Endocrinology 122:1472-1477.

Smith WGJ, Holden M, Benton M, Brown CB (1988). Carbamylated haemoglobin in chronic renal failure. Clin Chim Acta 178:297-304.

Spivak JL (1986). The mechanism of action of erythropoietin. Intl J Cell Clon 4:139-166.

Spivak JL, Barnes DC, Fuchs E, Quinn TC (1989). Serum immunoreactive erythropoietin in HIV-infected patients. JAMA 261:3104-3107.

Steinberg SE, Garcia JF, Matzke GR, Mladenovic J (1986). Erythropoietin kinetics in rats: generation and clearance. Blood 67:646-649.

Walle AJ, Wong GY, Clemons GK, Garcia JF, Niedermayer W (1987). Erythropoietin-hematocrit feedback circuit in the anemia of end-stage renal disease. Kid Intl 31:1205-1209.

Zappacosta AR, Caro J, Erslev A (1982). Normalization of hematocrit in patients with end-stage renal disease on continuous ambulatory peritoneal dialysis. Am J Med 72:53-57.

Zucker S, Lysik RM, Mohammad G (1985). Erythropoiesis in chronic renal disease. J Lab Clin Med 88:528-535.

The Biology of Hematopoiesis, pages 505–517

THE USE OF RECOMBINANT HUMAN ERYTHROPOIETIN [rHuEpo] IN MAN

J.W. Adamson and J.W. Eschbach

New York Blood Center, New York, New York, 10021 and University of Washington, Seattle, Washington, 98195

INTRODUCTION

A hypoproliferative anemia is an almost invariable consequence of chronic renal failure (CRF) (1). Most investigators believe that inadequate erythropoietin (Epo) production is the prime cause of the anemia. However, several other factors may contribute: (1) a mild to moderate shortening of red cell survival; (2) gastrointestinal and other blood loss associated with platelet dysfunction; (3) and the possible effect on erythropoiesis of inhibitors which are retained in CRF (4). Other factors which may contribute to the anemia are associated with specific complications and/or treatment of the dialysis patient. These factors include residual blood loss in the dialyzer, erythroid suppression from aluminum toxicity (brought about by the chronic ingestion of aluminum-containing phosphate binders), osteitis fibrosa from severe secondary hyperparathyroidism and, rarely, acute or chronic hemolysis (5).

While all of these mechanisms have at one time or another been raised as significant contributors to the anemia, Epo deficiency remains foremost. Consequently, one of the longstanding goals of both hematologists and nephrologists has been the application of Epo to the treatment of the anemia of CRF.

CORRECTION OF THE ANEMIA OF CRF WITH RECOMBINANT HUMAN EPO

The first published reports of the successful isolation, cloning and expression of the human Epo gene appeared in 1985 (6,7). This was rapidly confirmed and extended (8) and large amounts of recombinant human (rHu) Epo became available for clinical trials. Such clinical trials were initiated in December, 1985 in Seattle (9) and in March, 1986 in London (10), and were targeted to anemic patients on hemodialysis. Multicenter trials in the United States (11), Western Europe (12), and Japan (13), have been conducted and the results support the concept that Epo deficiency is the major mechanism responsible for the anemia.

In the initial United States trial, rHuEpo was administered as an intravenous bolus injection three times a week immediately following dialysis. Erythropoiesis was monitored by measurements of the reticulocyte count, quantitative ferrokinetics, transfusion requirements and hematocrit (9). The lowest rHuEpo doses used, 1.5 and 5 U/kg body weight, were ineffective. Initial responses were seen at 15 U/kg dose and, in some patients, this dose resulted in a cessation of transfusion reqirements and a partial correction of the anemia (Fig. 1). At all doses greater than 15 U/kg, effective responses were observed and the anemia was corrected. As shown in Figure 2, the rate of correction of the anemia was correlated directly with the initial dose of rHuEpo. At the highest doses employed, increases of as much as 10 hematocrit points were observed within two to three weeks after starting therapy.

Nearly 2,000 anemic hemodialysis patients have now been treated at centers in Canada, the United Kingdom, Western Europe, Japan and the United States. Although the dosage protocols have varied, the findings of the initial studies have been confirmed with a nearly 100% response rate. In the United States multicenter trial, the rate of rise of hematocrit was shown again to be dose dependent. In almost all patients, target hemoglobin and hematocrit levels were achieved within eight to twelve weeks after starting therapy. In this multicenter trial, only eight of 309 patients failed to respond to rHuEpo and, of those, several had complicating medical conditions which might have predicted a lack of response to the hormone. These included unrecognized iron deficiency, osteitis fibrosa, and infection. In Seattle, some patients have now received rHuEpo replacement therapy for more than three years. Patients who have entered maintenance therapy have continued to respond to rHuEpo without evidence of resistance and, at this writing, no patients have been reported who have developed antibodies to rHuEpo (11). Thus, rHuEpo is effective and well tolerated.

We have also treated seventeen patients with the anemia (hematocrit < 30) of progressive renal failure not yet requiring dialysis (14). These patients have responded to rHuEpo in a manner similar to hemodialysis patients. While most of the information available has been obtained with the intravenous administration of the drug, results in pre-dialysis patients (14) and from several dialysis centers (15, 16) indicate that subcutaneous dosing with rHuEpo may be more effective, although the precise correlation with intravenous dosing and details of pharmacokinetics have not been reported.

The use of rHuEpo has raised three issues related to management of anemic patients with CRF. These include iron availability, the management of hypertension, and the potential of inflammation to limit the effectiveness of rHuEpo.

IRON AVAILABILITY

The response to rHuEpo imposes a demand to mobilize iron from reticuloendothelial storage sites and to make it available to transferrin. Thus, during the initial period of response to rHuEpo, there is a one-way shunt of iron from stores, through the circulation, into the marrow and then into the circulation red cell mass. The amount of iron required for an effective response to rHuEpo can be calculated easily. If a patient weighing 70 kg raises his/her hematocrit from 18 to 40, the increase in red cell mass will be approximately 1,000 ml, equivalent to 1 gram of elemental iron. In addition, with rHuEpo treatment, iron accumulation from red cell transfusions ceases while residual dialyzer blood loss continues. Severely anemic individuals who begin therapy with rHuEpo, and who have iron stores less than 1 gram, are at risk of becoming iron deficient during the course of therapy. Currently, recommendations for managing patients during the acute or induction phase of therapy with rHuEpo include supplementing the diet with oral iron, or else supplementing reticuloendothelial stores more directly by the intravenous administration of iron dextran.

In individuals whose reponse to rHuEpo is so brisk that mobilization of iron from storage sites cannot keep pace with the demand, rHuEpo may become less effective despite the fact that some ferritin values clearly indicate that adequate iron stores are present. This is a condition of "relative" or "functional" iron deficiency. Relative iron deficiency, which we have arbitrarily defined as a transferrin saturation of less than 20 precent with a normal serum ferritin level, was seen in over 40 precent of the patients treated with rHuEpo in the multicenter trial conducted in the United States (11). While there are no obvious adverse effects of relative iron deficiency, it is a physiological state which reduces the effectiveness of rHuEpo.

HYPERTENSION

Correction of the anemia in CRF patients results in better tissue oxygenation. The clinical benefits of this improved oxygenation include improved exercise tolerance, skin circulation, central nervous system funtion, and increased peripheral vascular resistance (17). In the initial group of patients treated with rHuEpo, increases in blood pressure, including episodes of hypertensive encephalopathy, were observed with unexptected frequency, both in Seattle (9) and in the United Kingdom (10). In the United States multicenter trial, 35% of patients experienced an increase in diastolic blood pressure of > 10 mm Hg. In some patients, this increase in blood pressure did not achieve hypertensive proportions. In others, however, the increase in blood pressure exacerbated already existing hypertension or required the initiation of antihypertensive medication. Overall, approximately 25% of patients required new or increased blood pressure medications as they acutely responded to rHuEpo therapy (11). A similar increase in blood pressure was observed in hypertensive, pre-dialysis patients whose anemia was corrected with rHuEpo (14).

The mechanism underlying the increase in blood pressure may be related to an increase in total peripheral vascular resistance (17,18). Blood viscosity, which increases as the hematocrit increases, is similar in normotensive and hypertensive patients responding to rHuEpo (B.G. Danielson et al., unpublished paper, 1988 meeting Swedish Society of Nephrology) and, therefore, is not the sole cause. In studies from several centers, the increase in peripheral vascular resistance was associated with a decline in cardiac output (12), although these findings are not uniformly agreed upon (19). These observations are similar to data published by Neff and co-workers (20) which demonstrated that acutely raising the hematocrit with red cell transfusions in dialysis patients resulted in a progressive increase in diastolic and mean aterial blood pressure. These changes were mediated by an increase in peripheral vascular resistance which was associated with a decrease in cardiac output. It is believed that the increased vascular resistance results from the correction of the peripheral vasodilation which accompanies profound, sustained anemia (17). The blood pressure changes are not due to a direct pressor effect of rHuEpo since hypertension has not been observed in normal volunteers or in other patient groups receiving rHuEpo (21).

Since there is no way, at this time, to predict who will develop hypertension or become more hypertensive when rHuEpo therapy is initiated, our recommendation for the anemic, hemodialysis patient is to begin with a relatively low dose, i.e., 50-100 U/kg, thrice weekly, intravenously. As the hematocrit approaches 30, the dose should be reduced in order to more gradually reach the target hemo/globin/hematocrit. Reducing the dose allows more time to observe the blood pressure response and to initiate appropriate antihypertensive therapy. If, at any time, serious hypertension develops during the acute phase of therapy, rHuEpo should be witheld until the blood pressure is controlled. A rising blood pressure during the acute phase of treatment (i.e., when the hematocrit is increasing toward target levels) is more likely to precipitate seizures and/or hypertensive encephalopathy, than similar changes in blood pressure during the maintenance phase of therapy at at time when the hematocrit is relatively stable.

EFFECT OF INFLAMMATION ON RHUEPO RESPONSE

Considerable interest exists in using rHuEpo in patients with anemia associated with chronic inflammatory or infectious diseases or malignancies. There is a feature of inflammation which might blunt the response to rHuEpo, however. Specifically, chronic inflammatory diseases of many kinds are associated with a reduced release of iron from storage sites and a reduced percent transferrin saturation. This alteration in internal iron metabolism, referred to as reticuloendothelial iron blockade is one of the major criteria for the diagnosis of the anemia of chronic disease (22). Because this relative iron deficiency has been so refractory to simple manipulations such as oral or parenteral iron supplementation, it might be anticipated that rHuEpo will be less effective in this setting than in otherwise normal individuals. Figure 3 shows the effect of elective hip replacement in a dialysis patient who was receiving rHuEpo. The patient's hematocrit had been maintained by thrice weekly rHuEpo administration. With surgery, the hematocrit fell to below 20 and four to six weeks were required before the response to rHuEpo was re-established. As more data accumulate in patients with active inflammatory disease, a pattern of relative rHuEpo resistance may emerge, and it is possible that the doses required to maintain target hematocrit in these patients will be higher than the doses required in uncomplicated CRF patients.

USE OF RHUEPO IN PROMOTING BLOOD DONATIONS FOR AUTOLOGOUS USE

Because of the concerns for the safety of blood used in transfusions, a multicenter clinical trial was carried out to determine whether rHuEpo enhanced the ability of individuals to donate blood for self-use. The results of those studies have been published recently (23). The dose of rHuEpo was 600 U/kg, twice weekly, and the study was placebo-controlled and double-blinded. The mean number of units collected from the group receiving rHuEpo was 5.4 + 0.2 vs. 4.1 + 0.2 (SE) for the placebo-treated group. When the average hematocrit of the units drawn was taken into consideration, rHuEpo allowed the collection of 41% more red cells than was otherwise possible. Furthermore, the mean hematocrit of the two patient groups was significantly different at the end of the trial (38.6 vs 35.2 for the rHuEpo-treated and placebo control groups, respectively). Thus, rHuEpo has potential to increase the number of surgical procedures which can be carried out with the sole use of autologous blood. It is difficult to know how widespread the use of rHuEpo will become in this setting, however, because of the need for patients to travel multiple times from home to a donation site. As familiarity with the drug increases and strategies for optimizing iron delivery for erythropoiesis improve, it would be hoped that adjunctive therapy with rHuEpo in this setting would become increasingly important.

TREATMENT OF THE ANEMIA OF RHEUMATOID ARTHRITIS (RA)

Although the number of rHuEpo-treated RA patients reported to date is small, the drug has been shown to be effective in this group. The initial report included two patients whose hematocrits were normalized with doses of rHuEpo ranging from 150 to 200 U/kg given intravenously three times weekly (21). The degree of reticulocytosis was not as great as in patients with CRF and it is possible that the rate of response overall was somewhat blunted due to the inflammatory nature of the anemia. Furthermore, it was not clear that joint symptoms improved in these patients or that quality of life was enhanced as a result of rHuEpo treatment. More experience with rHuEpo in this group of patients will be necessary before firm conclusions can be drawn, but it is encouraging that at least the anemia of one form of chronic disease appears responsive to rHuEpo therapy.

USE OF RHUEPO IN THE ANEMIA OF PATIENTS WITH ACQUIRED IMMUNE DEFICIENCY SYNDROME (AIDS)

Anemia is common in patients with AIDS. The anemia is frequently much more severe in those individuals receiving Zidovudine therapy. Some patients develop red cell aplasia and become transfusion dependent. In a preliminary report, rHuEpo was shown to decrease by over 50% the number of red cell transfusions in selected groups of AIDS patients treated with AZT (24). Some patients not only became transfusion-independent, but also normalized their hemoglobin and hematocrit. Those patients whose plasma Epo levels were <500 mu/ml prior to rHuEpo therapy had a much greater likelihood of responding to the Epo than those whose endogenous Epo levels were >500 mu/ml. The improvement in hematocrit by rHuEpo in these patients was associated with an improved quality of life. The fact that rHuEpo will reduce the dependence of this group on red cell transfusions will save community resources in the form of blood and blood products.

USE OF RHUEPO IN OTHER CONDITIONS

Table 1 summarizes the known and proposed indications for the use of rHuEpo as a therapeutic. Clearly, patients with anemia associated with CRF or progressive renal failure are the prime candidates for rHuEpo treatment. One would also predict that some patients with myelodysplastic syndromes and, perhaps, chronic anemia associated with malignancy, would respond to rHuEpo with an improvement in hemoglobin and hematocrit and cessation of transfusion requirements. Elimination of transfusion dependency would be an important end-point for rHuEpo therapy in these patients but it is uncertain whether quality of life will be improved demonstrably. It is also uncertain that rHuEpo will be effective in patients with aplastic anemia or pure red cell aplasia. Nevertheless, the

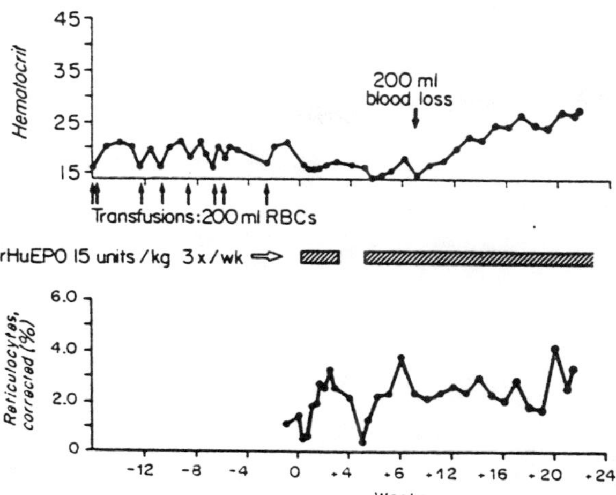

FIG. 1. Response of an anephric patient to rhEPO, 15 U/kg, given intravenously three times weekly. Transfusion requirements ceased after the onset of therapy. The reticulocyte count, corrected for the anaemia, rose with therapy and returned to baseline levels when therapy was interrupted for two weeks. The patient's haematocrit subsequently peaked at 25 with this dose.

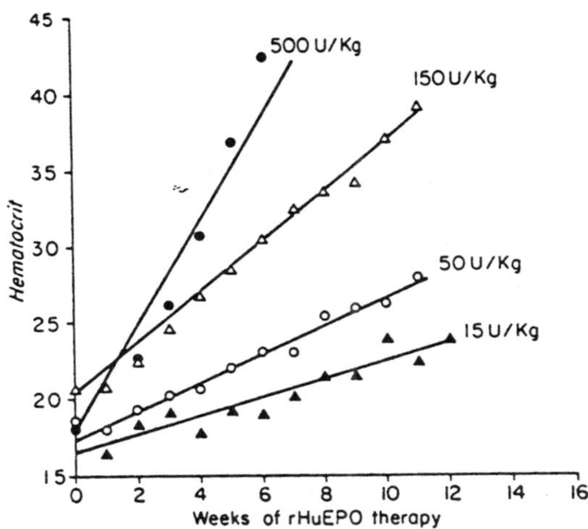

FIG. 2. The haematocrit response to various doses of rhEPO in haemodialysis patients. Each treatment group comprises four or five patients and the data represent the mean weekly haematocrits. (Reproduced from Eschbach et al 1987, with permission of the authors and the publishers.)

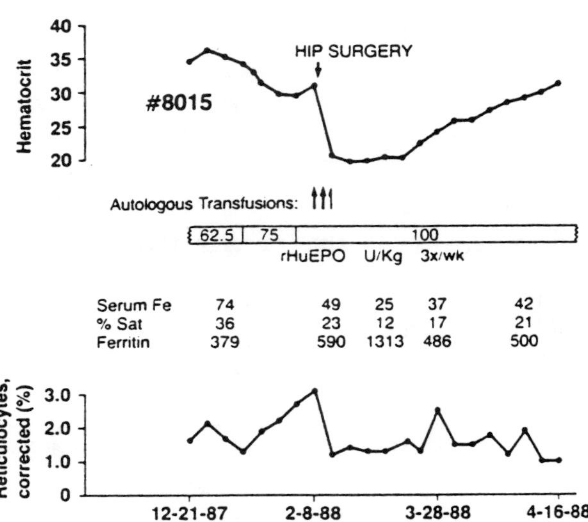

FIG. 3. The effect of the inflammation of surgery on the response to rhEPO. This dialysis patient's haematocrit was maintained at approximately 35 with 62.5 U/kg of rhEPO given intravenously three times per week. The dose was increased to 75 U/kg in order to allow the patient to donate three units of red cells for autologous use. Despite the patient receiving 2.5 units during hip-replacement surgery, the haematocrit fell to 18 where it remained for five weeks despite an rhEPO dose of 100 U/kg. Note that the serum ferritin concentration increased and the serum iron level decreased at the time of surgery and reversed when the patient began to respond again to rhEPO. (Reproduced from Adamson & Eschbach, Quarterly J. of Med., 1989, with permission of the authors and publishers.)

TABLE I. Potential Clinical Uses for rHuEpo.

1. Anemia of renal failure (both dialysis and pre-dialysis patients)
2. Autologous blood donation
3. Recovery from chemotherapy or radiation therapy
4. Chronic anemias
    a. Inflammation (e.g. rheumatoid arthritis)
    b. Infection (e.g. AIDS with or without AZT therapy)
    c. Neoplasia
    d. Aplastic anemia
    e. Myelodysplastic syndromes
    f. Hemoglobinopathies (e.g. sickle cell disease)
5. Anemia of prematurity

availability of rHuEpo promises to be a major therapeutic advance for nephrologists, hematologists and medical oncologists.

ACKNOWLEDGEMENTS

Portions of this work were supported by research grants DK 19410 and DK 33488 and Clinical Research Center grant FR-0037, all from the National Institutes of Health, DHHS, and patient support funds from AMGen Corporation, Thousand Oaks, California. This manuscript is reproduced in large part from a contribution to "Molecular Control of Haemopoiesis", a published symposium of the Ciba Foundation and is presented here with their permission.

REFERENCES

1. Adamson, J.W, Eschbach, J.W., and Finch, C.A.: The kidney and erythropoiesis. American Journal of Medicine 44:725-733, 1968.

2. Shaw, A.B.: Haemolysis in chronic renal failure. British Medical Journal 2:213-215, 1967.

3. Castaldi, P.A., Rozenberg, M.C., Stewart, J.H.: The bleeding disorder of uraemia. A qualitative platelet defect. Lancet 2:66-69, 1966.

4. Fisher, J.W.: Mechanism of the anemia of chronic renal failure. Editorial review. Nephron 25:106-111, 1980.

5. Eschbach, J.W., and Adamson, J.W.: Anemia of end-stage renal disease (ESRD). Kidney International 28:1- 5, 1985.

6. Jacobs, K., Shoemaker, C., Rudersdorf, R., Neill, S.D., Kaufman, R.J., Musfson, A., Seehra, J., Jones, S.S., Helwick, R., Fritsch, E.F., Kawakita, M., Shimizu, T., and Miyake, T.: Isolation and characterization of genomic and cDNA clones of human erythropoietin. Nature 313:806-810, 1985.

7. Lin, F.-K., Suggs, S., Lin, C.H., Browne, J.K., Smalling, R., Egrie, J.C., Chen, K.K., Fox, G.M., Martin, F., Stabinsky, Z., Badrawi, S.M., Lai, P.H., and Goldwasser, E.: Cloning and expression of the human erythropoietin gene. Proceedings of the National Academy of Sciences USA 92:7580-7585, 1985.

8. Powell, J.S., Berkner, K.L., Lebo, R.V., and Adamson, J.W.: Human erythropoietin gene: High level expression in stably transfected mammalian cells and chromosome localization. Proceedings of the National Academy of Sciences USA 83:6465-6469, 1986.

9. Eschbach, J.W., Egrie, J.C., Downing, M.R., Browne, J.K., and Adamson, J.W.: Correction of the anemia of end-stage renal disease with recombinant human erythropoietin: Results of a Phase I and II clinical trial. New England Journal of Medicine 316:73-78, 1987.

10. Winearls, C.G., Oliver, D.O., Pippard, M.J., Reid, C., Downing, M.R., and Cotes, P.M.: Effect of human erythropoietin derived from recombinant DNA on the anaemia of patients maintained by chronic haemodialysis. Lancet 2:1175-1178, 1986.

11. Eschbach, J.W., and Adamson, J.W.: Correction of the anemia of hemodialysis (HD) patients with recombinant human erythropoietin (rHuEpo): Results of a multi-center study. Kidney International 33:189(A), 1988.

12. Bommer, J., Kugel, M., Schoeppe, W., Brunkhorst, R. Samtleben, W., Bramsiepe, P., Scigalla, P: Dose-related effects of recombinant human erythropoietin on erythropoiesis: results of a multicenter trial in patients with end-stage renal disease. Treatment of Renal Anaemia with Recombinant Human Erythropoietin. Contributions to Nephrology 66:85-93, 1988.

13. Akizawa, T., Koshikawa, S., Takaku, F., Urabe, A., Akiyama, N., Mimura, N. Otsubo, O., Ninei, H., Suzuki, Y., Kawaguchi Y., Ota, K., Kubo, K., Marumo, F., Maseda, T.: Clinical effect of recombinant human erythropoietin on anemia associated with chronic renal failure. A multi-institutional study in Japan. International Journal of Artificial Organs. 11:343-350, 1988.

14. Eschbach, J.W., Kelly, M.R., Haley, N.R., Abels, R.I., Adamson, J.W.: Correction of anemia in progressive renal failure with recombinant human erythropoietin (rHuEpo). New England Journal of Medicine, 321:3 158-163, 1989.

15. Bommer, J., Ritz, E., Weinreich, T., Bommer, G., Ziegler, T.: Subcutaneous erythropoietin. Lancet 2:406, 1988.

16. Granolleras, C. Shaldon, S. Experience with daily subcutaneous rhEPO in haemodialysis patients maintained on IV rhEPO thrice weekly. Contributions to Nephrology, In press, 1989.

17. Nonnast-Daniel, B., Creutzig, A., Kuhn, K., Bahlmann, J., Reimers, E., Brunkhorst, R., Caspay, L., Koch, K.M.: Effect of treatment with recombinant human erythropoietin on peripheral hemodynamics and oxygenation. Contributions to Nephrology. Karger: Basel, 66:185-194, 1988.

18. Buckner, F.S., Eschbach, J.W., Haley, N.R., Davidson, R.R., Adamson, J.W.: Correction of the anemia in hemodialysis (HD) patients (PTS) with recombinant human erythropoietin (rHuEpo): Hemodynamic changes and risks for hypertension. Kidney Int. 35:190(A), 1989.

19. Paganini, E., Thomas, T., Fouad, F., Garcia, J., Bravo, E.: The correction of anemia in hemodialysis patients using recombinant human erythropoietin (rHuEpo): Hemodynamic effects. Kidney International 33:204, 1988.

20. Neff, M.S., Kim, K.E., Persoff, M., Onesti, G., Swartz, C.: Hemodynamics of uremic anemia. Circulation 63:876-883, 1971.

21. Means, R.T., Olsen, N.J., Krantz, S.B., Graber, S.E., Dessypris, E.N., Stone, W.J., O'Neil, V., Pincus, T.P.: Treatment of the anemia of rheumatoid arthritis with recombinant human erythropoietin: Clinical and in vitro studies. Arthritis and Rheumatism 32:638-642, 1989.

22. Douglas, S.W., Adamson, J.W.: The anemia of chronic disorders: Studies of marrow regulation and iron metabolism. Blood 45:55-65, 1975.

23. Goodnough, L.T., Rudnick, S., Price, T.H., Ballas, S.K., Collins, M.L., Crowley, J.P., Kosmin, M., Kruskall, M.S., Lenes, B.A., Menitove, J.E., Silberstein, L.E., Smith, K.J. Wallas, C.H., Abels, R., Von Tress, M.: Increased preoperative collection of Autologous blood with recombinant human erythropoietin therapy. New England Journal of Medicine 321:1163-1168, 1989.

24. Rarick, M., Wilson, E., Berstein-Singer, M., et al. Double blind placebo controlled study of recombinant human erythropoietin in AIDS patients with anemia caused by HIVinfection and Zidovudine. In: V International Conference on AIDS: the scientific and social challenge, Montreal, Quebec, Canada, June 4-9, 1989. Ottawa, Ont.: International Development Research Center, 1989:195. abstract.

25. Adamson, J.W., and Eschbach, J.W.: Management of the anaemia of chronic renal failure with recombinant erythropoietin. Quarterly Journal of Medicine, in press 1990.

The Biology of Hematopoiesis, pages 519–530

TARGET CELLS FOR GM-CSF AND KINETICS OF RESPONSE

Aglietta M., Bussolino F., Piacibello W., Apra' F., Sanavio F., Stacchini A., Monzeglio C., Carnino F., Stern A.C., Gavosto F. Clinica Medica A, Dipartimento di Scienze Biomediche ed Oncologia Umana (A.M., P.W., A.F., S.F., S.A., G.F.) Universita' di Torino; Dipartimento di Genetica, Biologia e Chimica Medica (B.F.), Universita' di Torino; Divisione di Ginecologia C, (M.C., C.F.) Ospedale S. Anna di Torino; Clinical Research Department Sandoz (S.A.C.), Basel, Switzerland.

Haemopoietic growth factors are cytokines whose activity is directed to the proliferation of myelopoietic progenitors and to mature cell function (Cannistra and Griffin, 1988; Sieff, 1987; Morstyn and Burgess, 1988; Metcalf, 1989). Their marked activity in vitro and in the experimental animal has quickly led to the launching of clinical trials to test their therapeutic potential in man. (Cannistra and Griffin, 1988; Sieff, 1987; Morstyn and Burgess, 1988; Metcalf, 1989; Aglietta and Gavosto, 1989; Steward and Scarffe, 1989).

The most obvious application is replacement management with growth factors of cases of altered myelopoiesis caused by the reduced production of one or more factors. With the exception of erythropoietin, whose plasma levels are reduced in renal failure and in other forms of chronic anaemia (Caro et al., 1979), there is no clear evidence of disease states derived from altered growth factor production, though this could be solely due to technical reasons. In the first place, exact dosages have only recently become available. In the second place, growth factors (once again with the exception of erythropoietin, which is almost entirely of renal origin) are primarily produced in the marrow microenviromment, where cytokines can act as short-distance mediators, with the result that their plasma levels do not provide an exact indication of what really occurs on the target cells.

Yet the possibilities opened up by the use of growth factors are not confined to replacement therapy. It is, in fact, possible (and the preliminary data are encouraging in this respect) that pharmacological doses can be employed in cases of altered myelopoiesis attributable not to insufficient production of growth factors, but to quantitative (e.g. secondary cytopenia) or qualitative (e.g. myeloproliferative disorders) alterations of the myelopoietic cells themselves. It is clear that the physiopathological implications of therapeutic approach of this type are completely different since the relation between self-maintenance and differentiation in the myelopoietic progenitors compartment might be modified.

Granulocyte-macrophage colony stimulating factor (GM-CSF) has been experimented in primary and secondary cytopenia on the strength of preclinical evidence that it is active on progenitors and mature cells. The initial clinical results are encouraging. They will be discussed in the light of what is currently known about the target cells and their response kinetics. In this connection, account is also taken of the fact that extramyelopoietic cells, too, are GM-CSF target cells.

GM-CSF receptors are expressed by all cells in the granulomonocyte line (Di Persio et al.,1988). GM-CSF on its own can induce the production of granulocytes and monocytes by granulomonocyte progenitors CFU-GM. Its action is either additive or synergic with that of other factors active on granulomonopoietic cells (i.e. G-CSF, M-CSF)(Strife et al., 1987; Tomonaga et al., 1986; Metcalf et al., 1986; Begley et al., 1988). In addition, it stimulates the proliferation of the other committed (BFU-E, CFU-Mk) and of multipotent (CFU-GEMM) myeloid progenitors: in the presence of other cytokines active on the intermediate and terminal stages of erythropoiesis and megakarycytopoiesis it induces the production of colonies composed of mature cells (Migliaccio et al., 1988; Sonoda et al., 1988).

In vivo investigations have confirmed many of the expectations raised by the in vitro findings. In patients with primary cytopenia (such as marrow aplasia, AIDS) GM-

CSF induces an increase in the number of circulating granulocytes and monocytes (Antin et al., 1988; Groopman et al., 1987; Nissen et al., 1988). In the same way, the stimulating effect of GM-CSF in cytopenia secondary to cytostatic chemotherapy or marrow tranplantation is demonstrated by the fact that recovery of granulomonopiesis occurs more quickly in patients treated with GM-CSF than in the controls (Nemunaitis et al., 1988; Brandt et al., 1988; Antman et al., 1988). While it is true that these are different pathological situations, the results thus obtained enable some interesting conclusions to be drawn with regard to the effect of GM-CSF in vivo.

In the first place, stimulation of granulomonopoiesis is linked to administration of the drug. On its discontinuation, there is a return to the basic situation in primary myelopathies, or to a picture similar to that which had occured without GM-CSF management in secondary cytopenia (Antin et al., 1988; Groopman et al., 1987; Nissen et al., 1988; Nemunaitis et al., 1988; Brandt et al., 1988; Antman et al., 1988), though here even a temporary effect resulting in drastic reduction of the granulomonocytopenia can be of major therapeutic significance since it reduces the risks of infection associated with chemotherapy.

The transient nature of the effect of GM-CSF suggests that it is unable to influence the self-maintenance potential of haemopoietic progenitors. The results of controlled clinical trials, however, must be awaited before a conclusion can be reached on this point.

Several points still remain to be established with regard to the action of GM-CSF on normal marrow cells.

To obtain a clearer definition of the granulo-monopoietic cells that form the targets of the molecule, we have investigated the effect of GM-CSF (human, recombinant, mammalian glycoylated, Sandoz/Schering Plough) on subjects with normal myelopoiesis, i.e. in a situation where its action could be evaluated with reference to constant baselines as opposed to the kinetically disturbed values produced by chemotherapy, and where other cytokines interacting with the molecule were at normal levels. In other words, the GM-CSF treatment was the only variable (Aglietta et al., 1989). It was found that GM-CSF administered for 3 days rapidly led to an approximately three-fold increase in the number of circulating leukocytes. Neutrophils, eosinophils and monocytes were elevated, whereas the absolute number of lymphocytes and the relation between the lymphocyte sub-populations were unchanged.

All the cells of the granulomonocyte differentiative line increase their proliferative activity following treatment with GM-CSF. The percentage of CFU-GM (day 14) in S phase (evaluated by means of the suicide tecnique) rises from 43±20 to 82±11%; that of the blasts, promyelocytes and mielocytes in S phase (evaluated autoradiographically) from 26±8 to 41±65.

These data, however, cannot be used to make an accurate quantitative assessment of the extent of the proliferative stimulus induced by GM-CSF, since no provision is made for calculation of any temporal variations in the cycle and its individual phases. They may be of greater importance than the number of cells in S phase in determining the cell production per unit of time.

Therefore, several kinetic parameters have been calculated by double-labeling of cells in S phase (in vivo with bromodesoxyruridine and in vitro with tritiated thymidine) so that a quantification of the stimulus has been achieved. During treatment with GM-CSF the number of cells produced per hour (Kb) is more than doubled, rising from 1.3 to 3.4 cells/100 following marked shortening of the Ts and above all of the Tc of the proliferating population.

GM-CSF is also a powerful activator of mature cells. It stimulates monocyte digestion of Leishmania Donovani in vitro (Weiser et al., 1987) and activates other monocyte functions, such as the production of TNF-alpha, IL-1 and prostaglandins E, this being the probable cause of its reduction of the monocyte IL-2 receptors (Hancock et al., 1988). GM-CSF increases the cytotoxic activity and prostaglandin E synthesis of the eosinophils and also enhances their survival (Owen et al., 1987; Silberstein et al., 1986).

GM-CSF in vitro enhances many neutrophil functions, such as the production of superoxides, antibody-dependent cell cytotoxicity, expression of receptors for complement, and expression of adhesion glycoproteins located on the cell membrane. Some of these effects have also been observed after the administration of GM-CSF in vivo (Weisbart et al., 1985; Fleischman et al., 1986; Arnaout et al., 1986; Mayer et al., 1987).

Our own work has shown that neutrophils from patients

undergoing GM-CSF treatment release 2-3 times more platelet activating factor (PAF) after stimulation with FMLP, tumor necrosis factor TNF-alpha, or during phagocytosis (Aglietta et al., submitted). In addition, smaller concentrations of FMLP or TNF-alpha are needed to induce the synthesis and release of PAF by neutrophils. As well as confirming the fact that GM-CSF is a neutrophil activator, these data are also of physiopatological interest in view of the role played by PAF in inflammation. Its powerful proinflammatory effect suggests that augmented PAF synthesis on the part of activated neutrophils may gradually boost a local inflammatory reaction.

It is clear from what has just been said that all the cells of the granulo-monocyte line are targets of the molecule. The effect of GM-CSF on other myelopoietic lines, however, is less evident. In cases of disturbed haemopoieis, treatment with GM-CSF results in an inconstant increase in platelet and red cell numbers. For this reason the in vivo action of GM-CSF on these differentiative lines is unclear.

Certain aspects of the question have been elucidated by our studies of patients with normal myelopoiesis. Treatment with GM-CSF does not enhance platelet and red cell production, nor does it alter the proliferative status of erythroblasts and megakarioblasts (Aglietta et al., 1989; and Aglietta et al., in preparation). During treatment, however, there is an increase in the proliferative activity of BFU-E and CFU-Mk. These findings suggest that the in vivo action of GM-CSF extends no further than the early stages of erythro and megakaryocytopoiesis and that other molecules (erythropoietin, TSH, TGF-beta, etc.) are crucial in the regulation of intermediate and terminal phases of thrombocytopoiesis and erythropoiesis, with the result that in normal subjects the GM-CSF stimulus cannot alter the production of mature cells. This interpretation also helps to explain why GM-CSF has an inconstant effect as a stimulator of red cell and platelet production when administered in a scenario of altered haemopoiesis (after chemotherapy, marrow transplantation, etc.), in other words in situations where the variability of the number of residual progenitors and of the levels of endogenous cytokines makes it less easy to predict its final effect.

GM-CSF is also active in transformed myeloid cells

(Griffin et al., 1986; Delwel et al., 1988; Aglietta et al., 1990). The possibility of inducing the differentiation of leukaemic cells and the risks associated with this approach have been extensively discussed (Antin et al., 1988; Vadhan-Raj et al., 1988; Ganser et al., 1989; Thompson et al., 1989). The enhanced proliferative activity of neoplastic cells after growth factor administration observed in myelodysplasia, and likely in myeloid leukaemia in the light of the preclinical data (Griffin et al., 1986; Delwen et al., 1988; Aglietta et al., 1989), could in theory be exploited to boost the effectiveness of chemotherapy. This therapeutic approach represents an attempt to overcome the kinetic resistances generated by the presence of quiescent neoplastic cells. It is supported by recent in vitro evidence of enhanced leukaemia progenitors sensitivity to cytostatics following preincubation with growth factor (Miyauchi et al.,1989). Even so, the great interest in theoretical terms of a chemotherapeutical approach to leukaemia based on recruitment and kinetic synchronisation must not make us forget the risk that the concomitant increase in the proliferative activity of the normal progenitors results in a serious and protracted aplastic phase. Controlled clinical trials now in progress offer the only way of defining the problem. Those undertaken in our Institute provide for the presence of a cryopreserved back-up marrow for infusion in the event of irreversible aplasia.

GM-CSF′s action on the myeloid cells is accompanied by relatively mild <u>toxicity</u> at doses of up to 5-10 ug/kg. At higher doses, substantial toxicity might appear, including thrombosis of major vessels with pulmonary embolism, pericardial or pleural effusion, and other signs of capillary leak syndrome. The reasons for these effects can possibly be sought in the action of GM-CSF on neutrophils (activation and priming for the response to chemotactic agents, increased release of PAF; enhanced expression of the CD 11b adhesion molecule), and on endothelial cells. The fact that higher levels of toxicity are present only with elevated doses that are not needed to obtain a significant biological effect is further evidence of the great therapeutic potential of growth factors, and of GM-CSF in particular, above all in oncology. Reduced marrow toxicity should improve the tolerance to current antineoplastic chemotherapeutic regimens. In the medium term, the possibility of speeding up the recovery of haemopoiesis could enable protocols to be reformulated so to permit the augmentation of the doses of myelotoxic drugs and their administration at shorter intervals. This therapeutic approach will enable an experimental check to be made of the value of Coldie and Goldman's somatic mutation theory (Goldie and Coldman, 1984). The prospect of a radical change in the chemoradiotherapeutic approach to the neoplastic patient thanks to the employement of growth factors will be rendered even more realistic if the synergic effect of the administration of several growth factors is also corroborated in man.

Enthusiasm for these substances, however, must be tempered by the consideration that no answer has been found to two extremely important questions namely:

1) What is the effect of protracted administration of growth factors?

It may be that they result in an eventual depletion of the stem compartment and hence persistent cytopenia. In addition to possible damage to this compartment, the likelihood of injury arising from an excessive production and activation of mature cells, if protracted, must also be born in mid. Nothing is know as yet in man. There are, however, data for transgenic mice whose macrophages constitutively produce GM-CSF. These animals die early from the effects of a wasting syndrome, including blindness, intestinal necrosis and the appearance of addominal nodules (Metcalf and Moore, 1988).

2) Do myelopoietic growth factors influence the growth of a neoplasm?

By contrast to what was believed unitil recently, the action of growth factors is not confined to the myelopoietic cells. Human endothelial cells have receptors for GM-CSF (and for G-CSF) and their proliferation and migration in vitro are stimulated by these molecules (Bussolino et al., 1989). It is possible that neovascularisation of both the primary tumour and its metastases is promoted by their administration. GM-CSF stimulate the proliferation of normal and neoplastic lymphoid cells in vitro. (Aglietta et al., 1989; Valtieri et al., 1987; Santoli et al., 1988). It has recently been reported that the proliferation of continuous human lung microcytoma and colon carcinoma cell lines is stimulated by growth factors, even though the concentrations of GM-CSF active on these cells might be greater than those active on myelopoietic cells (Baldwin et al., 1989; Berdel et al., 1989).In a recent phase I/II study the administration of GM-CSF had to be discontinued in two cases owing to increased bone metastasis pain (Herrmann et al., 1989) Although no clear evidence has as yet been produced to show that growth factors stimulate neoplastic progression one should not forget that the lack of evidence, might solely depend on the absence of controlled studies.

The conclusion to be drawn, therefore, is that growth factors may revolutionise the therapeutic approach to some haematological diseases and to chemo-and radiosensitive solid tumours. The many questions as yet unanswered, however, must not be forgotten and the use of these substances must at present be confined to controlled studies.

Acknowledgments: This work was supported with grants from CNR, Special Project Oncology, and from the Italian Association for Cancer Research.

REFERENCES

Aglietta M, De Felice L, Stacchini A, Sanavio A, Severino A, Piacibello W, Mandelli F (1990). Effect of hemopoietic growth factors on the proliferation of acute lymphoid and non lymphoid leukemias. Leukemia and Lymphoma, in press.

Aglietta M, Gavosto F (1989). CSFs, from basic science to clinical trials. Bone Marrow Transpl 4(suppl.1):16-19.

Aglietta M, Monzeglio C, Apra´ F, Mossetti C, Stern AC, Garibaldi G, Bussolino F. In vivo priming of human neutrophils by granulocyte-macrophage colony stimulating factor: effect on the production of platelet activating factor. Submitted for publication.

Aglietta M, Piacibello W, Sanavio F, Stacchini A, Apra´ F, Schena M, Mossetti C, Carnino F, Caligaris-Cappio F, Gavosto F (1989). Kinetics of human hemopoietic cells after in vivo administration of granulocyte-macrophage colony stimulating factor. J Clin Invest 83:551-557.

Antin JH, Smith BR, Holmes W, Rosenthal DS (1988). Phase

1/2 study of recombinant human granulocyte-macrophage colony stimulating factor in aplastic anemia and myelodysplastic syndrome. Blood 72:705-713.

Antman KS, Griffin JD, Elias A, Socinski MA, Ryan L, Cannistra SA, Oette D, Whitley M, Frei E, Schnipper LE (1988). Effect of recombinant human granulocyte-macrophage colony stimulating factor on chemotherapy induced myelosuppression. N Engl J Med 318:593-598.

Arnaout MA, Wang EA, Clark SC, Sieff CA (1986). Human recombinant granulocyte-macrophage colony stimulating factor increases cell to cell adhesion and surface expression of adhesion promoting surface glycoproteins on mature granulocytes. J Clin Invest, 78:597-601.

Baldwin GC, Gasson JC, Kaufman SE, Quan SG, Williams RE, Avalos BR, Gazdar AF, Golde DW, Dipersio JF (1989). Non hematopoietic tumor cells express functional GM-CSF receptors. Blood, 73:1033-1037.

Baldwin GC, Gasson JC, Quan SG, Fleischmann J, Weisbart R, Oette D, Mitsuyasu RT, Golde DW (1988). Granulocyte-macrophage colony stimulating factor enhances neutrophil function in acquired immunodeficiency patients. Proc Natl Acad Sci (USA),85:2763-2766.

Begley CG, Nicola NA, Metcalf D (1988). Proliferation of normal human promyelocytes and myelocytes after a single pulse stimulation by purified GM-CSF or G-CSF. Blood 71:640-645.

Berdel WE, Danhauser-Riedl S, Steinhauser G, Winton EF (1989). Various human hematopoietic growth factors (interleukin-3, GM-CSF, G-CSF) stimulate the clonal growth of nonhematopoietic tumor cells. Blood, 73:80-83.

Brandt SJ, Peters WP, Atwater Sk, Kurtzberg J, Borowitz MJ, Jones RB, Shpall EJ, Bast RC, Gilbert CJ, Oette DH (1988). Effect of recombinant human granulocyte-macrophage colony stimulating factor on hematopoietic reconstitution after high dose chemotherapy and autologous bone marrow transplantation. N Engl J Med 318:869-876.

Bussolino F, Wang JM, Defilippi P, Turrini F, Sanavio F, Edgell CJS, Aglietta M, Arese P, Mantovani A (1989). Granulocyte and granulocyte-macrophage colony stimulating factors induce human endothelial cells to migrate and proliferate. Nature 337:471-473.

Cannistra SA, Griffin JD (1988). Regulation of the production and function of granulocytes and monocytes. Sem Hematol 25:173-188.

Caro J, Brow S, Miller O, Murray T, Erslev AJ (1979).

Erythropoietin levels in uremic nephric and anephric patients. J Lab Clin Med 93:449-458.

Delwel R., Dalem M., Pellens C., Dorsser L., Wagemaker G., Clark SC, Lowenberg B (1988). Growth regulation of human myeloid leukemia: effects of five recombinant hematopoietic factors in serum free culture system. Blood 72:1944-1949.

Di Persio J, Billing P, Kaufman S, Eghtesady P, William RE, Gasson JC (1988). Characterization of the human granulocyte-macrophage colony stimulating factor receptor. J Biol Chem 263:1834-1841.

Fleischman J, Golde DW, Weisbart RH, Gasson JC (1986). Granulocyte-macrophage colony stimulating factor enhances phagocytosis of bacteria by human neutrophils. Blood, 68:708-711.

Ganser A, Volkers B, Greher J, Ottmann OG, Walther F, Becher R, Bergmann L, Schulz G, Hoelzer D (1989). Recombinant human granulocyte-macrophage colony stimulating factor in patients with myelodysplastic syndromes - a phase I/II trial. Blood, 73:31-37.

Goldie JH, Coldman AJ (1984). The genetic origin of drug resistance in neoplasms:implication for systemic therapy. Cancer Res 44:3643-3653.

Griffin JD, Young D, Hermann F, Wiper D, Wagner K, Sabbath KD (1986). Effect of recombinant human GM-CSF on proliferation of clonogenic cells in acute myeloblastic leukemia. Blood 67:1448-1453.

Groopman JE, Mitsuyasu RT, De Leo MJ, Oette DH, Golde DW (1987). Effect of recombinant human granulocyte-macrophage colony stimulating factor on myelopoiesis in the acquired immunodeficiency syndrome. N Engl J Med 317:593-598.

Hancock WW, Plean ME, Bobzik L (1988). Recombinant granulocyte-macrophage colony stimulating factor down regulates expression of Il-2 receptor on human mononuclear phagocytes by induction of prostaglandin E. J Immunol, 140:3021-3025.

Herrmann F, Schulz G, Lindemann A, Meyenburg W, Oster W, Krumwiek D, Mertelsmann R (1989). Hematopoietic responses in patients with advanced malignancy treated with recombinant human granulocyte-macrophage colony stimulating factor. J Clin Oncol, 7:159-167.

Mayer P, Lam C, Obenaus H, Liehl E, Besemer J (1987). Recombinant human GM-CSF induces leukocytosis and activates peripheral blood polymorphonuclear neutrophils in non human primates. Blood, 70:206-213.

Metcalf D (1989). The molecular control of cell division, differentiation and maturation in haemopoietic cells. Nature 339:27-30.

Metcalf D, Begley CG, Johnson GR, Nicola NA, Vadas MA, Lopez AF, Williamson DJ, Wong GG, Clark SC, Wang EA (1986). Biologic properties in vitro of a recombinant granulocyte-macrophage colony stimulating factor. Blood 67:37-45.

Metcalf D, Moore JG (1988). Divergent disease patterns in granulocyte-macrophage colony stimulating factor transgenic mice associated with different with different transgene insertion site. Proc Natl Acad Sci (USA), 85:7767-7771.

Migliaccio G, Migliaccio AR, Adamson JW (1988a). In vitro differentiation of human granulocyte-macrophage and erythroid progenitors: comparative analysis of the influence of recombinant human erythropoietin, G-CSF, GM-CSF and IL-3 in serum supplemented and in serum deprived cultures. Blood 72:248-256.

Morstyn G, Burgess AW (1988). Hemopoietic growth factors : a review. Cancer Res 48:5624-5637.

Miyauchi J, Kelleher CA, Wang C, Minkin S, McCulloch EA (1989). Growth factors influence the sensitivity of leukemic stem cells to cytosine arabinoside. Blood, 73:1272-1278.

Nemunaitis J, Singer JW, Buckner CD, Hill R, Storb R, Thomas ED, Appelbaum FR (1988). Use of recombinant human granulocyte-macrophage colony stimulating factor in autologous marrow tranbsplantation for lymphoid malignancies. Blood 72:834-836.

Nissen C, Tichelli A, Gratwohl A, Speck A, Milne A, Gordon-Smith EC, Schaedelin J (1988). Failure of recombinant human granulocyte-macrophage colony stimulating factor therapy in aplastic anemia patients with very severe neutropenia. Blood 72:2045-2047.

Owen WF Jr, Rothenberg ME, Silberstein DS, Gasson JC, Stevens RL, Austen KF, Soberman RJ (1987). Regulation of human eosinophil viability, density and function by granulocyte-macrophage colony stimulating factor in the presence of 3T3 fibroblasts. J Exp Med, 166:129-141.

Santoli D, Clark SC, Kreider BL, Maslin PA, Rovera G (1988). Amplification of IL-2 driven T cell proliferation by recombinant human IL-3 and granulocyte-macrophage colony stimulating factor. J Immunol, 141:519-526.

Sieff CA (1987). Hematopoietic growth factors. J Clin

Invest 79:1549-1557.

Silberstein DS, Owen WF, Gasson JC, Di Persio JF, Golde DW, Bina JC, Soberman R, Austen KF, David JR (1986) Enhancement of human eosinophil cytotoxicity and leukotriene synthesis by biosynthetic (recombinant) granulocyte-macrophage colony stimulating factor. J Immunol, 137:3290-3294.

Sonoda Y, Yang YC, Wong GG, Clark SC, Ogawa M (1988). Erythroid burst promoting activity of purified recombinant human GM-CSF and interleukin 3: studies with anti GM-CSF and anti IL-3 sera and studies in serum free cultures. Blood 72:1381-1386.

Steward WP, Scarffe JH (1989). Clinical trials with haemapoietic growth factors. Prog Growth Factor Res 1:1-12.

Strife A, Lambek C, Wisnienski D, Gulati S, Gasson JC, Golde DW, Welte K, Gabrilove JL, Clarkson B (1987). Activities of four purified growth factors on highly enriched human hematopoietic progenitor cells. Blood 69:1508-1523.

Tomonaga M, Golde DW, Gasson JC (1986). Biosynthetic (recombinant) human granulocyte macrophage colony stimulating factor: effect on normal bone marrow and leukemia cell lines. Blood 67:31-36.

Thompson JA, Lee DJ, Kidd P, Rubin E, Kaufman J, Bonnem EM, Fefer A (1989). Subcutaneous granulocyte-macrophage colony stimulating factor in patients with myelodysplastic syndrome: toxicity, pharmacokinetics, and hematological effects. J Clin Oncol, 7:629-637.

Vadhan-Raj S, Keating M, Le Maistre A, Hittelman W, Mc Credie K, Trujillo JM, Broxmeyer HE, Henney C, Gutterman JU (1988). Effects of recombinant human granulocyte-macrophage colony stimulating factor in patients with myelodysplastic syndromes. N Engl J Med 317:1545-1552.

Valtieri M, Santoli D, Caracciolo D, Kreider BL, Altmann SW, Tweardy DJ, Gemperlein I, Mavilio F, Lange B, Rovera G (1987). Establishment and charaterization of an undifferentiated human T leukemia cell line which requires granulocyte-macrophage colony stimulating factor for growth. J Immunol 138:4042-4045.

Weiser WY, van Niel A, Clark SC, David JR, Remold HG (1987). Recombinant human granulocyte-macrophage colony stimulating factor activates intracellular killing of Leishmania Donovani by human monocytes derived macrophages. J Exp Med 166:1436-1446.

Weisbart RH, Golde DW, Clark SC, Wong GG, Gasson JC (1985). Human granulocyte-macrophage colony stimulating factor is a neutrophil activator. Nature, 314:361-363.

The Biology of Hematopoiesis, pages 531–538

HEMATOPOIETIC GROWTH FACTORS IN BONE MARROW TRANSPLANTATION FOR HEMATOLOGIC MALIGNANCIES

Hillard M. Lazarus, M.D.

Department of Medicine, Ireland Cancer Center, University Hospitals of Cleveland, Case Western Reserve University, Cleveland, Ohio 44106

Ionizing radiation and many drugs exhibit a log-linear relationship between dose and tumor cell kill over a certain range, and small changes in dose can produce significant changes in anti-tumor response (Frei E III, et al., 1980). Bone marrow transplantation circumvents the problem of prolonged marrow suppression, permitting chemo-radiation therapy doses to be escalated to the "myeloablative" range and providing curative therapy in a variety of malignant and non-malignant disorders (O'Reilly RJ, 1983; Cheson BD, et al., 1989; Dicke KA, et al., 1986).

That successful marrow engraftment and expansion take place after intensive chemo-radiation therapy implies either that the regulatory systems controlling hemopoiesis are resistant to myeloablative therapy, or that the infused marrow itself contains populations of cells able to provide the necessary proliferative signals for hematopoietic tissue (Metcalf D, 1989). The "natural regeneration" after marrow infusion involves a period of delay during which the patient is seriously leukopenic and thrombocytopenic. It is during this period of transplantation that the greatest morbidity occurs. If the recovery of peripheral blood cell counts could be hastened by the use of hematopoietic growth factors to truncate the period of pancytopenia, the patient would benefit significantly.

In vitro analysis of the control of hematopoiesis has identified a group of glycoproteins that control the survival, proliferation, and differentiation of the various hematopoietic blood cell lineages (Metcalf D, 1988; Clark SC, et al., 1987). These hematopoietic growth factors not only act on committed progenitors but enhance the function of mature effector cells (Weisbart RH, 1989). The complementary DNA (cDNA) for each of the human gene analogues has been cloned and expressed in bacterial, yeast, or mammalian systems. Sufficient quantities of these agents have been produced and purified to evaluate their biological effects on hematopoiesis and host defense directly in patients with a variety of conditions including marrow transplant.

When to begin infusions of growth factors in the course of transplantation is unknown. The growth-supporting, growth-promoting, and growth-factor-like activities in the plasma of 34 patients were serially examined before, during, and after myeloablative therapy and marrow transplant (Yamasaki K, et al., 1988). Growth-promoting activity peaked 7 to 21 days after marrow transplant, the levels varying from patient to patient. Patients who had a longer delay before engraftment, however, had a longer duration of plasma-growth promoting activities. These data suggest that the optimal time for administration of growth factors would be during the first few weeks after marrow infusion.

Several studies have reported the administration of growth factors during autologous or allogeneic bone marrow rescue in patients with solid tumors or hematologic malignancies. In an early trial, colony stimulating factor derived from human urine (CSF-HU) was infused intravenously in 51 patients undergoing allogeneic (37 patients) or autologous (14 patients) marrow transplantation (Masaoka T, et al., 1988). Marrow recovery (increase in leukocytes over 1000/μl) occurred 16.7 days (mean) versus 25.4 days in a historical control group. Few side effects directly attributable to CSF-HU were noted, and no increase in the incidence of leukemic relapse or graft-versus-host disease were observed. Subsequently, most marrow transplant trials for hematologic malignancies have utilized recombinant hematopoietic growth factors (rhGF), (Table 1) ([a]Nemunaitis J, et al., 1988; [b]Devereaux S, et al., 1989; [c]Blazar BR, et al., 1989; [d]Spitzer G, et al., 1989; [e]Link H, et al., 1989; [f]Lazarus, et al.; [g]Masaoka T, et a., 1989). Infusions of granulocyte colony stimulating factor (G-CSF) or granulocyte-macrophage colony stimulating factor (GM-CSF) produced in yeast, _E. coli_, or Chinese hamster ovary cells, were begun the day of or shortly after marrow infusion. In most studies, growth factor therapy was continued for 14 to 21 days; all trials (except two) infused autologous marrow.

Table 1. Marrow Transplant Trials for Hematologic Malignancy Utilizing Recombinant Hematopoietic Growth Factors.

Ref	No. Pts.	Disease	Growth Factor	Dose Daily	Mean or Median Day PMN>500/µl Study	*Control	Bacteremia or Fungemia(%) Study	*Control
a	15	3 ALL 12 NHL	GM-CSF yeast	15-240 µg/m²	15	25	13	30
b	12	12 HD	G-CSF yeast& E.coli	100-400 µg/m	17.5	24.9	50	63
c	Φ25	25 ALL	GM-CSF yeast	16-256 µg/m²	Φ23	24	Φ40	44
d	26	26 HD	G-CSF E.coli	30-120 µg/m²	13	22	17	36
e	17	7 HD, 1 ALL, 9 ST	GM-CSF yeast& E.coli	250-500 µg/m²	13&15	21&23	-	-
f	8	8 NHL	GM-CSF CHO	11 µg/kg	13	22	25	39
g	+34	10 ALL, 8 AML, 9 CML, 4 SAA, 3 NHL	G-CSF E.coli	200-400 µg/m²	15.0- 16.9	26.1 27.4	-	-

*Historic controls, used as comparison.
+All patients received allogeneic marrow.
ΦAll study patients received marrow purged *in vitro*, while historic controls received unpurged marrow.
CHO=Chinese hamster ovary; ST=solid tumors (sarcoma, neuroblastoma); ALL=acute lymphocytic leukemia; AML=acute myelogenous leukemia; CML=chronic myelogenous leukemia; NHL=non-Hodgkin's lymphoma; HD=Hodgkin's Disease; SAA=severe aplastic anemia; PMN=neutrophils

One study (Masaoka T, et al., 1989) utilized allogeneic marrow in all patients. In another trial (Nemunaitis J, et al., 1988), 2 of the 15 patients received syngeneic marrow. *In vitro* purging was performed only in two studies. Monoclonal antibodies and/or chemotherapy were used to purge the marrow of all patients in one trial (Blazar BR, et al., 1989) and in 4 of 15 patients in another (Nemunaitis J, et al., 1988). In all these trials, manifestations of toxicity that may have been due to growth factor infusions have included low grade fever, bone pain, myalgias, macular rash, headaches, nausea, abdominal cramping, central venous catheter thrombosis, knee swelling, and mild edema. The capillary or vascular leak syndrome (edema, weight gain, and pleural, pericardial, or peritoneal effusions), reported in other marrow transplant trials (Brandt SJ, et al., 1988), was not observed. The rhGF infusions were associated with a significant shortening of the period of severe neutropenia (less than 500/µl) or leukopenia (less than 1000/µl) in comparison to a comparable historic control group. Randomized trials are now beginning to address this effect in a prospective fashion, but data are limited (Kwong YL, et al., 1989). In most trials no discernible effects have been observed upon recovery of reticulocyte or platelet count. One group (Nemunaitis J, et al., 1988) did observe that treated patients became independent of platelet transfusions about 19 days (mean) after transplant, compared to 38 days in a historic control group. The groups that received growth factor infusions generally had a marked decrease in documented infections, reported herein as bacteremias or fungemias (Table 1). Infections usually occurred within the first or second week after marrow infusion. These data are similar to those reported in breast and malignant melanoma patients treated by marrow transplantatation and growth factor infusions (Brandt SJ, et al., 1988; Oette D, et al.). Of 48 breast cancer or malignant melanoma patients who received infusions of GM-CSF (compared with a historic control population of 23 patients), the incidence of bacteremia was decreased from 35% (8 of 23 historical patients) to 18% (9 of 48 patients receiving recombinant GM-CSF). The occurrence of bacteremia generally was limited to the first week (1 in 47 patients) or second or third weeks (1 in 46 patients) after transplantation.

Discontinuance of growth factor infusions, however, has been associated in some patients with a mean drop in neutrophil count of 35% within 24 to 72 hours after stopping

GM-CSF therapy (range: 4-63%) (Nemunaitis J, et al., 1988). In our trial, 5 of 8 patients had a drop in absolute neutrophil count (mean: 26%; range: 7 - 54%) within 72 hours of discontinuing GM-CSF infusions (Lazarus HM, et al.). These data are similar to those obtained from solid tumor patients undergoing autologous marrow transplantation and growth factor infusions (Brandt SJ, et al., 1988). Apparent stem cell exhaustion was not observed in any of these trials. Still, the failure to achieve sustained engraftment in some patients raises the question of whether growth factors may cause differentiation of early stem cells and interfere with the self-renewal required for long-term reconstitution (Nemunaitis J, et al., 1988). Use of growth factors interestingly has led to significantly less renal, lung, and hepatic dysfunction, perhaps due to effective eradication of an early undetected systemic infection (Brandt SJ, et al., 1988). These findings need to be corroborated in other trials.

Complete engraftment after marrow transplantation uncommonly is a problem. Graft rejection, however, occurs in about 2% of unmanipulated HLA-identical transplants (Thomas ED, et al., 1975) and in as many as 21% of T-depleted matched or partially mismatched transplants (Anasetti C, et al., 1989; Martin PJ, et al., 1985; Beatty PG, et al., 1985; Storb R, et al., 1983). Significantly delayed engraftment may occur in up to 20% of autologous marrow transplant patients and 9% of allogeneic marrow transplant patients. Delayed engraftment may be the result of an abnormally small innoculum of stem cells, post-transplant viral infection, drug toxicity, or _in vitro_ marrow purging (Beatty PG, et al., 1985; Hill RS, et al., 1989; Winston DJ, et al., 1983; Kaizer H, et al., 1985). The prognosis for delayed engraftment or graft rejection is poor. An exception is the case of some aplastic anemia patients who receive a second marrow transplant for late engraftment failure after a successful initial graft (Bolger GB, et al., 1986; Champlin RE, et al., 1989). Infusions of recombinant human GM-CSF were given to 15 allogeneic, 21 autologous, and 1 syngeneic transplant patients who failed to engraft (Nemunaitis, et al., 1989). Graft failure was defined as failure to achieve an absolute neutrophil count of at least 100/µl by day 28 after transplant (or by day 21 in the setting of a life-threatening infection), or loss of engraftment (less than 500 neutrophils/µl) after successful engraftment had occurred. Patients received IV GM-CSF 60-1000 µg/m²/day for 14-21 days. Twenty-one of 37 patients achieved a neutrophil count greater than 500/µl within 2 weeks of beginning GM-CSF therapy. In those who responded, fever and infection resolved. Of note, none of 7 patients who received chemically-purged autologous bone marrow responded, while a number of patients who received unpurged or monoclonal antibody-purged marrow did respond.

Current issues that must be resolved regarding the use of rhGF infusions during marrow transplant include: the need for randomized trials, identifying the optimal dose and durations of therapy, finding effective strategies to deal with the decline in cell count after cessation of therapy, and sequential or combination rhGF studies. Regarding the latter, in a primate model IL-3 followed by GM-CSF was the most effective technique to stimulate hematopoiesis (Donahue, et al, 1988). As a result of answering such questions, bone marrow transplantation likely will occupy an even greater place in the therapeutic armamentarium for the treatment of hematologic malignancies.

REFERENCES

Frei E III, Canellos GP (1980). Dose: a critical factor in cancer chemotherapy. Am J Med 69:585-595.

O'Reilly RJ (1983). Allogeneic bone marrow transplantation: current status and future directions. Blood 62:941-964.

Cheson BD, Lacerna L, Leyland-Jones, B, et al (1989). Autologous bone marrow transplantation. Current status and future directions. Ann Intern Med 110:51-65.

Dicke KA, Spitzer G (1986). Evaluation of the use of high-dose cytoreduction with autologous marrow rescue in various malignancies. Transplantation 41:4-20.

Metcalf D (1989). Hematopoietic growth factors and marrow transplantation: an overview. Transpl Proc 21:2932-2933.

Metcalf D (1988). The Molecular Control of Blood Cells, Boston, Harvard University Press.

Clark SC, Kamen R (1987). The human hematopoietic colony-stimulating factors. Science 236:1229-1237.

Weisbart RH (1989). Colony-stimulating factors and host defense. Ann Intern Med 110:297-303.

Yamasaki K, Solberg LA, Jamal N, et al (1988). Hemopoietic colony growth-promoting activities in the plasma of bone marrow transplant recipients. J Clin Invest 82:255-261.

Masaoka T, Motoyoshi K, Takaku F, et al (1988). Administration of human urinary colony stimulating factor after bone marrow transplantation. Bone Marrow Transplant 3:121-127.

Nemunaitis J, Singer JW, Buckner CD, et al (1988). Use of recombinant human granulocyte-macrophage colony-stimulating factor in autologous marrow transplantation for lymphoid malignancies. Blood 72:834-836.

Devereaux S, Linch DC, Gribben JG, et al (1989). GM-CSF accelerates neutrophil recovery after autologous bone marrow transplantation for Hodgkin's disease. Bone Marrow Transplant 4:49-54.

Blazar BR, Kersey JH, McGlave PB, et al (1989). _In vivo_ administration of recombinant human granulocyte/macrophage colony-stimulating factor in acute lymphoblastic leukemia patients receiving purged autografts. Blood 73:849-857.

Spitzer G, Jagannath S, Taylor K, et al (1989). Studies of recombinant human granulocyte colony-stimulating factor (rhG-CSF) after high-dose cyclophosphamide, carmustine (BCNU), and etoposide (VP-16) (CBV therapy) with autologous bone marrow transplantation (ABMT) in relapsed Hodgkin's disease (abstr). Exp Hematol 17(suppl):710.

Link H, Burdach S, Seidel J, et al (1989). Use of recombinant human granulocyte-macrophage colony-stimulating factor after autologous bone marrow transplantation (abstr). Exp Hematol 17(suppl):709.

Lazarus HM, Oette D. Eastern Cooperative Oncology Group Study #P-Z488 (Sandoz Study #GMC 89-107/203): A Phase II Trial Examining GM-CSF Infusions After Autologous Bone Marrow Transplantation For Relapsed or Refractory Non-Hodgkin's Lymphoma. Unpublished observations.

Masaoka T, Shibata H, Takaku F, Kodera Y, Kato S (1989). Recombinant human granulocyte colony stimulating factor for allogeneic bone marrow transplantation (abstr). Exp Hematol 17(suppl):711.

Brandt SJ, Peters WP, Atwater SK, et al (1988). Effect of recombinant human granulocyte-macrophage colony-stimulating factor on hematopoietic reconstitution after high-dose chemotherapy and autologous bone marrow transplantation. N Engl J Med 318:869-876.

Kwong YL, Millar JL, Powles RL (1989). Recovery of circulating haematopoietic progenitor cells in patients in a clinical trial of the use of recombinant human granulocyte macrophage colony stimulating factor (GM-CSF) in allogeneic bone marrow transplantation (BMT) (abstr). Exp Hematol 17(suppl):709.

Oette D, Peters WP. Unpublished observations.

Thomas ED, Storb R, Clift RA, et al (1975). Bone marrow transplantation. N Engl J Med 292:832-843, 892-902.

Anasetti C, Amos D, Beatty PG, et al (1989). Effect of HLA compatibility on engraftment of bone marrow transplant patients with leukemia or lymphoma. N Engl J Med 320:197-204.

Martin PJ, Hansen JA, Buckner CD, et al (1985). Effects of in vitro depletion of T cells in HLA-identical allogeneic marrow grafts. Blood 66:664-672.

Beatty PG, Clift RA, Mickelson EM, et al (1985). Marrow transplantation from unrelated donors other than HLA-identical siblings. N Engl J Med 313:765-771.

Storb R, Prentice RL, Thomas ED, et al (1983). Factors associated with graft rejection after HLA-identical marrow transplantation for aplastic anemia. Br J Haematol 55:573-585.

Hill RS, Mazza P, Amos D, et al (1989). Engraftment in 86 patients with lymphoid malignancy after autologous marrow transplantation. Bone Marrow Transplant 4:69-74.

Winston DJ, Ho WG, Champlin RE, Gale RP (1983). Treatment and prevention of interstitial pneumonia associated with bone marrow transplantation. In Gale RP (ed): "Recent Advances in Bone Marrow Transplantation," New York: Alan R. Liss, pp 425-444.

Kaizer H, Stuart RK, Brookmeyer R, et al (1985). Autologous bone marrow transplantation in acute leukemia: A phase I study of in vitro treatment of marrow with 4-hydroperoxycyclophosphamide to purge tumor cells. Blood 65:1504-1510.

Bolger GM, Sullivan KM, Storb R, et al (1986). Second marrow infusion for poor graft function after allogeneic marrow transplantation. Bone Marrow Transplant 1:21-30.

Champlin RE, Horowitz MM, van Bekkum DW, et al (1989). Graft failure following bone marrow transplantation for severe aplastic anemia: Risk factors and treatment results. Blood 73:606-613.

Neumanaitis J, Singer JW, Epstein C, et al (1989). The use of RHGM-CSF for graft failure in patients after autologous or allogeneic bone marrow transplantation (BMT) (abstr). Exp Hematol 17:657.

Donahue RE, Seehra J, Metzger M et al (1988). Human IL-3 and GM-CSF act synergistically in stimulating hematopoiesis in primates. Science 241:1820-1823.

Index

Abbreviations, TPA, PDB, PDD, 260
Acetylcholinesterase, 216
Actinomycin–D, 235
Activator proteins, binding, 241
Acute leukocyte response, 367
Acute lymphoblastic leukemia (ALL), 407, 417, 418
  cases, U.S., 444
Acute myeloblastic leukemia, 441
  cases, U.S., 444
Acute myelogenous leukemia, 329
Acute myeloid leukemia (AML), 278, 279, 283
  193 cells, 273
    stimulation, 271
  human, 335
Acute radiation syndrome, hematological, 465
Adenosine deaminase (ADA), human, 287
Adenoviros E1A, 278
Adenylate cyclase system, 219, 220
Adjustment
  predictors, 429
  psychosocial, 431
Adult marrow, BFU–E, 23
Agar, 107
  colonies, 480
  cultures, 115
  overlay, 111
AIDS, 302, 309, 365
  neutrophil function, 377
  patients, rHuEpo use, 512
Albumin, 37–39, 44
  role, 45
ALL. *See* Acute lymphoblastic leukemia
Allogeneic bone marrow, 532
  grafting, 489
  transplant, 535
Allografts, 480
Alpha and beta chains, 182
Altered myelopoiesis, 519
AMGEM, 401
Amino acid
  protein, gene encoding, 282
  sequence
    comparison, 182
    data, 102
    derived, 243
AML. *See* Acute myeloid leukemia
Anabolic intracellular conversion, 411
ANC. *See* Peripheral neutrophil counts
Anemia, 496, 501, 506
  causes, listed, 505
  correction, CRF patients, 508
  hypoproliferative, 505
  mice strains, 136
  rheumatoid arthritis, 511
Anephric patient rHuEpo response, 513
Anion exchange, 110
Antibodies, second–step, 32
Anti IgM antibodies, 207
Antimouse platelet serum (APS), 134
Anti–phosphotyrosine antibody, 202
Anti–retroviral agents, HIV–infected states, 410
Antisense RNA inhibition, 305
Anti–viral dideoxynucleosides, 410
Aplastic anemia, 365, 381
APLR. *See* Autologous proliferative T cell response
APS. *See* Antimouse platelet serum
Astrocytes, 169

ATP
  analog, 172
  binding sites, 172
AU rich
  element, 235
  domains, 238
  motif, 238
  region, 235
  sequences, 263
  3′ untranslated regions, 235
Autocrine
  growth, 283
  regulation, 127
Autoimmune and inflammatory disorders, 375
Autologous adherent cell depleted MNC, 127
Autologous bone marrow, 532
  grafts, 483
  transplantation, 535
Autologous hematopoiesis suppression, 25
Autologous proliferative T cell response (APLR), 25, 26, 28
Autoradiography, 147

Background radiation effects, 443
Bacteremias, 534
Basic fibroblast growth factor (bFGF), 74
B cell
  growth factor (BCGF), mitogenic, 76
  malignant, 417
  precursor, 418
  specificity, 241, 247
BCGF. *See* B cell growth factor
$Beta_2$–adrenergic receptor, 282
Beta globin
  chains, 292
  human, 293
    expressed, 294
    genes transduced, 291
    mRNA identified, 295
    transduced, 29
  provirus, 289
BFGF. *See* Basic fibroblast growth factor
BFR–E suicide assay, 80
BFU–E. *See* Burst–forming units–erythroid
Bioethics, 340
BIOETHICSLINE data base, 339
BIOGEN, 401
Blastocysts, 388
Blood
  cell patterns, radiation exposure, 460
  donations autologous rHuEpo, 511
B lymphocytes, 57, 241
BM FH. *See* Bone marrow Ficoll–Hypaque
BMT. *See* Bone marrow transplantation
Bolus injection, 366
Bone marrow, 10, 449
  –derived, 419
    myeloid progenitor cells, 375
  ECM anion–exchange chromatography, 100
  FH cells, 13, 17
  human, 29
  labelling redifferential, 398
  lymphoid cells, 420
  population megakaryocytes, 123
  progenitors, 376
    enriched, 25
  transplantation (BMT), 423, 479, 484
    patients, 426
Bovine serum albumin (BSA), 10, 17, 37, 39, 42, 44, 87, 89
BPA. *See* Burst promoting activity
Bright cells, 2
BSA. *See* Bovine serum albumin
B6SUT cell line, 89
Burkitt's lymphoma, 277
Burst–forming units–erythroid (BFU–E), 9, 26, 39, 41, 79, 80, 85
  and CFU–Mk proliferative activity, 523
  derived colonies, 55
  fetal, 27
  growth, 15, 17
  late, 13
Burst promoting activity (BPA), 76
  Epo, 24

Ca^{++}
  and K^+ intracellular, 260
  liberation, 274
Ca^{2+}, 197
  antagonist effect, 206
  dependency, 198
CAAT boxes, 225
Cadmium, 40
CAFC. *See* Cobblestone area forming cells
cAMP, 219
Camptothecin, 252

Cancer
  patients off–treatment, 425
  psychosocial disruptions, 424
CAPD. *See* Continuous ambulatory
    peritoneal dialysis
Carboxyl
  deletion, 330
  –truncated c–myb gene product,
      330
CAT2, 245
CB–1/FIM3 locus, 333
CCAAT boxes, 316
  sequence, 315
CD3/antigen receptor, 201
CD34
  antigen human, 30, 31
  DR, 31
  –positive bone marrow cells, 32
CD71, 33
cDNA clone, 149
Cell
  –cell
    adhesion, bone marrow, 103
    contact, 97
    interactions, 71
  cycle parameters proliferating
      granulocytic cells, 402
  fraction frequency, 33
  line
    DA–1, 80
    growth, 83
    Pan B6, 84
  surface growth factor comparison, 57
  types listed, 58
Cellular immune responses, 302
CFC–Meg. *See* Colony forming cells–
    megakaryocyte
CF1 and PRF binding sites, 246
CFU. *See* Colony–forming units
CFU–E. *See* Colony–forming units–
    erythroid
CFU–GEMM. *See* Colony–forming units
    multipotent stem cells
CFU–GM. *See* Colony–forming units
    granulocyte-macrophage
CFU–S. *See* Colony–forming units spleen
    colony; *see also* Colony–forming units
    stem cells
Chemotaxis, 371
Chemotherapy, 534
Chimerism
  degree, 476
  long term, 4
Chinese hamster ovary cells (CHO), 228
2–chloro–ddA
  cell line effect, 414
  and 6–N–methyl–ddA comparison, 413
Chloroform, 40
CHO. *See* Chinese hamster ovary cells
Cholera toxin, 220
Chondroitin sulfate (CS), 92
  and FN interaction, 92
Chromatin lability, 251
Chromatographic separation, 210
Chromosome
  325, 334
  5, 281
Chronic granulocytic leukemia, cases U.S.,
    444
Chronic myelogenous leukemia, 277
Chronic renal failure (CRF), 505
Chx. *See* Cycloheximide
Class II antigen HLA–DR, 31
C–lectins calcium–dependent, 90
Clonal Rauscher lines, 161
Cloned stromal cell line, 89
Clone uEBP–E, 244
CMV infection, 302
c–myb hypothesis, 331
c–myc promoter, 247
  and IgH enhancer, common factor, 245
  regulatory elements, 246
Cobblestone area formation, 6
  cells (CAFC), 6
Co–creation, 344
Colonies, erythroid, myeloid, and
    multilineage, 23
Colony formation, 4
Colony forming cells–megakaryocyte
    (CFC–Meg), 123, 125
  cloning efficiency, 126
Colony–forming unit (CFU)
  –B1, 30, 34
  –D, human marrow, 9
  –erythroid (CFU–E), 9, 12, 18, 26
    cells, 146
    –F, 41
    growth, 13
    –like stage differentiation, 165
    progenitors, 39

purified, 15–17
serum–free medium, 11
progenitors, 39
–GEMM (multipotent stem cells)
growth, 43, 44
meylois progenitors, 520
–GM (granulocyte–macrophage), 33, 41, 88
formation, 5
neoglycoprotein agglutination, 89
6 –M, 5
–S (spleen colony), 3, 88
assay, 29
content, 451, 457
pluripotent, 391
structural distributions, 392
Colony–stimulating factor (CSF), 71, 115, 141, 189, 205, 258, 261, 280, 365
–1, 108, 110, 112, 191
R, tyrosine kinase activity, 196
action outcome, 117
biological function, 116
and IL, 385
inducement, 521
low target cell specificity, 120
major species, 116
production, 393
regulation, 264
subclasses, 205
Combination chemotherapy, 423
Compton electron, 442
Concanavalin A (Con A), 183
affinity chromatography, 110
Continuous ambulatory peritoneal dialysis (CAPD), 493
treatment, 500
COS cell supernatants, 194
Covalent coupling proteins, 151
CRF. *See* Chronic renal failure
Cross–linking
analyses, 153
FVA cell membranes, 149
CS. *See* Chondroitin sulfate
CsA. *See* Cyclosporin A
CSF. *See* Colony stimulating factor
Current issues listed, rhGF infusions, 536
Cyclic AMP, 219
Cycloheximide (Chx), 174, 210
cell stabilization, 211
Cyclophosphamide, nonlethal dose, 484
Cyclosporin A (CsA), 207, 209
production inhibition, 208
Cysteine–rich region, 200
Cytokines, 125, 189, 269
induction IL–1, 238
receptor families, 190, 195
regulation, CFU-B1 system, 30
synthesis, CsA block, 208
transcription, 235, 263
Cytoplasmic domain, 195
Cytosolic proteins, 201

DA–1 cells, 80
growth, 83
action, 85
IL–3
exposed, 81
repeated exposure, 82
DC. *See* Double copy
ddA. *See* Dideoxyadenosine
ddNs. *See* Dideoxynucleosides
Degranulation, 377
Deletion breakpoints, 280
Deletion mutants, 229
EPO, 231
Deoxyribonucleotides polymerization, 409
Dexter
culture, murine, 109
long–term marrow system, 107
stroma, 109
cells, 107
DHFR genes, 302
Diacylglycerol, 197
Dialysis patients, 509
Diastolic and mean aterial blood pressure, 509
Dibutyryl cyclic AMP, 219, 220
Dideoxyadenosine (ddA), 410, 415
cytotoxicity, 412
Dideoxynucleosides (ddNs), 410
Dimerization motifs uEBP–C2, 245
Dimethylsufoxide (DMSO), 102, 161, 162, 217, 254
primed Rauscher cells, 165
priming, 162–166
treatment, 167
Disease and treatment–related variables, 426
Disulfide
bonds, 228
bridges, 149, 150, 170, 171

–linked subunits, 153
DMSO. *See* Dimethylsulfoxide
DNA
  binding activity, 241
  methylation and globin gene switching, 324
  polymerase alpha, 410
Dominant negative mutants, 308
Double copy (DC) vectors, 306, 307
DR–specific, 26
Drug resistance genes, 301
DUTPase (dut), 228

EC. *See* Endothelial cells
ECFC. *See* Erythroid colony–forming cells
ECM. *See* Extracellular matrix
EL–4 cells, 209
  mouse thymoma cell line, 197
Elevated serum erythropoietin, 500
Endocytosis, receptor–mediated, 148
Endometrial carcinoma cell line, 333
Endothelial cell growth factor (FGFA), 282
Endothelial cells (EC), 259
  L–cells, 237
  vascular, 233
  role, IL–1/CSF network, 234
End stage renal disease, 493, 494, 501
  causes, 496
  patients, 495
Enhancer–binding proteins renamed (EPB), 242
  uEBP–C2 protein sequence, 244
  uEBP–E, 243
Eosinophils, 367, 376, 377
EP. *See* Erythropoietin
Epidermal growth factor, 71
EPO. *See* Erythropoietin
EPO–R. *See* Erythropoietin resident progenitor cell
Erythroblasts, 153, 250, 253
  chromatin structure, 254
  sequence content, 252
  sm–sol DNA, 251
Erythrocytes, 145
Erythroin BFU–Es, 50, 79
Erythroid bursts, 23, 217
Erythroid cells
  normal human, 149
  surrogate, 324
Erythroid chromosomes, adult, 325
Erythroid colonies, 9, 12, 13, 24
  growth, 18
Erythroid colony–forming cells (ECFC), 10, 17
  capacity, 14
  growth, 15
Erythroid progenitors, 376
  cells, 392
Erythroleukemia cell differentiation, 161
Erythropoiesis, 26, 499, 506, 520
  and erythropoietin levels, 499
Erythropoietin (EP, EPO, rEp), 7, 9, 10, 23, 24, 42, 43, 145, 153, 162, 166, 227, 505, 519
  3^+, 3^-, 26
    degradation, 148
    receptors, 146, 150
    survival dependency, 147
  assay, 494
  ^{125}EPO binding studies, 154
  deficiency, 496, 506
  and DMSO synergism, 163
  elevated levels, 500
  expression, 225
  gene, 226
    codes, 227
  human recombinant, 44
  information, 161
  kidney, 493
  levels
    elevated, 499
    log serum, 497
  normal and mutant COS7 cells, 230
  production, 501
  receptor, 154
    density, 163
    doublet observed, 157
    polypeptide, 155, 157
    structure, 158
  resident progenitor cell (EPO–R), 153, 154
    cDNA, 153
    polypeptide size determination, 156
    studies conflicting results, 153
  response, 161, 165, 166
    cells, 162
  responsive progenitor cells, 21
  signal pathway, 163
  specific cells, 166
  structural features, 227

Ethical issues, genetic research, and application, 364
Eucaryotic cells, 310
Evi–1
- and CB–1/FIM3 loci genetic link, 332
- common integration site, 331
- gene mapping, 334
- locus, 333

Extracellular domain, 195
- homology, 196

Extracellular matrix (ECM), 74
- adhesion, 103
- components, 99
- isolation, 99
- role, 91

Factor V
- antigen levels, 129
- expression, 130
- steady state, 127
- synthesis, 128

False primers, 309
Family
- context, 429
- milieu, 428

F–BSA. *See* Fucosyl–BSA
Feeder population, 415
Fetal bovine serum titration, 42
Fetal hemoglobin, 313
Fetal and hepatic marrow response, 23
Fetal hepatic progenitors, 28
- cells, purification, 21

Fetal splenic T cells, 28
FGFA. Endothelial cell growth factor
FH. *See* Ficoll–Hypaque
Fibrin clot culture, 38
Fibroblasts, 258, 259, 385
- line, stable, 154
- transfectants, 153
  - stable development, 157, 158

Fibronectin (FN), 97
- membrane-associated, 92

Ficoll–Hypaque (FH), 9, 10, 22, 32
- density gradient centrifugation, 366

FIM3 locus, 331
FITC, 32
5–fluorouracil (5FU), 288, 289
F–Met–Leu–Phe, 377
FN. *See* Fibronectin
Folic acid deficiency, 496
Forskolin, 219, 220
FOS–JUN family member, 242
Friend MEL cells, 146
Friend virus (FVA) cells, 145, 146, 148
5FU. *See* 5–fluorouracil
Fucosyl–BSA (F–BSA), 88
Fungemias, 534
FVA. *See* Friend virus

Galactosyl
- and mannosyl
  - groupings, 90
  - moieties, 88
- specificities, 89

Ganglion neurons, 72
G cells, 458
G–CSF. *See* Granulocyte inducers
Gel electrophoresis
- HN purification steps, 101
- SDS, 98

Gel mobility shift assays, 246
Gene
- inhibition, 304
- research ethics, 356
- therapy, 301, 347, 350
  - human, 352

Genetic engineering, 347
Genetic manipulation, 342
Genetic research, social goals, 361
Genetic therapy types identified, 348
GF. *See* Growth factors
Glial cells, 76
Glioma brain cells, 169
Global
- and illness–specific quality, 431
- psychological distress, 426, 427
- Severity Index (GSI), 426

Globin, 254
- adult, 324
- coding region, 252
- gene
  - activation sequential, 323
  - adult, 318
  - expression, 316
  - regulation, 318
- normal human, 317
- switch developmental, 327

Glucocorticoid receptor (GRL), 281
Glocoprotein adult kidney, 493
Glucose phosphate isomerase A (GPI–A), 450
- mice, 454, 455

Glutathione, 443
Glycoconjugate ligand, 90
Glycoproteins, 116, 258, 365
  inducers, 115
  regulation, 205
  stromal cells, 103
Glycosaminoglycan, 150
GM–CFU–C. *See* Granulocyte–macrophage colony forming unit cultures
GM–CSF. *See* Granulocyte–macrophage colony stimulating factor (GM–CSF)
GNBP. *See* Homologous guanine nucleotide binding regulatory proteins
God, playing, 339
GPI–A. *See* Glucose phosphate isomerase A
Graft–versus–Host–Disease (GvHD), 480, 481
Granulocyte, 365
  concentration, 461
  inducers (G–CSF), 109, 110, 115, 191, 399, 473
    accelerated recovery, 484
    and CSF–1, 189
    and GM–CSF recombinant human, 483
    and Il–6, 112
    induced neutrophilia, 397
    and M–CSF genes, 262
    production, 400
  recovery, 462
Granulocyte–macrophage colony forming units culture (GM–CFU–C), 108
Granulocyte–macrophage colony stimulating factor (GM–CSF), 18, 108, 110, 112, 117, 129, 191, 197, 208, 261, 365, 375, 376, 473, 534
  action myeloid cells, 524
  activity, 237
  baseline neutrophil superoxide release, 370
  early response gene expression, 381
  effect, 523
    mice, 400
  and G–CSF, 190
    mRNA molecules, 234
  gene, 209
  human recombinant, 521
  and IL–3, 23, 24, 192
    action, 189
    response to, 269
    tyrosine phosphorylation, 274
  induction
    B cells, 206
    T cells, 207
  major effect, 372
  management, secondary cytopenia, 521
  molecules, 215, 216
  mRNA, 199, 235, 238
    response, 237
  powerful activator, 522
  presence, 377, 378
  primary response gene expression, 380
  production, 525
    control B and T cells, 208
  receptors, 379, 520
  stimulatory effect, 485
  transcription, 209, 210
    EL–4 cells, 210
Granulocytic cells, 398
  binding, 99
  maturing, 401
  renewal, 462
Granulocytopenia amelioration, 395
Granulocytopoiesis
  kinetics, 440
  model, 463
Granulocytosis, 462
Granulomonopoietic cells, 521
Granulopoiesis
  G–CSF–stimulated, 398
  GM–CSF response, 365
GRL. *See* Glucocorticoid receptor
Growth factors (GFs), 393
  /cytokine–independent differentiation, 420
  effectiveness, 44
  infusions, 535
    discontinuance, 534
Growth regulators, cell–surface associated, 59
GSI. *See* Global Severity Index
GvHD. *See* Graft–versus–Host–Disease
HCD 33 and HCD 57 cells, 147, 148
Helix, 229
Hematocrit
  level, 499
  response rHuEpo, 513
Hematologic malignancy, 533
Hematopoiesis, 25, 97
  active, 107
  adult, 385
  control, 531
  in culture, 119

  fetal and adult, 28
  long term, 32
  regulation levels, 120
  sustaining, 32
Hematopoietic
  adhesion strategy, 103
  cells, 97
    growth control mechanism, 76
    maturation and positioning, 115
    proliferation, 85
  colonies, 25
    growth reduced oxygen, 41
  growth factor (HGF), 23, 166, 376
    cytokines, 519
    stromal cells, 386
    and T cells, 28
  homing receptor, 90
  precursor cells, 29
  process, regulatory factors, 189
  progenitor cells, 21
  progenitor purification protocol, 22
  stem cell (HSC), 29
    assay, 5
    maturation, 205
    proliferation, 116
    reports, 38
  system, 115
  tissue, 401
Hematopoietin 1 activity, 474
Hemizygosity, 277
Hemodialysis, 493, 494
  patients, 506
Hemoglobin, 496
  and circulating erythropoietin, 501
  erythropoietin relationship, 497
  fetal, 313
  level, 499
  switching, 318
Hemonectin, 101
  cell attachment, 98
  derived peptide, 103
  identification, 97
  mediated adhesion, 101
  mouse bone marrow, 98
  tissue distribution, 99
Heparan, 74, 75
  –affinity chromatography, 75
  binding cell surface, 57
  –like molecules, 74
  sulfate proteoglycan (HSPG), 73
Hereditary persistence fetal hemoglobin (HPFH), 313, 314
  genes, 318
  mutation locations and types, 315
  nondeletion, 318
Herpes simplex virus, 314
Heterodimers jun and fos oncogene, 202
HGF. *See* Hematopoietic growth factor
Hierarchical setwise multiple regression, 430
Higher levels erythropoietin hematocrit, 500
High proliferative potential colony forming cells (HPP–CFC), 108
HIV
  –infected persons ddNs, 412
  replication, 309
HL–60, 101, 191, 274
  binding, 102
HLA–DQ, 22
HLA–DR, 26
  and CD33, 32
  –identical transplants unmanipulated, 535
  /PE fluorescence, 31
H_2O_2, 37
Homing
  inhibition, 88
  lectin–carbohydrate mediated, 88
  multiple interactions, 92
  receptor
    binding, 91
    purification, 90
Homoglobinized cells, 164
Homologous guanine nucleotide binding regulatory proteins (GNBP), 218, 220
Homozygosity, 277
Host defense cell function enhancement, 377
HPFH. *See* Hereditary persistence fetal hemoglobin
HPP–CFC. *See* High proliferative potential colony forming cells
HSC. *See* Hematopoietic stem cell
HSPG, *See* Heparan sulfate proteoglycan
$_3$HTdR labelling, 398
Human actin, 307
Human blood BFU–E, 11
Human Epo gene, 506
Human germ line therapy, 350
Human/mouse discrepancy, 400
Human urine (CSF–HU), 532

Humic acid, organic, 40
Humoral immune responses, 302
Hybridoma antibodies, 27
Hydrocortisone, 18
Hydroxyurea, 138
  suicide, 85
Hypertension, 509
Hypothesis, protein binding, 192

^{125}I, 87
  –EP, 146
    FVA cell binding, 147
    preparation, 145
  –EPO binding untransfected cells, 155
  –erythropoietin binding, 162
  –labeled
    G–BSA use, 89
    GM–CSF, 378
ICAM–1, 97
IES. *See* Impact of Events Scale
IFN–gamma. *See* Interferon–gamma
Ig. *See* Immunoglobulin
IGF. *See* Insulin–like growth factor
IL. *See* Interleukin
Immunocompetant cells role, 124
Immunofluorescent
  analysis, 290
  microscopy, 98
Immunoglobulin (Ig), 417
  A, 375
  E receptor–mediated activation, 169–170
  heavy chain (IgH) genes, 240
    enhancer, 241, 243
    transcription, 243, 246
  /TCR gene rearrangements, 419
Immunoprecipitation EPO–receptor, 156
Immunoreactive erythropoietin, 500
Immunoselection by panning negative, 22
Immunothrombocytopenia, acute, 134, 140
Impact of Events Scale (IES), 426
Inhomogenous radiation exposure, 461
Injured cell hypothesis, 467
Inorganic contaminants deleterious, 40
Insulin, 17
  human, 13
  –like growth factor (IGF)–I, 9, 15–17
    I and II, 18
Integral protein, 51
Interferon, 129, 130, 372
  –gamma (IFN–gamma), 261
    treated NK cells, 126
Interleukin (IL), 4
  /CSF network complexity, 233
  IL–1, 5, 71, 108, 197, 235, 259, 263, 385, 471, 472
    cytokine gene transcription, 234
    GM–CSF expression EC, 238
    hematopoiesis promotion, 476
    hematopoietic activity, 233
    radioprotective effect, 474
    recombinant human, 236
    responsive genes, 238
    treatment, 475
  IL–2, 179, 181, 183, 197, 209, 303
    gene, 200
    and GM–CSF CsA sensitivity difference, 209
    receptors, 179, 194
    receptors classes, 180
  IL–2R, alpha and beta, 181
  IL–3, 110, 117, 197, 218, 219, 280, 288, 329, 330
    binding, 191
    cDNA, 118
    circulating molecule detection, 401
    dependence NRP relation, 84
    dependent cell lines, 330
    –dependent myeloid leukemia cell lines, 331, 335
    effect, mice, 400
    and GM–CSF stimulation, 272
    or GM–CSF tyrosine kinase activation, 271
    growth dependence, 80
    growth inhibition, 83
    and IL–6 combination, 34, 295, 296, 300
    and NRP antagonism, 85
    plus Pan B6 exposure, 81, 82
    production inhibition, 207
    receptors, 190
    recombinant, 215, 216
  IL–4, 117, 193
    and IL–5, 282, 283
    receptor, 189, 190, 194
  IL–6, 117, 385, 386
    and LIF, 389
    mRNA, 109
  IL–7, 387–388
Intracellular immunization, 304

Iodination EP, 145
Iodotyrosine, 148
Ionizing radiation, 442, 459, 469, 471, 531
Iron
  mobilization, 508
  .otoporphyrin, 42
ıradiated host, 457
Irradiated mice survival, 472
Irreversible bone marrow aplasia, 479
Irreversible hematopoietic failure, 460
Irreversible stem cell pool change, 467
Isozyme–specific antibodies, 198

JM–1 cell line, 191
Jun–jun homodimers, 202

140 kDa protein phosphorylated, 274
60kD protein, 98
KG–1 cells, 191, 192

Laminin, 97
LAR. *See* Locus Activation Region
Large granular lymphocytes (LGLs), 181
L–cells, 246
  transfection, 236
Lectin, 109
  assignment progenitor cells, 89
Leukemias, 277
  cells characterized, 283, 524
  inhibitory factor (LIF), 387
  patients, young adult, 426
  process, 440
Leukemogenesis, 439, 441
Leukocyte
  regeneration time, 491
  responses, GM–CSF infusion, 368
Leukopoiesis effects, 371
LGL. *See* Large granular lymphocyte
LIF. *See* Leukemia inhibitory factor
Linker scanning mutants, 231
Lipids cell membrane biogenesis, 39
Lipopolysacharides (LPS) bacterial, 471
  addition, 212
Lipoproteins, 39
Lithium, 108
Liver release erythropoietin, 500
Locus Activation Region (LAR), 326
Long term hematopoiesis, 34
Long–term marrow culture, (LTMC), 97, 393
Loosely associated protein (LRP), 51
LPS. *See* Lipopolysacharides
LTMC. *See* Long–term marrow culture
LTR sequences, 225
Lymph vessels, 115
Lymphoblastic leukemia, 278
Lymphoblastic lymphoma, 409
Lymphoblasts, sequence content, 252
Lymphocytes, CSF production, 263
Lymphohematopoietic
  cell growth, 269
  factors receptors, 274
Lymphokine
  IL–3, 42
  production
    dependence, 199
    potential steps, 202
    T cell, 197
  transcription, 199
Lymphomas, 277
Lymphopoiesis, 118
  IL–7 regulator, 193
Lymphotoxin and TNF alpha lung fibroblasts, 259

Macrocytic megakaryocytes, 139
Macrocytosis, 141
Macromegakaryocytosis, 139
Macrophage colony stimulating factor (M–CSF), 63, 67, 280
  cDNAz
    amino acid encoding, 68
    coding regions, 64
  clones, 69
  mRNA, 258
  protein cell surface, 66
  recombinant, CAS–7 cells, 67
  specific proteins synthesized, 65
  transcription, 68
Macrophages, 117, 365, 376
  inducers (M–CSF), 115, 117
  pivotal, 261
Malignant diseases treatment, 278
Mannosyl specificities, 89
MANOVA. Multivariate analysis of variance
Marrow
  adherent stromal elements, 107
  macrophages, 112
  microenvironment, 520

repopulating ability (MRA), 3
transplantation, 87
trials, 533
Mast cells, 169
mBPA. *See* Membrane–associated erythroid burst–promoting activity
MC. *See* Methylcellulose
M–CSF. *See* Macrophage colony stimulating factor; *see also* Macrophage inducers
MEDLARS, 339
Megakarycytopoiesis, 520
Megakaryocytes, 124, 376
colonies, 127
burst, 218
frequency, 219
proliferation, 220
stimulatory factor (Meg–CSF), 129
development, 129
Factor V content, 128
low frequency, 217
macrocytic, 137
mean size, 135
measurements, 134
–platelet dyscrasia, 216
progenitor cells, 123
signal transduction, 216
size, 142
stimulatory factor (MSF), 129
Megakaryocytic lineage, 215
Megakaryocytic macrocytosis, 140
Megakaryocytopenia, 134, 139–141
delayed effects, 138
effects, 142
Megakaryocytopenic mice, 137
Megakaryocytopoiesis, 123
adjustments, 133
Meg–CSF. *See* Megakaryocyte colony stimulatory factor
MEL (adult murine)
cell environment, 325
explained, 324
erythroid, 326
hybrids, 325
Melanoma cells, 379
Melopoiesis, 118
Membrane–associated CSF–1, 71
Membrane–associated erythroid burst–promoting activity (mBPA), 50, 53
expression, 55
extraction and purification, 52
interaction lipid bilayer, 52
and neurite membrane–derived mitogen, 54
protein lymphocyte surface presence, 56
Membrane glycoconjugates, 87, 89
Membrane lectin, 87
absence, 89
Membrane preparations, 55
Membrane proteins, 49, 50
phase separation, 53
Membrane ruffling, 377
Mesenchymal cells, 263
origin, 257
Metallothionein production, 472
Metastatic carcinoma, 366
Methotrexate (MTX), 300
Methylcellulose (MC), 10, 27, 38
cultures, 25, 26
erythroid bursts, large, 12
FH cells, 13, 14, 16
MHR. *See* Myc homology region
Microarchitectural relationship, 392
Microenvironment
irradiated, 449
tissue functioning, 401
regulation hemopoiesis, 393
stroma, 393
MIL–3. *See* Murine interleukin–3
Mitogen
bound to HSPG, 75
cell sensitivity to, 41
membrane–associated, 71
MØ. *See* Monocyte–macrophages
Moncytes, 367
Monoclonal antibodies, 534
Monocyte, 376
activity, 366
ADCC, 368, 369, 372
TNF and IFN secretion, 369
Monocyte–macrophages (MØ), 124, 127
Monomeric glycoproteins, small, 63
Monosaccarides, pyranose form, 87
Moral issures, 350
Morphologic subsets AML, 279
Mouse
cell line, Pan B6 bone marrow–derived, 79
studies, 399
MRA. *See* Marrow repopulating ability

mRNA
coding, 260
Factor V level changes, 129
MSF. *See* Megakaryocyte stimulatory factor
MTX. *See* Methotrexate
Multiple hematopoietic lineages, 30
Multiple growth factors, 112
Multipotent stem cells (CFU–GEMM), 42
Multivariate analysis of variance (MANOVA), 426
Murine
CFU–E, 165
CFU–S, 30
erythroid colony forming units, 37
GM–CSF, 287
interleukin–3 (mIL–3), 169, 174–176, 287
binding, 172, 173
dependent cell lines, 169, 170, 174
receptor, 170, 171, 173, 174
L cells, 236
models, 134
monoclonal antibodies, 22
myeloid leukemias, 335
progenitor cells, 219
pulmonary cells, 217
myc homology
family, 243
region (MHR), 244
Myeloblast promyelocyte compartment doubling, 399
Myelodysplasia, 365
Myelofibrosis experimental, 391
Myeloid
cell, 329
line, human, 271, 376
differentiation, 330
leukemias, 330
cell lines, 269, 378
leukemogenesis, 279
progenitor cells, 33
stimulation, 376
Myelopoiesis, 257, 371
normal, 521

NaF, 261
National Council of Churches policy, 342
National Library of Medicine, 339
Natural killer (NK) cells, 125
megakaryocyte colony effect, 125
mediated stimulation, CFUuMeg cloning, 126
Natural radiation, 439, 446
Natural regeneration, 531
N–CAM, 97
homology, 103
NDGF. *See* Neuron–derived growth factor
NECA. *See* 5–N–ethyl–carboxyamidoadenosine
Negative cooperactivity, 146
Negative Regulatory Protein (NRP), 79, 85
explained, 80
growth inhibition, 80, 83
toxicity, 82
5–N–ethyl–carboxyamidoadenosine, 219, 220
Neurite mitogen, 51
Neuron
–derived growth factor (NDGF), 71, 74, 75
and Schwann cells, interactions, 72
Neutropenia, 484
Neutrophils, 366, 367, 376
chemotaxis, 371
count drop, 534
evaluation, 366
labelled emergence, 397
receptors, 377
superoxide release, 370
Neutrophilic granulocytes and monocytes, 375
N–glycanase studies, 171
NK. *See* Natural killer
2 N–linked carbohydrate moieties, 171
N–linked glycosylation, 67
N–linked sugars, 73
Non–helical turns, 229
Nondeletion HPFH, 314
Nonthrombocytopenic megakaryocytopenias, 133
Normal B cell precursors, 420
Normal hemopoietic cell proliferation, 439
Northern analysis, 198, 209, 236, 243, 260
N–ras oncogene, 441
NRP. *See* Negative Regulatory Protein
Nuclear
energy, 446
PKC substrates, nuclei isolated, 201

Oligonucleotide multimer IgH enhancer B site, 245
Oncogenes recessive, 278
Orbital electron, 442
Oxygen reduced, 41

PAF. *See* Platelet activating factor
Pan B6, 83
PE. *See* Phorbol ester
Pediatric ALL, 417
Peptides
  amino acid synthetic, 155
  growth factors, 190
Peripheral membrane proteins, 50
Peripheral neutrophil counts (ANC), 396
Peripheral protein, 51
PF4. *See* Platelet factor 4
PFGE. *See* Pulsed field gel electrophoresis
PGK–A. *See* Phosphoglycerate kinase A
PGK–B. *See* Phosphoglycerate kinase B
Phenol, 40
Phorbol
  dibutyrate, 218
  diesters, 216, 218
  ester (PEs), 197
    GM–CSF and M–CSF expression, 260
    –induced proteins, 199
    responsive element (TRE), 199
  myristate acetate, 217, 219
Phosphoglycerate kinase A (PGK–A), 450
  A and B enzyme markers, 450
  BMC, 455
  mice, 453–456
Phosphoglycerate kinase B (PGK–B), 450
  BMC, 453–456
  mice, 455
Phosphorylated ddA, 411
Phosphorylation kinetics, 270
Phosphotidylinositol groups, 49
PHSC. *See* Pluripotent hemopoietic stem cells
Phthalate ester, 40
Psychosocial difficulties, 425
Physphatidylserine binding, 201
PKC. *See* Protein kinase C
Plasma membrane proteins, 49, 53, 55
Platelet
  activating factor (PAF), 523
  –derived growth factor, 18
  factor 4 (PF4), 127, 128
  and megakaryocyte numbers, 137
Playing God, 341–345
  role, biomedical activity, 340
  see also Bioethics
Pleated sheet, 229
Pleiotropic cytokine, 473
Ploidy
  cells, 139
  distribution, 133
  increase, 141
Pluripotent hemopoietic stem cells (PHSC), 1–7, 29, 287, 329
  infection frequency, 292
  purification, 1
Pluripotent progenitor cells, 376
Pluripotent stem cells, 115, 169, 480
PMA. *See* Tumor promoting phorbol diesters
PMUE. *See* Pregnant mouse uterus extract
Poisson statistics, 445
Polyacrylamide gel electrophoresis, 90
Polyclonal
  anti–peptide antibodies, 155
  antisera, 158
Polycystic kidney disease, 499
Polyploid megakaryocytes, 123
Post–irradiation treatment, 486
Post–translational glycosylation, 227
P140 protein, 272
Pre–B and pre–T cell populations, 415
Pregnant mouse uterus extract, 4
Primary response genes induction, 380
Procaryotic system, 310
Proerythroblasts, 145
Progenitor cells (CFU–GM), 88
  binding stroma, 89
Progenitor–specific antibodies, 27
Proliferating granulocytic cells, 399
Proliferating synkaryons, 324
Prostaglandins, 117
Protein kinase C (PKC), 129, 173, 174, 197, 220, 260, 274
  activation, 197
  calcium–mediated, 216
  depletion effects, 273
  isozymes EL4 cells, 198
  –mediated phosphorylation, 201
  stimulators, 258

substrates, 201
identified, 200
type II, 198
type III, 199
Proteins, 129
c–myb carboxyl–truncated, 330
cross–linking identified differences, 149
cytokines and matrix, 32
IL–2 receptor associated, 184
140 kDa, 272
migrates SDS–PAGE, 151
murine, IL–2 receptor associated, 183
phosphorylation, 129, 174
properties, 277
Proteoglycan, 91, 97, 110
binding and target cells, 112
Proteolyzed integral proteins, (M–CSFs), 51
Protooncogene, 440
Protoporphyrins, hemin and hematin, 44
Psychosexual adjustment, 428
Psychosocial
adjustment, 427
functioning, 431
intervention, 431
Pulsed field gel electrophoresis (PFGE), 282
Purification procedure protocol, 171

Rabbit beta–globin
gene, 236
RNA, 237, 238
Radiation
accidents, 459
management, 468
induced
leukemia, 441
myelotoxicity reversal, 474
medical, 446
Radioprotection IL–1, 471
Rauscher
cells, EPO–sensitivity, 166
erythroleukemia cell differentiation, 163
murine erythroleukemia cells, 161
subclone, 161
RB1 locus, 278
Receptor–mediated endocytosis, 148
Recombinant cytokines, 473
Recombinant DNA technology, 342
Recombinant hematopoietic growth factors, 533
Recombinant human Epo (rHuEpo), 506, 508
anemia correction, 509
and blood pressure, 510
doses, 506
in man, 505
potential clinical uses, 513
replacement therapy, 507
response
inflammation effect, 509
surgery inflammation, 513
therapy, 509
use, 511
Renal disease end–stage, 493
rEp. *See* Erythropoietin
Reporter gene, 202, 258
Restrictin–P, 120
putative factors, 121
Reticuleoendothelial storage, 507
Reticulocyte
recovery, 479
regeneration time, 491
Retinoblastoma prototypic model, 278
Retroviral
gene transfer, 304
integrations, 333
vectors, 306, 349
Reversible damage stem cell pool, 467, 468
Rhodamine 123 (Rh123), 2
–bright cells, 6, 7
–bright fraction, 5
–dull cells, 6, 7
–dull fraction, 5
rHuEpo. *See* Recombinant human Epo
Ribosome binding site, 225
Ribozymes, 308
Risk–free environment, 439
RNA
binding decoys, 309
polymerase
II, 307
III, 308
RNase protection analysis, 291

S.I.E. *See* Serum immunoreactive erythropoietin
Schwann cells
division, 72
proliferation, 71

SDS–PAGE, 171, 172
Sequences
  G–C rich, 314
  protein, 277
  treatment, 253
Serine
  phosphorylation, 204
  /threonine
    kinase coactivation, 273–274
    and tyrosine kinase, 269
Serum
  albumin
    role, 44
    titration, 45
  creatinine, 496
    and log serum erythropoietin, 498
  erythropoietin, 499
  immunoreactive erythropoietin (S.I.E.), 495, 496
Severe bone marrow aplasia, 372
Slippery Slope argument, 344
Sm–sol DNA, 251
  sequence content, 254
Social goals, genetic research, 361
Sociodemographic patient characteristics, 425
Somatic mutation theory, 525
Southern blot analysis, 283, 293
  peripheral blood DNA, 291
Spatial distribution, 394
Spleen cells phenotypic analysis, 475
Spleen colony (CFU–S), 2
  formation, 3
Splenocytes activated, 183
Spontaneous hemopoietic recovery, 461
Spontaneous leukemia incidence, 440
Stem cells (CFU–S), 88
  division alternative pathways, 116
  pool, 116
    damage irreversible, 465
    irreversible, 466
    size calculations, 464, 469
  self–renewal, 29
  substitution therapy, 466
Stochastic differentiation explained, 7
Stroma–dependent bone marrow, 5
Stromal cells, 97, 118
  colonies, 109
  factors
    functions, 119
    growth production, 111
  inhibitory signals, 120
  layers, 107
Sulfated glycan structures, 91
Sulfhydryl groups results, 150
Surface molecules and cellular differentiation, 51
SV40 large T oncoproteins, 278
Swiss 3T3 cells, 380
Synergistic
  co–regulators, 217, 219
  effects, IL–3 and IL–6, 296
  interactions, calcium–PKC, 217
Syngeneic transplant patients, 535
Synthetic neoglycoprotein, 88
  probes, 87
  specific, 88

TATA box, 225
Tat and rev gene products, 309
TBI. *See* Total Body Irradiation
TCR. *See* T cell receptor
T cells, 25, 201, 209
  depletion, 310, 481, 483
  double negative, 117
  factors, 76
  gene rearrangement, 420
  receptor (TCR), 417
  response, 303
    immune, 179
TdT. *See* Terminal deoxynucleotidyl transferase
Terminal deoxynucleotidyl transferase (TdT), 409–411
  cellular function, 414–415
  –negative precurson compartments, 415
  –positive cells, 415
    leukemia, 412
  –positive populations, 415
  therapeutic target, 415
Terminal differentiation, 116
Testosterone, 18
Tetradecanoyl–phorbol–13–acetate (TPA), 205, 208, 209
  addition, 210
  treatment, 209
  tumor promotor, 380
  –stimulated T cells, 207

Thrombocyte, 479
Thrombocytopenia, 133–135, 137, 139–141
  acute, 135
Thrombocytosis, 133, 134
  transfusion–induced, 137
Thrombopenic values, 462
Thrombopoietin, 141
Thrombospondin, 74
Thymoma EL–4, 207
Thyroid, 18
TIS gene expression, 381
Titrations interleukin–3, 43
T lymphocyte, 385, 480
  activated, 169
  autologous, CFC–Meg effect, 126
  interleukins produce, 263
  secrete IL–3, 263
  stimulation, 271
T–lymphoid cells, 310
TMB–8. *See* Trimethoxybenzoate hydrochloride
TNF. *See* Tumor necrosis factor
Topoisomerase inhibitors, 253, 255
  effects, 252
  Type II, 250
Total Body Irradiation (TBI), 479, 480, 483, 484
  dose, 482, 484
  stem cell kill, 486
Total body x–irradiation fractionation, 490
Total peripheral vascular resistance, 509
TPA. *See* Tetradecanoyl–phorbol–13–acetate
Trans–acting factor, 314, 315, 316
Transcription
  factors, 323
  initiation inhibitor, 209
  response requirement, 200
Transfection PKC catalytic fragment, 202
Transferrin, 17, 42
  human, 10, 11
  iron–saturated, 13, 37
  serum–deprived cultures, 39
Transforming growth factor, 71
  –beta, 129, 130
Transfusion–induced thrombocytosis, 138, 142
Transgenic
  mice, 317, 318
  organisms, 343
Transmembrane
  domain, 195
  proteins, 49
Trimethoxybenzoate hydrochloride (TMB–8), 207
Tritiated thymidine, 138
  incorporation, 80
Trypan blue staining, 83
Trypsin passage, 109
Tumor
  cell kill, 531
  necrosis factor (TNF), 259, 263
    alpha, 369, 372
    and IL–1B, 262
    rapid alkalination, 259
    role host defenses, 262
  promoting
    compounds, 217
    phorbol diesters (PMA), 216–219, 272, 273
  suppressor genes, 278
Type 4 collagen, 97
Tyrosine
  kinase, 202, 275
    activity, 172, 201, 271
    signal, PKC role, 273
  phosphorylate, 172, 173, 182
  residues, 183
Tyr–phosphorylated proteins, 201

Untransfected COS cells, 151
Uracil N–glycolase (ung), 228
3′ UT, 237

Vaccinia virus growth factor, 71
Vascular endothelial, 258
V_{H1} promoter, 242, 244
VM26, 253, 254

Western blotting, 198
  probed, 202
Wheat germ agglutinin (WGA), 2, 4, 5
Wild type EPO cDNA, 230

Young adult leukemia patient characteristics, 433

Zinc fingers, 282